Respiratory Medicine

Series Editors

Sharon I.S. Rounds
Alpert Medical School of Brown University
Providence, RI, USA

Anne Dixon
University of Vermont, Larner College of Medicine
Burlington, VT, USA

Lynn M. Schnapp
University of Wisconsin - Madison
Madison, WI, USA

MW01200943

More information about this series at http://www.springer.com/series/7665

Stephanie Duggins Davis • Margaret Rosenfeld
James Chmiel
Editors

Cystic Fibrosis

A Multi-Organ System Approach

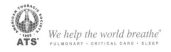

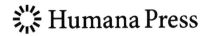

Editors
Stephanie Duggins Davis
The University of North Carolina at
Chapel Hill
Department of Pediatrics
UNC Children's Hospital
Chapel Hill, NC
USA

Margaret Rosenfeld
Department of Pediatrics
University of Washington School
of Medicine
Division of Pulmonary and Sleep Medicine
Seattle Children's Hospital
Seattle, WA
USA

James Chmiel
Department of Pediatrics
Indiana University School of Medicine
Division of Pediatric Pulmonology, Allergy
and Sleep Medicine, Riley Hospital for
Children at IU Health
Indianapolis, IN
USA

ISSN 2197-7372   ISSN 2197-7380   (electronic)
Respiratory Medicine
ISBN 978-3-030-42384-1   ISBN 978-3-030-42382-7   (eBook)
https://doi.org/10.1007/978-3-030-42382-7

This Humana imprint is published by the registered company Springer Nature Switzerland AG
The registered company address is: Gewerbestrasse 11, 6330 Cham, Switzerland

Preface

This is an exciting time in the care of people with cystic fibrosis (CF). There are now more adults than children living with CF, and highly effective modulator therapies are poised to dramatically improve outcomes. We offer this book to medical students, residents, and seasoned clinicians wishing for state-of-the-art reviews on all aspects of CF care. Unique features of the book include patients and parents' perspectives in many of the chapters, as well as chapters on health disparities and mental health. The book covers major pulmonary and non-pulmonary manifestations of CF as well as advanced lung disease and lung transplantation. There is also a section on the molecular genetics of CF and treatment of the basic defect. Because many excellent reviews on CFTR modulators are readily available, this section covers gene editing and small molecules instead. We dedicate this book to our patients and their families who have inspired and taught us so much.

Chapel Hill, NC, USA   Stephanie Duggins Davis, MD
Seattle, WA, USA   Margaret Rosenfeld, MD
Indianapolis, IN, USA   James Chmiel, MD, MPH, ATSF

Acknowledgments

I am truly grateful for Sam, Harrison, Jackson, and Parker for their incredible love and support.

-Stephanie Duggins Davis

To my patients for helping me to understand life with CF, and to my colleagues and family for their enduring support.

-Margaret Rosenfeld

To Jennifer, Abigail, James, Michael, my siblings, and my parents for all of the love and support.

-James Chmiel

Contents

Contributors

Micheál Mac Aogáin, BSc, PhD Translational Respiratory Research Laboratory, Lee Kong Chian School of Medicine, Nanyang Technological University, Singapore, Singapore

Kathryn L. Behrhorst, MS Virginia Commonwealth University, Department of Psychology, Richmond, VA, USA

Anna Bertolini, BSc Medicine Department of Pediatrics, University Medical Center Groningen, Groningen, The Netherlands

Frank A. J. A. Bodewes, MD, PhD Pediatric Gastroenterology, Department of Pediatrics, University Medical Center Groningen, Groningen, The Netherlands

Cynthia D. Brown, MD Indiana University School of Medicine, Division of Pulmonary, Critical Care, Occupational and Sleep Medicine, Indianapolis, IN, USA

Jennifer L. Butcher, PhD Michigan Medicine C.S. Mott Children's Hospital, Department of Pediatrics, Ann Arbor, MI, USA

Sanjay H. Chotirmall, MD, PhD Translational Respiratory Research Laboratory, Lee Kong Chian School of Medicine, Nanyang Technological University, Singapore, Singapore

Jonathan D. Cogen, MD, MPH Division of Pulmonary & Sleep Medicine, Department of Pediatrics, Seattle Children's Hospital, Seattle, WA, USA

Erin Crowley, MD Indiana University School of Medicine, Division of Pulmonary, Critical Care, Occupational and Sleep Medicine, Indianapolis, IN, USA

Garry R. Cutting, MD Johns Hopkins University School of Medicine, Institute of Genetic Medicine, Baltimore, MD, USA

Matthew J. DiMagno, MD University of Michigan School of Medicine, Department of Internal Medicine, Division of Gastroenterology and Hepatology, Ann Arbor, MI, USA

Mitchell L. Drumm, PhD Case Western Reserve University, Department of Genetics and Genome Sciences, Cystic Fibrosis Research Center, Cleveland, OH, USA

Isabelle Durieu, MD, PhD Centre de Reference de la Mucoviscidose, Centre Hospitalier Lyon Sud, Lyon, France

Robin S. Everhart, PhD Virginia Commonwealth University, Department of Psychology, Richmond, VA, USA

Patrick A. Flume, MD Department of Medicine, Medical University of South Carolina, Charleston, SC, USA

Department of Pediatrics, Medical University of South Carolina, Charleston, SC, USA

Bryan Garcia, MD Department of Medicine, Medical University of South Carolina, Charleston, SC, USA

Alex H. Gifford, MD Dartmouth Institute for Health Policy and Clinical Practice, Dartmouth-Hitchcock Medical Center, Department of Pulmonary and Critical Care Medicine, Lebanon, NH, USA

Andrea Granados, MD Washington University School of Medicine in St. Louis, St. Louis Children's Hospital, Department of Pediatrics, Division of Pediatric Endocrinology and Diabetes, One Children's Place, St. Louis, MO, USA

Nicole Green, MD Division of Gastroenterology and Hepatology, Department of Pediatrics, Seattle Children's Hospital-University of Washington, Seattle, WA, USA

Sophie Guérin Service de Pneumologie et Allergologie Pédiatrique, Hôpital Necker Enfants Malades, Paris, France

Jennifer S. Guimbellot, MD, PhD Department of Pediatrics, Division of Pediatric Pulmonary and Sleep Medicine, Gregory Fleming James Cystic Fibrosis Research Center, University of Alabama at Birmingham (UAB), Birmingham, AL, USA

Sangwoo T. Han, PhD Johns Hopkins University School of Medicine, Institute of Genetic Medicine, Baltimore, MD, USA

Kara S. Hughan, MD, MHSc Department of Pediatrics, Pittsburgh Heart, Lung, Blood and Vascular Medicine Institute, University of Pittsburgh, UPMC Children's Hospital of Pittsburgh, Division of Pediatric Endocrinology and Diabetes, Pittsburgh, PA, USA

Allison A. Lambert, MD, MHS University of Washington, Department of Medicine, Division of Pulmonary and Critical Care Medicine, WWAMI Spokane Foundations, UW at Schoenberg Center—Gonzaga, Spokane, WA, USA

John J. LiPuma, MD Department of Pediatrics, University of Michigan Medical School, Ann Arbor, MI, USA

Amar Mandalia, MD University of Michigan Hospital and Health Systems, Department of Internal Medicine, Division of Gastroenterology and Hepatology, Ann Arbor, MI, USA

Peter J. Mogayzel Jr, MD The Johns Hopkins Medical Institutions, Department of Pediatrics, Baltimore, MD, USA

Kristina Montemayor, MD Johns Hopkins University, Department of Medicine, Division of Pulmonary and Critical Care Medicine, Baltimore, MD, USA

Emily F. Muther, PhD University of Colorado School of Medicine, Children's Hospital Colorado, Department of Psychiatry, Aurora, CO, USA

Dave Nichols, MD Seattle Children's Hospital, University of Washington School of Medicine, Department of Pediatrics, Seattle, WA, USA

Gabriela R. Oates, PhD Division of Pulmonary and Sleep Medicine, Department of Pediatrics, University of Alabama at Birmingham, Birmingham, AL, USA

Shruti M. Paranjape, MD Johns Hopkins School of Medicine, Eudowood Division of Pediatric Respiratory Sciences, Baltimore, MD, USA

Joseph M. Pilewski, MD University of Pittsburgh, Pittsburgh, PA, USA

Pulmonary, Allergy, and Critical Care Medicine Division, University of Pittsburgh Medical Center, Pittsburgh, PA, USA

Cystic Fibrosis Center, UPMC Children's Hospital of Pittsburgh, Pittsburgh, PA, USA

Deepika Polineni, MD, MPH The University of Kansas Health System, Department of Internal Medicine, Kansas City, KS, USA

Andrew Prayle, BMedSci, BMBS, PhD The University of Nottingham, Child Health, Obstetrics and Gynaecology, Queens Medical Centre, Nottingham, UK

Bradley S. Quon, MD, MSc, MBA St. Paul's Hospital, University of British Columbia, Department of Medicine, Vancouver, BC, Canada

Bonnie W. Ramsey, MD Department of Pediatrics, University of Washington, School of Medicine, Seattle, WA, USA

Center for Clinical and Translational Research, Seattle Children's Research Institute, Seattle, WA, USA

Seattle Children's Hospital, Center for Clinical and Translational Research, Seattle, WA, USA

Sarath C. Ranganathan, MBChB, PhD, ATSF Department of Respiratory and Sleep Medicine, Royal Children's Hospital, Parkville, VIC, Australia

Respiratory Diseases Group, Murdoch Children's Research Institute, Parkville, VIC, Australia

Department of Paediatrics, University of Melbourne, Melbourne, VIC, Australia

Amanda Reis, MD Saint Louis Children's Hospital, Department of Pediatrics, Washington University School of Medicine, Saint Louis, MO, USA

Clement L. Ren, MD, MBA Division of Pediatric Pulmonology, Allergy and Sleep Medicine, Riley Hospital for Children and Indiana University School of Medicine, Indianapolis, IN, USA

Kristin A. Riekert, PhD Johns Hopkins School of Medicine, Department of Medicine, Baltimore, MD, USA

Steven M. Rowe, MD, MSPH Department of Medicine, Department of Pediatrics, Department of Cell Developmental and Integrative Biology, Gregory Fleming James Cystic Fibrosis Research Center, University of Alabama at Birmingham (UAB), Birmingham, AL, USA

Thomas Ruffles, MBBS, BSc, MRCPCH Queensland Children's Hospital, Department of Respiratory & Sleep Medicine, South Brisbane, QLD, Australia

Child Health Research Centre, The University of Queensland Brisbane QLD Australia, Brisbane, QLD, Australia

Michael S. Schechter, MD, MPH Division of Pulmonary Medicine, Department of Pediatrics, Virginia Commonwealth University, Children's Hospital of Richmond at VCU, Richmond, VA, USA

Sarah Jane Schwarzenberg, MD University of Minnesota Masonic Children's Hospital, Department of Pediatrics, Minneapolis, MN, USA

Isabelle Sermet-Gaudelus, MD, PhD Service de Pneumologie et Allergologie Pédiatrique, Hôpital Necker Enfants Malades, Paris, France

Institut Necker Enfants Malades, INSERM U1151, Paris, France

Mordechai Slae, MD Pediatric Gastroenterology Unit, Department of Pediatrics, Hadassah Hebrew University Medical Center, Jerusalem, Israel

Adam C. Stein, MD Division of Gastroenterology and Hepatology, Northwestern Medicine, Chicago, IL, USA

Caroline S. Thomas, MD The Monroe Carell Jr. Children's Hospital at Vanderbilt and Vanderbilt University Medical Center, Department of Pediatric Allergy, Immunology, and Pulmonary Medicine, Nashville, TN, USA

Céline Vidaillac, PharmD, PhD Translational Respiratory Research Laboratory, Lee Kong Chian School of Medicine, Nanyang Technological University, Singapore, Singapore

Claire Wainwright, MBBS, MRCP, FRACP, MD Queensland Children's Hospital, Department of Respiratory & Sleep Medicine, South Brisbane, QLD, Australia

Child Health Research Centre, The University of Queensland Brisbane QLD Australia, Brisbane, QLD, Australia

Valerie J. Waters, MD, MSc Division of Infectious Diseases, Department of Pediatrics, Hospital for Sick Children, University of Toronto, Toronto, ON, Canada

Natalie E. West, MD, MHS Johns Hopkins University, Department of Medicine, Division of Pulmonary and Critical Care Medicine, Baltimore, MD, USA

Andrew J. White, MD Saint Louis Children's Hospital, Department of Pediatrics, Washington University School of Medicine, Saint Louis, MO, USA

Michael Wilschanski, MBBS Pediatric Gastroenterology Unit, Department of Pediatrics, Hadassah Hebrew University Medical Center, Jerusalem, Israel

Part I
Introduction

Chapter 1
The Changing Face of Cystic Fibrosis

Jonathan D. Cogen and Bonnie W. Ramsey

Introduction

Cystic Fibrosis (CF) is a progressive genetic disease thought to affect over 70,000 people worldwide. It is associated with chronic lung infection, gastrointestinal abnormalities including malabsorption, and numerous additional comorbidities that require lifelong treatments and shorten life expectancy. The story of CF over the past 75 years is truly remarkable and inspiring. From the original description of the disease in the 1930s [1, 2] to the elucidation of the basic physiological defect [3] and identification of the CF gene [4–6], the international CF community has witnessed a rapid expansion of scientific knowledge about the pathophysiology of this life-shortening disease. In the past 15 years, this knowledge has been successfully translated into new therapies to correct or replace the abnormal protein function which are improving patient care. These advances are also associated with increased survival; in fact, in 2014, for the first time the majority of people with CF in the United States are adults rather than children [7] (Fig. 1.1), a testament to the power of worldwide collaborative efforts among researchers, foundations, pharmaceutical companies, healthcare providers, and patients and their families to work towards a common goal of improving the lives of patients with CF [8].

J. D. Cogen (✉)
Division of Pulmonary & Sleep Medicine, Department of Pediatrics,
Seattle Children's Hospital, Seattle, WA, USA
e-mail: jonathan.cogen@seattlechildrens.org

B. W. Ramsey
Department of Pediatrics, University of Washington, School of Medicine, Seattle, WA, USA

Center for Clinical and Translational Research, Seattle Children's Research Institute,
Seattle, WA, USA

Seattle Children's Hospital, Center for Clinical and Translational Research, Seattle, WA, USA

© Springer Nature Switzerland AG 2020
S. D. Davis et al. (eds.), *Cystic Fibrosis*, Respiratory Medicine,
https://doi.org/10.1007/978-3-030-42382-7_1

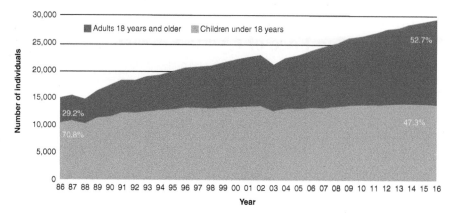

Fig. 1.1 Number of children and adults with CF in the United States, 1986–2016. (From Cystic Fibrosis patients under care at CF Foundation-accredited care centers in the United States, who consented to have their data entered)

Brief History of Earliest Descriptions

CF appears to have been recognized as early as the Middle Ages and Renaissance period; a medical account from eighteenth century modern-day Switzerland in an Almanac of Children's Songs and Games, for example, likely describes a child with CF: "Woe to the child who tastes salty from a kiss on the brow, for he is cursed and soon must die" [9]. In the 1930s, both an American pathologist named Dorothy Andersen and an Italian pediatrician named Guido Fanconi characterized cystic fibrosis of the pancreas and correlated it with CF-related lung and intestinal disease [1, 2]. Dr. Paul di Sant' Agnese in the 1950s paved the way for diagnostic sweat chloride testing (Gibson-Cooke Sweat Test) [10] by demonstrating that people with CF have elevated salt in their sweat [11]. With the availability of the diagnostic sweat test, standardized, multidisciplinary clinical care was established in the 1960s based upon three treatment pillars: (1) optimizing nutrition and pancreatic enzyme replacement, (2) the initiation of airway clearance, and (3) antimicrobial treatment of lung infections [12]. Nevertheless, with only limited treatment options available, the majority of people with CF born in the early to mid-1900s did not survive into adulthood [13].

Work by pioneers, such as Drs. Quinton [3] and Knowles [14], in the 1980s led to research uncovering the basic physiological defect that would unify the known clinical findings of the disease. It was demonstrated in multiple organs, including the sweat gland, respiratory tract and gastrointestinal tract, that there was a lack of anion (Cl^- and HCO_3^-) conductance across epithelial cells, and this impermeability was likely regulated by cyclic-AMP phosphorylation. These important physiological clues were further enhanced by the collaborative discovery of the CFTR gene in 1989 by Drs. Lap-Chee Tsui and John Riordan at Toronto Hospital for Sick Children and Dr. Francis Collins at the University of Michigan [4]. These researchers utilized a combination of "chromosome jumping" (a technique that accelerates mapping of a given genetic region) and DNA cloning to determine the location of the CFTR gene and also illustrated that a deletion of three base pairs of a phenylalanine residue (so-called Phe508del mutation) was detected in a majority of people with CF [4–6]. This combination of discoveries transformed the CF research field permitting scientists to identify a wide range of genetic mutations and to understand how these mutations impacted protein biogenesis and the function of mature CFTR [15]. Ultimately, this knowledge would expand understanding of the pathophysiology of the clinical disease and eventually provide potential therapeutic targets.

CFTR Gene/Protein Structure

Since the 1990s, it has been known that the Cystic Fibrosis Transmembrane Regulator (CFTR) is an anion channel that helps to manage fluid and electrolyte absorption/secretion within the epithelia of many body organs [16]. When CFTR function is reduced or absent in organs, such as the respiratory tract, alterations in airway surface liquid lead to a lowered pH, which inhibits antimicrobial activity and abnormal biophysical properties of mucus, leading to impaired mucociliary clearance and obstructive lung disease, a hallmark clinical manifestation of the disease [17]. Initial work with the Phe508del mutation illustrated that the CFTR protein failed to progress through its normal stages of development within the cell (a processing defect) and never made it to the cell surface to serve its function [15]. Additional studies evaluating CFTR mutations have revealed six unique mutation classes, though some mutations (such as Phe508del) exhibit defects across multiple mutation classes. Over 2000 CFTR mutations have been identified, though to date only ~300 have been established to be disease-causing [18]. An improved understanding of how CFTR mutations cause disease ultimately set the stage for the introduction of CFTR modulators, therapies designed to correct the underlying defect (malfunctioning protein) in CF.

Changes in CF Diagnosis

Over the last 30 years, remarkable progress has been made in CF screening and diagnosis. Today the diagnosis of CF is based upon a positive sweat chloride test, identification of 2 disease causing CFTR variants, or a positive nasal potential difference test [19]. Even if the diagnosis is made by a positive sweat test, genetic testing is also recommended to identify the specific disease causing mutations and determine eligibility for the newly available CFTR modulators. Since 2010, universal newborn screening (NBS) has been available in all 50 U.S. states and the District of Columbia based upon the evidence provided by an important prospective randomized NBS study initiated in Wisconsin in 1985 demonstrating improvements in long-term growth and a reduction in the prevalence of severe malnutrition [20]. These results helped to inform a 2004 report from the U.S. Centers for Disease Control and Prevention that recommended universal newborn screening for CF based on long-term benefits [21]. The implementation of universal newborn screening in the United States has aided in lowering the median age of CF diagnosis from 1.1 years in 1992 to 4 months in 2016 [7, 22]. In 2016, 62.4% of new CF diagnoses and 86% of diagnoses among infants <6 months were detected via newborn screening in the United States [7]. Additional newborn screening programs are currently in place in Canada, Australia, and much of Europe [23–25].

Changes in Clinical Management of CF

From the 1950s to 2011, all treatment of patients with CF was focused on treating consequences of abnormal CFTR function, including malabsorption, malnutrition, recurrent pulmonary infections and other comorbidities, such as liver disease and CF-related diabetes. Through the principles developed with the CF care centers of multidisciplinary, multisystem preventative care, significant advances in survival and improved quality of life occurred over this 60-year period. Pancreatic insufficiency and malnutrition have been treated with enzyme replacement and nutritional supplements. The introduction of NBS permitted the identification of people with CF prior to symptom onset and allowed CF care teams the opportunity to focus on early nutritional outcomes. A recent study found that U.S. infants with CF diagnosed by NBS were able to correct weight deficit by 12 months of age, although some remained stunted [26]. High-fat, high-calorie diets have been associated with improved nutrition, growth, and long-term survival as early as the 1980s [27], and numerous studies since have described improvements in clinical outcomes, quality of life, and overall survival with better nutritional status [28–30]. CF infant and toddler nutrition continues to improve (Fig. 1.2), with an overall median weight-for-length percentile of 64.4% (IQR 13.8–96.7%) in the United States reported in 2016 [7]. CF Foundation nutrition guidelines target normal growth and recommend that a body mass index percentile ≥50% be maintained [31].

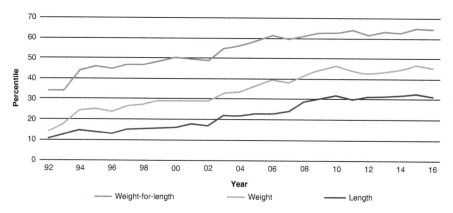

Fig. 1.2 Weight for length percentile, 1992–2016. (From Cystic Fibrosis patients under care at CF Foundation-accredited care centers in the United States, who consented to have their data entered)

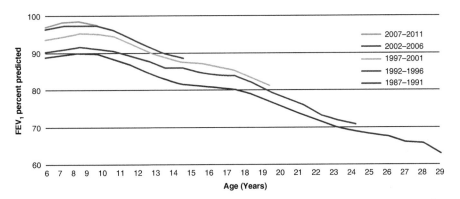

Fig. 1.3 Median FEV$_1$ percent predicted, by age and birth cohort. (From Cystic Fibrosis patients under care at CF Foundation-accredited care centers in the United States, who consented to have their data entered)

The management of lung disease continues to focus on optimizing airway clearance and aggressive treatment of endobronchial bacterial infections and inflammation, as discussed in detail in Chaps. 3, 4, 5, 6, 7, 8, 10, and 11. For example, dornase alfa and hypertonic saline are inhaled medications utilized to enhance mucus clearance and are recommended by the CF Foundation to improve lung function and quality of life and to reduce pulmonary exacerbations [32]. Equally important, optimizing treatment of lung infections with chronic inhaled antibiotics and anti-inflammatory (e.g., azithromycin and ibuprofen) medications has also contributed to improved quality of life and lung function.

It is well documented in the United States and other national registries that pulmonary function (routinely measured as forced expiratory volume in one second (FEV$_1$) percent predicted) in people with CF for a given age continues to increase. This finding is important because lung disease is a primary driver of morbidity and mortality in CF. Mean FEV$_1$% predicted in adolescents, for example, is currently >90%, a remarkable change from the 1980s and 1990s when average FEV$_1$% predicted in this age group was <80% [7] (Fig. 1.3).

Changes in Survival/CF Registries

Excitingly, these improvements in CF diagnosis, nutrition, and therapeutics are likely direct contributors to the rapidly increasing CF survival seen over the last 30 years. The median age of death (i.e. the age at which exactly half of the deaths of people with CF in a given calendar year were below and half were above) and median predicted survival (the age beyond which 50% of infants born with CF during a given year are expected to live, assuming that no change over their lifetimes in mortality rates occurs) for people with CF has increased all over the world. In the United States in 2016, the median age of death and median predicted survival were 29.6 years and 47.7 years, respectively [7] (Fig. 1.4). In Canada, the median predicted survival eclipsed 50 years in 2012 and in 2016 was 53.3 years [33].

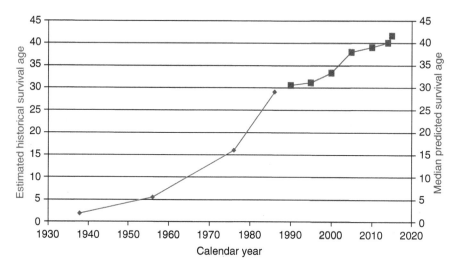

Fig. 1.4 The change in survival in the United States is displayed from the 1930s to 2017. (Reprinted with permission of the American Thoracic Society. Copyright © 2018 American Thoracic Society. Cite: Ramsey and Welsh [63])

These survival data are captured in CF registries—information warehouses that store large amounts of demographic and clinical data from registry-consented patients. The first CF-specific registry was created in 1966 by the CF Foundation, and currently registries exist all over the world, including the United States, Canada, Australia, the United Kingdom, and several European countries [34]. Registries enable researchers to undertake studies related to CF health and disease, such as to describe the natural progression of lung function decline, to monitor for changes in the microbiology of the CF airway, or to evaluate the impact of new or existing therapies. Results from registry-based studies can and have directly influenced care. A 2012 study that examined CF Foundation Patient Registry data, for example, found that inhaled antibiotic use for chronic *Pseudomonas aeruginosa* (*Pa*) infection was associated with decreased mortality compared to no reported use [35], and these results were used to inform the creation of chronic inhaled antibiotic use guidelines. As CF care enters the CFTR modulator era, CF registries have an extremely important role in gathering clinical outcomes from the use of these therapies to determine the most effective treatment strategies moving forward for all patients with CF.

CF Care Centers/Quality Improvement

In 1961, the CF Foundation created a care network with the establishment of two CF-specific care centers [7], and by 1978, more than 100 CFF-accredited care centers existed. Currently, the CF Foundation care network is made up of over 280 pediatric, adult, and affiliate programs within ~120 care centers [36]. In Canada, 42 pediatric and adult CF care centers exist [37], and specialized CF centers are present in Australia, the United Kingdom, and in many countries around Europe. These centers are frequently made of up multidisciplinary teams consisting of experienced clinicians, nurses, dieticians, social workers, respiratory therapists, and child-life specialists. The creation of these multidisciplinary CF care teams has not only facilitated the implementation of guideline-based care into clinical practice, but it has also been associated with improvements in nutrition and lung health for people with CF [38].

CF care teams also play a key role in the implementation of quality improvement (QI) to improve center-specific CF outcomes. The QI model focuses on the healthcare system rather than an individual patient, with the goal of improving healthcare processes in a timely, cost-effective, and efficient manner [39]. Common QI methodologies include the use of plan-do-study-act (PDSA) cycles, lean principles, and process mapping with the choice of methodology dependent on the QI project aims and outcomes [40]. QI requires continuous data collection to determine if a given intervention (e.g., preclinic phone calls to improve clinic attendance) is deemed a success. The ability of CF registries to collect demographic and clinical data over time has aided in the creation of CF-related QI projects. In 2003, for example, the CF Foundation Patient Registry released a web-based data entry system (PortCF) that allows CF care centers to access data in real time. These data can be used to develop new QI projects, to track existing efforts, and to facilitate patient recruitment for prospective QI or clinical studies [41].

More recently, added emphasis has been placed on the incorporation of QI principles into the care of people with CF. In 2002, for example, the CF Foundation launched the Learning and Leadership Collaborative, a 12-month curriculum designed to train QI leaders, to teach individual care teams how to identify areas of improvement, and to develop strategies that ultimately improve health outcomes [42]. The CF Learning Network created in 2016 currently has 26 U.S. participating care centers and follows a Model for Improvement framework (such as PDSA cycles) to address clinical care outcomes and quality of life and reduce cost of care [43]. In France, a collaborative QI program (known as the PHARE-M initiative) was recently established to strengthen quality of care and collaborations among parents and families within French CF care centers [44]. The use of QI systems has undoubtedly contributed to advances in CF care, and QI is likely to remain an important tool for care teams in the future.

Changing the Lives of Patients with CF by Treating the Basic Defect: Abnormal CFTR and Its Sequelae

Since the discovery of the CFTR gene in 1989, researchers have been searching for drugs that could correct the basic defect that contributes to clinical disease. Initial efforts focused on gene therapy, the goal of which is to replace the ineffective CFTR gene in the CF lung with a functional gene that would produce a normal CFTR protein. In the early 1990s, using viral and nonviral vectors researchers had successfully inserted functional CFTR mRNA into rats and mice and documented at least partial correction of the malfunctioning protein [45, 46]. By the mid-1990s, research was underway in humans; these trials were small and designed around molecular and electrophysiological outcomes, but several did illustrate partial CFTR correction in the nasal epithelia of people with CF [47–49]. While these and other studies have established a "proof of principle" for CFTR gene transfer, significant barriers remained, including determining how to overcome the lung host defense mechanisms that limit the effectiveness of gene transfer [50] (more on this in Chap. 22). To date, gene therapy is not part of CF clinical care.

Thus, in the late 1990s, 10 years after the discovery of the CF gene, there were no new therapeutic approaches to correct dysfunctional CFTR. In response, the Cystic Fibrosis Foundation launched an audacious program, the Therapeutics Development Program, to catalyze efforts across academic investigators, industry partners, and its own programs to begin screening small molecule chemical compounds that might modulate CFTR function. Also key to this focused approach on therapeutic development was the establishment in 1999 of the Therapeutics Development Network (CF-TDN) to provide the necessary scientific expertise and infrastructure to assist industry through the process of new drug development [8]. This partnership paved the way for high-throughput screening for CFTR modulators and the development of ivacaftor and is a wonderful example of the power of collaboration among academic centers, industry, and disease-specific foundations to advance care.

High-throughput screening is an automated process that tests for chemical compounds that may have activity as either an activator or inhibitor of a given biologic target, such as the CFTR protein [51]. This technique has since been used in the discovery of CFTR potentiators (compounds that increase chloride channel gating of CFTR) and correctors (compounds that enhance protein folding and trafficking to the cell surface). Over 228,000 compounds were screened prior to the discovery of the first CFTR potentiator therapy (VX-770 or ivacaftor) [52].

In 2011, results of the Phase 3 trial testing ivacaftor in people with CF and the G551D mutation were published in *The New England Journal of Medicine* [53]. This study randomized 161 patients $\geq$12 years of age with CF and at least one G551D mutation to ivacaftor or placebo. Strikingly, by 24 weeks, when compared to placebo, people on ivacaftor had a 10.6% greater improvement in $FEV_1\%$ predicted and at 48 weeks were 55% less likely to have had a pulmonary exacerbation (Fig. 1.5). A subsequent study in children 6–11 years of age showed similarly impressive improvements in $FEV_1\%$ predicted and weight gain in the ivacaftor-treated group compared to placebo [54]. On January 31, 2012, the US Food and Drug Administration (FDA) approved ivacaftor (Kalydeco) for people aged 6 years and older with CF and at least one G551D *CFTR* mutation [55]. The FDA has since expanded ivacaftor approval to treat additional CFTR mutations, and on August 15, 2018, ivacaftor was approved to treat children with CF as young as 12 months [56].

For the first time in the history of CF care, a treatment was now available to target the underlying defect in CF. However, only a small number of people with CF (<10%) can benefit from ivacaftor monotherapy, so researchers quickly focused on the creation of a CFTR corrector—a molecule that can rescue misfolded CFTR

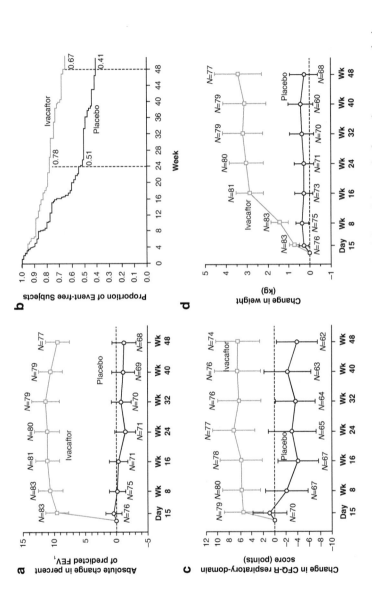

Fig. 1.5 Changes from baseline in percent of predicted FEV_1, respiratory symptoms, and weight, and time to the first pulmonary exacerbation, according to study group. Panel A shows the absolute mean change from baseline in the percent of predicted forced expiratory volume in 1 second (FEV_1), through week 48. Panel B shows the time to the first pulmonary exacerbation, expressed as estimates of the proportion of subjects free from events. Panel C shows the absolute mean change from baseline in the score on the respiratory domain of the Cystic Fibrosis Questionnaire–revised (CFQ-R), a quality-of-life questionnaire that is scored on a 100-point scale, with higher numbers indicating a lower effect of symptoms on the patient's quality of life. The established minimum clinically important difference of the CFQ-R respiratory domain is 4 points. Panel D shows the absolute mean change from baseline in weight, through week 48. The values and the 95% confidence intervals (indicated by I bars) in Panels A, C, and D are unadjusted. The first data points in Panels A, C, and D are baseline data. (From Ramsey et al. [53]. Copyright © 2011 Massachusetts Medical Society. Reprinted with permission)

protein within the cell and bring it to the cell surface [57]—that could be used for people with CF who have the most common mutation (Phe508del). The first combined potentiator-corrector (lumacaftor-ivacaftor) in people with CF who are Phe508del homozygous was shown to improve lung function and reduce pulmonary exacerbations [58] and is currently approved in the United States for people with CF aged 2 years and older who are homozygous for the Phe508del mutation. A second-generation potentiator-corrector (tezacaftor-ivacaftor) is also available for people with CF ≥12 years who are either Phe508del homozygous or have at least one mutation in the *CFTR* gene that is responsive to tezacaftor-ivacaftor based on in vitro data and/or clinical studies (see Chap. 21 for more details on CFTR modulators).

These first-generation correctors (lumacaftor and tezacaftor) in combination with the potentiator ivacaftor are efficacious in approximately 50–60% of patients with CF. A large portion of the remaining people with CF have one copy of Phe508del and a second minimal function mutation not responsive to these first-generation correctors. Laboratory studies [59] have demonstrated that a second corrector is required to augment CFTR trafficking in these patients. Two next-generation triple combination therapies with ivacaftor, tezacaftor, and a second corrector (either VX-445 or VX-659) are currently being tested in phase 2 and 3 studies. The phase 2 study results [59, 60] have demonstrated with both triple combinations a rapid and remarkable decrease in sweat chloride values (> 40 mmol/Liter) and improvement in FEV_1% predicted of >12%. With these encouraging findings, phase 3 trials are currently underway for both triple combinations. If successful, this triple combination approach could be available to over 90% of patients with CF over 12 years of age.

What Does the Next Decade Bring?

Since the discovery of the CFTR gene in 1989, unprecedented improvements in clinical care, quality of life, and survival have been achieved in people with CF. However, CFTR modulators are not as of yet available to treat class I mutations (premature stop codons that result in no protein production) and other rare mutations, such as splice mutations. Thus, more work is needed to increase the availability of CFTR modulators to all people with CF. Furthermore, concerns remain regarding adherence to these and other chronic maintenance therapies [61]. The daily burden of care for persons living with CF is high and withdrawal studies are needed to evaluate the safety of removing certain chronic therapies in patients on effective modulators. Furthermore, these disease-modifying medications are extremely expensive (in the United States in 2017, ivacaftor had a list price of >$300,000 per patient per year while lumacaftor-ivacaftor was >$250,000 per person per year [62]) and in some cases may be cost-prohibitive. Healthcare systems around the world will have to address the growing costs of care to make these novel therapies readily accessible to eligible people with CF. Survival outcomes differ globally, suggesting that significant variations in care need to be addressed through better access to care and therapies, quality improvement initiatives, and other comparative effectiveness research.

While CF in the 1950s–1960s was a devastating diagnosis in which few afflicted survived past adulthood, it is now a chronic disease that can frequently be managed well into adulthood and beyond. A child born with CF today will almost certainly benefit from the substantial contributions made by researchers, clinicians, and care teams towards improving CF clinical care and outcomes, with the ultimate goal of improving the lives of all people with CF.

References

1. Andersen DH. Cystic fibrosis of the pancreas and its relation to celiac disease: a clinical and pathologic study. Am J Dis Child. 1938;56(2):344–99.
2. Fanconi G, Uehlinger E, Knauer C. Das Coeliakie-syndrom bei angeborener zystischer Pankreasfibromatose und Bronchiektasien. Wien Med Wchnschr. 1936;86:753–6.
3. Quinton PM, Bijman J. Higher bioelectric potentials due to decreased chloride absorption in the sweat glands of patients with cystic fibrosis. N Engl J Med. 1983;308:1185–9.
4. Rommens JM, Iannuzzi MC, Kerem B, Drumm ML, Melmer G, Dean M, Rozmahel R, Cole JL, Kennedy D, Hidaka N, Zsiga M, Buchwald M, Riordan JR, Tsui L, Collins FS. Identification of the cystic fibrosis gene: chromosome walking and jumping. Science. 1989;245(4922):1059–65.
5. Riordan JR, Rommens JM, Kerem B, Alon N, Rozmahel R, Grzelczak Z, Zielenski J, Lok S, Plavsic N, Chous J, Drumm ML, Iannuzzi MC, Collins FS, Tsui L. Identification of the cystic fibrosis gene: cloning and characterization of complementary DNA. Science. 1989;245(4922):1066–73.
6. Kerem B, Rommens JM, Buchanan JA, Markiewicz D, Cox TK, Chakravarti A, Buchwald M, Tsui L. Identification of the cystic fibrosis gene: genetic analysis. Science. 1989;245(4922):1073–80.
7. Cystic Fibrosis Foundation Patient Registry 2016 Annual Data Report. Bethesda. ©2016 Cystic Fibrosis Foundation. https://www.cff.org/Research/Researcher-Resources/Patient-Registry/2014-Patient-Registry-Annual-Data-Report.pdf
8. Ramsey BW, Nepom GT, Lonial S. Academic, foundation, and industry collaboration in finding new therapies. N Engl J Med. 2017;376(18):1762–9.
9. Busch R. On the history of cystic fibrosis. Acta Univ Carol Med. 1990;36(1–4):13–5.
10. Gibson LE, Cooke RE. A test for concentration of electrolytes in sweat in cystic fibrosis of the pancreas. Pediatrics. 1959;23(3):545–9.
11. di Sant-Agnese PA, Darling RC, Perera GA, Shea E. Abnormal electrolyte composition of sweat in cystic fibrosis of the pancreas. Clinical significance and relationship to disease. Pediatrics. 1953;12:549–63.
12. Matthews LW, Doershuk CF, Wise M, Eddy G, Nudelman H, Spector S. A therapeutic regimen for patients with cystic fibrosis. J Pediatr. 1964;65(4):558–75.
13. Andersen DH. Cystic fibrosis of the pancreas. J Chronic Dis. 1958;7(1):58–90.
14. Knowles MR, Stutts MJ, Spock A, Fischer N, Gatzy JT, Boucher RC. Abnormal ion permeation through cystic fibrosis respiratory epithelium. Science. 1983;221(4615):1067–70.
15. Welsh MJ, Smith AE. Molecular mechanisms of CFTR chloride channel dysfunction in cystic fibrosis. Cell. 1993;73:1251–4.
16. Sheppard DN, Welsh MJ. Structure and function of the CFTR chloride channel. Physiol Rev. 1999;79:S23–45.
17. Stoltz DA, Meyerholz DK, Welsh MJ. Origins of cystic fibrosis lung disease. N Engl J Med. 2015;372:351–62.

18. US CF Foundation, Johns Hopkins University, The Hospital for Sick Children. The Clinical and Functional Translation of CFTR (CFTR2). http://www.cftr2.org. Accessed 7 Aug 2018.
19. Farrell PM, White TB, Ren CL, Hempstead SE, Accurso F, Derichs N, Howenstine M, McColley SA, Rock M, Rosenfeld M, Sermet-Gaudelus I, Southern KW, Marshall BC, Sosnay PR. Diagnosis of cystic fibrosis: consensus guidelines from the Cystic Fibrosis Foundation. J Pediatr. 2017;181S:S4–15.
20. Farrell PM, Kosorok MR, Rock MJ, Laxova A, Zeng L, Lai HC, Hoffman G, Laessig RH, Splaingard ML, The Wisconsin Cystic Fibrosis Neonatal Screening Study Group. Early diagnosis of cystic fibrosis through neonatal screening prevents severe malnutrition and improves long-term growth. Pediatrics. 2001;107(1):1–13.
21. Grosse SD, Boyle CA, Botkin CA, Comeau AM, Kharrazi M, Rosenfeld M, Wilfond BS. Newborn screening for cystic fibrosis. Evaluation of benefits and risks and recommendations for State Newborn Screening Programs. MMWR. 2004;53(RR13):1–36.
22. Gregg RG, Simantel A, Farrell PM, Koscik R, Kosorok MR, Laxova A, Laessig R, Hoffman G, Hassemer D, Mischler EH, Splaingard M. Newborn screening for cystic fibrosis in Wisconsin: comparison of biochemical and molecular methods. Pediatrics. 1997;99(6):819–24.
23. Cystic Fibrosis Canada. https://www.cysticfibrosis.ca/our-programs/advocacy/cf-newborn-screening. Accessed 8 Aug 2018.
24. Massie J, Clements B, the Australian Paediatric Respiratory Group. Diagnosis of cystic fibrosis after newborn screening: the Australasian experience—twenty years and five millions babies later: a consensus statement from the Australasian Paediatric Respiratory Group. Pediatr Pulmonol. 2005;39:440–6.
25. Castellani C, Massie J, Sontag M, Southern KW. Newborn screening for cystic fibrosis. Lancet Respir Med. 2016;4:653–61.
26. Leung DH, Heltshe SL, Borowitz D, Gelfond D, Kloster M, Heubi JE, Stalvey M, Ramsey BW. Effects of diagnosis by newborn screening for cystic fibrosis on weight and length in the first year of life. J Am Med Assoc. 2017;171(6):546–54.
27. Corey M, Mclaughlin FJ, Williams M, Levkon H. A comparison of survival, growth, and pulmonary function in patients with cystic fibrosis in Boston and Toronto. J Clin Epidemiol. 1988;41(6):583–91.
28. Konstan MW, Butler SM, Wohl ME, et al. Growth and nutritional indexes in early life predict pulmonary function in cystic fibrosis. J Pediatr. 2003;142:624–30.
29. Shoff SM, Tluczek A, Laxova A, Farrell PM, Lai HJ. Nutritional status is associated with health-related quality of life in children with cystic fibrosis aged 9-19 years. J Cyst Fibros. 2013;12:746–53.
30. Yen EH, Quinton H, Borowitz D. Better nutritional status in early childhood is associated with improved clinical outcomes and survival in patients with cystic fibrosis. J Pediatr. 2013;162(2):530–5.
31. Lahiri T, Hempstead SE, Brady C, Cannon CL, Clark K, Condren ME, Guill MF, Guillerman RP, Leone CG, Maguiness K, Monchil L, Power SW, Rosenfeld M, Schwarzenberg SJ, Tompkins CL, Zemanick E, Davis SD. Pediatrics. 2016;137(4):e20151784.
32. Mogayzel PJ, Naureckas ET, Robinson KA, Mueller G, Hadjiliadis D, Hoag JB, Lubsch L, Hazle L, Sabadosa K, Marshall B. Cystic fibrosis pulmonary guidelines: chronic medications for maintenance of lung health. Am J Respir Crit Care Med. 2013;187(7):680–9.
33. Cystic Fibrosis Canada. The Canadian Cystic Fibrosis Registry 2016 annual report. Available from: http://www.cysticfibrosis.ca/blog/2016-registry-annual-data-report/. Accessed date: 16 Aug 2018.
34. Jackson AD, Goss CH. Epidemiology of CF: how registries can be used to advance our understanding of the CF population. J Cyst Fibros. 2018;17:297–305.
35. Sawicki GS, Signorovitch JE, Zhang J, et al. Reduced mortality in cystic fibrosis patients treated with tobramycin inhalation solution. Pediatr Pulmonol. 2012;47(1):44–52.
36. Cystic Fibrosis Foundation. Care Centers. Available from https://www.cff.org/Care/Care-Centers/. Accessed date: 17 Aug 2018.

37. Cystic Fibrosis Canada. Care Centers. Available from https://www.cysticfibrosis.ca/our-pro-grams/healthcare/how-cf-care-is-delivered/cf-clinics-in-canada?province=SK. Accessed date: 18 Aug 2018.
38. Mahadeva R, Webb K, Westerbeek RC, Carroll NR, Dodd ME, Bilton D, Lomas DA. Clinical outcome in relation to care in centres specialising in cystic fibrosis: cross sectional study. BMJ. 1998;316:1771–5.
39. Varkey P, Reller K, Resar RK. Basics of quality improvement in health care. Mayo Clin Proc. 2007;82(6):735–9.
40. U.S. Department of Veteran Affairs. QUERI-quality enhancement research initiative. Available from https://www.queri.research.va.gov/implementation/quality_improvement/default.cfm. Accessed date: 21 Aug 2018.
41. Schechter MS, Fink AK, Homa K, Goss CH. The Cystic Fibrosis Foundation patient registry as a tool for use in quality improvement. BMJ Qual Saf. 2014;23:i9–i14.
42. Godfrey MM, Oliver BJ. Accelerating the rate of improvement in cystic fibrosis care: contributions and insights of the learning and leadership collaborative. BMJ Qual Saf. 2014;23:i23–32.
43. CF Learning Network. Available from https://www.cflearningnetwork.org/what-we-do/. Accessed date: 21 Aug 2018.
44. Bertrand DP, Minguet G, Lombrail P, Rault G. Introduction of a collaborative quality improvement program in the French Cystic Fibrosis Network: the PHARE-M initiative. Orphanet J Rare Dis. 2018;13(S1):14–26.
45. Rosenfeld MA, Yoshimura K, Trapnell BC, Yoneyama K, Rosenthal ER, Dalemans W, Fukayama M, Bargon J, Stier LE, Stratford-Perricaudet L. In vivo transfer of the human cystic fibrosis transmembrane conductance regulator gene to the airway epithelium. Cell. 1992;68:143–55.
46. Hyde SC, Gill DR, Higgins CF, Trezise AE, MacVinish LJ, Cuthbert AW, Ratcliff R, Evans MJ, Colledge WH. Correction of the ion transport defect in cystic fibrosis transgenic mice by gene therapy. Nature. 1993;362:250–5.
47. Zabner J, Couture LA, Gregory RJ, Graham SM, Smith AE, Welsh MJ. Adenovirus-mediated gene transfer transiently corrects the chloride transport defect in nasal epithelia of patients with cystic fibrosis. Cell. 1993;75:207–16.
48. Hay JG, McElvaney NG, Herena J, Crystal RG. Modification of nasal epithelial potential differences of individuals with cystic fibrosis consequent to local administration of a normal CFTR cDNA adenovirus gene transfer vector. Hum Gene Ther. 1995;6(11):1487–96.
49. Wagner JA, Messner AH, Moran ML, et al. Safety and biological efficacy of an adeno-associated virus vector-cystic fibrosis transmembrane regulator (AAV-CFTR) in the cystic fibrosis maxillary sinus. Laryngoscope. 1999;109(2 Pt 1):266–74.
50. Griesenbach U, Alton E. Moving forward: cystic fibrosis gene therapy. Hum Mol Genet. 2013;22(1):R52–8.
51. Broach JR, Thorner J. High-throughput screening for drug discovery. Nature. 1996;384(7):14–6.
52. Van Goor F, Hadid S, Grootenhuis PDJ, Burton B, Cao D, Neuberger T, Turbull A, Singh A, Joubran J, Hazlewood A, Zhou J, McCartney J, Arumugam V, Decker C, Yang J, Young C, Olson ER, Wine JJ, Frizzell RA, Ashlock M, Negulescu P. Rescue of CF airway epithelial cell function in vitro by a CFTR potentiator, VX-770. PNAS. 2009;106(44):18825–30.
53. Ramsey BW, Davies J, McElvaney NG, Tullis E, Bell SC, Drevinek P, Griese M, McKone EF, Wainwright CE, Konstan MW, Moss R, Ratjen F, Sermet-Gaudelus I, Rowe SM, Dong Q, Rodriguez S, Yen K, Ordonez C, Elborn JS. A CFTR potentiator in patients with cystic fibrosis and the G551D mutation. N Engl J Med. 2011;365(18):1663–72.
54. Davies JC, Wainwright CE, Canny GJ, Chilvers MA, Howenstine MS, Munck A, Mainz JG, Rodriguez S, Li H, Yen K, Ordonez CL, Ahrens R. Efficacy and safety of ivacaftor in patients aged 6 to 11 years with cystic fibrosis with a G551D mutation. Am J Respir Crit Care Med. 2013;187(11):1219–25.
55. FDA Approves Kalydeco. Available from https://www.drugs.com/newdrugs/fda-approves-kalydeco-rare-cystic-fibrosis-3078.html. Accessed date: 6 Sept 2018.

56. FDA Approval History. Available from https://www.drugs.com/history/kalydeco.html. Accessed date: 6 Sept 2018.
57. Solomon GM, Marshall SG, Ramsey BW, Rowe SM. Breakthrough therapies: cystic fibrosis (CF) potentiators and correctors. Pediatr Pulmonol. 2015;50:S3–S13.
58. Wainwright CE, Elborn JS, Ramsey BW, Marigowda G, Huang X, Cipolli M, Colombo C, Davies JC, De Boeck K, Flume PA, Konstan MW, McColley SA, McCoy K, McKone EF, Munck A, Ratjen F, Rowe SM, Waltz D, Boyle MP. Lumacaftor-ivacaftor in patients with cystic fibrosis homozygous for Phe508del CFTR. N Engl J Med. 2015;373(3):220–31.
59. Davies JC, Moskowitz SM, Brown C, Horsley A, Mall MA, McKone EF, Plant BJ, Prais D, Ramsey BW, Taylor-Cousar JL, Tullis E, Uluer A, McKee CM, Robertson S, Shilling RA, Simard C, Van Goor F, Waltz D, Xuan F, Young T, Rowe SM. X-659-tezacaftor-ivacaftor in patients with cystic fibrosis and one or two Phe508del alleles. N Engl J Med. 2018;379:1599–611.
60. Keating D, Marigowda G, Burr L, Daines C, Mall MA, McKone EF, Ramsey BW, Rowe SM, Sass LA, Tullis E, McKee CM, Moskowitz SM, Robertson S, Savage J, Simard C, Van Goor F, Waltz D, Xuan F, Young T, Taylor-Cousars JL. VX-445-tezacaftor-ivacaftor in patients with cystic fibrosis and one or two Phe508del alleles. N Engl J Med. 2018;379:1612–20.
61. Quittner AL, Zhang J, Marynchenko M, Chopra PA, Signorovitch J, Yushkina Y, Riekert KA. Pulmonary medication adherence and health-care use in cystic fibrosis. Chest. 2014;146(1):142–51.
62. For Vertex Pharmaceuticals, Can one billion-dollar breakthrough beget another? Available from https://www.forbes.com/sites/matthewherper/2017/08/08/vertex-pharmaceuticals-and-the-price-of-inspiration/#6c035ca65del. Accessed date: 16 Oct 2018.
63. Ramsey BW, Welsh MJ. Progress along the pathway of discovery leading to treatment and cure of cystic fibrosis. AJRCCM. 2017;195(9):1092–9. The American Journal of Respiratory and Critical Care Medicine is an official journal of the American Thoracic Society.

Chapter 2
Diagnosis of Cystic Fibrosis

Caroline S. Thomas and Clement L. Ren

Patient Perspective
A Mother's Words

My name is Laura Spiegel, and shortly before noon on August 13, 2013, my daughter Emily was diagnosed with cystic fibrosis. In that moment, my professional and personal worlds collided. The before forever separated from the after. And the most pervasive emotion I felt on that hot August day was the whisper in my heart that everything had changed.

I knew of cystic fibrosis but had contained it to a mental dumping ground of facts accumulated from high school and college biology classes. The disease had never manifested itself in my family. The idea of conducting genetic testing in utero or batting an eyelash in anticipation of my daughter's heel prick results was absurd. Cystic fibrosis was something that impacted a small group of souls in this world. It had nothing to do with me. Until it did…

The night that my husband Jon and I received our daughter's diagnosis, we huddled together and scoured the Internet for insights to help us make sense of our new reality. The pediatrician who had delivered the diagnosis had suggested we consult Google. I can safely say that was the worst advice we have ever been given. Fortunately, we stumbled upon the Cystic Fibrosis Foundation's web page, and by the time we arrived at our first appointment at the Riley Children's Hospital Cystic Fibrosis Center, we were armed with factual and practical information about our daughter's disease.

C. S. Thomas
The Monroe Carell Jr. Children's Hospital at Vanderbilt and Vanderbilt University Medical Center, Department of Pediatric Allergy, Immunology, and Pulmonary Medicine, Nashville, TN, USA

C. L. Ren (✉)
Division of Pediatric Pulmonology, Allergy and Sleep Medicine, Riley Hospital for Children and Indiana University School of Medicine, Indianapolis, IN, USA
e-mail: clren@iu.edu

© Springer Nature Switzerland AG 2020
S. D. Davis et al. (eds.), *Cystic Fibrosis*, Respiratory Medicine,
https://doi.org/10.1007/978-3-030-42382-7_2

I will never forget the moment that I handed our pediatric pulmonologist a document that I had printed from the Cystic Fibrosis Foundation's web site. It was titled Evidence-Based Guidelines for Cystic Fibrosis Care in Infants and Preschoolers. I had dog-eared pages and highlighted key sections that I wished to discuss. The pulmonologist looked at me, looked down at the paper, and looked back at me again. She asked with a smile if I had recognized her name on the list of leading authors. I had not. It was the first and only time a family had presented our pulmonologist with her own work upon diagnosis.

Several moments into the conversation, our pulmonologist did something that has stuck with me to this day. She pulled her chair alongside me, took my hands in hers, and told me that my daughter was going to live a long and full life. That it was her job as a physician and mine as a parent to help enable this. Those words imprinted on my heart and enabled me to truly hear everything else that day. Because what parent can absorb hours of information on nutrition, respiratory therapy, infection control, and research opportunities when a voice is whispering in the back of her head that one day she will have to bury her child?

A different physician might have seen the peer-reviewed documents and prioritized lists of questions that my husband and I clutched and plunged right into a checklist of clinical care. Our physician recognized that despite our preparation; despite my decade of professional experience in chronic illness; despite our Notre Dame educations; and despite our solid socioeconomic status, we were shaken to the core. Her words and physical gestures that day were a true tipping point for us. They blasted through barriers of fear and enabled us to truly hear what the rest of the care team was saying that day. They put the first building block in place for a lasting foundation of empathy and trust. They helped us take the first step in accepting our new reality and moving forward with hope.

Five years later, our daughter is undoubtedly living a full life. She is in kindergarten, plays on a soccer team, takes gymnastics and dance lessons, and loves to draw. She has no shortage of neighborhood friends who sit with her on the front porch as she does her respiratory treatments. She swallows fistfuls of enzymes with no prodding and is the first to tell visitors to take off their shoes and wash their hands. She is the kindest, silliest, and strongest girl that I know. She accepts that she has cystic fibrosis, but she is in no way defined by it.

Our daughter's diagnosis has taught our family several important lessons over the years. First and foremost, it has given us a new sense of perspective. When your child's life has been called into question, more trivial worries tend to evaporate. Her diagnosis has also helped to shape our life choices. When Emily was born, I was on a leadership track at the world's largest biotech company. Two years later, I came to the abrupt realization that I needed to focus on my family and myself. What I spend my time doing – and who I spend it with – are two of the most important drivers of fulfillment in my life. I now soak up time with Emily and her older brother Joseph, blog about my family's experiences, and have even written a memoir about our journey. These choices have enriched my life and helped me to be more mindful of the beauty and blessings that are all around. Cystic fibrosis has been an unlikely prompter of this new reality.

Finally, Emily's diagnosis has given me a fierce desire to control what I can control. If cystic fibrosis management were limited to self-care alone, it would be an easier beast to slay. Take enzymes before eating? Fine. Do a few hours of respiratory therapy? A hassle but still doable. The hardest part is navigating the outside forces beyond my control. The bacteria that looms in the sandbox, the garden, and the shower head. The person in the check-out line who has a wet cough. The classmate who shows up covered in snot. My fight-or-flight response kicks into high gear the minute cold and flu season arrives. But I've come to realize that short of locking my daughter in a tower, there is only so much I can do to protect her from the outside world. I want her to live a full life without fear. I also want her to be healthy enough to benefit from new therapies coming down the pipeline over the coming decade. It is a delicate balancing act to say the least.

I continue to comfort myself by directing my energies toward that which I can control. I maintain a PowerPoint that tracks all of Emily's illnesses, her symptoms, and the medications that address these issues. This same document follows her BMI percentiles, her bacteria cultures, and the answers to questions we ask in clinic. I participate on two family advisory boards at our children's hospital and proactively communicate opportunities for quality improvement. These efforts give me a sense of control and enable me to feel like I am contributing to my daughter's long-term health beyond the nuts and bolts of her day-to-day self-care.

If I could speak directly to other parents who are experiencing a new diagnosis, I would tell them that it is normal to mourn the loss of the life that you thought you would lead. Parenting a child with cystic fibrosis will not be as simple as parenting a child that is healthy. You will be faced with a host of new and different challenges. But that doesn't mean that your child can't live a long and full life. Control what you can control and figure out how to let go of the rest. It's okay to seek help here. I blog as a means of catharsis, and I take medication to manage my anxiety. I am a better parent for it.

If I could speak to other cystic fibrosis care team members, I tell them that above all, words matter. You don't need to be perfect, but you do need to see us as real families who are doing our best to manage cystic fibrosis as just one part of our busy and harried lives. We may have psychosocial barriers that are getting in our way. We may be depressed. We may be worried about how in the world we are going to afford yet another medication. We may be on pins and needles because the teenager in the waiting room pulled down her protective mask to suck on a lollipop when she was less than 6 feet from our daughter.

Whatever the case may be, help us to address not just the clinical aspects of cystic fibrosis care, but the emotional aspects as well. Recognize when we are struggling. Tell us when we are doing a good job. Remind us not to build walls around our kids no matter what our instincts may tell us. And always remember that our children are more than their cystic fibrosis. They are smart, strong, brave, and kind individuals who, just like you, are doing their best to navigate this wonderfully chaotic journey we call life.

– Laura Spiegel

Historical Background

Several landmark developments have occurred throughout history leading to earlier and improved diagnostic testing in cystic fibrosis (CF). Andersen first differentiated between CF and celiac disease in 1938 following an autopsy study of children with pancreatic insufficiency [1, 2]. Several years later, in 1946, Andersen and Hodges postulated that CF was a heritable disease based on the study of families of infants with pancreatic fibrosis [2, 3]. In 1953, di Sant'Agnese published his findings that individuals with CF have abnormal sweat chloride levels in response to a thermal stimulus, which sparked interest in using sweat chloride measurements for CF diagnosis [2, 4]. Then, in the late 1950s, Gibson and Cooke developed the quantitative pilocarpine iontophoresis test (QPIT) for measurement of sweat chloride concentrations (the sweat test), a technique that is still used today [2, 5]. Abnormalities in chloride transport and increased sodium reabsorption, the electrolyte defects characteristic of CF, were described in the early 1980s [2]. CF newborn screening (NBS) began in the United States (US) in 1982, but it would take almost 3 decades before becoming universal in all states [6]. Finally, the era of genetic testing for CF was ushered in by the identification of the gene coding for the cystic fibrosis transmembrane conductance regulator (CFTR) protein in 1989 [2].

As sweat testing gained popularity, the US CF Foundation (CFF) recognized the importance of standardizing criteria for diagnosis, thereby leading to diagnostic guidelines in 1963. Since that time, the US CFF has convened several consensus expert groups to develop and revise guidelines for the standardization of diagnosis in US CF centers [7]. The most recent consensus guidelines were written by an international committee and published in 2017 [8, 9]. The recommendations address sweat testing guidelines, diagnostic evaluation of infants with a positive CF NBS, evaluation of infants with a positive CF NBS and inconclusive diagnostic testing, application of genetic testing to CF diagnosis, role of CFTR functional testing, diagnosis of CF in non-screened populations, and CFTR-related disorders [9].

Sweat Chloride Testing

CFTR regulates chloride flux in the sweat ducts. In the presence of CFTR dysfunction, Cl- has low permeability and resorption resulting in higher concentrations of NaCl in the sweat of CF patients [10]. Historical methods for sweat collection have included placing individuals in heated rooms, wrapping patients in occlusive plastic, and using silver nitrate to react with sweat in fingertips. Contemporary methods for sweat collection utilize filter paper, gauze, or the Macroduct® system (a plastic disk attached to coiled plastic tubing) applied to an extremity (e.g., the forearm) to collect sweat. QPIT is the current preferred method for sweat testing and the only valid method recognized by the CFF. Iontophoresis uses a small electrical current to move topically applied pilocarpine through the epidermis, which then allows pilocarpine to stimulate muscarinic receptors in sweat glands to secrete sweat [11]. There are four basic steps to sweat testing: pilocarpine iontophoresis to stimulate sweat production, sweat collection as described above, quantification of the sweat collected by weight or volume, and measurement of sweat chloride concentration [12, 13]. Clinical laboratories that perform sweat testing should follow the published guidelines in order to ensure accurate testing; this includes both sweat collection and analysis [9].

All individuals with a positive CF NBS or positive prenatal testing should be referred to a CF center for sweat testing. Sweat testing is also the preferred method to diagnose individuals with clinically suspected CF who were not identified by newborn screening [9]. Additionally, siblings of CF individuals should undergo sweat chloride testing.

There are several potential causes of false-positive sweat tests although clinically these individuals are usually easily distinguished from individuals with CF (Table 2.1) [14, 15]. Other potential sources of error in sweat testing include inadequate sweat collection or errors in sweat electrolyte analysis [12, 16, 17].

The most recent 2017 CF Foundation consensus guidelines for diagnosis provide sweat chloride thresholds for interpretation of test results. A sweat chloride concentration ≥60 mmol/L is elevated, and a diagnosis of CF can be made for individuals with this result and a positive NBS, compatible clinical features, or a positive family history of CF. A sweat chloride concentration <30 mmol/L suggests that CF is unlikely, although a repeat sweat chloride test and CFTR mutation analysis can be considered if clinical suspicion remains high. This recommendation represents a change from the 2008 CF Foundation consensus guidelines, which listed a threshold of <40 mmol/L as the cutoff for an unlikely diagnosis of CF in individuals >6 months

Table 2.1 Causes for false-positive sweat test results	
	Adrenal insufficiency
	Autonomic dysfunction
	Congenital adrenal hyperplasia
	Ectodermal dysplasia
	Eczema
	Fucosidosis
	Glucose-6-phosphate dehydrogenase (G6PD) deficiency
	Glycogen storage disease type 1
	Human immunodeficiency virus (HIV)
	Hypoparathyroidism
	Hypothyroidism
	Klinefelter's syndrome
	Malnutrition including anorexia nervosa
	Mauriac syndrome
	Nephrogenic diabetes insipidus
	Pseudohypoaldosteronism

Adapted from O'Sullivan et al. [14] and Wallis [15]

old. Finally, a sweat chloride test result of 30–59 mmol/L is an intermediate result. Individuals with an intermediate test result should have a repeat sweat chloride test. If the test result remains in the intermediate range, individuals should have CFTR gene mutation analysis as well as potential evaluation of CF clinical features (e.g., exocrine pancreatic function) [9].

Sweat test results are part of the national CFF Patient Registry (CFFPR) and should be included for all confirmed diagnoses. The CF Foundation consensus guidelines continue to recommend sweat testing as the gold standard diagnostic test to confirm CFTR dysfunction and diagnosis. Interestingly, the number of individuals with recorded sweat test results in the CFFPR has declined over time; this may reflect a reliance by clinicians on genotype data only for diagnosis. However, sweat testing is important to confirm genetic findings reported through CF NBS. In addition, sweat chloride, a biomarker of CFTR function, has been demonstrated to respond (decrease) when patients undergo treatment with CFTR restoration therapies.

Other Methods to Assess CFTR Function

In individuals with intermediate sweat chloride concentrations and a positive NBS, CF symptoms, or positive family history, and fewer than two known CF-causing mutations, additional CFTR functional testing may be needed [9]. Intestinal current measurements (ICM) and nasal potential difference (NPD) measurements are two alternative methods to evaluate CFTR function. ICM is performed using ex vivo samples obtained from rectal suction biopsy. The rectal biopsy tissue is placed in an Ussing chamber where it is stimulated with Cl^- secretory agents, enabling measurement of transepithelial tissue current. CFTR is highly expressed in rectal tissue, and ICM are specific and sensitive assays for CFTR activity [18, 19]. NPD is a minimally invasive in vivo test that measures the bioelectric potential across the nasal epithelium when the nasal epithelium is bathed in solutions that inhibit the epithelial sodium channel and enhance Cl- transport through CFTR [20]. NPD has been successfully performed in young infants [21]. ICM and NPD require specialized equipment and skilled technicians, neither of which is widely available throughout centers. These tests also lack clearly defined reference ranges for clinical use [9].

Recent research has explored the use of theratyping, which is a form of personalized medicine that matches therapies to specific mutations. Theratyping can be particularly helpful when trying to predict the potential efficacy of a CFTR modulator for a rare mutation. Researchers have used the rectal epithelium and nasal epithelium of CF individuals to develop rectal organoids and nasal epithelioid cell spheroids, respectively. These organoids and spheroids are in vitro models that assess CFTR function and could be used for diagnostic purposes, although at this point, they are mainly research tools for evaluating response to CFTR modulator therapy [22–25].

Newborn Screening

Early diagnosis of CF through NBS is associated with better nutritional outcomes compared with diagnosis through clinical features alone [26]. In turn, better nutritional outcomes have been associated with improved lung function and mortality [27]. Many countries worldwide now conduct CF NBS [28]. CF NBS in the United States began in Colorado in 1982. Over the next two decades, debate continued regarding the long-term benefits of early diagnosis through NBS. However, as accumulating evidence of the benefits of CF NBS began to accrue, a consensus emerged that the benefits outweighed the small risk of harm. By 2010, CF NBS was available in all 50 states in the United States [29].

CF NBS algorithms vary by country and state. In the US, all CF NBS begins with the detection of serum immunoreactive trypsinogen (IRT), a pancreatic proenzyme that is elevated in almost all infants with CF [30]. A dried blood spot assay for IRT was first developed in 1979 for use in screening [31]. However, an elevated IRT is not specific for CF. Some infants without CF can have transiently elevated IRT levels, and perinatal stress can also increase these levels. IRT can also be elevated in African-American newborns without CF [32, 33]. To improve the sensitivity of CF NBS, a second or third tier of testing is performed, the choice of which is state-specific. In the US, three different CF NBS algorithms are most commonly used. One approach is to repeat the IRT testing 2–4 weeks later (IRT/IRT algorithm). In infants without CF, the IRT level is usually normal, whereas in infants with CF, it is persistently elevated. This approach was employed in Colorado, the first state to perform CF NBS, prior to the discovery of the CFTR gene. The IRT/IRT diagnostic algorithm is now used less frequently than algorithms that include DNA analysis (IRT/DNA) because the latter has increased sensitivity, improved positive predictive value, led to fewer false positives, and decreased time to diagnosis [34–36]. Under an IRT/DNA algorithm, if the IRT is elevated, then CFTR gene mutation analysis is performed on the dried NBS blood spot. Usually, a panel of 23–45 mutations is tested; the exact composition of the mutation panel varies from state to state [9]. Some states, such as California and New York, perform gene sequencing [37, 38]. To increase the sensitivity and specificity of screening and decrease the rate of carrier identification, some states have employed an IRT/IRT/DNA algorithm [34]. With this algorithm, IRT testing is repeated 1–2 weeks after the initial IRT testing reveals elevated levels. If the IRT level is persistently elevated, then DNA analysis is performed. Although using an IRT/IRT/DNA algorithm can increase the time to diagnosis, the use of this algorithm still allows for CF diagnosis within the first month of life [34]. Some NBS algorithms recommend sweat testing for infants with very high IRT. The very high IRT algorithm can be helpful in detecting infants with rare mutations, particularly in populations with high racial and ethnic diversity, who may be missed with a standard DNA mutation panel [39]. However, this approach is also associated with a high false-positive rate.

Similar to programs in the US, the European programs also use IRT as the first step in CF NBS. A few European countries include pancreatitis-associated protein (PAP) analysis as part of the second step in their screening algorithm. PAP is a protein released by the pancreas during times of inflammation and is elevated in neonates with CF, but it is not a specific marker for this disease. Benefits of IRT/PAP analysis compared to IRT/DNA analysis include decreased incidence of carrier detection as well as an estimated decrease in cost of screening [40].

Regardless of the choice of algorithm, NBS is only a screen and is not diagnostic of CF. NBS does not abrogate the need for sweat testing. All patients with positive NBS should receive confirmatory testing with sweat chloride testing to demonstrate evidence of CFTR dysfunction. The CFF diagnostic guidelines recommend sweat testing even for infants with two CF-causing mutations through NBS, since laboratory errors can occur [9]. Patients with negative NBS but clinical suspicion for CF should always undergo sweat testing.

Prenatal Screening

The American College of Obstetricians and Gynecologists currently recommends offering CF carrier screening to all women considering pregnancy or who are pregnant. This testing is also offered to their partners. A 23-mutation panel is recommended for screening. Expanded panels are available and can increase the sensitivity of carrier screening, particularly for non-Caucasian patients. A history of a newborn with a negative NBS does not mean that parents are not carriers, so prenatal screening should still be offered [38]. If prenatal testing does show two CF-causing CFTR mutations, the diagnosis should still be confirmed postnatally with sweat testing [9]. Conversely, negative prenatal results do not rule out CF, since the fetus could have two rare mutations that are not on the testing panel.

Genetic Testing

CF is an autosomal recessive disease caused by two *in trans* CFTR mutations (i.e., each mutation on separate alleles). As of 2018, gene sequencing has identified over 2000 CFTR mutations, but not all of these are disease-causing. In an effort to categorize mutations and describe their clinical relevance, the US CFF gathered an international research team to develop a database for CFTR mutations. The Clinical and Functional Translation of CFTR (CFTR2) database is a repository of information that provides information about the most common mutations. By 2013, researchers were able to successfully describe the pathogenicity of 127 variants using a combination of clinical features, functional assessment of each variant, and population penetrance information [41]. As of December 2017, the database has expanded to include 374 disease-causing variants [42]. The CFTR2 database divides mutations into four categories: (1) CF-causing, (2) varying clinical consequence, (3) non-CF-causing, and (4) unknown significance. These categories allow for easier interpretation of genetic results. Evidence of CFTR dysfunction via sweat testing is still required to confirm a diagnosis of CF, even in the presence of two CF-causing mutations. Genotyping is used to support the diagnosis of CF, but it is not confirmatory, particularly given the abundance of CFTR mutations with varying clinical consequence or unknown significance. Additionally, not detecting two CF-causing mutations does not exclude a diagnosis of CF [43].

States that use DNA as part of their NBS algorithm select mutation panels for genotyping. Panels are state-specific, and the choice of panel can be influenced by population demographics and the prevalence of mutations in that population. [43]. California and New York also use third-tier CFTR sequencing as part of the NBS algorithm [37, 38]. As previously mentioned, obstetricians also rely on mutation panels for CF prenatal screening.

The 2017 CF diagnostic guidelines do not contain a statement recommending routine genotyping for individuals diagnosed with CF; however, the supplemental material states that CFTR genotyping should be performed for all individuals with CF. In the era of CFTR modulator therapy, knowledge of an individual's genotype will help determine eligibility for treatment [43]. Genotyping is typically performed with next-generation sequencing technology. With this technology, the full coding region of the gene can be sequenced, but there is an option to only report variants of known clinical consequence based on targeted assays. However, if clinically indicated, the laboratory can supply the full report of variants [43, 44]. Other laboratory methods may be required to detect large deletions, duplications, or variants in the noncoding region of genes, all of which may be missed by sequencing [43]. However, even sequencing with del/dup will not detect deep intronic mutations or large deletions in the CFTR gene that can cause disease [45]. Also, as discussed above, the disease liability of some CFTR mutations has not been determined.

CF genotyping has resulted in an increased identification of carriers through false-positive NBS results or through positive prenatal screening. Parents of infants identified as CF carriers have reported decreased anxiety after speaking with a genetic counselor even before receiving a negative sweat test result [46]. When recommending CF NBS, the Centers for Disease Control and Prevention recognized that parents of CF carriers may experience psychological distress and may also be at risk for misunderstanding the implications of carrier status. Furthermore, parents are faced with the decision to disclose their child's carrier status to the extended family. Genetic counseling can be helpful for parents to better understand a CF carrier diagnosis [6]. The American College of Obstetricians and Gynecologists recommends genetic counseling if both parents are found to be CF carriers [38].

Diagnosis of CF in the Non-screened Population

With the advent of NBS, the majority of new CF diagnoses in the US are identified during infancy. Although data from the CFFPR show that 60–65% percent of new CF diagnoses are detected through NBS, a substantial proportion are diagnosed because of clinical signs and symptoms (Table 2.2) [47–49]. These patients are typically older pediatric patients who were born before CF NBS was implemented in their states, pediatric patients with false-negative newborn screening results, or adults. Some of these late diagnoses have residual function CFTR mutations

Table 2.2 Clinical features of CF

Respiratory signs and symptoms
Chronic cough with sputum production
Digital clubbing
Persistent wheezing
Recurrent pneumonia
Persistent chest radiograph abnormalities such as bronchiectasis, atelectasis, and infiltrates
Respiratory cultures positive for typical CF pathogens
Hemoptysis
Nasal polyps
Chronic sinusitis
Gastrointestinal signs and symptoms
Meconium ileus
Prolonged neonatal jaundice
Failure to thrive
Rectal prolapse
Recurrent intussusception
Pancreatic insufficiency
Steatorrhea
Fat-soluble vitamin deficiencies
Recurrent pancreatitis
Chronic hepatic disease
Reproductive signs and symptoms
Male reproductive tract abnormalities such as congenital bilateral absence of the vas deferens
Other signs and symptoms
Salty tasting skin
Chronic metabolic alkalosis
Acute hyponatremic dehydration

Adapted from Filbrun et al. [48] and Rosenstein et al. [49]

associated with a milder phenotype [50]. If there is clinical suspicion for CF, patients should have sweat testing performed to demonstrate CFTR dysfunction and confirm diagnosis. CFTR genetic analysis should be performed if the sweat chloride results are ≥30 mmol/L on two separate occasions [51].

Cystic Fibrosis Transmembrane Conductance Regulator-Related Metabolic Syndrome and Cystic Fibrosis Screen-Positive/Inconclusive Diagnosis

Cystic fibrosis transmembrane conductance regulator-related metabolic syndrome (CRMS) and cystic fibrosis screen-positive/inconclusive diagnosis (CFSPID) are terms used for individuals with positive NBS but inconclusive diagnostic testing. CRMS is typically used in the US while CFSPID is more often used in other countries. The diagnosis of CRMS/CFSPID is given to an individual without signs or symptoms of CF who have a positive CF NBS with (1) normal sweat test results and two CFTR mutations with at least one mutation having an unclear significance or (2) intermediate sweat test results and zero or one CF-causing mutations [52]. CRMS/CFSPID can be a challenging diagnosis for healthcare providers and families particularly regarding the risk of developing features of CF and need for follow-up. Although recent studies have helped better describe prevalence and outcomes, long-term outcome data are still lacking [52]. Guidelines in the US and Europe discuss recommendations for care of these individuals, including establishing care at a CF center, but optimal frequency of follow-up visits has not been determined [52–54].

Several recent studies conducted across the world have provided some insight into the prevalence and outcomes of CRMS/CFSPID. Although the population and study design differ among the various investigations, some common themes have emerged. The ratio of CF diagnoses to CRMS/CFSPID diagnoses has ranged from 0.67:1 to 7.8:1 [37, 55–58]. This wide range may be a reflection of differences among NBS algorithms and diversity in patient populations. A ratio of 0.67 CF diagnosis for every 1 CRMS/CFSPID diagnosis occurred in California, where gene sequencing is part of the NBS algorithm. This algorithm has resulted in the identification of several novel CFTR variants of uncertain significance leading to a higher incidence of CRMS/CFSPID [37]. Some studies have analyzed individuals initially diagnosed with CRMS/CFSPID who were later diagnosed with CF. In the California cohort, 3.7% of CRMS/CFSPID infants eventually received a diagnosis of CF [37]. The Canadian/Italian study reported that 10.9% of CRMS/CFSPID individuals were later diagnosed with CF after their mutations were determined to be disease-causing; this highlights the importance of performing complete genetic analysis in CRMS/CFSPID infants and keeping up to date on advances in CF genetics. Infants whose diagnosis was changed to CF had significantly higher IRT and sweat chloride levels compared to patients whose diagnosis did not change [56]. The Australian study had the highest percent of CRMS/CFSPID individuals later diagnosed with CF at 48%. However, many of these patients had nonspecific respiratory symptoms (e.g., cough) [55]. With the exception of the data from Australia, the studies from California and Canada/Italy did not look at data for the past 5 years. In all the studies, the vast majority of CRMS/CFSPID patients were pancreatic sufficient [37, 55–58]. The percent of individuals with respiratory cultures positive for *Pseudomonas aeruginosa* ranged from 10.7% to 78.6% [55–58], and the percent of individuals with *Stenotrophomonas maltophilia*-positive cultures ranged from 4.9% to 9.4% [56, 58]. Although not diagnostic of CF, these microbiologic findings do raise concerns that CRMS/CFSPID infants can develop manifestations of the disease. While these studies provide insight into CRMS/CFSPID, ultimately more research is needed to better answer the question of whether or not an individual will progress to a diagnosis of CF.

Table 2.3 CFTR-related disorders

Idiopathic chronic pancreatitis (ICP)
Congenital bilateral absence of the vas deferens (CBAVD)
Disseminated bronchiectasis
Chronic sinusitis and/or nasal polyposis

CFTR-Related Disorders

In contrast to patients with CRMS/CFSPID, patients with CFTR-related disorders are symptomatic at diagnosis. CFTR-related disorders are clinical conditions associated with CFTR dysfunction that do not fulfill diagnostic criteria for CF. CFTR-related disorders are usually diagnosed in adult patients with monosymptomatic disease. These monosymptomatic, single-organ disorders include idiopathic chronic pancreatitis (ICP), congenital bilateral absence of the vas deferens (CBAVD), disseminated bronchiectasis, and chronic sinusitis and/or nasal polyposis (Table 2.3) [51, 59].

CFTR is thought to have a role in ICP for several reasons. Patients with ICP have inspissated secretions that plug their pancreatic ducts, similar to CF patients with pancreatic disease. Additionally, ICP can be associated with an elevated sweat chloride result. Finally, pancreatitis sometimes occurs in patients with CF. Indeed, an association was found between ICP and CFTR mutations [60]. It is estimated that 30% of patients with ICP have CFTR mutations [59].

CBAVD is usually diagnosed in males undergoing evaluation for infertility, and it is typically an autosomal recessive disorder associated with CFTR gene mutations. Some males with CBAVD have normal spermatogenesis and can have children through the use of assisted reproductive technologies (ART). Prenatal screening should be offered to males and their female partners prior to ART [59].

Disseminated bronchiectasis can be a diagnostic dilemma, and disagreement exists regarding the classification of disseminated bronchiectasis as a CFTR-related disorder rather than CF. It has been reported that 10–50% of patients with bronchiectasis have at least one CFTR mutation. However, in the absence of other organ involvement as is typical for CF, it is difficult to determine whether CFTR dysfunction is the driving force behind bronchiectasis development. Workup for patients with bronchiectasis should include evaluation for other clinical features of CF (e.g., semen analysis in men) as well as consideration for other diagnoses such as primary ciliary dyskinesia, immunodeficiency, congenital lung abnormalities, and recurrent aspiration [51, 59].

Additional Testing

Rare cases exist where clinical suspicion for CF is high, but sweat testing is normal or inconclusive and CFTR analysis is not definitive. In these instances, additional workup to assess for clinical features of CF may be helpful depending on the signs

Table 2.4 Additional diagnostic testing for CF

Pulmonary
Chest computed tomography
Oropharyngeal, sputum, or bronchoalveolar cultures for typical CF pathogens
Pulmonary function testing
Nasal nitric oxide testing
Genetic analysis for mutations associated with primary ciliary dyskinesia
Gastrointestinal
Fecal elastase
Abdominal imaging
Fat-soluble vitamin levels
Evaluations for celiac disease, inflammatory bowel disease, or recurrent pancreatitis
Immunity
Immunodeficiency evaluation
Reproductive
Male infertility workup

Adapted from reference [51]

and symptoms and other potential diagnoses. Additional workup may include but is not limited to chest computed tomography to look for bronchiectasis; oropharyngeal, sputum, or bronchoalveolar lavage cultures to assess for *Pseudomonas aeruginosa* or other typical CF pathogens; pulmonary function tests; fecal elastase testing; abdominal imaging; fat-soluble vitamin levels; male infertility workup; and specific testing for alternative diagnoses including primary ciliary dyskinesia, immunodeficiencies, celiac disease, inflammatory bowel disease, and recurrent pancreatitis (Table 2.4) [51].

Fecal elastase (FE) testing is used as a noninvasive measure of pancreatic function. Pancreatic elastase is produced by the pancreas, and levels can be measured in the stool. A FE level that is <200 µg/g is abnormal and suggests pancreatic insufficiency. Testing is specific for human elastase, which allows for interpretation of results in individuals who are receiving porcine-derived pancreatic enzyme replacement therapy. Longitudinal data from infants have shown that FE values can vary during the first year of life with some infants having fluctuations between the abnormal and normal ranges [61]. Fecal elastase testing can be a particularly helpful ancillary test while waiting for repeat sweat testing in infants whose sweat chloride levels are not sufficient. Evidence of pancreatic insufficiency supports initiating pancreatic enzyme replacement therapy in these individuals and helps prevent malabsorption. FE testing, however, does not confirm a diagnosis of CF and would miss diagnosing individuals with CF who are pancreatic sufficient at birth.

Male infertility workup can lead to a diagnosis of CF in adults. Approximately 95% of males with CF are infertile due to azoospermia, which is the absence of sperm in ejaculated semen. Azoospermia in CF usually occurs due to absence of the vas deferens. Males with CF typically have normal spermatogenesis, but their CBAVD results in obstructive azoospermia [62]. Genetic testing for CFTR is indicated for men with the following abnormal testing: (1) semen analysis with no or low sperm concentrations and at least one absent vas deferens or (2) semen analysis without any sperm who still have evidence of normal spermatogenesis [63].

Summary

The development of sweat testing, advances in prenatal and newborn screening, and the genetic analysis of CFTR have transformed the path to CF diagnosis. Now, many CF individuals are identified prior to the appearance of clinical signs and symptoms. Despite the many tools available, however, not all diagnoses are straightforward. CRMS/CFSPID and CFTR-related disorders are diagnoses in particular that can be difficult for clinicians and patients. Published guidelines from the US CFF have been instrumental in helping to standardize CF diagnosis and address challenges in the process. The accurate and timely diagnosis of CF is paramount in order to provide appropriate care for individuals with this disease.

References

1. Andersen DH. Cystic fibrosis of the pancreas and its relation to celiac disease: a clinical and pathologic study. Am J Dis Child. 1938;56(2):344–99.
2. Davis PB. Cystic fibrosis since 1938. Am J Respir Crit Care Med. 2006;173(5):475–82.
3. Andersen DH, Hodges RG. Celiac syndrome; genetics of cystic fibrosis of the pancreas, with a consideration of etiology. Am J Dis Child (1911). 1946;72:62–80.
4. Di Sant'Agnese PA, Darling RC, Perera GA, Shea E. Abnormal electrolyte composition of sweat in cystic fibrosis of the pancreas; clinical significance and relationship to the disease. Pediatrics. 1953;12(5):549–63.
5. Gibson LE, Cooke RE. A test for concentration of electrolytes in sweat in cystic fibrosis of the pancreas utilizing pilocarpine by iontophoresis. Pediatrics. 1959;23(3):545–9.
6. Grosse SD, Boyle CA, Botkin JR, Comeau AM, Kharrazi M, Rosenfeld M, et al. Newborn screening for cystic fibrosis: evaluation of benefits and risks and recommendations for state newborn screening programs. MMWR Recomm Rep. 2004;53(RR-13):1–36.
7. Farrell PM, White TB, Derichs N, Castellani C, Rosenstein BJ. Cystic fibrosis diagnostic challenges over 4 decades: historical perspectives and lessons learned. J Pediatr. 2017;181s:S16–s26.
8. Farrell PM, White TB. Introduction to "Cystic Fibrosis Foundation consensus guidelines for diagnosis of cystic fibrosis". J Pediatr. 2017;181s:S1–s3.
9. Farrell PM, White TB, Ren CL, Hempstead SE, Accurso F, Derichs N, et al. Diagnosis of cystic fibrosis: consensus guidelines from the Cystic Fibrosis Foundation. J Pediatr. 2017;181:S4–S15.e1.
10. Quinton PM. Chloride impermeability in cystic fibrosis. Nature. 1983;301(5899):421–2.
11. Collie JT, Massie RJ, Jones OA, LeGrys VA, Greaves RF. Sixty-five years since the New York heat wave: advances in sweat testing for cystic fibrosis. Pediatr Pulmonol. 2014;49(2):106–17.
12. LeGrys VA, Yankaskas JR, Quittell LM, Marshall BC, Mogayzel PJ Jr. Diagnostic sweat testing: the Cystic Fibrosis Foundation guidelines. J Pediatr. 2007;151(1):85–9.

13. Hammond KB, Turcios NL, Gibson LE. Clinical evaluation of the macroduct sweat collection system and conductivity analyzer in the diagnosis of cystic fibrosis. J Pediatr. 1994;124(2):255–60.
14. O'Sullivan BP, Freedman SD. Cystic fibrosis. Lancet. 2009;373(9678):1891–904.
15. Wallis C. Diagnosis and presentation of cystic fibrosis. In: Wilmott RW, Boat TF, Bush A, Chernick V, Deterding RR, Ratjen F, editors. Kendig and Chernick's disorders of the respiratory tract in children. 8th ed. Philadelphia: Elsevier Saunders; 2012. p. 763–9.
16. LeGrys VA, McColley SA, Li Z, Farrell PM. The need for quality improvement in sweat testing infants after newborn screening for cystic fibrosis. J Pediatr. 2010;157(6):1035–7.
17. LeGrys VA, Applequist R, Briscoe DR, Farrell P, Hickstein R, Lo SF, Passarell R, Rheinheimer DW, Rosenstein BJ, Vaks JE. Sweat testing: sample collection and quantitative chloride analysis; approved guideline. 3rd ed. Wayne: Clinical and Laboratory Standards Institute (CLSI); 2009.
18. Clancy JP, Szczesniak RD, Ashlock MA, Ernst SE, Fan L, Hornick DB, et al. Multicenter intestinal current measurements in rectal biopsies from CF and non-CF subjects to monitor CFTR function. PLoS One. 2013;8(9):e73905.
19. Derichs N, Sanz J, Von Kanel T, Stolpe C, Zapf A, Tummler B, et al. Intestinal current measurement for diagnostic classification of patients with questionable cystic fibrosis: validation and reference data. Thorax. 2010;65(7):594–9.
20. Rowe SM, Clancy J-P, Wilschanski M. Nasal potential difference measurements to assess CFTR ion channel activity. Methods Mol Biol (Clifton, NJ). 2011;741:69–86.
21. Sermet-Gaudelus I, Girodon E, Roussel D, Deneuville E, Bui S, Huet F, et al. Measurement of nasal potential difference in young children with an equivocal sweat test following newborn screening for cystic fibrosis. Thorax. 2010;65(6):539–44.
22. Dekkers JF, Berkers G, Kruisselbrink E, Vonk A, de Jonge HR, Janssens HM, et al. Characterizing responses to CFTR-modulating drugs using rectal organoids derived from subjects with cystic fibrosis. Sci Transl Med. 2016;8(344):344ra84.
23. Dekkers JF, Wiegerinck CL, de Jonge HR, Bronsveld I, Janssens HM, de Winter-de Groot KM, et al. A functional CFTR assay using primary cystic fibrosis intestinal organoids. Nat Med. 2013;19(7):939–45.
24. Brewington JJ, Filbrandt ET, LaRosa FJ 3rd, Moncivaiz JD, Ostmann AJ, Strecker LM, et al. Generation of human nasal epithelial cell spheroids for individualized cystic fibrosis transmembrane conductance regulator study. J Vis Exp. 2018;134.
25. Brewington JJ, Filbrandt ET, LaRosa FJ 3rd, Ostmann AJ, Strecker LM, Szczesniak RD, et al. Detection of CFTR function and modulation in primary human nasal cell spheroids. J Cyst Fibros. 2018;17(1):26–33.
26. Farrell PM, Kosorok MR, Laxova A, Shen G, Koscik RE, Bruns WT, et al. Nutritional benefits of neonatal screening for cystic fibrosis. Wisconsin cystic fibrosis neonatal screening study group. N Engl J Med. 1997;337(14):963–9.
27. Rosenfeld M. Overview of published evidence on outcomes with early diagnosis from large US observational studies. J Pediatr. 2005;147(3 Suppl):S11–4.
28. Therrell BL, Padilla CD, Loeber JG, Kneisser I, Saadallah A, Borrajo GJ, et al. Current status of newborn screening worldwide: 2015. Semin Perinatol. 2015;39(3):171–87.
29. Wagener JS, Zemanick ET, Sontag MK. Newborn screening for cystic fibrosis. Curr Opin Pediatr. 2012;24(3):329–35.
30. Farrell PM, White TB, Howenstine MS, Munck A, Parad RB, Rosenfeld M, et al. Diagnosis of cystic fibrosis in screened populations. J Pediatr. 2017;181s:S33–S44.e2.
31. Crossley JR, Elliott RB, Smith PA. Dried-blood spot screening for cystic fibrosis in the newborn. Lancet (London, England). 1979;1(8114):472–4.
32. Rock MJ, Mischler EH, Farrell PM, Bruns WT, Hassemer DJ, Laessig RH. Immunoreactive trypsinogen screening for cystic fibrosis: characterization of infants with a false-positive screening test. Pediatr Pulmonol. 1989;6(1):42–8.
33. Giusti R. Elevated IRT levels in African-American infants: implications for newborn screening in an ethnically diverse population. Pediatr Pulmonol. 2008;43(7):638–41.

34. Sontag MK, Lee R, Wright D, Freedenberg D, Sagel SD. Improving the sensitivity and positive predictive value in a cystic fibrosis newborn screening program using a repeat immunoreactive trypsinogen and genetic analysis. J Pediatr. 2016;175:150–8.e1.
35. Sanders DB, Lai HJ, Rock MJ, Farrell PM. Comparing age of cystic fibrosis diagnosis and treatment initiation after newborn screening with two common strategies. J Cyst Fibros. 2012;11(2):150–3.
36. Gregg RG, Simantel A, Farrell PM, Koscik R, Kosorok MR, Laxova A, et al. Newborn screening for cystic fibrosis in Wisconsin: comparison of biochemical and molecular methods. Pediatrics. 1997;99(6):819–24.
37. Kharrazi M, Yang J, Bishop T, Lessing S, Young S, Graham S, et al. Newborn screening for cystic fibrosis in California. Pediatrics. 2015;136(6):1062–72.
38. Caggana M. Changes to the New York Newborn Screening Program's Cystic Fibrosis (CF) Screening Protocol New York: New York State Department of Health; 2017. Available from: https://www.wadsworth.org/news/changes-to-the-new-york-newborn-screening-programs-cystic-fibrosis-cf-screening-protocol.
39. Kay DM, Langfelder-Schwind E, DeCelie-Germana J, Sharp JK, Maloney B, Tavakoli NP, et al. Utility of a very high IRT/No mutation referral category in cystic fibrosis newborn screening. Pediatr Pulmonol. 2015;50(8):771–80.
40. Sarles J, Berthezene P, Le Louarn C, Somma C, Perini JM, Catheline M, et al. Combining immunoreactive trypsinogen and pancreatitis-associated protein assays, a method of newborn screening for cystic fibrosis that avoids DNA analysis. J Pediatr. 2005;147(3):302–5.
41. Sosnay PR, Siklosi KR, Van Goor F, Kaniecki K, Yu H, Sharma N, et al. Defining the disease liability of variants in the cystic fibrosis transmembrane conductance regulator gene. Nat Genet. 2013;45(10):1160–7.
42. The Clinical and Functional TRanslation of CFTR (CFTR2): US CF Foundation Johns Hopkins University The Hospital for Sick Children; 2011. Available from: http://cftr2.org.
43. Sosnay PR, Salinas DB, White TB, Ren CL, Farrell PM, Raraigh KS, et al. Applying cystic fibrosis transmembrane conductance regulator genetics and CFTR2 data to facilitate diagnoses. J Pediatr. 2017;181S:S27–S32.e1.
44. Baker MW, Atkins AE, Cordovado SK, Hendrix M, Earley MC, Farrell PM. Improving newborn screening for cystic fibrosis using next-generation sequencing technology: a technical feasibility study. Genet Med. 2016;18(3):231–8.
45. Wine JJ, Kuo E, Hurlock G, Moss RB. Comprehensive mutation screening in a cystic fibrosis center. Pediatrics. 2001;107(2):280–6.
46. Lang CW, McColley SA, Lester LA, Ross LF. Parental understanding of newborn screening for cystic fibrosis after a negative sweat-test. Pediatrics. 2011;127(2):276–83.
47. Cystic Fibrosis Foundation Patient Registry 2016 Annual Data Report. Bethesda, Maryland; 2017.
48. Filbrun AG, Lahiri T, Ren CL. Diagnosis of cystic fibrosis. In: Handbook of cystic fibrosis. Cham: Adis; 2016. p. 43–63.
49. Rosenstein BJ, Cutting GR. The diagnosis of cystic fibrosis: a consensus statement. Cystic Fibrosis Foundation Consensus Panel. J Pediatr. 1998;132(4):589–95.
50. Nick JA, Nichols DP. Diagnosis of adult patients with cystic fibrosis. Clin Chest Med. 2016;37(1):47–57.
51. Sosnay PR, White TB, Farrell PM, Ren CL, Derichs N, Howenstine MS, et al. Diagnosis of cystic fibrosis in nonscreened populations. J Pediatr. 2017;181S:S52–S7.e2.
52. Ren CL, Borowitz DS, Gonska T, Howenstine MS, Levy H, Massie J, et al. Cystic fibrosis transmembrane conductance regulator-related metabolic syndrome and cystic fibrosis screen positive, inconclusive diagnosis. J Pediatr. 2017;181S:S45–S51.e1.
53. Mayell SJ, Munck A, Craig JV, Sermet I, Brownlee KG, Schwarz MJ, et al. A European consensus for the evaluation and management of infants with an equivocal diagnosis following newborn screening for cystic fibrosis. J Cyst Fibros. 2009;8(1):71–8.

54. Borowitz D, Parad RB, Sharp JK, Sabadosa KA, Robinson KA, Rock MJ, et al. Cystic Fibrosis Foundation practice guidelines for the management of infants with cystic fibrosis transmembrane conductance regulator-related metabolic syndrome during the first two years of life and beyond. J Pediatr. 2009;155(6 Suppl):S106–S16.
55. Groves T, Robinson P, Wiley V, Fitzgerald DA. Long-term outcomes of children with intermediate sweat chloride values in infancy. J Pediatr. 2015;166(6):1469–74.e3.
56. Ooi CY, Castellani C, Keenan K, Avolio J, Volpi S, Boland M, et al. Inconclusive diagnosis of cystic fibrosis after newborn screening. Pediatrics. 2015;135(6):e1377–85.
57. Levy H, Nugent M, Schneck K, Stachiw-Hietpas D, Laxova A, Lakser O, et al. Refining the continuum of CFTR-associated disorders in the era of newborn screening. Clin Genet. 2016;89(5):539–49.
58. Ren CL, Fink AK, Petren K, Borowitz DS, McColley SA, Sanders DB, et al. Outcomes of infants with indeterminate diagnosis detected by cystic fibrosis newborn screening. Pediatrics. 2015;135(6):e1386–92.
59. Bombieri C, Claustres M, De Boeck K, Derichs N, Dodge J, Girodon E, et al. Recommendations for the classification of diseases as CFTR-related disorders. J Cyst Fibros. 2011;10(Supplement 2):S86–S102.
60. Cohn JA, Friedman KJ, Noone PG, Knowles MR, Silverman LM, Jowell PS. Relation between mutations of the cystic fibrosis gene and idiopathic pancreatitis. N Engl J Med. 1998;339(10):653–8.
61. O'Sullivan BP, Baker D, Leung KG, Reed G, Baker SS, Borowitz D. Evolution of pancreatic function during the first year in infants with cystic fibrosis. J Pediatr. 2013;162(4):808–12. e1
62. Ong T, Marshall SG, Karczeski BA, Sternen DL, Cheng E, Cutting GR. Cystic fibrosis and congenital absence of the vas deferens. In: Adam MP, Ardinger HH, Pagon RA, Wallace SE, Bean LJH, Stephens K, et al., editors. GeneReviews((R)). Seattle: University of Washington, Seattle University of Washington, Seattle. GeneReviews is a registered trademark of the University of Washington, Seattle. All rights reserved; 1993.
63. Turek PJ. Chapter 24 – male infertility. In: Strauss JF, Barbieri RL, editors. Yen & Jaffe's reproductive endocrinology. 7th ed. Philadelphia: W.B. Saunders; 2014. p. 538–50.e2.

Chapter 3
Health Disparities

Gabriela R. Oates and Michael S. Schechter

Abbreviations

BMI	Body mass index
CF	Cystic fibrosis
CFF	Cystic Fibrosis Foundation
CFFPR	Cystic Fibrosis Foundation Patient Registry
CFQ-R	Cystic Fibrosis Questionnaire-Revised
CFTR	Cystic fibrosis transmembrane regulator
CI	Confidence interval
ECFSPR	European Cystic Fibrosis Society Patient Registry
EU	European Union
FEV_1	Forced expiratory volume in 1 second
HR	Hazard ratio
OR	Odds ratio
SD	Standard deviation
SES	Socioeconomic status

G. R. Oates (✉)
Division of Pulmonary and Sleep Medicine, Department of Pediatrics, University of Alabama
at Birmingham, Birmingham, AL, USA
e-mail: goates@uab.edu

M. S. Schechter
Division of Pulmonary Medicine, Department of Pediatrics, Virginia Commonwealth
University, Children's Hospital of Richmond at VCU, Richmond, VA, USA
e-mail: mschechter@vcu.edu

© Springer Nature Switzerland AG 2020
S. D. Davis et al. (eds.), *Cystic Fibrosis*, Respiratory Medicine,
https://doi.org/10.1007/978-3-030-42382-7_3

Patient Perspective

My name is Svetlana. I have a 22-year-old daughter with CF, Alexandra, who is about to graduate from college. At home we call her Sasha. We live in a small town in Bulgaria, about 80 kilometers from a larger city with a university hospital. We don't have CF centers in Bulgaria. Until she was 18 years old, Sasha was followed at the pediatric clinic of the university hospital. Now we go to our local general practitioner in town. He is not a specialist, but we try our best to stay on top of things at home.

In Bulgaria, children are usually diagnosed with CF after a series of recurring pneumonias. Since we don't have CF Centers, CF care consists of labs every 6 months – blood work, urine, sputum culture, and pulmonary function testing – on the basis of which a doctor issues a medication protocol. In the university hospital, we would see the doctor in the general pulmonary ward where people are admitted with all kinds of infections. I always felt that going there exposes my daughter to huge risks. But anyhow, every 6 months we get our medication protocol.

The National Health Insurance Fund covers three medications for patients with CF: Creon, Pulmozyme, and Tobi. All other medicines – oral and IV antibiotics, every vitamin, every nutritional supplement – have to be purchased by the patient. Nebulizers, oxygen, and equipment are not covered either. Not every family has the means to buy these medicines and supplies. Bulgaria is the poorest country in Europe; people are not wealthy here. That's why many resort to public fundraising to afford a month's worth of medication.

As for inpatient care, four hospitals in the country can admit CF patients, but that's only if the patient's health is "sufficiently deteriorated" and there is space on the floor. People with CF are admitted in rooms with 3–4 beds per room along with patients who have various respiratory infections. Admission is for a maximum of 7 days, and treatment is the same as for a regular person with pneumonia. Often, the hospital cannot cover a course of expensive IV antibiotics, so we have to pay for them if we want them administered.

The other problem is the life of CF patients after 18 years old. It's hard to find work they can do. Typically, there is no understanding or sympathy from the employer, so people with CF hide their disease. Of course, this can only work for a while because their health gets worse and then they just have to quit. I have to say though that the Bulgarian patients with CF are warriors! They are brave and smart, never giving up, always believing they could live longer.

Sasha has a nonsense mutation and we are fortunate that she is still in relatively good health and hasn't suffered the severe consequences this disease has unleashed on others. It's hard work, but we've managed. My fear as a parent is that we won't manage for a very long time. Many Bulgarian patients with CF have immigrated to countries with better health care so they can take control of their disease. Here it's different. Our doctors tell us, "Oh, she is fine for someone with CF." Or "Well, it's from the disease...." This doesn't reassure me. It makes me feel doomed and completely powerless.

Many people with CF who are Sasha's age are so sick that their only chance is a lung transplant. That's only a dream though, because lung transplantation is not done in our country. If someone wanted to get it abroad, the Bulgarian Ministry of Health would need to sign a contract with the foreign clinic and pay for the procedure since the family cannot afford it out of pocket. Just in the past month, two young people with CF died while hoping the Ministry would send them for a lung transplantation abroad.

That's what inequality is: inhumane, unjust, and painful. For us, it's a bleak, inescapable reality.

– Svetlana

Defining Health Disparities

The term "health disparities" denotes the potentially avoidable differences in health and health risks between disadvantaged social groups and the general population [1, 2]. Although the term is often used to indicate health differences based on race or ethnicity, disparities exist across many other dimensions, including socioeconomic status, geographic location, sexual orientation, and disability [3]. The importance of these dimensions is particularly apparent in cystic fibrosis (*CF*).

Measuring Health Disparities in *CF*

The examination of potential contributors to health disparities is typically driven by models or theories of disparities. Modifiable factors such as education, income, and environmental exposures may interact with each other and with fixed biological variables such as mutation class or gender. Some proximal variables with direct causal link may be markers for other, more distant factors that are underlying causes of disparities. Several conceptual models have been developed to explain the complex pathways by which genetic, socio-environmental, behavioral, and health-care factors shape the health of individuals and groups [4–7]. These models, which are applicable to the study of *CF* health disparities, underscore that such influences operate on multiple levels, from the individual to the family to the community to the larger socioeconomic and political context, and have direct, indirect, and interactive effects on health. Their timing and duration is critical, and they result in an intergenerational transmission of health. *CF* health disparities research should be informed by models that explicate disease-specific mechanisms of disparities and identify variables that offer the greatest potential for mitigating existing inequalities through health system interventions and policy approaches.

Factors Contributing to Health Disparities in *CF*

Although life expectancy and quality of life for patients with *CF* have improved steadily over the past five decades, significant variation in *CF* progression exists even among individuals with identical CFTR genotypes [8–10]. While the impact of gene modifiers continues to be a subject of intense research [11], a number of nongenetic factors also contribute to this variability [12]. Collaco et al. [8] estimate that they account for approximately 50% of the clinical variation in *CF*. The influence of the *socioeconomic context,* including access to financial resources, family structure, social support, and cultural and community influences, has been established. In the past decade, disparities by *race/ethnicity* have also been reported, as well as variation associated with *health-care* access and quality. Similarly, a body of literature has documented the role of *environmental influences,* including exposures related to the physical environment. The following section describes these nongenetic determinants, which have both direct and indirect effect on *CF* outcomes and interact with fixed biological variables such as CFTR mutation classes, gene polymorphisms, and gender to promote or mitigate their influence, thereby generating health disparities.

Socioeconomic Factors

An individual's socioeconomic status (SES), assessed by indicators such as income, education, and occupation, is linked to a range of health outcomes [13–15]. Typically, lower SES is associated with poorer health and higher mortality at every point of the life course and across all health conditions. Moreover, health disparities follow a gradient pattern, with health improving incrementally as income, education, and occupational prestige increase [16–19].

Mortality One of the earliest studies that showed independent effect of SES in *CF* was conducted by Britton [20]. Using mortality data for England and Wales from 1959 to 1986, he found that median age at death from *CF* was higher in nonmanual vs. manual occupations (OR 2.75, 95% CI 2.16 to 3.52). This work was later updated with data from 1959 to 2008 [21], which after 2001 categorized SES into three groups: professional and managerial, intermediate, and routine and manual occupation. Results showed that individuals in the highest socioeconomic group are more likely to die above the median age of death from *CF* than those in the lowest socioeconomic group (OR 2.50, 95% CI 2.16 to 2.90 for 1959–2000; OR 1.89, 95% CI 1.20 to 2.97 for 2001–2008) [21].

In the United States, Schechter et al. [22, 23] used Medicaid coverage as an easily accessible proxy for low SES. Analyzing *CF* Foundation Patient Registry (CFFPR) data for 1986–1994, they reported that the adjusted risk of death was 3.65 times higher for *CF* patients on Medicaid than for those not on Medicaid. Similarly, O'Connor et al. [24] evaluated *CF* mortality at five levels of median family income using ZIP code data from the US Census. They found a 44% increased risk of death for *CF* patients in the lowest-income ZIP codes (<$20,000/year) compared to the highest-income ZIP codes (>$50,000/year). Equally interesting was their finding of a monotonic successive relationship between the five income categories and mortality, illustrating that the relationship between SES and *CF* outcomes is incremental rather than dichotomous.

Lung Function The effects of SES on *CF* health are evidenced not only in mortality but in outcome measures such as lung function and nutrition. The aforementioned study by Schechter et al. [22] found that the $FEV_1\%$ of Medicaid patients was lower by 9.1% (95% CI 6.9 to 11.2) than that of non-Medicaid patients. Similarly, CFFPR data on 20,351 US patients from 1986 to 2011 showed that those in areas with lower income had a $FEV_1\%$ 3–10% lower than those in higher-income areas and those privately insured [25]. Taylor-Robinson et al. [26] assessed the correlation between social deprivation and *CF* outcomes in a longitudinal study of the UK *CF* population younger than 40 years of age between 1996 and 2009. The authors evaluated data for weight, height, BMI, $FEV_1\%$ predicted, and risk of *P. aeruginosa* colonization. The results showed that *CF* patients residing in disadvantaged areas have worse growth and lung function than *CF* patients from affluent areas. Compared with *CF* patients in the least deprived areas, those in the most deprived areas weighed less (standard deviation [SD] score − 0.28; 95% CI -0.38 to −0.18), were shorter (SD score − 0.31; −0.40 to −0.21), had a lower BMI (SD score − 0.13; −0.22 to −0.04), and were more likely to have lower $FEV_1\%$ predicted (−4.12%; −5.01 to −3.19) and chronic *P. aeruginosa* infection (OR 1.89; 1.34 to 2.66).

Socioeconomic inequalities in *CF* health are not limited to the United States and the United Kingdom. A retrospective longitudinal cohort study of all children and adults in the Danish *CF* patient registry between 1969 and 2010 who could be linked to the national administrative register ($N = 442$) showed that, even in the context of the Danish health and welfare system, *CF* patients from disadvantaged backgrounds have worse lung function than those who were not socially disadvantaged [27]. Specifically, low parental educational was associated with a 0.5% greater annual decline in $FEV_1\%$ predicted (95% CI 0.58 to 0.39) after adjustment for demographic, genetic, and clinical factors.

The disparity in *CF* outcomes based on socioeconomic status has an early onset [22–24, 26, 28]. Maternal educational attainment of high school or less was significantly associated with lower mean $FEV_1\%$ predicted (−4.2 [−7.3, −1.2]) at age $6 \geq 7$ in a large US multicenter cohort of children with *CF* enrolled in the Early Pseudomonas Infection Control (EPIC) Observational Study before age 4 [29]. A significant association between paternal education and lung function has been demonstrated as early as 12 months of age in infants diagnosed with *CF* through newborn screening [30].

Life-course models that promote the notion of "critical periods" in a person's biological and social development emphasize the importance of timing of health risks and demonstrate that exposures during particular biological or developmental stages can have long-lasting health impacts. Two such critical periods are pregnancy and early childhood. Maternal stress during pregnancy has been linked to preterm birth, low birth weight, and reduced cognitive ability [31–36], and early-life economic deprivation has been shown to set a child on a trajectory toward diminished health [37, 38]. Children with *CF* are not an exception when exposed to the health risks of poverty, deprivation, and social disadvantage. In the cross-sectional study of US data by Schechter et al. [22], large inequalities in $FEV_1\%$ predicted by Medicaid status were evident at 5 years of age (9% difference) and widened only slightly up to 20 years of age. In the longitudinal study of U.S. data by O'Connor et al. [24], a difference of 5.5% between the most and least deprived income quintiles were evident in first spirometry at 6 years of age and persisted until 18 years of age without increasing significantly over time. Similarly, in the longitudinal study of UK data by Taylor-Robinson et al. [26], disparities in $FEV_1\%$ predicted (-4.12%, 95% CI–5.01 to -3.19) were present at 5 years of age and did not increase over time. By contrast, in the aforementioned Danish epidemiologic study [27], a similar gap of 4% in $FEV_1\%$ predicted between the most and least disadvantaged based on parental education did not develop until approximately 17 years of age. Besides methodological differences between the studies, including different measures of socioeconomic exposure, it is possible that these differences are reflective of societal differences between the three countries, including health-care delivery. Specifically, Taylor-Robinson et al. suggest that "the Danish welfare system, coupled with lower levels of child poverty, and universal access to high quality healthcare may reduce social differences in outcomes in early childhood" [27]. The authors further acknowledge the potential contribution of monthly follow-up and aggressive treatment of infections in Denmark, which may protect the most disadvantaged in the early years.

Nutrition In the United States, about 8% of *CF* patients age 2–19 and 18% of *CF* patients age 20 and older are below the fifth percentile for weight [39]. Individuals with *CF* require a high-fat, high-protein diet and nutritional supplements that are costly and likely less affordable to lower-income families. Additionally, it has been shown that mothers with low educational attainment are less likely to understand the nutritional aspects of *CF*, which impacts the dietary adherence and overall nutritional status of their children with *CF* [40].

A relationship between SES and diet quality has been shown for the general population [41]. Although such relationship in *CF* is underexplored, there is evidence that the nutritional status of *CF* patients is correlated with their socioeconomic status [26, 42, 43]. The previously mentioned study by Schechter et al. [22] found that Medicaid patients were 2.19 times more likely to be below the fifth percentile for weight (95% CI 1.91 to 2.51) and 2.22 times more likely to be below the fifth percentile for height (95% CI 1.95 to 2.52) than non-Medicaid patients. The UK study by Taylor-Robinson et al. [26] found that *CF* patients in the most deprived geographic areas weighed less (SD–0.28; 95% CI–0.38 to -0.18), were shorter (-0.31; -0.40 to -0.21), and had a lower BMI (-0.13; -0.22 to -0.04) when compared to those residing in the most affluent areas.

Balmer et al. [44] examined the relationship between financial capital (household income), human capital (educational attainment of the primary caregiver), and social capital (number of caregivers in the household), on the one side, and growth and pulmonary status, on the other, in *CF* preadolescents with pancreatic insufficiency. They found that each social risk factor – low income, limited education, or single caregiver – was associated with suboptimal growth and pulmonary function at baseline or a decline in growth over 24 months. The composite score of the three dimensions, termed Advantage Index, was the strongest predictor of growth in this sample. In fact, the growth status of preadolescent *CF* children who were socially advantaged was comparable to that of a healthy population.

Stress SES is associated with differential exposure to chronic stressors [45, 46], a primary mechanism of socioeconomic inequalities in health [47]. Among the factors that contribute to greater stress at lower SES levels are economic strain, job insecurity, employment with low levels of control, residential crowding, noise exposure, and social isolation [45, 48–53]. Disproportionate stress exposure affects health through elevated stress responses. Moreover, continuous and repeated stressors have a cumulative effect on the allostatic load, the burden placed on the organism and its biological functions in responding to hardship [54, 55]. Multiple studies show that the distribution of allostatic load is patterned by SES [54, 56]. Children with *CF* are affected by stress also indirectly, through the toll it takes on their parents/caregivers [57–59]. Macpherson et al. [28] report that children with *CF* who are cared for by single mothers have worse health outcomes than children with dual caregivers. Mothers of children with *CF* report high levels of stress related to decision-making and responsibility for parenting [60, 61]. Time-consuming treatments, altered diet and difficult mealtime behaviors, frequent clinic visits or hospitalizations, and uncertainty about disease progression disrupt family life, limit employment opportunities, affect relationships, and negatively impact the physical and mental health of caregivers [62–66]. A third of *CF* parents are clinically depressed [67], and low SES is associated with a higher prevalence of depressive symptoms [68]. Depression, in turn, is associated with an increased likelihood of worse health outcomes, including quality of life and lung function [59, 69, 70]. In a study by Quittner et al. [71], low SES was associated with significantly lower quality of life for *CF* children and their parents on the majority of domains of the CFQ-R.

The harmful effects of stress on health can be buffered by sense of control, self-esteem, and stress-mitigating resources [47]. A number of studies report on the importance of social support [72, 73] in *CF*. Additionally, Reynolds et al. [74] found that positive spiritual coping plays a key role in maintaining long-term health of adolescent patients with *CF*.

Behavioral Factors Goldman and Smith [75] consider a different mechanism of the link between SES and health outcomes – better self-management of disease by the more educated. A relationship between SES and adherence to treatment has been reported in several chronic diseases, including asthma [76] and juvenile rheumatoid arthritis [77]. Worse adherence may also be a contributor to poorer outcomes among *CF* children of low SES [78, 79]. Knowledge of the treatment regimen and an understanding of its rationale are a prerequisite for adherence [80, 81]. Quittner et al. [82] found that nonadherence was explained by patients' misunderstanding of the prescribed regimen, while Anthony et al. [40] reported that caloric intake and growth outcomes in children with *CF* are associated with maternal nutritional knowledge specific to *CF*.

In summary, multiple studies report an association between socioeconomic disadvantage and worse *CF* outcomes, which begins in early childhood and persists throughout the life course. The mechanisms by which socioeconomic status influence *CF* health are varied and complex. Improved understanding of these mechanisms will require increased inclusion of socioeconomic data in *CF* patient registries, as well as linking of patient registry data with administrative data sets, such as Census data. Such studies are fundamental for advancing *CF* health equality as they can provide critical evidence for policy, social, and health-care initiatives to reduce disparities within countries and between countries.

Race and Ethnicity

Members of racial or ethnic minorities make up a growing proportion of US patients with *CF*. Between 2001 and 2016, the CFFPR reported an increase in minorities from 3.9% to 4.6% for African Americans, from 5.4% to 8.5% for Latinos, and from 1.6% to 3.5% for others [83]. An increase in the proportion of racial/ethnic minorities to a total of 7.2% of all *CF* patients is also observed in the Canadian *CF* Registry [84].

Analysis of US CFFPR data from 2007 to 2012 revealed significant geographic differences in the racial distribution of the *CF* population, including that half of African Americans with *CF* reside in the South [85]. *CF* patients from racial/ethnic minority backgrounds experience greater burden of disease and worse outcomes that parallel the disparities by race/ethnicity in the general population. For example, African Americans with *CF* have lower lung function than Caucasians [86], and in the South they also have a higher risk of future hospitalization compared with Caucasians [87]. Both African Americans and Hispanics had increased Medicaid usage (52.2% and 41.8%, respectively). In the previously mentioned study by Quittner et al. [71], after controlling for disease severity and SES, African American and Hispanic patients reported worse emotional and social functioning. Additionally, it has been reported [88] that Hispanic *CF* patients in California have 2.81 times the mortality rate of their non-Hispanic counterparts. Low median household income on the neighborhood level, although associated with a higher rate of death (adjusted HR 2.93; 95% CI 1.04–8.24), did not completely attenuate the difference in mortality rates. In contrast, a study of the Hispanic *CF* population in Texas found no differences in mortality or other *CF* outcomes by Hispanic origin. Regional differences in Hispanic outcomes became evident in a retrospective analysis of national US CFFPR data from 2010 to 2014 [89], which showed that, after adjusting for genetic mutations and clinical and sociodemographic covariates, Hispanic *CF* patients had 1.27 times higher rate of death than non-Hispanics in the Midwest, Northeast, and West, but not in the South. These findings illustrate the limitation of lumping together all persons of Spanish descent into one ethnic category regardless of variations in country of origin, immigration patterns, socioeconomic status, language, religion, and culture. The lack of difference in access to care and clinical and biologic measures between Hispanic and non-Hispanic individuals points to the potential role of adherence to treatment, self-management, health literacy, and English proficiency as contributing factors to health disparities.

It has been suggested that Hispanics with *CF* may have a unique CFTR mutation pattern [88], although its contribution to observed phenotype has not been thoroughly investigated. It is also possible that Hispanic patients may have CFTR variants of unknown functional consequence that may place them at a disadvantage in the era of targeted CFTR modulators. To understand the determinants of disparate *CF* phenotypes among different racial/ethnic groups and intervene in disease progression, it is critical to expand both bench research and research into environmental and lifestyle factors that interact with genetically determined biological variables. However, racial/ethnic minorities are inadequately represented in *CF* clinical trials. Between 1999 and 2015, less than a fifth of 147 phase 1, 2, and 3 clinical trials of *CF* therapies reported the race or ethnicity of study subjects [90]. In the 29 that did, the percentage of subjects from minority background was 2% for Latinos, 1% for Blacks, and 0.1% for Asians, indicating a significant underrepresentation [90]. Inadequate inclusion of racial/ethnic minorities in research and failure to report the racial/ethnic background of subjects in clinical trials limit our understanding of factors that influence drug response and may contribute to health disparities for racial/ethnic minorities with *CF*.

Current methodologies of newborn screening (NBS) also have implications for racial/ethnic health disparities. As discussed by Ross [91], the most prevalent method of screening in the Unites States (IRT/DNA) is very effective in non-Hispanic Caucasians, but false negatives may include a disproportionate number of racial/ethnic minorities, as their *CFTR* mutations are less likely to be included in newborn screening panels. In order to minimize disparities, the IRT/IRT method may be justifiable, even if it is more expensive or cumbersome. However, it may also delay diagnosis. It is therefore important to consider the impact of NBS methodologies on racial/ethnic communities, to prevent embedding health-care disparities into public health programs such as NBS. The issue of *CF* racial/ethnic disparities is additionally complicated by differences in access to care in the United States where, in the absence of universal health system, differences in health-care systems, payer systems, and practice patterns create conditions for racial/ethnic discrimination and inequity.

Health Care

The Institute of Medicine report, "Unequal Treatment: Confronting Racial and Ethnic Disparities in Healthcare," defines health-care disparities as "differences in the quality of health care that are not due to access-related factors or clinical needs, preferences or appropriateness of intervention" [92]. While the overall impact of health-care disparities is small relative to other determinants of health, it is often deemed most relevant to the medical community as it is amenable to changes within the health-care system. Health care is also the most salient aspect of health in the United States today, where lack of health insurance or access to quality medical care remain serious problems.

To determine whether SES-related disparities in *CF* outcomes in the United States can be explained by differences in medical treatment, Schechter et al. [93] performed a cross-sectional analysis of data on patients age <18 years from the Epidemiologic Study of Cystic Fibrosis. Disease severity showed a similar inverse correlation with all three SES measures. However, the number of stable clinic visits was unrelated to SES, and low-SES patients were prescribed more rather than less chronic therapies. The authors concluded that while *CF* health outcomes are correlated with SES, the disparity is not explained by differential use of health services or prescription of therapy in pediatric patients with *CF*. In a later study, Schechter et al. [94] used the same data to determine if SES influences the likelihood of antibiotic treatment of pulmonary exacerbations and again found more, rather than less, antibiotic treatments prescribed to low-SES pediatric patients. Recently, a similar study with CFFPR data from 2005 to 2013 was completed in *CF* patients >18 years of age [95]. Just as in the pediatric *CF* population, public insurance was associated with equal or greater use of *CF* care compared to private insurance. However, lack of insurance was a major barrier to receiving recommended care. Among patients with moderate to severe disease, it was also associated with lower adherence to medications [95]. Transition from pediatric to adult *CF* care is a high-risk period for losing health insurance [96], and the group of 18–25-year-olds have the highest uninsured rate of any *CF* patient age group [83]. Therefore, universal health coverage is critical for improving access to *CF* care.

Although generally there are no socioeconomic differences in prescribed therapies, treatment of pulmonary exacerbations, or hospitalization for *CF* [93, 94, 97], a notable exception is lung transplantation. Low SES as measured by ZIP code median household income, education level, and Medicaid insurance has been independently associated with not being referred to evaluation for lung transplantation [98] or accepted for lung transplantation [99] despite meeting all the criteria. *CF* patients with Medicaid insurance have higher risk of death while awaiting lung transplantation compared to those with Medicare or private insurance [100]. Additionally, US patients with Medicare/Medicaid insurance have worse survival after lung transplantation than those with private insurance (HR 0.78, 0.68–0.90, $p = 0.001$) as well as in comparison with UK patients (HR 0.63, 0.41–0.97, $p = 0.03$) [101]. Further studies are needed to determine barriers to equal access to and outcomes of lung transplantation for all *CF* patients.

A recent study by Stephenson et al. reported that *CF* patients in Canada have a 10-year survival advantage compared to US counterparts (median survival 50.9 vs. 40.6 years, respectively) and 34% lower adjusted risk of death [102]. Survival differences varied according to US patients' insurance status, without significant difference in risk of death among Canadians and US patients with private coverage. The Canadian survival advantage is likely explained by the greater socioeconomic heterogeneity in the United States and stronger focus on addressing the social determinants of health in Canada [103] rather than by differences in health care, except possibly in the context of lung transplantation.

Previous studies of socioeconomic barriers to treatment care were done prior to the widespread use of CFTR modulator drugs, whose cost-effectiveness is well beyond thresholds considered acceptable by US insurers. For example, it has been estimated that the effect of lumacaftor/ivacaftor (Orkambi) costs over $3 million per each additional quality-adjusted life year [104]. A recent retrospective analysis of claims data showed that per-patient expenditures for privately insured US *CF* patients have doubled from 2010 to 2016, largely due to the cost of CFTR modulator drugs. During 2014–2016, the years in which lumacaftor/ivacaftor was introduced, pharmaceutical spending rose by 33.1% [105]. In addition to the CFTR modulator drugs currently on the market, triple-combination CFTR modulators that target the mutations of more than 90% of people with *CF* will soon become available. The growing pipeline of CFTR drugs and increasing number of mutation-eligible *CF* patients will likely lead to payer concerns and scrutiny of costs [106] in both the private and public sector. This economic pressure might shift to patients, resulting in decreased access due to the increased cost-sharing and out-of-pocket expenses [107], or arbitrary limitations that restrict use in the Medicaid population. It is imperative that the pharmaceutical industry, insurers, health-care providers, policy makers, and *CF* stakeholders engage in a deliberate process to address the affordability of CFTR modulators and find solutions to make *CF* precision medicine available to all.

Environmental Exposures

Environmental exposures, such as tobacco smoke, indoor and outdoor air quality, allergens, and infectious agents, are important influences on *CF* lung health. As environmental exposures are highly correlated with SES, it is hypothesized that they mediate the link between SES and *CF* outcomes.

Tobacco Smoke Exposure Because of persistent differences in the prevalence of smoking according to SES [18], tobacco smoke exposure has been proposed as a primary mechanism by which SES affects *CF* lung health [10, 108]. Exposure to tobacco smoke is associated with poorer growth and lung function in *CF* [79]. A dose-dependent association between tobacco smoke exposure and overall disease severity and growth in *CF* was first reported by Rubin [109]. His findings have been corroborated in subsequent publications. More recently, analysis of data from the Early Pseudomonas Infection Control (EPIC) Observational Study also found that smoke exposure had an additive effect on SES-related disparities in lung function and anthropometric measures in children with *CF* [110].

Few studies have attempted to disentangle tobacco smoke and SES and define the effects of these complementary yet distinct exposures on *CF* lung function trajectory over time. A retrospective assessment of the US Cystic Fibrosis Twin and Sibling Study found an association between diminished lung function and both TSE and SES, reporting a 6.1% longitudinal decrease in mean $FEV_1\%$ at age 20 [10]. Since the relationship between lung function and TSE was unaffected by adjustment for SES, and the effect of SES on lung function was no longer significant after adjustment for TSE, the authors concluded that SES does not confound the relationship between TSE and reduced lung function. On the other hand, an analysis of the EPIC Study, which reported a 4-year decrease in mean $FEV_1\%$ (6.0% if mother smoked after birth, 4.6% if mother smoked during pregnancy, 3.2% if child ever around smokers, 2.6% if a household member smokes), showed that TSE and income have independent effects on lung function. In that study, the effect of SES changed minimally after adjustment for TSE, whereas the effect of TSE was attenuated after adjusting for SES [111]. The two studies used different measures of SES (e.g., ZIP code income derived from US Census data vs. individual-level income) and different samples (older *CF* population regardless of health status vs. *CF* children who had been *P. aeruginosa* negative for at least 2 years). Although further research is needed, routine sociodemographic assessments may present an opportunity to identify socio-environmental risk factors and prioritize children who are both low-income and smoke-exposed for targeted interventions.

Air Pollution In general, people of low SES are more likely to live in areas with greater environmental pollution [112]. Although exposure to industrial air toxins has decreased dramatically over the past decades, it remains highly correlated with social class [113]. Similarly, people in poor neighborhoods have higher exposure to long-term air pollution and short-term nitrogen dioxide concentrations than people in affluent neighborhoods [114]. Exposure to air pollution compromises lung growth in children [115] and leads to increased mortality in adults [114, 116]. A study that followed 204 Belgian *CF* patients over 12 years reported a significant correlation between ambient concentrations of particulate matter, nitrogen dioxide, and ozone and prescriptions of IV antibiotics for pulmonary exacerbations [117]. Similarly, a longitudinal study of 103 Brazilian *CF* showed that exposure to short-term air pollution nearly doubles the risk of a pulmonary exacerbation. Analysis of CFFPR data of air pollution by residence ZIP code showed that increased exposure to ambient ozone and particulate matter is associated both with an increase in pulmonary exacerbations and a decrease in lung function [118]. Exposure to fine particulate matter based on air pollution monitors within 30 miles of place of residence was associated with an increased risk of *P. aeruginosa* acquisition as well, in a cohort of 3,575 children age 6 or younger [119].

Infectious Agents The acquisition of *P. aeruginosa* leads to a more rapid decline in lung function and growth status in *CF* patients [120–122], especially once it takes on mucoid characteristics [123]. The UK study by Taylor-Robinson et al. [30] found that patients living in the most deprived geographic areas were 1.89 times more likely (CI 1.34–2.66) to have chronic *P. aeruginosa* infection than comparators in the most affluent areas. The likelihood of *P. aeruginosa* acquisition has also been shown to be increased in US children with low maternal education [124].

Geographic Disparities in *CF*

The United States has significant regional variations in *CF* demographics, insurance, pathogens, medication usage, and comorbidities [85]. For example, the South has the highest proportion of patients with methicillin-resistant *Staphylococcus aureus* (41.9%), *P. aeruginosa* (71.2%), and nontuberculous mycobacterium

(10.0%), as well as the lowest mean BMI and FEV_1. The Midwest has the highest percentage of depressed *CF* patients (18.3%), while inhaled dornase alfa is most prevalent in the West (84.7%). Although mean regional *CF* mortality rates are not statistically different among regions, the South has the highest mortality rates in each age grouping [85], which parallel the greater mortality and morbidity among the general population in the Southeast [125]. It should also be noted that average ambient temperature is associated with *CF* lung function in both the United States and Australia, an effect that seems to be mediated by the increased presence of *P. aeruginosa* and MRSA in *CF* patients living in warmer climates [126, 127].

Rural Disparities There is some evidence of disparities between rural and urban *CF* populations. For example, a cross-sectional study in Iran from 2001 to 2014 reported that the risk of mortality was 50% higher in rural than in urban patients with *CF* ($p = 0.03$) in an Azeri Turkish population [128]. In contrast, studies from Australia generally report lack of rural/urban disparities, likely due to extensive outreach care supported by academic *CF* centers [129] as well as the adoption of telehealth clinics [130]. However, adult patients with *CF* in British Columbia who lived more than 2.5 hours from a *CF* center were less likely to attend quarterly clinic visits than those within 45 minutes' travel distance [131]. Those in the farthest group (>6 hours) were also at risk for more rapid $FEV_1\%$ decline (-3.1% per year [95% CI -5.1 to -1.1] vs. -0.9% per year [95% CI -1.6 to 0.1], $p = 0.04$). Telehealth approaches may help ensure equitable access to care for all people with *CF*.

Global Disparities On a global level, there is a glaring gap in *CF* median age of survival between countries based on gross domestic product or level of industrialization, ranging from more than 40 years of age in Canada, United States, and Western Europe to 20 years in Brazil [132] to less than 15 years in El Salvador, India, and East European countries such as Bulgaria (https://www.cfww.org). A 35-country European *CF* registry (EuroCareCF) with 29,095 patients was developed to compare *CF* outcomes between countries. The disparate country-specific prevalence of *CF* in EuroCareCF could not be explained by differential population frequency of CFTR mutations or case under-ascertainment; rather, it is indicative of excess premature childhood *CF* mortality in non-West European countries [133]. Another analysis of EuroCareCF data showed a median age difference of 4.9 years (95% CI 4.4 to 5.1; $p < 0.0001$) between *CF* patients in European Union (EU) vs. non-EU countries. The proportion of patients older than 40 years was 5% vs. 2%, with an odds ratio of 2.4 (95% CI 1.9 to 3.0, $p < 0.0001$). The study estimated that the *CF* population in non-EU countries would increase by 84% if patients had a demographic profile comparable to that of patients in EU countries [134]. Disparities in *CF* mortality based on country-level income were most recently corroborated with data from the European Cystic Fibrosis Society Patient Registry (ECFSPR) [135].

Describing and understanding the international differences in *CF* survival is only possible through robust national *CF* patient registries. High-quality registry data are vital for identifying epidemiologic trends in *CF* and monitoring the impact of interventions over time. Although advancements in *CF* care have led to dramatic improvements in survival on a population level, there are both individual patient-level factors that can impact survival as well as national differences in survival. It is important to understand such factors to ensure that each *CF* individual and population group is able to achieve their full health potential.

Achieving Health Equality in *CF*

With advancements in early diagnosis and medical treatment, survival in *CF* has improved rapidly, yet variations in disease progression persist. People with *CF* from socioeconomically disadvantaged backgrounds die younger than those in more advantaged positions. Multiple mechanisms are responsible for generating and sustaining disparities in *CF* health, and our discussion outlined some of the ways by which financial, human, and social resources are translated into health advantages in people with *CF*. As mentioned previously, the health effect of SES is not dichotomous [136]. A stepwise gradient relationship between wealth and *CF* health has been described both in the United Kingdom [26] and the United States [24]. The next step is to develop approaches and test interventions that may not only reduce disparities but optimize *CF* outcomes across the entire socioeconomic spectrum [137]. Population-level policy, system, and environmental interventions will be more impactful than individual patient-level interventions [138, 139]. To achieve equality in *CF* health, therefore, population-wide policies that address the root causes of health inequalities are necessary, as well as health policies that ensure equal access to high-quality health care for all.

References

1. Braveman P. Health disparities and health equity: concepts and measurement. Annu Rev Public Health. 2006;27:167–94. https://doi.org/10.1146/annurev.publhealth.27.021405.102103.
2. NIH Health Disparities Strategic Plan and Budget, Fiscal Years 2009–2013: National Institute of Health; 2009.
3. Healthy People 2020: Office of Disease Prevention and Health Promotion 2010.
4. Brunner E, Marmot M. Social organization, stress and health. In: Marmot M, Wilkinson RG, editors. Social determinants of health. 2nd ed. Oxford, UK: Oxford University Press; 2006. p. 6–30.
5. House JS. Understanding social factors and inequalities in health: 20th century progress and 21st century prospects. J Health Soc Behav. 2002;43(2):125–42.
6. House JS, Williams DR. Understanding and reducing socioeconomic and racial/ethnic disparities in health. In: Smedley BD, Syme SL, editors. Promoting health: intervention strategies from social and behavioral research. Washington, DC: National Academy Press; 2000. p. 81–124.
7. Kaplan GA. What is the role of the social environment in understanding inequalities in health? In: Adler NE, Marmot M, McEwen BS, Stewart J, editors. Socioeconomic status and

health in industrialized nations. New York: Annals of the New York Academy of Sciences; 1999. p. 116–9.

8. Collaco JM, Blackman SM, McGready J, Naughton KM, Cutting GR. Quantification of the relative contribution of environmental and genetic factors to variation in cystic fibrosis lung function. J Pediatr. 2010;157(5):802–7.e1-3. https://doi.org/10.1016/j.jpeds.2010.05.018.

9. Ratjen F, Doring G. Cystic fibrosis. Lancet. 2003;361(9358):681–9. https://doi.org/10.1016/S0140-6736(03)12567-6.

10. Collaco JM, Vanscoy L, Bremer L, et al. Interactions between secondhand smoke and genes that affect cystic fibrosis lung disease. JAMA. 2008;299(4):417–24. https://doi.org/10.1001/jama.299.4.417.

11. Corvol H, Blackman SM, Boelle PY, et al. Genome-wide association meta-analysis identifies five modifier loci of lung disease severity in cystic fibrosis. Nat Commun. 2015;6:8382. https://doi.org/10.1038/ncomms9382.

12. Wolfenden LL, Schechter MS. Genetic and non-genetic determinants of outcomes in cystic fibrosis. Paediatr Respir Rev. 2009;10(1):32–6. https://doi.org/10.1016/j.prrv.2008.04.002.

13. Krieger N, Williams DR, Moss NE. Measuring social class in US public health research: concepts, methodologies, and guidelines. Annu Rev Public Health. 1997;18:341–78. https://doi.org/10.1146/annurev.publhealth.18.1.341.

14. Oakes JM, Rossi PH. The measurement of SES in health research: current practice and steps toward a new approach. Soc Sci Med. 2003;56(4):769–84.

15. Spilerman S. Wealth and stratification processes. Ann Rev Soc. 2000;26:497–524. https://doi.org/10.1146/annurev.soc.26.1.497.

16. Braveman PA, Cubbin C, Egerter S, Williams DR, Pamuk E. Socioeconomic disparities in health in the United States: what the patterns tell us. Am J Public Health. 2010;100(Suppl 1):S186–96.

17. Kitagawa EM, Hauser PM. Differential mortality in the United States: a study in socioeconomic epidemiology. Cambridge, MA: Harvard University Press; 1973.

18. Pappas G, Queen S, Hadden W, Fisher G. The increasing disparity in mortality between socioeconomic groups in the United States, 1960 and 1986. N Engl J Med. 1993;329(2):103–9. https://doi.org/10.1056/NEJM199307083290207.

19. Adler NE, Ostrove JM. Socioeconomic status and health: what we know and what we don't. Ann N Y Acad Sci. 1999;896:3–15. https://doi.org/10.1111/j.1749-6632.1999.tb08101.x.

20. Britton JR. Effects of social class, sex, and region of residence on age at death from cystic fibrosis. BMJ. 1989;298(6672):483–7.

21. Barr HL, Britton J, Smyth AR, Fogarty AW. Association between socioeconomic status, sex, and age at death from cystic fibrosis in England and Wales (1959 to 2008): cross sectional study. Br Med J. 2011;343 https://doi.org/10.1136/Bmj.D4662.

22. Schechter MS, Shelton BJ, Margolis PA, Fitzsimmons SC. The association of socioeconomic status with outcomes in cystic fibrosis patients in the United States. Am J Respir Crit Care Med. 2001;163(6):1331–7.

23. Schechter MS, Margolis PA. Relationship between socioeconomic status and disease severity in cystic fibrosis. J Pediatr. 1998;132(2):260–4.

24. O'Connor GT, Quinton HB, Kneeland T, et al. Median household income and mortality rate in cystic fibrosis. Pediatrics. 2003;111(4):e333–9.

25. Johnson B, Ngueyep R, Schechter MS, Serban N, Swann J. Does distance to a cystic fibrosis center impact health outcomes? Pediatr Pulmonol. 2018;53(3):284–92. https://doi.org/10.1002/ppul.23940.

26. Taylor-Robinson DC, Smyth RL, Diggle PJ, Whitehead M. The effect of social deprivation on clinical outcomes and the use of treatments in the UK cystic fibrosis population: a longitudinal study. Lancet Respir Med. 2013;1(2):121–8. https://doi.org/10.1016/S2213-2600(13)70002-X.

27. Taylor-Robinson DC, Thielen K, Pressler T, et al. Low socioeconomic status is associated with worse lung function in the Danish cystic fibrosis population. Eur Respir J. 2014;44(5):1363–6. https://doi.org/10.1183/09031936.00063714.

28. Macpherson C, Redmond AO, Leavy A, McMullan M. A review of cystic fibrosis children born to single mothers. Acta Paediatr. 1998;87(4):397–400.
29. Sanders DB, Emerson J, Ren CL, et al. Early childhood risk factors for decreased FEV1 at age six to seven years in young children with cystic fibrosis. Ann Am Thorac Soc. 2015;12(8):1170–6. https://doi.org/10.1513/AnnalsATS.201504-198OC.
30. Britton LJ, Mims C, Harris WT, Brown J. Predictors of patient outcomes at 12 months of age in patients diagnosed by newborn screening (abstract). Pediatr Pulmonol. 2013;48(S36):372–3.
31. Sandman CA, Davis EP. Neurobehavioral risk is associated with gestational exposure to stress hormones. Expert Rev Endocrinol Metab. 2012;7(4):445–59. https://doi.org/10.1586/eem.12.33.
32. Lu MC, Halfon N. Racial and ethnic disparities in birth outcomes: a life-course perspective. Matern Child Health J. 2003;7(1):13–30.
33. Brunton PJ. Programming the brain and behaviour by early-life stress: a focus on neuroactive steroids. J Neuroendocrinol. 2015;27(6):468–80. https://doi.org/10.1111/jne.12265.
34. Zhu P, Sun MS, Hao JH, et al. Does prenatal maternal stress impair cognitive development and alter temperament characteristics in toddlers with healthy birth outcomes? Dev Med Child Neurol. 2014;56(3):283–9. https://doi.org/10.1111/dmcn.12378.
35. Sandman CA. Fetal exposure to placental corticotropin-releasing hormone (pCRH) programs developmental trajectories. Peptides. 2015;72:145. https://doi.org/10.1016/j.peptides.2015.03.020.
36. Smith R, Nicholson RC. Corticotrophin releasing hormone and the timing of birth. Front Biosci. 2007;12:912–8.
37. Hayward MD, Gorman BK. The long arm of childhood: the influence of early-life social conditions on men's mortality. Demography. 2004;41(1):87–107.
38. Lynch J, Smith GD, Hillemeier M, Shaw M, Raghunathan T, Kaplan G. Income inequality, the psychosocial environment, and health: comparisons of wealthy nations. Lancet. 2001;358(9277):194–200. https://doi.org/10.1016/S0140-6736(01)05407-1.
39. Cystic Fibrosis Foundation Patient Registry. 2013 Annual data report to center directors. Bethesda: Cystic Fibrosis Foundation; 2014.
40. Anthony H, Paxton S, Bines J, Phelan P. Psychosocial predictors of adherence to nutritional recommendations and growth outcomes in children with cystic fibrosis. J Psychosom Res. 1999;47(6):623–34.
41. James WP, Nelson M, Ralph A, Leather S. Socioeconomic determinants of health. The contribution of nutrition to inequalities in health. BMJ. 1997;314(7093):1545–9.
42. Taylor-Robinson D, Whitehead M, Diggle P, Smyth R. The effect of social deprivation on weight in the UK cystic fibrosis population. J Epidemiol Community Health. 2011;65:A389-A. https://doi.org/10.1136/jech.2011.142976n.30.
43. Pinto IC, Silva CP, Britto MC. Nutritional, clinical and socioeconomic profile of patients with cystic fibrosis treated at a referral center in northeastern Brazil. J Bras Pneumol. 2009;35(2):137–43.
44. Balmer DF, Schall JI, Stallings VA. Social disadvantage predicts growth outcomes in preadolescent children with cystic fibrosis. J Cyst Fibros. 2008;7(6):543–50. https://doi.org/10.1016/j.jcf.2008.06.004.
45. Pearlin L. The sociological study of stress. J Health Soc Behav. 1989;30(3):241–56.
46. Turner RJ, Wheaton B, Lloyd DA. The epidemiology of social stress. Am Sociol Rev. 1995;60(1):104–25. https://doi.org/10.2307/2096348.
47. Thoits PA. Stress and health: major findings and policy implications. J Health Soc Behav. 2010;51(Suppl):S41–53. https://doi.org/10.1177/0022146510383499.
48. Pearlin L, Schieman S, Fazio EM, Meersman SC. Stress, health, and the life course: some conceptual perspectives. J Health Soc Behav. 2005;46(2):205–19. https://doi.org/10.1177/002214650504600206.
49. Evans GW, Kim P. Multiple risk exposure as a potential explanatory mechanism for the socioeconomic status-health gradient. Ann N Y Acad Sci. 2010;1186:174–89. https://doi.org/10.1111/j.1749-6632.2009.05336.x.

50. Thoits PA. Stress, coping, and social support processes: where are we? What next? J Health Soc Behav. 1995;Spec No:53–79.
51. Marmot MG, Bosma H, Hemingway H, Brunner E, Stansfeld S. Contribution of job control and other risk factors to social variations in coronary heart disease incidence. Lancet. 1997;350(9073):235–9.
52. Harper S, Lynch J, Hsu WL, et al. Life course socioeconomic conditions and adult psychosocial functioning. Int J Epidemiol. 2002;31(2):395–403.
53. Berkman LF, Kawachi I. Social epidemiology. New York: Oxford University Press; 2000.
54. Seeman TE, McEwen BS, Rowe JW, Singer BH. Allostatic load as a marker of cumulative biological risk: MacArthur studies of successful aging. Proc Natl Acad Sci U S A. 2001;98(8):4770–5. https://doi.org/10.1073/pnas.081072698.
55. McEwen BS, Seeman T. Protective and damaging effects of mediators of stress. Elaborating and testing the concepts of allostasis and allostatic load. Ann N Y Acad Sci. 1999;896:30–47.
56. Kubzansky LD, Kawachi I, Sparrow D. Socioeconomic status, hostility, and risk factor clustering in the Normative Aging Study: any help from the concept of allostatic load? Ann Behav Med. 1999;21(4):330–8.
57. Patterson JM, Budd J, Goetz D, Warwick WJ. Family correlates of a 10-year pulmonary health trend in cystic fibrosis. Pediatrics. 1993;91(2):383–9.
58. Everhart RS, Fiese BH, Smyth JM, Borschuk A, Anbar RD. Family functioning and treatment adherence in children and adolescents with cystic fibrosis. Pediatr Allergy Immunol Pulmonol. 2014;27(2):82–6. https://doi.org/10.1089/ped.2014.0327.
59. Cruz I, Marciel KK, Quittner AL, Schechter MS. Anxiety and depression in cystic fibrosis. Semin Respir Crit Care Med. 2009;30(5):569–78. https://doi.org/10.1055/s-0029-1238915.
60. Hodgkinson R, Lester H. Stresses and coping strategies of mothers living with a child with cystic fibrosis: implications for nursing professionals. J Adv Nurs. 2002;39(4):377–83.
61. Quittner AL, Opipari LC, Regoli MJ, Jacobsen J, Eigen H. The impact of caregiving and role strain on family life: comparisons between mothers of children with cystic fibrosis and matched controls. Rehabil Psychol. 1992;37:275–90.
62. Bittman M, Hill T, Thomson C. The impact of caring on informal carers' employment, income and earnings: a longitudinal approach. Aust J Soc Issues. 2007;42(2):255–72.
63. Vitaliano PP, Zhang J, Scanlan JM. Is caregiving hazardous to one's physical health? A meta-analysis. Psychol Bull. 2003;129:946–72.
64. Pinquart M, Sorensen S. Differences between caregivers and noncaregivers in psychological health and physical health: a meta-analysis. Psychol Aging. 2003;18:250–67.
65. Schulz R, Beach SR. Caregiving as a risk factor for mortality: the Caregiver Health Effects Study. JAMA. 1999;282(23):2215–9.
66. Hatzmann J, Heymans HS, Ferrer-i-Carbonell A, van Praag BM, Grootenhuis MA. Hidden consequences of success in pediatrics: parental health-related quality of life–results from the Care Project. Pediatrics. 2008;122(5):e1030–8. https://doi.org/10.1542/peds.2008-0582.
67. Neri L, Lucidi V, Catastini P, Colombo C, Group LS. Caregiver burden and vocational participation among parents of adolescents with CF. Pediatr Pulmonol. 2016;51(3):243–52. https://doi.org/10.1002/ppul.23352.
68. Schechter MS, Cruz I, Blackwell LS, Quittner AL. Risk factors for anxiety and depression in cystic fibrosis. Pediatr Pulmonol. 2010;45(Suppl 33):109–10.
69. Besier T, Goldbeck L. Anxiety and depression in adolescents with CF and their caregivers. J Cyst Fibros. 2011;10(6):435–42. https://doi.org/10.1016/j.jcf.2011.06.012.
70. Yohannes AM, Willgoss TG, Fatoye FA, Dip MD, Webb K. Relationship between anxiety, depression, and quality of life in adult patients with cystic fibrosis. Respir Care. 2012;57(4):550–6. https://doi.org/10.4187/respcare.01328.
71. Quittner AL, Schechter MS, Rasouliyan L, Haselkorn T, Pasta DJ, Wagener JS. Impact of socioeconomic status, race, and ethnicity on quality of life in patients with cystic fibrosis in the United States. Chest. 2010;137(3):642–50. https://doi.org/10.1378/chest.09-0345.

72. Foster C, Eiser C, Oades P, et al. Treatment demands and differential treatment of patients with cystic fibrosis and their siblings: patient, parent and sibling accounts. Child Care Health Dev. 2001;27(4):349–64.

73. Barker DH, Driscoll KA, Modi AC, Light MJ, Quittner AL. Supporting cystic fibrosis disease management during adolescence: the role of family and friends. Child Care Health Dev. 2012;38(4):497–504. https://doi.org/10.1111/j.1365-2214.2011.01286.x.

74. Reynolds N, Mrug S, Britton L, Guion K, Wolfe K, Gutierrez H. Spiritual coping predicts 5-year health outcomes in adolescents with cystic fibrosis. J Cyst Fibros. 2014;13(5):593–600. https://doi.org/10.1016/j.jcf.2014.01.013.

75. Goldman DP, Smith JP. Can patient self-management help explain the SES health gradient? Proc Natl Acad Sci U S A. 2002;99(16):10929–34. https://doi.org/10.1073/pnas.162086599.

76. Apter AJ, Reisine ST, Affleck G, Barrows E, ZuWallack RL. Adherence with twice-daily dosing of inhaled steroids. Socioeconomic and health-belief differences. Am J Respir Crit Care Med. 1998;157(6 Pt 1):1810–7. https://doi.org/10.1164/ajrccm.157.6.9712007.

77. Rapoff MA, Belmont JM, Lindsley CB, Olson NY. Electronically monitored adherence to medications by newly diagnosed patients with juvenile rheumatoid arthritis. Arthritis Rheum. 2005;53(6):905–10. https://doi.org/10.1002/Art.21603.

78. Pendleton DA, David TJ. The compliance conundrum in cystic fibrosis. J R Soc Med. 2000;93(Suppl 38):9–13.

79. Schechter MS. Non-genetic influences on cystic fibrosis lung disease: the role of sociodemographic characteristics, environmental exposures, and healthcare interventions. Semin Respir Crit Care Med. 2003;24(6):639–52. https://doi.org/10.1055/s-2004-815660.

80. Ievers CE, Brown RT, Drotar D, Caplan D, Pishevar BS, Lambert RG. Knowledge of physician prescriptions and adherence to treatment among children with cystic fibrosis and their mothers. J Dev Behav Pediatr. 1999;20(5):335–43.

81. Lask B. Non-adherence to treatment in cystic fibrosis. J R Soc Med. 1994;87:25–7.

82. Quittner AL, Drotar D, Ievers-Landis C. Adherence to medical treatments in adolescents with cystic fibrosis: the development and evaluation of family based interventions. In: Drotar D, editor. Promoting adherence to medical treatment in childhood chronic illness: concepts, methods, and interventions. Erlbaum Associates, Inc: Hillsdale; 2000.

83. Cystic Fibrosis Foundation Patient Registry. 2016 annual data report. Bethesda: Cystic Fibrosis Foundation. p. 2017.

84. The Canadian Cystic Fibrosis Registry. 2016 annual data report. Toronto, ON: Cystic Fibrosis Canada; 2017.

85. Kopp BT, Nicholson L, Paul G, Tobias J, Ramanathan C, Hayes D Jr. Geographic variations in cystic fibrosis: an analysis of the U.S. CF Foundation Registry. Pediatr Pulmonol. 2015;50(8):754–62. https://doi.org/10.1002/ppul.23185.

86. Hamosh A, FitzSimmons SC, Macek M Jr, Knowles MR, Rosenstein BJ, Cutting GR. Comparison of the clinical manifestations of cystic fibrosis in black and white patients. J Pediatr. 1998;132(2):255–9.

87. Kopp BT, Nicholson L, Paul G, Tobias J, Ramanathan C, Hayes D Jr. The geographic impact on hospitalization in patients with cystic fibrosis. J Pediatr. 2016;170:246–52.e1-4. https://doi.org/10.1016/j.jpeds.2015.11.012.

88. Buu MC, Sanders LM, Mayo JA, Milla CE, Wise PH. Assessing differences in mortality rates and risk factors between hispanic and non-hispanic patients with cystic fibrosis in California. Chest. 2016;149(2):380–9. https://doi.org/10.1378/chest.14-2189.

89. Rho J, Ahn C, Gao A, Sawicki GS, Keller A, Jain R. Disparities in mortality of hispanic patients with cystic fibrosis in the United States. A National and Regional Cohort Study. Am J Respir Crit Care Med. 2018;198(8):1055–63. https://doi.org/10.1164/rccm.201711-2357OC.

90. McGarry ME, McColley SA. Minorities are underrepresented in clinical trials of pharmaceutical agents for cystic fibrosis. Ann Am Thorac Soc. 2016;13(10):1721–5. https://doi.org/10.1513/AnnalsATS.201603-192BC.

91. Ross LF. Newborn screening for cystic fibrosis: a lesson in public health disparities. J Pediatr. 2008;153(3):308–13. https://doi.org/10.1016/j.jpeds.2008.04.061.

92. Smedley BD, Stith AY, Nelson AR, Institute of Medicine (U.S.). Committee on Understanding and Eliminating Racial and Ethnic Disparities in Health Care. Unequal treatment: confronting racial and ethnic disparities in health care. Washington, DC: National Academy Press; 2003.

93. Schechter MS, McColley SA, Silva S, et al. Association of socioeconomic status with the use of chronic therapies and healthcare utilization in children with cystic fibrosis. J Pediatr. 2009;155(5):634–9.e1-4. https://doi.org/10.1016/j.jpeds.2009.04.059.

94. Schechter MS, McColley SA, Regelmann W, et al. Socioeconomic status and the likelihood of antibiotic treatment for signs and symptoms of pulmonary exacerbation in children with cystic fibrosis. J Pediatr. 2011;159(5):819–24. e1. https://doi.org/10.1016/j.jpeds.2011.05.005.

95. Li SS, Hayes D Jr, Tobias JD, Morgan WJ, Tumin D. Health insurance and use of recommended routine care in adults with cystic fibrosis. Clin Respir J. 2018;12(5):1981–8. https://doi.org/10.1111/crj.12767.

96. Tuchman LK, Schwartz LA, Sawicki GS, Britto MT. Cystic fibrosis and transition to adult medical care. Pediatrics. 2010;125(3):566–73. https://doi.org/10.1542/peds.2009-2791.

97. Stephenson A, Hux J, Tullis E, Austin PC, Corey M, Ray J. Socioeconomic status and risk of hospitalization among individuals with cystic fibrosis in Ontario. Canada Pediatr Pulmonol. 2011;46(4):376–84. https://doi.org/10.1002/ppul.21368.

98. Ramos KJ, Quon BS, Psoter KJ, et al. Predictors of non-referral of patients with cystic fibrosis for lung transplant evaluation in the United States. J Cyst Fibros. 2016;15(2):196–203. https://doi.org/10.1016/j.jcf.2015.11.005.

99. Quon BS, Psoter K, Mayer-Hamblett N, Aitken ML, Li CI, Goss CH. Disparities in access to lung transplantation for patients with cystic fibrosis by socioeconomic status. Am J Respir Crit Care Med. 2012;186(10):1008–13. https://doi.org/10.1164/rccm.201205-0949OC.

100. Krivchenia K, Tumin D, Tobias JD, Hayes D Jr. Increased mortality in adult cystic fibrosis patients with Medicaid insurance awaiting lung transplantation. Lung. 2016;194(5):799–806. https://doi.org/10.1007/s00408-016-9927-7.

101. Merlo CA, Clark SC, Arnaoutakis GJ, et al. National healthcare delivery systems influence lung transplant outcomes for cystic fibrosis. Am J Transplant. 2015;15(7):1948–57. https://doi.org/10.1111/ajt.13226.

102. Stephenson AL, Sykes J, Stanojevic S, et al. Survival comparison of patients with cystic fibrosis in Canada and the United States: a population-based cohort study. Ann Intern Med. 2017;166(8):537–46. https://doi.org/10.7326/M16-0858.

103. Stankiewicz A, Herel M, DesMeules M. Report summary–Rio political declaration on social determinants of health: a snapshot of Canadian actions 2015. Health Promot Chronic Dis Prev Can. 2015;35(7):113–4.

104. Sharma D, Xing S, Hung YT, Caskey RN, Dowell ML, Touchette DR. Cost-effectiveness analysis of lumacaftor and ivacaftor combination for the treatment of patients with cystic fibrosis in the United States. Orphanet J Rare Dis. 2018;13(1):172. https://doi.org/10.1186/s13023-018-0914-3.

105. Grosse SD, Do TQN, Vu M, Feng LB, Berry JG, Sawicki GS. Healthcare expenditures for privately insured US patients with cystic fibrosis, 2010–2016. Pediatr Pulmonol. 2018;53(12):1611–8. https://doi.org/10.1002/ppul.24178.

106. Hyde R, Dobrovolny D. Orphan drug pricing and payer management in the United States: are we approaching the tipping point? Am Health Drug Benefits. 2010;3(1):15–23.

107. Kanavos P, Nicod E. What is wrong with orphan drug policies? Suggestions for ways forward. Value Health. 2012;15(8):1182–4. https://doi.org/10.1016/j.jval.2012.08.2202.

108. Schechter MS. Nongenetic influences on cystic fibrosis outcomes. Curr Opin Pulm Med. 2011;17(6):448–54. https://doi.org/10.1097/MCP.0b013e32834ba899.

109. Rubin BK. Exposure of children with cystic fibrosis to environmental tobacco smoke. N Engl J Med. 1990;323(12):782–8. https://doi.org/10.1056/NEJM199009203231203.

110. Schechter M, Emerson J, Rosenfeld M. The relationship of socioeconomic status and environmental tobacco smoke exposure with disease outcomes in the EPIC observational cohort. Pediatr Pulmonol. 2012;47(S35):379.

111. Ong T, Schechter M, Yang J, et al. Socioeconomic status, smoke exposure, and health outcomes in young children with cystic fibrosis. Pediatrics. 2017;139(2) https://doi.org/10.1542/peds.2016-2730.

112. Wheeler BW, Ben-Shlomo Y. Environmental equity, air quality, socioeconomic status, and respiratory health: a linkage analysis of routine data from the Health survey for England. J Epidemiol Community Health. 2005;59(11):948–54. https://doi.org/10.1136/jech.2005.036418.

113. Ard K. Trends in exposure to industrial air toxins for different racial and socioeconomic groups: a spatial and temporal examination of environmental inequality in the U.S. from 1995 to 2004. Soc Sci Res. 2015;53:375–90. https://doi.org/10.1016/j.ssresearch.2015.06.019.

114. Deguen S, Petit C, Delbarre A, et al. Neighbourhood characteristics and long-term air pollution levels modify the association between the short-term nitrogen dioxide concentrations and all-cause mortality in Paris. PLoS One. 2015;10(7):e0131463. https://doi.org/10.1371/journal.pone.0131463.

115. Gauderman WJ, Avol E, Gilliland F, et al. The effect of air pollution on lung development from 10 to 18 years of age. N Engl J Med. 2004;351(11):1057–67. https://doi.org/10.1056/NEJMoa040610.

116. Pope CA, Thun MJ, Namboodiri MM, et al. Particulate air-pollution as a predictor of mortality in a prospective-study of us adults. Am J Respir Crit Care Med. 1995;151(3):669–74.

117. Goeminne PC, Kicinski M, Vermeulen F, et al. Impact of air pollution on cystic fibrosis pulmonary exacerbations: a case-crossover analysis. Chest. 2013;143(4):946–54. https://doi.org/10.1378/chest.12-1005.

118. Goss CH, Newsom SA, Schildcrout JS, Sheppard L, Kaufman JD. Effect of ambient air pollution on pulmonary exacerbations and lung function in cystic fibrosis. Am J Respir Crit Care Med. 2004;169(7):816–21. https://doi.org/10.1164/rccm.200306-779OC.

119. Psoter KJ, De Roos AJ, Mayer JD, Kaufman JD, Wakefield J, Rosenfeld M. Fine particulate matter exposure and initial Pseudomonas aeruginosa acquisition in cystic fibrosis. Ann Am Thorac Soc. 2015;12(3):385–91. https://doi.org/10.1513/AnnalsATS.201408-400OC.

120. Kosorok MR, Zeng L, West SE, et al. Acceleration of lung disease in children with cystic fibrosis after Pseudomonas aeruginosa acquisition. Pediatr Pulmonol. 2001;32(4):277–87.

121. Nixon GM, Armstrong DS, Carzino R, et al. Clinical outcome after early Pseudomonas aeruginosa infection in cystic fibrosis. J Pediatr. 2001;138(5):699–704. https://doi.org/10.1067/mpd.2001.112897.

122. Emerson J, Rosenfeld M, McNamara S, Ramsey B, Gibson RL. Pseudomonas aeruginosa and other predictors of mortality and morbidity in young children with cystic fibrosis. Pediatr Pulmonol. 2002;34(2):91–100. https://doi.org/10.1002/ppul.10127.

123. Li Z, Kosorok MR, Farrell PM, et al. Longitudinal development of mucoid Pseudomonas aeruginosa infection and lung disease progression in children with cystic fibrosis. JAMA. 2005;293(5):581–8. https://doi.org/10.1001/jama.293.5.581.

124. Kosorok MR, Jalaluddin M, Farrell PM, et al. Comprehensive analysis of risk factors for acquisition of Pseudomonas aeruginosa in young children with cystic fibrosis. Pediatr Pulmonol. 1998;26(2):81–8.

125. Goldhagen J, Remo R, Bryant T 3rd, et al. The health status of southern children: a neglected regional disparity. Pediatrics. 2005;116(6):e746–53. https://doi.org/10.1542/peds.2005-0366.

126. Collaco JM, McGready J, Green DM, et al. Effect of temperature on cystic fibrosis lung disease and infections: a replicated cohort study. PLoS One. 2011;6(11):e27784. https://doi.org/10.1371/journal.pone.0027784.

127. Collaco JM, Raraigh KS, Appel LJ, Cutting GR. Respiratory pathogens mediate the association between lung function and temperature in cystic fibrosis. J Cyst Fibros. 2016;15(6):794–801. https://doi.org/10.1016/j.jcf.2016.05.012.

128. Vahedi L, Jabarpoor-Bonyadi M, Ghojazadeh M, Hazrati H, Rafeey M. Association between outcomes and demographic factors in an Azeri Turkish population with cystic fibrosis: a cross-sectional study in Iran from 2001 through 2014. Iran Red Crescent Med J. 2016;18(4):e29615. https://doi.org/10.5812/ircmj.29615.

129. Thomas CL, O'Rourke PK, Wainwright CE. Clinical outcomes of Queensland children with cystic fibrosis: a comparison between tertiary centre and outreach services. Med J Aust. 2008;188(3):135–9.
130. Wood J, Mulrennan S, Hill K, Cecins N, Morey S, Jenkins S. Telehealth clinics increase access to care for adults with cystic fibrosis living in rural and remote Western Australia. J Telemed Telecare. 2017;23(7):673–9. https://doi.org/10.1177/1357633X16660646.
131. Roberts JM, Wilcox PG, Quon BS. Evaluating adult cystic fibrosis care in BC: disparities in access to a multidisciplinary treatment Centre. Can Respir J. 2016;2016:8901756. https://doi.org/10.1155/2016/8901756.
132. The Brazilian Cystic Fibrosis Patient Registry 2015; 2016.
133. Mehta G, Macek M Jr, Mehta A, European Registry Working G. Cystic fibrosis across Europe: EuroCareCF analysis of demographic data from 35 countries. J Cyst Fibros. 2010;9(Suppl 2):S5–S21. https://doi.org/10.1016/j.jcf.2010.08.002.
134. McCormick J, Mehta G, Olesen HV, et al. Comparative demographics of the European cystic fibrosis population: a cross-sectional database analysis. Lancet. 2010;375(9719):1007–13. https://doi.org/10.1016/S0140-6736(09)62161-9.
135. Zolin A, Bossi A, Cirilli N, Kashirskaya N, Padoan R. Cystic fibrosis mortality in childhood. Data from European Cystic Fibrosis Society Patient Registry. Int J Environ Res Public Health. 2018;15(9) https://doi.org/10.3390/ijerph15092020.
136. Adler NE, Stewart J. Health disparities across the lifespan: meaning, methods, and mechanisms. Ann N Y Acad Sci. 2010;1186:5–23. https://doi.org/10.1111/j.1749-6632.2009.05337.x.
137. Schechter MS. Wealth as a disease modifier in cystic fibrosis. Lancet Respir Med. 2013;1(2):93–5. https://doi.org/10.1016/S2213-2600(13)70014-6.
138. Final Report of the Commission on Social Determinants of Health. Geneva. Geneva, Switzerland World Health Organization; 2008.
139. Taylor-Robinson D, Schechter MS. Health inequalities and cystic fibrosis. BMJ. 2011;343:d4818. https://doi.org/10.1136/bmj.d4818.

Part II
Pulmonary Manifestations

Chapter 4
Early Cystic Fibrosis Lung Disease

Sarath C. Ranganathan

Patient Perspective
New Frontiers in CF Research and Treatment

I've lived with cystic fibrosis for 56 years, but was not diagnosed with the disease until I was eight. My diagnosis was via *a sweat test, the gold standard for* CF *diagnosis then. Despite having an older sibling who was diagnosed at birth, I somehow slipped through undiagnosed, there being no routine neonatal screening process available in subtropical Brisbane, Australia in the 1960s.*

Medical knowledge about CF *was rudimentary back then and largely a one-size-fits-all affair. Most children born with* CF *didn't live to adulthood. But somehow this ominous cloud failed to cast a bleak shadow on my spirit. Instead, like most kids my age, I dreamt mostly of having my own swimming pool as well as one day getting a good job, finding a partner and having a family of my own. Perhaps it was my youthful innocence or perhaps I was influenced by the desperate optimism of my parents, but having* CF *did not limit my dreams for the future, at that young age at least. This was despite a rigorous and frequently unpleasant regimen of medications, hospital admissions and therapies, such as daily physiotherapy. I grew up, went to university and became a newspaper reporter and later a freelance writer.*

My mother was a gentle, religious woman. She made every effort to make my life as normal and my treatments as comfortable as possible. While she was very respectful of my doctors, as an extra assurance she would buy my medications and place them at the altar at our local church, praying they would keep me well.

S. C. Ranganathan (✉)
Department of Respiratory and Sleep Medicine, Royal Children's Hospital, Parkville, VIC, Australia

Respiratory Diseases Group, Murdoch Children's Research Institute, Parkville, VIC, Australia

Department of Paediatrics, University of Melbourne, Melbourne, VIC, Australia
e-mail: sarath.ranganathan@rch.org.au

© Springer Nature Switzerland AG 2020
S. D. Davis et al. (eds.), *Cystic Fibrosis*, Respiratory Medicine,
https://doi.org/10.1007/978-3-030-42382-7_4

Much like today, when I was growing up families of CF children hoped advances in medical knowledge, technology and treatments would help relieve the suffering of children and give them a brighter and healthier future. This is not surprising because just 2 years before my diagnosis, astronaut Neil Armstrong walked on the moon. If science could send a man to the moon, the potential for finding treatments and cures for human diseases on planet earth must have seemed limitless to my parents.

I found out I had the most common inherited CF genetic mutation in 1990 when I was newly married and living in Scotland. F508del, the cystic fibrosis transmembrane conductance regulator (CFTR) gene, had been discovered the year before and I was given the opportunity to be tested at a hospital in Edinburgh.

Today's emerging CF research and treatment technologies can at times seem like something out of a futuristic novel. But I guess this was also true when I was young. The first human lung transplantation procedure was performed in Mississippi in 1963, the year I was born, but outcomes remained poor for decades because of complications and the lack of immunosuppressive drugs to prevent rejection. Lung transplantation programs did not begin in earnest in Australia until the 1990s. I was fortunate to receive a life-saving double lung transplant in Melbourne in 2001.

I was also very fortunate that the eight-year delay in my CF diagnosis did not cause a significant decline in my lung function as a child. It's now been established that lung damage in people with CF begins very early, often without symptoms or signs. Specialists in Australia believe early childhood is a critical period for intervention to delay or stop irreversible damage. Very early treatment of children with cystic fibrosis is seen as key if doctors are to help them live longer and have a better quality of life.

A few years ago I joined the Australian Respiratory Early Surveillance Program for Cystic Fibrosis (AREST CF), headed by Professor Sarath Ranganathan, as a volunteer consumer representative. One of my tasks is to assess proposed research projects for potential detrimental impacts on CF children and families. Already I have noticed advances in research and treatment possibilities. Until recently, generalized therapies were recommended for the majority of infants and children with CF because of an inability to predict a child's individual risk of disease progression. Now, new research is aimed at detecting markers of future outcomes so treatment can be customised for each child in the hope it will maximise their life expectancy and quality of life. All this points to a better prognosis for most people born with CF today. Already researchers are turning to advanced tools such as Artificial Intelligence to analyze the complex array of information already known about a patient in the hope of better predicting their progression of lung disease. By having faster and more accurate ways of predicting the future, doctors hope to better meet individual patient needs through the customization of disease monitoring, treatments and therapies. By initiating appropriate therapies earlier, before lung damage begins, doctors hope patients will live longer and have a better quality of life.

As well as future research strategies, doctors in Australia are also considering immediate changes to their clinical practice based on these recent findings. They believe it's not feasible to await the results of future studies before intervening.

Logic and experience, they contend, mean certain initiatives can be started to improve the care of babies and children with CF, even if direct evidence is not yet available. This means parents may face having their healthy-looking infants undergo increased surveillance and new therapy regimens. Parents want the very best for their children and such intervention may bring about fresh challenges for families. Because of this, CF care teams believe they have an obligation to provide better CF education and support for parents and families after diagnosis.

While using therapies earlier and more intensively seems an appropriate response to current scientific evidence, there are always potential risks of treatment-related side effects and increasing health costs. These risks will need to be balanced against the unfortunate fact that lung inflammation, infection and structural lung damage are common in infants and preschool children who have CF. Current clinical approaches have so far failed to stop most children with CF from having permanent lung scarring by the age of five.

In the future, studies will be designed to find innovative new ways to halt early disease progression. There will be an increased focus on treating lung inflammation, minimising lung function decline and preventing infection. The exact mechanisms linking the basic CF defect to organ damage, including irreversible damage to the lungs, are still unclear, but information from intensive CF early surveillance programs, such as those developed by the Australian Respiratory Early Surveillance Program for Cystic Fibrosis, has provided important insights into the biological mechanisms and natural history of lung disease in early life.

My brother is the oldest person I know with CF still living. I have known at least 50 people with CF who have died, most of them much younger than me. Next year (2020) I will be 57, the same age my mother was when she died from breast cancer. It seems strange, given the grim prognosis for children born with CF in the 1960s, that I may live longer than my mother. I believe better prediction of disease progression and the early implementation of protective therapies are essential if we are to improve the longevity and quality of life for the next generation of people born with CF. Patients, parents and medical staff will now have the challenge of navigating the complicated and sometimes emotional impacts of this new frontier.

– Helen Lester

Introduction

The discovery of the CF gene in 1989 and the subsequent widespread introduction of CF genetic-based screening programs offer us the potential to intervene early in infancy, thereby potentially preventing many of the multisystem consequences of this disease. The concept of early nutritional intervention is well recognised with pancreatic enzyme supplementation being introduced immediately following diagnosis to provide early rescue and subsequent normalised growth trajectories during infancy in the majority who are pancreatic insufficient. However, appropriate interventions at a similar time frame to prevent respiratory consequences of CF, which, of all systems involved, is the most important as these are ultimately the cause of death in 90% of individuals, are less clear. With the advent of disease-modifying medications, such as CFTR modulators, there is now potential to intervene as soon as a diagnosis is made, but this practice has not generally been adopted. In order to do so, improved understanding of early aspects of respiratory disease, its trajectories, the longer-term consequences and how best to monitor progress during the preschool years is required. The fact that lung function when first measured using spirometry in populations recorded in CF registries has improved consistently over the past decades highlights that early interventions, irrespective of the evidence base that supports modern treatment regimes, has been beneficial and has improved respiratory health in people with CF. As the preschool years represent the time of most rapid lung development during the life course, future outcomes would seem to depend critically on how the first few years of life are managed. This chapter will review what we know about infection, inflammation, lung structural destruction and the approaches being deployed to treat these manifestations within the context of early CF lung disease.

Pathogenesis of CF

The exact mechanisms linking the basic gene defect in CF via abnormalities in CFTR production, trafficking and function to actual organ damage, including irreversible damage to the lungs, is unclear. The earliest post-mortem studies in human infants identified relatively normal airways but abnormal mucus glands [1, 2]. Recent data from the CF pig model highlight a number of defects identifiable at birth that may be relevant to human infants with CF. These include congenital airway abnormalities of the trachea, increased acidity of the airway surface liquid that results in inhibition of the function of antimicrobial peptides, failure of mucus to detach from submucosal gland ducts and increase in airway mucins and mucin flakes [3–5]. These basic defects lead to the clinical consequences of infection, inflammation, functional abnormalities and lung structural damage, all of which can be identified when first studied shortly after diagnosis and within the first few months of life [6], but which are often ignored or not aggressively treated in an asymptomatic infant.

Early Pulmonary Infection

Based on standard microbiological culture techniques, typical respiratory infections in CF are most often due to *Staphylococcus aureus*, *Haemophilus influenzae* and *Pseudomonas aeruginosa*. *S. aureus* is commonly cultured shortly after diagnosis and in up to 30% of infants during the first 6 months of life. When cultured from the lower respiratory tract in infants and young children, these organisms are associated with pulmonary inflammation even in the absence of clinical symptoms or signs. Aspergillus species are also associated with pulmonary inflammation in young children with CF [7], but the role of Aspergillus in the development and progression of early structural lung disease and lung function decline in CF remains unknown. A significant difference in prevalence of early infection in the lower respiratory tract with these organisms may occur at geographically distinct CF centres, leading to worse early outcomes [8]. To a certain extent therefore, there may be a geographical context to early trajectories in terms of lung disease severity in relation to these infections.

P. aeruginosa is a significant pathogen in terms of early clinical decline. Initial infection with P. aeruginosa occurs with a median age of first detection at around 2 years in the lower respiratory tract and as early as 3 months of age [6, 9]. Environmental factors, in addition to host and bacterial factors, play a part in acquiring infection with this organism [10]. Residence in a rural versus a metropolitan area is a significant risk factor for the first acquisition of P. aeruginosa [11]. Temperature, rainfall, dew point, latitude, longitude and elevation of residence have all been implicated in the first acquisition of P. aeruginosa, as has exposure to particulate environmental pollution [12].

Successful eradication of lower respiratory P. aeruginosa infection is achievable in the majority of preschool children and infants [13]. However again, environmental and climatic factors appear to play a role in its reacquisition following eradication [14]. Whether P. aeruginosa is detected in upper or lower airway samples during clinical surveillance does not seem to influence clinical outcomes [15], and it appears appropriate to treat P. aeruginosa when detected in upper airway samples rather than scheduling bronchoscopy with broncho-alveolar lavage for surveillance of this organism.

Detection and eradication of P. aeruginosa during the preschool years may prevent the morbidity and mortality associated with chronic P. aeruginosa infection but does not prevent the development of associated structural lung disease or lower lung function as high rates of bronchiectasis occur despite eradication [15]. In children diagnosed either clinically, or following newborn screening, prior eradication of P. aeruginosa was associated with ongoing increased pulmonary inflammation following eradication [13] and lower lung function measured by spirometry through preschool and school age, compared with those never infected [16, 17]. These data suggest functional, structural and inflammatory changes occur despite aggressive treatment and eradication of P. aeruginosa and that newer approaches for prevention and treatment of this organism are indicated in order to prevent the respiratory consequences of infection with P. aeruginosa, including much earlier and more aggressive surveillance of early respiratory exacerbations.

When cultured, the eradication of S. aureus (methicillin-sensitive or methicillin-resistant organisms) or H. influenzae is not usually attempted even in symptomatic patients even though both organisms are associated with lung function decline [16]. De novo S. aureus acquisition at age 3 in those receiving anti-staphylococcal prophylaxis until age 2 years is associated with later bronchiectasis and lower FEF_{25-75} in children with CF [18]. Whether eradication is feasible or impacts on subsequent lung function decline, or attenuates lung damage, is worthy of further study but such attempts at eradication need to be considered in the context of how this might impact on the evolving early gut and lung microbiota. Although BAL does not improve outcomes when used for detection and treatment of infection with *P. aeruginosa*, this might not be the case for *S. aureus* and *H. influenza*e as these are more routinely found in the upper respiratory tract even in healthy individuals and are poorly associated with pulmonary inflammation when cultured from this location. Eradication regimes designed for these two organisms are likely to require detection specifically in the lower airways in order to improve risk/benefit ratios. It is likely that treatment of traditional CF pathogens, including attempts at eradicating them in early life, will have impact on the microbiota and its constituency meaning that distinguishing between colonisation by organisms in the upper respiratory tract versus detecting lower respiratory infection associated with inflammation is crucial.

Early Lung Microbiome

The use of culture-independent techniques for microbiological analysis of airway specimens has to a certain extent altered our understanding of microbial organisms in CF lung disease, such that infection is now understood to be polymicrobial [19].

Although it is currently difficult to implicate the respiratory microbiota in disease progression in CF, there are emerging data to suggest that the microbiota are very different in this condition. Alpha diversity appears reduced in infants with CF and compositional differences are apparent between infants with CF and those without CF. These differences appear to be driven by increased *Staphylococcus* and decreased *Fusobacterium* and are most apparent in symptomatic infants with CF [20]. Bacterial biomass, a measure of the quantity of bacteria present, is associated with inflammation in infants and so the influence of antibiotics on this relationship is likely. These differences in lower airway microbial community composition and structure are established by 6 months of age [20]. Bacterial diversity continues to decrease during the preschool years in CF with a dominance of a CF pathogen being associated with increased pulmonary inflammation and pathogens that are detected by standard microbiological culture [19]. As predicted, the microbiota of infants treated with anti-staphylococcal antibiotic prophylaxis is significantly less diverse than infants receiving only intermittent antibiotics, and in contrast to the cohort studies of Frayman et al. that preceded the use of antibiotic prophylaxis, the reduced diversity is associated with decreased inflammation, at least in the short term [21]. The longer-term outcomes of treatment with anti-staphyloccocal antibiotics in terms of their impact on the lung microbiota is not yet known, but its impact on the early lung microbiota suggests that bacterial diversity and biomass are significantly affected.

Characterisation of the lower airway microbiome using lower respiratory samples obtained from clinically stable infants and preschool children who underwent bronchoscopy and chest computed tomography (CT) suggests a progression of the lower airway microbiome with age, beginning with relatively sterile airways in infancy. By age 2, bacterial sequences typically associated with the oral cavity dominate lower airway samples. The presence of an oral-like lower airway is associated with increased pulmonary inflammation, but it is not yet clear whether this follows aspiration from the upper airway into the lower airway or how this relates to the ontogeny of the developing gut microbiota. The majority of CF subjects older than 4 in the study by Muhlebach et al. harboured a pathogen-dominated airway microbiome with significantly greater pulmonary inflammation, suggesting that changes within the CF lower airway microbiome occur during the first years of life and that distinct microbial signatures are associated with the progression of early CF lung disease [22].

Factors associated with chronicity of infection include the recently studied implications of bile acid reflux in CF [23]. Gastro-oesophageal reflux is common in infants and in CF may be exacerbated by cough and chest physical therapy. The aspiration specifically of bile acids into the lungs of patients correlates with a markedly reduced microbiome diversity in patients with CF. Bile elicits chronic colonisation with several prominent respiratory pathogens, including *P. aeruginosa*. This includes a switch towards biofilm formation and suppression of virulence factors associated with the acute phase of infection. From a clinical perspective, tolerance to the polymyxin and macrolide classes of antibiotics is observed in the presence of bile. Research into this area has the potential to inform therapies relevant to infants following first acquisition of CF pathogens and efforts aiming to prevent their colonisation [24].

Inflammation

Lung disease in CF is characterised by neutrophil-dominated inflammation. We have known for decades that this can be detected within the first few weeks of life, even in asymptomatic infants without evidence of pulmonary infection [25], but this knowledge has not really led to any effective medications or interventions. The presence of pulmonary inflammation in infancy and the preschool years is associated with worse nutritional status [26], the presence of organisms cultured from the lower respiratory airways [7], bronchiectasis on chest CT [27] and lung function abnormalities [28]. While infection is the main contributor to early inflammation, the increase in pulmonary inflammation with age during the preschool years appears to be relatively independent of current or past infection status detected by BAL and instead may be due to the acquisition of a pathogen-dominated airway microbiome as discussed [22]. There appears to be a role for both neutrophil-derived serine proteases and reactive oxygen species in the evolution of early lung disease [29]. Free neutrophil elastase activity is detectable in BAL in up to 30% of infants and is associated with CT scan-diagnosed bronchiectasis by age 3 years [30]. The serine anti-protease host defence mechanisms are therefore overwhelmed in CF, creating the potential for enzymatic degradation of the lung structure. Pulmonary infection is also associated with increased oxidative loss of glutathione and biomarkers of oxidative stress [29]. Therapies targeting oxidative stress pathways (e.g. anti-myeloperoxidase agents) may boost antioxidant defence and potentially slow the onset and progression of lung disease in CF but no trials have been initiated yet in early lung disease. In addition to characterising the impact of CFTR dysfunction on numerous immune pathways in the aetiology of pulmonary inflammation, identifying potential therapeutic strategies for reducing inflammation and infection is likely critical for preventing early CF lung disease [31].

In a study that aimed to characterise the inflammatory profiles of airway epithelial cells from children with CF compared with cells from healthy control subjects, CF and healthy airway epithelial cells had similar basal expression of IL-8 in response to pro-inflammatory stimuli, but elevated IL-8 release in response to infection with human rhinovirus was noted in CF. The elevated IL-8 response, together with dampened apoptotic responses by CF cells to human rhinovirus, could contribute to augmented airway inflammation in the setting of recurrent viral infections early in life. Recurrent viral infections early in life could therefore contribute to the pulmonary inflammation identified in infants with CF [32]. In a prospective observational study of infants with CF, viral infections were associated with increased airway neutrophilic inflammation and more bacterial isolates, including classic CF bacterial pathogens, in the lower airway. Human rhinovirus was the most common virus detected, found at least once in 66% of participants and isolated more frequently in those with symptoms including cough and nasal congestion. In 52% of cases where antibiotics were prescribed for respiratory-related indications, a virus was detected [33]. Future studies will show whether antiviral precautions, and treatments, will play a role in the prevention or attenuation of early lung disease.

Metabolites and pathways altered in association with neutrophilic inflammation and the development of destructive lung disease have also been studied recently. Ninety-three metabolites were associated with early neutrophilic inflammation, representing pathways involved in metabolism of adenyl purines, amino acids and small peptides, cellular energy and lipids [34]. These were detected in BAL fluid. If these findings can be replicated in samples obtained by less invasive means, then such metabolites may serve as relatively non-invasive biomarkers of pulmonary inflammation in CF.

Protease-activated receptor 1 (PAR1) is a cell surface receptor, activated by serine proteases including neutrophil elastase, which is well recognised as a modulator of inflammation. While PAR1 is known to play an important role in regulating inflammation, virtually nothing is known about its potential importance in CF pathogenesis. Expression of PAR1 in BAL cells from young children with CF is strongly correlated with neutrophil elastase. PAR1 activation suppressed the IL-8 response of BAL cells from patients stimulated ex vivo with *P. aeruginosa*. PAR1 exerts complex and multifaceted influences on various aspects relevant to CF pathogenesis (Ranganathan et al. submitted). Endogenous anti-inflammatory, and potentially protective, pathways therefore also warrant further investigation. Clinical translation of such novel research findings into trials of tolerable anti-inflammatory agents that effectively modulate the immune response present a unique challenge in young children but are worthy of study as they may have a significant therapeutic role in addition to, or instead of, CFTR modulation, in the treatment of early lung disease in CF.

Structural Changes

Structural damage to the lung is the end point of the pathophysiological injury incurred through infection and inflammation, but due to difficulty in its assessment during the preschool years and perhaps due to failure until recently to recognise its existence, detecting or preventing it has not generally been the main target for clinicians. Many studies now identify infancy and the early preschool years as the period when structural changes in the CF lung begin [6, 35, 36]. Advances in CT technology, the advent of low-dose radiation acquisition protocols, adaptation of CT technology that was initially designed chiefly for adults and improved algorithms for acquisition of chest CT images have markedly improved the sensitivity with which lung disease can be detected [37]. Although radiation doses should always be as low as reasonably achievable, the risk of performing chest CT is not incalculable, and cumulative radiation doses provide risk akin to a single larger exposure to radiation, although it is estimated that current low-dose protocols are associated only with a very small cancer risk [38]. Recent studies suggest that bronchiectasis, defined as a bronchus to arterial ratio of >1.0, can be identified in many asymptomatic infants shortly after diagnosis [6]. Indeed, use of the artery to airway ratio itself as an objective outcome measure has been proposed [39]. This and other new quantitative scoring systems designed for use in early mild lung disease in CF will significantly enhance the study of the pathogenesis of lung structural abnormalities and interventions designed to prevent them [40]. However, investigations into non-ionising radiation modalities such as magnetic resonance imaging are underway.

Although the radiological abnormalities seen during the preschool years are generally mild in comparison to the end-stage lung findings that impact survival in CF [41], these early changes are the likely precursors of the bronchiectasis identified routinely in adolescent and adult patients with CF. Unfortunately, even as survival improves, the majority of children with CF have bronchiectasis by the time they attend school. CT scan-diagnosed bronchiectasis can be detected in up to 30–40% of children with CF between the ages of 3 and 4 years old [27] and in up to 80% of children by the age of 5 years [15, 42, 43]. Air trapping, defined as hypolucent areas on expiratory chest CT scans, is seen more commonly than bronchiectasis. Air trapping is reliably identified with excellent inter-observer agreement [27, 44]. The cause of early air trapping is unknown, but it could result from airway developmental abnormalities, severe bronchial wall thickening and mucus impaction leading to airway closure and hypoperfusion. Airway structural abnormalities, for example, congenital tracheomalacia, are unlikely to be amenable to

CF therapies, whereas inflammation and abnormal mucus might be modifiable. Air trapping on CT scan in infancy is also a risk factor for bronchiectasis at 3 years of age [30].

Infant and Preschool Lung Function

Lung function in infants with CF is characterised by reduced forced expiratory flows and volumes measured by forced expiration, increased functional residual capacity measured by plethysmography and elevated lung clearance index (LCI) measured by multiple gas washout [45, 46]. These lung function findings likely reflect the underlying structural findings of airway obstruction, air trapping and ventilation inhomogeneity, respectively [45–48]. Longitudinal studies of lung function suggest that those infants that remain free of pulmonary infections during infancy experience lung growth similar to that of healthy infants [49]. In infants, LCI was associated with lower respiratory infection with *P. aeruginosa* and pulmonary inflammation [48], but not with early bronchiectasis [47]. In preschoolers and older children, LCI is much better at predicting underlying lung structural changes [50]. It is likely that LCI may be a useful surveillance tool to monitor structural lung disease in preschool and school-age children with CF.

Implications and Conclusions

Recognition that lung disease starts early in CF and leads to bronchiectasis during the first years of life has resulted in a change in paradigm in treatment of the seemingly well preschool child [51]. An example of strategies that have been and could be adopted consequently is shown in Table 4.1. As recent clinical approaches failed to prevent the majority of children with CF having established bronchiectasis by 5 years of age, a shift of focus towards prevention of this early disease progression has occurred, with opportunities for future studies to inform modification of the early disease trajectory. Such studies have commenced and the future is bright in terms of our ability to maximise the benefits and opportunities afforded by newborn screening programs. Early introduction of disease-modifying therapies and implementation of new CF treatment paradigms will improve longevity and quality of life for the next generation of infants and preschool children born with CF.

Table 4.1 Strategies targeting improvement of outcomes in early childhood

Required activity	Remarks
Move routine treatments into the preschool era	Where there is no direct evidence of efficacy but no expectations of significant side effects, it may be safe to move existing treatments and strategies directly into early care, for example, early and aggressive treatment of pulmonary exacerbations, even if these are considered clinically mild
Assess efficacy of routine treatments in the preschool era	Existing treatments commonly used in older subjects, such as inhaled hypertonic saline and Rh DNAse, should be assessed in clinical studies in younger children as risk versus benefit is unlikely to be the same in younger children. Trials of these specific therapies are being conducted. An example is the saline hypertonic in Preschoolers (SHIP) study (NCT02378467) in which 7% hypertonic saline was associated with a significant improvement in lung clearance index measured by the multiple breath washout technique [52]
Intervention trials in infants with CF	An increasing number of trials are being conducted in infants and preschool children with CF. the inhaled hypertonic saline study in infants (ISIS) trial indicated that such trials are feasible with appropriate end points [53] SHIP-CT (ACTRN 12615001067561) is assessing the impact of hypertonic saline on lung structure and function. Studies of CFTR modulators (e.g. NCT02742519) in 3- to 5-year-old children are being conducted. At least eight trials of CFTR modulator therapy in preschool children are registered on clinical trials.gov indicating that preschool children are no longer denied access to trials and that disease-modifying medications will not bypass this age group. Future intervention studies of new anti-infective strategies, such as *S. aureus* and *H. influenzae* eradication protocols, and studies of anti-proteases and anti-oxidants are also urgently required
Intervention trials specifically aiming to prevent or delay onset of bronchiectasis	The first such trial is nearing completion (COMBAT: NCT01270074) and could become the template for further trials that introduce interventions from diagnosis aiming to decrease the prevalence of bronchiectasis during the preschool years. More studies predicated on prevention of bronchiectasis are required
Develop national and international clinical trial networks for evaluation of programmed therapeutic activities	Trial networks are required in order to achieve the larger numbers of subjects required to study treatment programs that provide incremental benefits in terms of preschool outcomes. Novel, adaptive trial designs should be considered to facilitate the large number of interventions and clinical program variations available

References

1. Bedrossian CW, Greenberg SD, Singer DB, Hansen JJ, Rosenberg HS. The lung in cystic fibrosis. A quantitative study including prevalence of pathologic findings among different age groups. Hum Pathol. 1976;7(2):195–204.
2. Sturgess J, Imrie J. Quantitative evaluation of the development of tracheal submucosal glands in infants with cystic fibrosis and control infants. Am J Pathol. 1982;106(3):303–11.
3. Stoltz DA, Meyerholz DK, Welsh MJ. Origins of cystic fibrosis lung disease. N Engl J Med. 2015;372(4):351–62.

4. Hoegger MJ, Fischer AJ, McMenimen JD, Ostedgaard LS, Tucker AJ, Awadalla MA, et al. Impaired mucus detachment disrupts mucociliary transport in a piglet model of cystic fibrosis. Science. 2014;345(6198):818–22.

5. Esther CR Jr, Muhlebach MS, Ehre C, Hill DB, Wolfgang MC, Kesimer M, et al. Mucus accumulation in the lungs precedes structural changes and infection in children with cystic fibrosis. Sci Transl Med. 2019;11(486):pii: eaav3488.

6. Sly PD, Brennan S, Gangell C, de Klerk N, Murray C, Mott L, et al. Lung disease at diagnosis in infants with cystic fibrosis detected by newborn screening. Am J Respir Crit Care Med. 2009;180(2):146–52.

7. Gangell C, Gard S, Douglas T, Park J, de Klerk N, Keil T, et al. Inflammatory responses to individual microorganisms in the lungs of children with cystic fibrosis. Clin Infect Dis. 2011;53(5):425–32.

8. Ramsey KA, Hart E, Turkovic L, Padros-Goossens M, Stick SM, Ranganathan SC. Respiratory infection rates differ between geographically distant paediatric cystic fibrosis cohorts. ERJ Open Res. 2016;2(3):00014-2016.

9. Emerson J, Rosenfeld M, McNamara S, Ramsey B, Gibson RL. Pseudomonas aeruginosa and other predictors of mortality and morbidity in young children with cystic fibrosis. Pediatr Pulmonol. 2002;34(2):91–100.

10. Psoter KJ, DE Roos AJ, Wakefield J, Mayer JD, Bryan M, Rosenfeld M. Association of meteorological and geographical factors and risk of initial Pseudomonas aeruginosa acquisition in young children with cystic fibrosis. Epidemiol Infect. 2016;144(5):1075–83.

11. Ranganathan SC, Skoric B, Ramsay KA, Carzino R, Gibson AM, Hart E, et al. Geographical differences in first acquisition of Pseudomonas aeruginosa in cystic fibrosis. Ann Am Thorac Soc. 2013;10(2):108–14.

12. Psoter KJ, De Roos AJ, Mayer JD, Kaufman JD, Wakefield J, Rosenfeld M. Fine particulate matter exposure and initial Pseudomonas aeruginosa acquisition in cystic fibrosis. Ann Am Thorac Soc. 2015;12(3):385–91.

13. Douglas TA, Brennan S, Gard S, Berry L, Gangell C, Stick SM, et al. Acquisition and eradication of P. aeruginosa in young children with cystic fibrosis. Eur Respir J. 2009;33(2):305–11.

14. Warrier R, Skoric B, Vidmar S, Carzino R, Ranganathan S. The role of geographical location and climate on recurrent Pseudomonas infection in young children with cystic fibrosis. J Cyst Fibros. 2019;18(6):817–822.

15. Wainwright CE, Vidmar S, Armstrong DS, Byrnes CA, Carlin JB, Cheney J, et al. Effect of bronchoalveolar lavage-directed therapy on Pseudomonas aeruginosa infection and structural lung injury in children with cystic fibrosis: a randomized trial. JAMA. 2011;306(2):163–71.

16. Ramsey KA, Ranganathan SC, Gangell CL, Turkovic L, Park J, Skoric B, et al. Impact of lung disease on respiratory impedance in young children with cystic fibrosis. Eur Respir J. 2015;46(6):1672–9.

17. Kozlowska WJ, Bush A, Wade A, Aurora P, Carr SB, Castle RA, et al. Lung function from infancy to the preschool years after clinical diagnosis of cystic fibrosis. Am J Respir Crit Care Med. 2008;178(1):42–9.

18. Caudri D, Turkovic L, Ng J, de Klerk NH, Rosenow T, Hall GL, et al. The association between Staphylococcus aureus and subsequent bronchiectasis in children with cystic fibrosis. J Cyst Fibros. 2018;17(4):462–9.

19. Frayman KB, Armstrong DS, Carzino R, Ferkol TW, Grimwood K, Storch GA, et al. The lower airway microbiota in early cystic fibrosis lung disease: a longitudinal analysis. Thorax. 2017;72(12):1104–12.

20. Frayman KB, Wylie KM, Armstrong DS, Carzino R, Davis SD, Ferkol TW, et al. Differences in the lower airway microbiota of infants with and without cystic fibrosis. J Cyst Fibros. 2018;18(5):646–52.

21. Pittman JE, Wylie KM, Akers K, Storch GA, Hatch J, Quante J, et al. Association of Antibiotics, airway microbiome, and inflammation in infants with cystic fibrosis. Ann Am Thorac Soc. 2017;14(10):1548–55.

22. Muhlebach MS, Zorn BT, Esther CR, Hatch JE, Murray CP, Turkovic L, et al. Initial acquisition and succession of the cystic fibrosis lung microbiome is associated with disease progression in infants and preschool children. PLoS Pathog. 2018;14(1):e1006798.
23. Reen FJ, Woods DF, Mooij MJ, Chroinin MN, Mullane D, Zhou L, et al. Aspirated bile: a major host trigger modulating respiratory pathogen colonisation in cystic fibrosis patients. Eur J Clin Microbiol Infect Dis. 2014;33(10):1763–71.
24. Reen FJ, Flynn S, Woods DF, Dunphy N, Chroinin MN, Mullane D, et al. Bile signalling promotes chronic respiratory infections and antibiotic tolerance. Sci Rep. 2016;6:29768.
25. Khan TZ, Wagener JS, Bost T, Martinez J, Accurso FJ, Riches DW. Early pulmonary inflammation in infants with cystic fibrosis. Am J Respir Crit Care Med. 1995;151(4):1075–82.
26. Ranganathan SC, Parsons F, Gangell C, Brennan S, Stick SM, Sly PD, et al. Evolution of pulmonary inflammation and nutritional status in infants and young children with cystic fibrosis. Thorax. 2011;66(5):408–13.
27. Mott LS, Park J, Murray CP, Gangell CL, de Klerk NH, Robinson PJ, et al. Progression of early structural lung disease in young children with cystic fibrosis assessed using CT. Thorax. 2012;67(6):509–16.
28. Pillarisetti N, Williamson E, Linnane B, Skoric B, Robertson CF, Robinson P, et al. Infection, inflammation, and lung function decline in infants with cystic fibrosis. Am J Respir Crit Care Med. 2011;184(1):75–81.
29. Kettle AJ, Turner R, Gangell CL, Harwood DT, Khalilova IS, Chapman AL, et al. Oxidation contributes to low glutathione in the airways of children with cystic fibrosis. Eur Respir J. 2014;44(1):122–9.
30. Sly PD, Gangell CL, Chen L, Ware RS, Ranganathan S, Mott LS, et al. Risk factors for bronchiectasis in children with cystic fibrosis. N Engl J Med. 2013;368(21):1963–70.
31. Cantin AM, Hartl D, Konstan MW, Chmiel JF. Inflammation in cystic fibrosis lung disease: pathogenesis and therapy. J Cyst Fibros. 2015;14(4):419–30.
32. Sutanto EN, Kicic A, Foo CJ, Stevens PT, Mullane D, Knight DA, et al. Innate inflammatory responses of pediatric cystic fibrosis airway epithelial cells: effects of nonviral and viral stimulation. Am J Respir Cell Mol Biol. 2011;44(6):761–7.
33. Deschamp AR, Hatch JE, Slaven JE, Gebregziabher N, Storch G, Hall GL, et al. Early respiratory viral infections in infants with cystic fibrosis. J Cyst Fibros. 2019;18(6):844–50.
34. Esther CR Jr, Turkovic L, Rosenow T, Muhlebach MS, Boucher RC, Ranganathan S, et al. Metabolomic biomarkers predictive of early structural lung disease in cystic fibrosis. Eur Respir J. 2016;48(6):1612–21.
35. Brody AS. Early morphologic changes in the lungs of asymptomatic infants and young children with cystic fibrosis. J Pediatr. 2004;144(2):145–6.
36. VanDevanter DR, Kahle JS, O'Sullivan AK, Sikirica S, Hodgkins PS. Cystic fibrosis in young children: a review of disease manifestation, progression, and response to early treatment. J Cyst Fibros. 2016;15(2):147–57.
37. Simpson SJ, Mott LS, Esther CR Jr, Stick SM, Hall GL. Novel end points for clinical trials in young children with cystic fibrosis. Expert Rev Respir Med. 2013;7(3):231–43.
38. Rosenow T, Oudraad MC, Murray CP, Turkovic L, Kuo W, de Bruijne M, et al. Reply: excess risk of cancer from computed tomography scan is small but not so low as to be incalculable. Am J Respir Crit Care Med. 2015;192(11):1397–9.
39. Kuo W, Soffers T, Andrinopoulou ER, Rosenow T, Ranganathan S, Turkovic L, et al. Quantitative assessment of airway dimensions in young children with cystic fibrosis lung disease using chest computed tomography. Pediatr Pulmonol. 2017;52(11):1414–23.
40. Rosenow T, Oudraad MC, Murray CP, Turkovic L, Kuo W, de Bruijne M, et al. PRAGMA-CF. A quantitative structural lung disease computed tomography outcome in young children with cystic fibrosis. Am J Respir Crit Care Med. 2015;191(10):1158–65.
41. Loeve M, Hop WC, de Bruijne M, van Hal PT, Robinson P, Aitken ML, et al. Chest computed tomography scores are predictive of survival in patients with cystic fibrosis awaiting lung transplantation. Am J Respir Crit Care Med. 2012;185(10):1096–103.

42. Owens CM, Aurora P, Stanojevic S, Bush A, Wade A, Oliver C, et al. Lung clearance index and HRCT are complementary markers of lung abnormalities in young children with CF. Thorax. 2011;66(6):481–8.

43. Gustafsson PM, De Jong PA, Tiddens HA, Lindblad A. Multiple-breath inert gas washout and spirometry versus structural lung disease in cystic fibrosis. Thorax. 2008;63(2):129–34.

44. Stick SM, Brennan S, Murray C, Douglas T, von Ungern-Sternberg BS, Garratt LW, et al. Bronchiectasis in infants and preschool children diagnosed with cystic fibrosis after newborn screening. J Pediatr. 2009;155(5):623–8.e1.

45. Linnane BM, Hall GL, Nolan G, Brennan S, Stick SM, Sly PD, et al. Lung function in infants with cystic fibrosis diagnosed by newborn screening. Am J Respir Crit Care Med. 2008;178(12):1238–44.

46. Hoo AF, Thia LP, Nguyen TT, Bush A, Chudleigh J, Lum S, et al. Lung function is abnormal in 3-month-old infants with cystic fibrosis diagnosed by newborn screening. Thorax. 2012;67(10):874–81.

47. Hall GL, Logie KM, Parsons F, Schulzke SM, Nolan G, Murray C, et al. Air trapping on chest CT is associated with worse ventilation distribution in infants with cystic fibrosis diagnosed following newborn screening. PLoS One. 2011;6(8):e23932.

48. Belessis Y, Dixon B, Hawkins G, Pereira J, Peat J, MacDonald R, et al. Early cystic fibrosis lung disease detected by bronchoalveolar lavage and lung clearance index. Am J Respir Crit Care Med. 2012;185(8):862–73.

49. Ramsey KA, Ranganathan S, Park J, Skoric B, Adams AM, Simpson SJ, et al. Early respiratory infection is associated with reduced spirometry in children with cystic fibrosis. Am J Respir Crit Care Med. 2014;190(10):1111–6.

50. Ramsey KA, Rosenow T, Turkovic L, Skoric B, Banton G, Adams AM, et al. Lung clearance index and structural lung disease on computed tomography in early cystic fibrosis. Am J Respir Crit Care Med. 2016;193(1):60–7.

51. Ranganathan SC, Hall GL, Sly PD, Stick SM, Douglas TA. Australian respiratory early surveillance team for cystic F. early lung disease in infants and preschool children with cystic fibrosis. What have we learned and what should we do about it? Am J Respir Crit Care Med. 2017;195(12):1567–75.

52. Ratjen F, Davis SD, Stanojevic S, Kronmal RA, Hinckley Stukovsky KD, Jorgensen N, et al. Inhaled hypertonic saline in preschool children with cystic fibrosis (SHIP): a multicentre, randomised, double-blind, placebo-controlled trial. Lancet Respir Med. 2019;7(9):802–809.

53. Rosenfeld M, Ratjen F, Brumback L, Daniel S, Rowbotham R, McNamara S, et al. Inhaled hypertonic saline in infants and children younger than 6 years with cystic fibrosis: the ISIS randomized controlled trial. JAMA. 2012;307(21):2269–77.

Chapter 5
Bacterial Infections and the Respiratory Microbiome

Valerie J. Waters and John J. LiPuma

Introduction

Cystic fibrosis (CF) is a genetic, multisystem disease due to defects in the cystic fibrosis transmembrane conductance regulator (CFTR) protein, an anion channel responsible for chloride and bicarbonate trafficking [1, 2]. Although this channel is expressed in many tissues, its impaired function in airway epithelial cells leads to hyperviscous mucous secretions impeding effective mucociliary clearance. Impaired clearance of inhaled microorganisms results in the establishment of chronic infection, triggering an overexaggerated inflammatory response [3]. The resulting release of inflammatory cytokines and enzymes causes pulmonary damage in the form of bronchiectasis, further impairing mucociliary action, forming a vicious cycle. Subsequent respiratory failure remains the leading cause of death in individuals with CF [4].

The epidemiology of bacterial pulmonary infections in CF follows a typical pattern (Fig. 5.1) [5]. The airways of young children are typically colonized early in life with organisms such as *Staphylococcus aureus* and *Haemophilus influenzae*. Over time, these bacteria are gradually replaced with opportunistic, Gram-negative organisms such as *Pseudomonas aeruginosa* (most commonly), *Stenotrophomonas maltophilia*, *Burkholderia cepacia* complex, and *Achromobacter* species. More recently, there has also been increasing identification of infection due to nontuberculous

V. J. Waters (✉)
Division of Infectious Diseases, Department of Pediatrics, Hospital for Sick Children,
University of Toronto, Toronto, ON, Canada
e-mail: Valerie.Waters@sickkids.ca

J. J. LiPuma
Department of Pediatrics, University of Michigan Medical School, Ann Arbor, MI, USA
e-mail: jlipuma@med.umich.edu

© Springer Nature Switzerland AG 2020
S. D. Davis et al. (eds.), *Cystic Fibrosis*, Respiratory Medicine,
https://doi.org/10.1007/978-3-030-42382-7_5

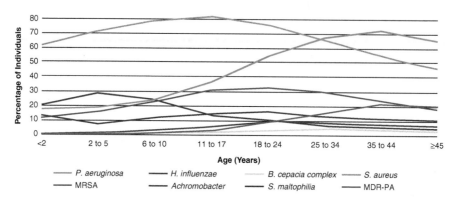

Fig. 5.1 Prevalence of respiratory microorganisms by age cohort in cystic fibrosis patients in 2017. (Cystic Fibrosis Foundation Patient Registry, 2017 Annual Data Report, Bethesda, Maryland ©2018 Cystic Fibrosis Foundation)

mycobacterial species in patients with CF. Furthermore, although much of the focus has traditionally been on bacterial pulmonary infection, the role of fungal and viral infections of CF airways have increasingly been studied as well.

The aim of this chapter is to review the microbiological diagnosis and epidemiology of CF airway infections. Fungal and atypical mycobacterial infections are covered in more detail in Chaps. 5 and 6, respectively. Infection prevention and control recommendations [6] as well as treatment guidelines for these infections [7] are outside the scope of this chapter and are extensively reviewed elsewhere.

Cystic Fibrosis Airway Microbiome

Much of what is known about the microbiology of airway infection in CF has been learned through the use of in vitro culture of respiratory specimens from affected individuals. While early studies (1940–1970) focused on the recovery in culture of known human pathogenic bacteria (e.g., *S. aureus* and *H. influenzae*), refined bacterial taxonomy and the use of selective culture media in subsequent studies (1970–2000) led to the recognition that several opportunistic bacterial species, in particular *P. aeruginosa*, are also involved in CF airway infection. In the early 2000s, so-called "culture-independent" methods of profiling mixed bacterial communities began to be applied to the study of CF airway microbiology [8]. These methods, which rely on amplification and analysis of bacterial DNA to identify species present in a particular site (or biologic specimen), demonstrated that the airways of persons with CF most often harbor rich microbial communities that are poorly reflected in selective culture. In addition to providing a less biased and sensitive means of detecting microbial species, culture-independent analyses also allow an estimation of the relative abundances of the species in a polymicrobial community. Applying these methods to CF respiratory specimens has shown that beyond the species typically associated with infection in CF based on routine culture, a variety of "nonpathogenic" bacteria, especially anaerobic species, are both prevalent and often present in relatively high abundances [9].

Studies of the CF airway microbiome using culture-independent methods have challenged several tenets of CF microbiology conventional wisdom [10]. For example, the commonly held beliefs that exacerbation of pulmonary symptoms results from an increase in the density of *P. aeruginosa* or reflects the acquisition of a "new" pathogen by an individual with CF have not been borne out by DNA sequence-based analyses. Another unexpected finding, demonstrated in several studies of the CF airway microbiome, is that the diversity of the bacterial communities in airways *decreases* with advancing patient age and lung disease progression [11]. That is, at younger ages, during the early stages of lung disease, CF airways typically harbor rich polymicrobial communities that include high relative abundances of anaerobic species derived from the oropharynx. As lung disease progresses with age, and as the administration of antimicrobials accelerates, airway bacterial communities become increasingly less diverse. With advanced lung disease, these communities often constrict markedly, becoming dominated by a single species (most often *P. aeruginosa*, but occasionally *B. cepacia* complex or an *Achromobacter* species).

Perhaps the most important development reshaping current views of CF microbiology is the increasing appreciation that myriad interspecies interactions – as well as complex interactions with the human host – likely have profound effects on lung disease and clinical response to therapy. In this sense, the polymicrobial community in CF airways, including bacteria, viruses, and fungi, may be considered the "pathogenic unit." The structure and activity of this microbial consortium in the context of the host's response to infection is the major determinant of CF respiratory disease.

While studies of the CF microbiome hold promise to translate into novel therapies and improved management of patients, our understanding of this complex ecology requires additional investigation. What has been learned about the epidemiology of CF airway infections, as described in the following sections, provides a foundation for these studies.

Diagnostics

Airway Sampling

The identification of bacterial organisms in the airways is dependent on the type of respiratory tract specimen sent for culture. Spontaneously expectorated sputum is the most common sample used for bacterial culture in both adults and children of sufficient age. In children who are too young to expectorate, oropharyngeal swabs (or "cough swabs") are used and have been shown, in the case of *P. aeruginosa* infection, to have a good negative predictive value but poor positive predictive value compared to lower respiratory tract sampling [12, 13]. Specimens from bronchoal-veolar lavage (BAL) may also be used for bacterial culture and have a higher sensitivity for detecting *P. aeruginosa* in the lower airway compared to oropharyngeal swabs [14]. However, this type of airway sampling is invasive and has not been shown to result in a lower prevalence of *P. aeruginosa* infection or less structural lung disease when compared to the use of oropharyngeal swabs in the diagnosis and management of CF pulmonary infections [15].

Bacterial Identification

Once a respiratory tract sample is sent for bacterial culture, it is then plated on selective media to enhance the growth of specific, well-known CF pathogens [16]. These media include mannitol salt agar, using sodium chloride as a selective agent and phenol red as an indicator of mannitol utilization, to recover *S. aureus* and *B. cepacia* selective agar (BCSA) and chocolate agar (incubated anaerobically) to recover *H. influenzae* [17]. Special sputum processing is required to improve recovery of nontuberculous mycobacteria by decontaminating sputum with N-acetyl-L-cysteine and sodium hydroxide followed by oxalic acid [18]. Identification of bacterial growth has traditionally been done using microscopy and biochemical testing. However, the introduction of matrix-assisted desorption ionization-time of flight mass spectrometry (MALDI-TOF) in the clinical microbiology laboratory has significantly accelerated the bacterial identification process [19]. Molecular methods using polymerase chain reaction (PCR) can also be used to speciate certain bacterial organisms such as *B. cepacia* complex (by amplification and sequencing of the *recA* gene) [20] and *Achromobacter* species (by *nrdA* gene sequencing) [21].

Antimicrobial Susceptibility Testing

Once a bacterial organism has been identified, antimicrobial susceptibility testing may be done to guide antibiotic therapy. Microbroth dilution assay is often considered the gold standard for antimicrobial susceptibility testing of CF bacterial isolates; however, agar-based diffusion assays, such as antibiotic disks or E-tests (antibiotic impregnated strips), are also accurate and comparable to the reference method [17]. In contrast, commercial automated microbroth dilution assays, such as Microscan and Vitek, have unacceptably high error rates when compared with reference broth dilution assay for antimicrobial susceptibility testing of CF bacterial isolates [22]. The minimum inhibitory concentration (MIC) obtained for each drug is interpreted according to interpretive criteria outlined by the Clinical Laboratory Standards Institute, which sets breakpoints for determining resistance [23]. There are no interpretive criteria for many antibiotics for multidrug-resistant CF organisms, such as *B. cepacia* complex, *S. maltophilia*, and *Achromobacter* spp.

Bacterial Infections

Staphylococcus aureus (Including MRSA)

S. aureus is a Gram-positive coccus that is nonmotile, non-spore-forming, and coagulase positive. It is a frequent colonizer of the skin and mucosa of humans and animals and, in contrast to most other CF pathogens, is well known to cause infections in non-CF individuals as well [24]. It has a host of virulence factors including Staphylococcal protein A (SpA) (a potent IgG binder) and more than 30 adhesin and toxin genes [25]. Antimicrobial resistance occurs through the expression of penicillinases, drug efflux pumps, and ribosome modification (mediated by the *erm* gene), for example [26]. Upon exposure to antibiotics such as trimethoprim-sulfamethoxazole, *S. aureus* may also grow as small colony variants [27]. Small colony variants are slow-growing secondary to metabolic defects and are associated with resistance to many antibiotics and persistence of infection [28]. Methicillin-resistant *S. aureus* (MRSA) is resistant to methicillin through the expression of an altered penicillin-binding protein (PBP2a) encoded by the *mecA* gene [29].

S. *aureus* is an early colonizer and the most frequent bacterial organism isolated from CF patients [5]. The prevalence of infection peaks in childhood with approximately 70% of CF children ages 11–17 having *S. aureus*-positive respiratory tract culture. As the reservoir for *S. aureus* are humans/animals, initial infection is thought to occur from direct contact, with family members, for example [30]. As *S. aureus* is an early colonizer in CF, it is often difficult to measure its impact on clinical outcomes as children under 6 may not reproducibly perform pulmonary function testing. In a multicenter observational study of CF patients (average age 16 yrs) with *S. aureus* infection, a higher density of *S. aureus* on throat swab was associated with accelerated lung function decline [31]. Similarly, in CF children undergoing bronchoalveolar lavage, those with *S. aureus* infection had higher levels of pulmonary inflammation (as measured by neutrophil counts, IL-8, and neutrophil elastase levels in bronchoalveolar lavage fluid) compared to those without *S. aureus* infection [32].

The prevalence of MRSA infection in CF is considerably less than the prevalence of methicillin-susceptible *S. aureus* (MSSA) infection, and ranges from 5% to 26% depending on the country of origin [5, 33]. Acquisition is through direct contact and patient to patient transmission of MRSA infection has been well described [34]. MRSA strains can be either hospital-acquired MRSA (HA-MRSA) or community-acquired MRSA and are distinguished by the type of *mecA* gene they carry [35]. Studies have reported that approximately 14% of CF patients with MRSA infection harbor CA-MRSA, while the remainder harbor HA-MRSA strains [36]. The impact of MRSA infection on clinical outcomes in individuals with CF has been well defined. Using data from the US CF Patient Registry, investigators showed that chronic MRSA infection (3 or more positive cultures in the preceding year) in CF patients ages 8–21 years was associated with increased lung function decline (as measured by forced expiratory volume in 1 second [FEV_1]) compared to those without chronic infection [37]. Furthermore, after adjusting for other markers of disease severity, MRSA infection was independently associated with an earlier time to death in CF patients [38]. MRSA infection has also been demonstrated to be a risk factor for failing to recover baseline lung function following antibiotic treatment for a pulmonary exacerbation [39].

Pseudomonas aeruginosa

P. aeruginosa is a non-lactose-fermenting Gram-negative bacterium, commonly found in water sources such as rivers, lakes, and municipal water systems [24]. It has both flagella, conferring motility, and pili, important for initial attachment to airway epithelial cells [40, 41]. *P. aeruginosa* expresses three main exopolysaccharides, alginate, Pel, and Psl, which are important in the establishment and maintenance of a biofilm structure (see below) [42]. It is an aerobe but can survive under anaerobic conditions and grows selectively at 42 ° C [16]. It is intrinsically resistant to many ß-lactam antibiotics and can acquire resistance through either chromosomal mutation or horizontal gene transfer. Some of the antimicrobial resistance mechanisms in *P. aeruginosa* include the expression of aminoglycoside-modifying enzymes, multidrug efflux pumps, and carbapenamase production, to name a few [43].

Approximately 40% of individuals with CF have *P. aeruginosa* infection [5, 33]. *P. aeruginosa* has a predilection for causing pulmonary infection in individuals with CF and is considered a criteria in the diagnosis of CF disease [44]. *P. aeruginosa* infection may be a consequence of impaired mucociliary clearance but others have suggested that *P. aeruginosa* flagella may bind directly to defective CFTR protein [4, 45]. Children with CF are likely most often initially colonized with *P. aeruginosa* strains acquired from their environment [46]. Genotypic studies of incident CF *P. aeruginosa* isolates have found sharing of strains with those isolated from environmental sources, suggesting a mode of initial acquisition [47]. However, patient to patient transmission of *P. aeruginosa* infection has been documented in infants identified through newborn screening who attended an unsegregated CF clinic, prior to the implementation of current infection prevention guidelines [48]. Once *P. aeruginosa* enters the CF airways through inhalation, it can establish chronic infection. Randomized controlled trials have demonstrated that antibiotic treatment, with inhaled tobramycin, for example, improves the clearance rate of incident *P. aeruginosa* compared to no treatment [49, 50]. Thus, it is standard of care to treat first time *P. aeruginosa* infection with antibiotic therapy with the goal of eradication.

Without eradication, *P. aeruginosa* will adapt itself to the environment of the CF airway [51]. After initial colonization, *P. aeruginosa* will downregulate its acute virulence factors, such as flagella, to evade detection and clearance by cells of the immune system [52]. Furthermore, it will upregulate genes involved in quorum sensing (*las/rhl* genes) leading to biofilm formation [53]. *P. aeruginosa* biofilms are microbial communities encased in a matrix composed primarily of its exopolysaccharides: alginate, Psl, and Pel [54]. Biofilms are antibiotic resistant due to impairment of antibiotic diffusion through the matrix as well as slowed bacterial growth [55].

Additional bacterial adaptations permitting the establishment of chronic infection include the development of persister cells (metabolically dormant cells) and alginate hyperproduction (also known as mucoidy status) impairing neutrophil phagocytosis [56–58].

Chronic *P. aeruginosa* infection is associated with increased pulmonary inflammation as *P. aeruginosa* stimulates IL-8 production by airway epithelial cells, leading to neutrophil recruitment and neutrophil elastase release [4, 59]. Sputum neutrophil elastase levels have been shown to most closely correlate with the development of bronchiectasis in CF patients [60]. CF patients with chronic *P. aeruginosa* infection will thus experience worse clinical outcomes in the form of accelerated lung function decline and earlier death [61, 62]. Supporting this fact, studies using the US CF Patient Registry have demonstrated that treatment of chronic *P. aeruginosa* infection (with inhaled tobramycin) is associated with prolonged survival in individuals with CF [63].

While *P. aeruginosa* is appropriately considered the major opportunistic bacterial pathogen in CF, its role in lung disease within the broader context of the airway microbiome is the subject of current investigation. For example, the commonly held belief that exacerbation of pulmonary symptoms results from an increase in the density of *P. aeruginosa* has not been borne out by DNA-sequence-based analyses. In fact, it appears that *P. aeruginosa* density *decreases* with exacerbation, while the relative abundance of anaerobic species increases [64, 65]. Further, recent studies have suggested that myriad interspecies interactions likely play critical roles in influencing *P. aeruginosa* virulence in vivo [66]. Interactions between *P. aeruginosa* and *S. aureus*, in particular, are of considerable interest and hold promise to advance our understanding of how complex polymicrobial communities in CF airways act in concert to impact lung disease [67–70].

Burkholderia cepacia *Complex*

The *Burkholderia cepacia* complex is comprised of over 23 *Burkholderia* species, with *Burkholderia multivorans* and *Burkholderia cenocepacia* being the most common species isolated from CF patients [71]. *Burkholderia gladioli* is a closely related species that is the third most common *Burkholderia* species isolated in CF, but it is not part of the *B. cepacia* complex. *Burkholderia* are aerobic, Gram-negative bacteria that are motile due to the presence of flagella. Like *P. aeruginosa*, *B. cepacia* complex are frequently found in moist environments and in the soil, including in plant material [72]. *B. cepacia* complex species exhibit a number of different virulence factors including pili that facilitate epithelial cell attachment, extracellular proteases resulting in tissue damage, quorum sensing genes facilitating biofilm formation, and a type III secretion system promoting cellular invasion [73–77]. *B. cepacia* complex are intrinsically resistant to a number of different antimicrobial classes including aminoglycosides due to efflux pumps and penicillin derivatives secondary to inducible chromosomally encoded ß-lactamases [78, 79].

The prevalence of *B. cepacia* complex infection in CF patients is approximately 3–5% according to American and Canadian Registry data [5, 33]. The distribution of infection by species has changed over the last several decades, shifting from a predominance of *B. cenocepacia* to *B. multivorans* in many CF populations [80]. This is likely due to the recognition of patient to patient transmission of *B. cenocepacia*, leading to changes in infection control practices and subsequent decline in new *B. cenocepacia* infections [17, 81, 82]. The majority of new *B. cepacia* complex infections are now most commonly acquired from environmental sources, although the potential for patient to patient transmission still exists [83]. Infection with *B. cepacia* complex has been associated with worse lung function and is a risk factor for earlier death [84–86]. Infection with *B. cenocepacia* in particular has been associated with decreased survival in CF patients post lung transplantation compared to CF patients without *B. cepacia* complex infection or with infection with other *Burkholderia* species [87]. *B. cenocepacia* has the ability to angio-invade leading to necrotizing pneumonia and sepsis, known as "cepacia syndrome" [88]. Although this has been most commonly described with *B. cenocepacia*, it can occur with other *Burkholderia* species as well, such as *B. dolosa* [89]. CF patients with cepacia syndrome have high markers of inflammation, commonly develop diffuse pulmonary infiltrates, and are often bacteremic. The associated mortality can be as high as 80% [78].

Stenotrophomonas maltophilia

In addition to *P. aeruginosa* and *B. cepacia* complex, there are a number of other non-lactose-fermenting Gram-negative bacilli that are known to infect the airways of CF patients. One of the most common is *Stenotrophomonas maltophilia*. *S. maltophilia* is an aerobic, motile bacteria commonly found in water supplies and known to cause infections in immunocompromised individuals as well as CF pulmonary infections [90]. *S. maltophilia* produces a variety of extracellular enzymes, such as alkaline serine proteases, which cause tissue necrosis. Their outer membrane lipopolysaccharides are also a potent inducer of cytokine-mediated inflammation [91]. *S. maltophilia* can form biofilms as well and are inherently resistant to a number different classes of antimicrobials [92, 93]. Resistance occurs through the expression of multidrug efflux pumps, ß-lactamases, aminoglycoside-modifying enzymes, and reduced outer membrane permeability [94].

The prevalence of *S. maltophilia* infection in the CF population ranges from 12% to 30% [5, 33, 95, 96]. Initial infection is likely from environmental sources with little evidence of patient to patient transmission. Risk factors for acquisition include intravenous and oral antibiotic use [97]. Epidemiologic studies using the CF Foundation Patient Registry found that CF patients with *S. maltophilia* infection were older and had worse lung function compared to those without *S. maltophilia*, but after controlling for confounders, they did not have a steeper FEV_1 decline or worse short-term survival (3 years) [98, 99]. However, studies focusing on CF patients with chronic *S. maltophilia* infection (2 or more positive cultures in preceding year) have noted that it is an independent risk factor for pulmonary exacerbations treated with intravenous antibiotics as well as a risk factor for death or lung transplantation [100, 101]. In a multicenter study examining survival post lung transplantation, infection with multidrug-resistant (MDR) organisms including *S. maltophilia* (but excluding *B. cepacia* complex) was associated with worse survival in CF patients compared to those without MDR infection, although many MDR organisms were included in the analyses [102].

Achromobacter Species

Achromobacter species are Gram-negative, non-sporulating straight rods. The *Achromobacter* genus has undergone many taxonomic reclassifications [103, 104]. Currently, a total of 23 species are identified within the *Achromobacter* genus. Within CF populations, *A. xylosoxidans* and *A. ruhlandii* are the two most common *Achromobacter* species identified, accounting for 42% and 23% of infections, respectively [21]. *Achromobacter* species are generally aerobic and non-fermentative, with growth occurring between 25 and 37 °C. They are widely distributed in the environment, particularly in water and soil. In addition to being motile due to the presence of flagella, certain strains of *Achromobacter* have the ability to bind to mucin, collagen, and fibronectin, which may facilitate initial infection in the airways [105, 106]. As with the other aforementioned Gram-negative organisms, *Achromobacter* species can also form biofilms and are intrinsically resistant to several classes of antimicrobials through the expression of efflux pumps, ß-lactamases, and aminoglycoside-modifying enzymes [107–109]. They are generally resistant to narrow-spectrum penicillins, cephalosporins such as cefotaxime and ceftriaxone, aztreonam, and aminoglycosides.

The average prevalence of *Achromobacter* infection is approximately 5–6% although rates as high as 29% have been reported in certain CF centers [5, 33, 110, 111]. Most patients harbor unique strains acquired from the environment, although cross-contamination between patients has rarely been described [111–114]. Epidemiologic studies that have examined the effect of *Achromobacter* infection on clinical outcomes in CF have generally been limited by small sample size. The study by De Baets et al. demonstrated that CF individuals with chronic *Achromobacter* infection had lower lung function and more pulmonary exacerbations, than age-, gender-, and *P. aeruginosa*–matched controls, representing a sicker patient population [110]. Only one study, using serum antibodies to *Achromobacter* to define chronic infection, showed worsening lung function upon the development of chronic *Achromobacter* infection [115]. In a registry-based epidemiologic study of over 1000 CF patients, chronic *Achromobacter* infection (defined as 2 or more positive cultures in the previous 12 months) was associated with a twofold increased risk of death or transplant compared to those with no history of *Achromobacter* infection, even after adjusting for other known confounders [116].

Anaerobes

The bacterial species discussed in the preceding sections are aerobic organisms, although some can survive under anaerobic conditions. With the advent of molecular methods of identification, there has been an increasing recognition of the presence and potential role of anaerobic bacteria in CF lung disease [117, 118]. An anaerobe is an organism that requires reduced oxygen for growth, failing to grow on the surface of solid media in 10% CO_2 in air [119]. Anaerobes can be both Gram-positive and Gram-negative and are part of the normal human microbiota of many mucosal surfaces including the upper airways, the gastrointestinal tract, and the female genital tract. They can cause serious infections such as brain abscesses, sinusitis, necrotizing pneumonia, liver abscess, and bacteremia, to name a few [24]. A number of virulence factors are associated with pathogenic anaerobes including capsular polysaccharide, hemolysins, proteases, and lipopolysaccharides [120]. Anaerobes that commonly cause human infection (e.g., *Bacteroides fragilis*, *Prevotella melaninogenica*, *Fusobacterium nucleatum*) are generally aerotolerant (tolerating 2–8% oxygen) [121].

Respiratory specimens obtained from CF airways are not routinely cultured under anaerobic conditions, and the culture and identification of anaerobic species can be both difficult and time-consuming [16]. Thus, the general prevalence of anaerobic infections in CF patients is not known. However, studies that have specifically cultured CF sputum samples under anaerobic conditions have identified obligate anaerobes in approximately 60–90% of samples, predominantly in the genera *Prevotella*, *Veillonella*, *Propionibacterium*, and *Peptostreptococcus* [122–124]. Culture-independent microbial detection methods, such as 16S-rRNA-based analysis, generally have shown higher prevalence rates of anaerobes in CF respiratory specimens and have identified a vast diversity of anaerobic species in CF. In a study of CF children undergoing bronchoscopic alveolar lavage, Harris et al. found 65 different anaerobic species in BAL samples by rRNA sequence analysis [125]. Given the fact that the upper airways are colonized by anaerobic bacteria, identifying lower airway infection by anaerobes (rather than contamination passing through the oral cavity) can be difficult. Furthermore, the association between the presence of anaerobic organisms and CF lung disease is somewhat controversial [126]. In vitro studies have demonstrated that anaerobic bacteria can produce short-chain fatty acids that mediate the release of pro-inflammatory cytokines from human bronchial epithelial cells [127]. These pro-inflammatory cytokines lead to neutrophil recruitment into CF lungs [128]. Anaerobes can also interact with other organisms within the CF airways, increasing the virulence of *P. aeruginosa*, for example, and producing extended-spectrum ß-lactamases conferring antimicrobial resistance to *P. aeruginosa* [129, 130]. In contrast, both cross-sectional and longitudinal studies have noted an association between anaerobes and lower pulmonary inflammation as well as better lung function [118, 124, 131–134]. This association has been demonstrated using culture-based methods (increased bacterial density) as well as molecular-based methods (increased relative abundance). Higher loads of anaerobes in airway secretions may represent greater microbial community diversity in CF patients with milder lung disease who have received less antimicrobial therapy.

Viral Infections

In addition to bacterial organisms, a significant number of CF patients will harbor viruses in their airways [135]. Viruses are not detected by traditional culturing techniques of sputum and, thus, both the correct specimen and test must be requested in order to diagnose a viral infection [24]. In the past, viral culture and serologic testing (acute and convalescent serology) were used to identify viral infection, but these methods are expensive and relatively insensitive and time-consuming [136]. The introduction of direct immunofluorescence for viruses in respiratory tract samples improved the sensitivity and turnaround time of testing. The advent of molecular methods, based on polymerase chain reaction (PCR), led to more reliable, rapid, and cost-effective viral diagnostics [137].

The overall prevalence of viral infections during exacerbations in individuals with CF is estimated to be between 13% and 60% [135, 138]. Respiratory syncytial virus (RSV) and influenza A and B virus are the most common viruses identified in CF patients. However, sensitive multiplex molecular diagnostics assays have detected a great diversity of respiratory viruses in people with CF including rhinovirus, human metapneumovirus, picornavirus, coronavirus, and coxsackie/echovirus [139–143]. Although viruses are detected more frequently in CF children, a significant proportion of adults with CF also develop respiratory viral infections [144]. CF and non-CF children (including infants) are equally likely to acquire viral infections; however, CF children are more likely to suffer viral-related morbidity [136, 139, 145, 146]. Viral infections in both adults and children with CF are associated with an increased risk of pulmonary exacerbation [142, 147]. These viral-associated exacerbations are characterized by greater drops in lung function at the time of presentation, higher markers of systemic inflammation, longer duration of intravenous antibiotic therapy, and poorer lung function response [148, 149]. RSV in particular has been associated with failure to recover to baseline FEV_1 following antibiotic treatment for a pulmonary exacerbation. Infants with CF who are infected with RSV not only have a higher rate of respiratory exacerbations but also prolonged hospitalizations and prolonged symptoms over the ensuing 2 years [150]. Similarly, influenza virus infection has also been associated with significant morbidity in children with CF, specifically an increased risk of hospital admission [151]. A large epidemiologic study using the CF Foundation Patient Registry determined that there was an estimated excess of 2.1% of total exacerbations during the influenza season [152]. The exact mechanism through which viral infections lead to worse lung function in CF patients is not fully understood but may involve interactions with bacteria such as *P. aeruginosa*. Epidemiologic studies have demonstrated that new *P. aeruginosa* infection occurs more commonly in the winter season and is often preceded by a viral infection [153]. RSV has been shown to enhance *P. aeruginosa* adherence to epithelial cells [154]. In addition, RSV infection of airway epithelium induces antiviral IFN signaling leading to enhanced *P. aeruginosa* biofilm growth [155]. Less is known about other viral-induced mechanisms of CF lung disease.

Summary

In summary, the microbiology of CF pulmonary infections is complex, characterized by a polymicrobial environment and changing with age and varying lung disease severity. Infection with opportunistic, environmental Gram-negative organisms is typical in CF due to defective mucociliary clearance and contributes to the ongoing inflammation and tissue destruction within the lung. Our understanding of the CF pulmonary microbiome continues to evolve and has the potential to inform the infectious disease management of CF patients in the future.

References

1. Ratjen F, Doring G. Cystic fibrosis. Lancet. 2003;361:681–9.
2. Tsui LC, Buchwald M, Barker D, Braman JC, Knowlton R, Schumm JW, et al. Cystic fibrosis locus defined by a genetically linked polymorphic DNA marker. Science. 1985;230:1054–7.
3. Cohen TS, Prince A. Cystic fibrosis: a mucosal immunodeficiency syndrome. Nat Med. 2012;18:509–19.
4. Gibson RL, Burns JL, Ramsey BW. Pathophysiology and management of pulmonary infections in cystic fibrosis. Am J Respir Crit Care Med. 2003;168:918–51.
5. Cystic Fibrosis Foundation. Patient registry report. In: CFF, editor. Bethesda; Cystic Fibrosis Foundation and Cystic Fibrosis Canada; 2016.
6. Saiman L, Siegel JD, LiPuma JJ, Brown RF, Bryson EA, Chambers MJ, et al. Infection prevention and control guideline for cystic fibrosis: 2013 update. Infect Control Hosp Epidemiol. 2014;35(Suppl 1):S1–S67.
7. Waters V. New treatments for emerging cystic fibrosis pathogens other than Pseudomonas. Curr Pharm Des. 2012;18:696–725.
8. Rogers GB, Hart CA, Mason JR, Hughes M, Walshaw MJ, Bruce KD. Bacterial diversity in cases of lung infection in cystic fibrosis patients: 16S ribosomal DNA (rDNA) length heterogeneity PCR and 16S rDNA terminal restriction fragment length polymorphism profiling. J Clin Microbiol. 2003;41:3548–58.
9. Huang YJ, LiPuma JJ. The microbiome in cystic fibrosis. Clin Chest Med. 2016;37:59–67.
10. O'Toole GA. Cystic fibrosis airway microbiome: overturning the old, opening the way for the new. J Bacteriol. 2018;200:pii: e00561-17.
11. Zhao J, Schloss PD, Kalikin LM, Carmody LA, Foster BK, Petrosino JF, et al. Decade-long bacterial community dynamics in cystic fibrosis airways. Proc Natl Acad Sci U S A. 2012;109:5809–14.

12. Saiman L. Microbiology of early CF lung disease. Paediatr Respir Rev. 2004;5(Suppl A):S367–9.
13. Rosenfeld M, Emerson J, Accurso F, Armstrong D, Castile R, Grimwood K, et al. Diagnostic accuracy of oropharyngeal cultures in infants and young children with cystic fibrosis. Pediatr Pulmonol. 1999;28:321–8.
14. Breuer O, Caudri D, Akesson L, Ranganathan S, Stick SM, Schultz A, et al. The clinical significance of oropharyngeal cultures in young children with cystic fibrosis. Eur Respir J. 2018;51:pii: 1800238.
15. Wainwright CE, Vidmar S, Armstrong DS, Byrnes CA, Carlin JB, Cheney J, et al. Effect of bronchoalveolar lavage-directed therapy on Pseudomonas aeruginosa infection and structural lung injury in children with cystic fibrosis: a randomized trial. JAMA. 2011;306:163–71.
16. Gilligan P, et al. Cumitech 43, cystic fibrosis microbiology. Washington, DC: ASM Press; 2006.
17. Saiman L, Siegel J. Infection control recommendations for patients with cystic fibrosis: microbiology, important pathogens, and infection control practices to prevent patient-to-patient transmission. Infect Control Hosp Epidemiol. 2003;24:S6–52.
18. Whittier S, Olivier K, Gilligan P, Knowles M, Della-Latta P. Proficiency testing of clinical microbiology laboratories using modified decontamination procedures for detection of nontuberculous mycobacteria in sputum samples from cystic fibrosis patients. The Nontuberculous Mycobacteria in Cystic Fibrosis Study Group. J Clin Microbiol. 1997;35:2706–8.
19. Homem de Mello de Souza HA, Dalla-Costa LM, Vicenzi FJ, Camargo de Souza D, Riedi CA, Filho NA, et al. MALDI-TOF: a useful tool for laboratory identification of uncommon glucose non-fermenting Gram-negative bacteria associated with cystic fibrosis. J Med Microbiol. 2014;63:1148–53.
20. Vermis K, Coenye T, Mahenthiralingam E, Nelis HJ, Vandamme P. Evaluation of species-specific recA-based PCR tests for genomovar level identification within the Burkholderia cepacia complex. J Med Microbiol. 2002;51:937–40.
21. Spilker T, Vandamme P, Lipuma JJ. Identification and distribution of Achromobacter species in cystic fibrosis. J Cyst Fibros. 2013;12:298–301.
22. Burns JL, Saiman L, Whittier S, Krzewinski J, Liu Z, Larone D, et al. Comparison of two commercial systems (Vitek and MicroScan-WalkAway) for antimicrobial susceptibility testing of Pseudomonas aeruginosa isolates from cystic fibrosis patients. Diagn Microbiol Infect Dis. 2001;39:257–60.
23. Clinical Laboratory Standards Institute. M-100S. 28th ed.; 2018.
24. Mandell GL, Bennett JE, Dolin R. Principles and practice of infectious diseases. 7th ed. Philadelphia: Elsevier Churchill Livingstone; 2015.
25. O'Gara JP. Into the storm: chasing the opportunistic pathogen Staphylococcus aureus from skin colonisation to life-threatening infections. Environ Microbiol. 2017;19:3823–33.
26. Foster TJ. Antibiotic resistance in Staphylococcus aureus. Current status and future prospects. FEMS Microbiol Rev. 2017;41:430–49.
27. Kriegeskorte A, Lore NI, Bragonzi A, Riva C, Kelkenberg M, Becker K, et al. Thymidine-dependent Staphylococcus aureus small-colony variants are induced by trimethoprim-sulfamethoxazole (SXT) and have increased fitness during SXT challenge. Antimicrob Agents Chemother. 2015;59:7265–72.
28. Proctor RA, von Eiff C, Kahl BC, Becker K, McNamara P, Herrmann M, et al. Small colony variants: a pathogenic form of bacteria that facilitates persistent and recurrent infections. Nat Rev Microbiol. 2006;4:295–305.
29. Wielders CL, Vriens MR, Brisse S, de Graaf-Miltenburg LA, Troelstra A, Fleer A, et al. In-vivo transfer of mecA DNA to Staphylococcus aureus [corrected]. Lancet. 2001;357:1674–5.
30. Goerke C, Kraning K, Stern M, Doring G, Botzenhart K, Wolz C. Molecular epidemiology of community-acquired Staphylococcus aureus in families with and without cystic fibrosis patients. J Infect Dis. 2000;181:984–9.

31. Junge S, Gorlich D, den Reijer M, Wiedemann B, Tummler B, Ellemunter H, et al. Factors associated with worse lung function in cystic fibrosis patients with persistent Staphylococcus aureus. PLoS One. 2016;11:e0166220.
32. Sagel SD, Gibson RL, Emerson J, McNamara S, Burns JL, Wagener JS, et al. Impact of Pseudomonas and Staphylococcus infection on inflammation and clinical status in young children with cystic fibrosis. J Pediatr. 2009;154:183–8.
33. Cystic Fibrosis Canada. Canadian patient data registry report. In: Canada CF, editor. Cystic Fibrosis Foundation and Cystic Fibrosis Canada; 2016.
34. Givney R, Vickery A, Holliday A, Pegler M, Benn R. Methicillin-resistant Staphylococcus aureus in a cystic fibrosis unit. J Hosp Infect. 1997;35:27–36.
35. Daum RS, Ito T, Hiramatsu K, Hussain F, Mongkolrattanothai K, Jamklang M, et al. A novel methicillin-resistance cassette in community-acquired methicillin-resistant Staphylococcus aureus isolates of diverse genetic backgrounds. J Infect Dis. 2002;186:1344–7.
36. Goodrich JS, Sutton-Shields TN, Kerr A, Wedd JP, Miller MB, Gilligan PH. Prevalence of community-associated methicillin-resistant Staphylococcus aureus in patients with cystic fibrosis. J Clin Microbiol. 2009;47:1231–3.
37. Dasenbrook EC, Merlo CA, Diener-West M, Lechtzin N, Boyle MP. Persistent methicillin-resistant Staphylococcus aureus and rate of FEV1 decline in cystic fibrosis. Am J Respir Crit Care Med. 2008;178:814–21.
38. Dasenbrook EC, Checkley W, Merlo CA, Konstan MW, Lechtzin N, Boyle MP. Association between respiratory tract methicillin-resistant Staphylococcus aureus and survival in cystic fibrosis. JAMA. 2010;303:2386–92.
39. Sanders DB, Bittner RC, Rosenfeld M, Hoffman LR, Redding GJ, Goss CH. Failure to recover to baseline pulmonary function after cystic fibrosis pulmonary exacerbation. Am J Respir Crit Care Med. 2010;182:627–32.
40. Feldman M, Bryan R, Rajan S, Scheffler L, Brunnert S, Tang H, et al. Role of flagella in pathogenesis of Pseudomonas aeruginosa pulmonary infection. Infect Immun. 1998;66:43–51.
41. Mahenthiralingam E, Campbell ME, Speert DP. Nonmotility and phagocytic resistance of Pseudomonas aeruginosa isolates from chronically colonized patients with cystic fibrosis. Infect Immun. 1994;62:596–605.
42. Chew SC, Kundukad B, Seviour T, van der Maarel JR, Yang L, Rice SA, et al. Dynamic remodeling of microbial biofilms by functionally distinct exopolysaccharides. MBio. 2014;5:e01536–14.
43. Lister PD, Wolter DJ, Hanson ND. Antibacterial-resistant Pseudomonas aeruginosa: clinical impact and complex regulation of chromosomally encoded resistance mechanisms. Clin Microbiol Rev. 2009;22:582–610.
44. Farrell PM, Rosenstein BJ, White TB, Accurso FJ, Castellani C, Cutting GR, et al. Guidelines for diagnosis of cystic fibrosis in newborns through older adults: Cystic Fibrosis Foundation consensus report. J Pediatr. 2008;153:S4–S14.
45. Bryan R, Kube D, Perez A, Davis P, Prince A. Overproduction of the CFTR R domain leads to increased levels of asialoGM1 and increased Pseudomonas aeruginosa binding by epithelial cells. Am J Respir Cell Mol Biol. 1998;19:269–77.
46. Ranganathan SC, Skoric B, Ramsay KA, Carzino R, Gibson AM, Hart E, et al. Geographical differences in first acquisition of Pseudomonas aeruginosa in cystic fibrosis. Ann Am Thorac Soc. 2013;10:108–14.
47. Kidd TJ, Ritchie SR, Ramsay KA, Grimwood K, Bell SC, Rainey PB. Pseudomonas aeruginosa exhibits frequent recombination, but only a limited association between genotype and ecological setting. PLoS One. 2012;7:e44199.
48. Kosorok MR, Jalaluddin M, Farrell PM, Shen G, Colby CE, Laxova A, et al. Comprehensive analysis of risk factors for acquisition of Pseudomonas aeruginosa in young children with cystic fibrosis. Pediatr Pulmonol. 1998;26:81–8.
49. Ratjen F, Doring G, Nikolaizik WH. Effect of inhaled tobramycin on early Pseudomonas aeruginosa colonisation in patients with cystic fibrosis. Lancet. 2001;358:983–4.

50. Schelstraete P, Haerynck F, Van daele S, Deseyne S, De Baets F. Eradication therapy for Pseudomonas aeruginosa colonization episodes in cystic fibrosis patients not chronically colonized by P aeruginosa. J Cyst Fibros. 2013;12:1–8.
51. Winstanley C, O'Brien S, Brockhurst MA. Pseudomonas aeruginosa evolutionary adaptation and diversification in cystic fibrosis chronic lung infections. Trends Microbiol. 2016;24:327–37.
52. Hogardt M, Heesemann J. Adaptation of Pseudomonas aeruginosa during persistence in the cystic fibrosis lung. Int J Med Microbiol. 2010;300:557–62.
53. D'Argenio DA, Wu M, Hoffman LR, Kulasekara HD, Deziel E, Smith EE, et al. Growth phenotypes of Pseudomonas aeruginosa lasR mutants adapted to the airways of cystic fibrosis patients. Mol Microbiol. 2007;64:512–33.
54. Colvin KM, Irie Y, Tart CS, Urbano R, Whitney JC, Ryder C, et al. The Pel and Psl polysaccharides provide Pseudomonas aeruginosa structural redundancy within the biofilm matrix. Environ Microbiol. 2012;14:1913–28.
55. Prince AS. Biofilms, antimicrobial resistance, and airway infection. N Engl J Med. 2002;347:1110–1.
56. Hentzer M, Teitzel GM, Balzer GJ, Heydorn A, Molin S, Givskov M, et al. Alginate overproduction affects Pseudomonas aeruginosa biofilm structure and function. J Bacteriol. 2001;183:5395–401.
57. Leid JG, Willson CJ, Shirtliff ME, Hassett DJ, Parsek MR, Jeffers AK. The exopolysaccharide alginate protects Pseudomonas aeruginosa biofilm bacteria from IFN-gamma-mediated macrophage killing. J Immunol. 2005;175:7512–8.
58. Bigger J. Treatment of staphylococcal infections with penicillin by intermittent sterilisation. Lancet. 1944;244:497–500.
59. Cantin A. Cystic fibrosis lung inflammation: early, sustained, and severe. Am J Respir Crit Care Med. 1995;151:939–41.
60. Sly PD, Gangell CL, Chen L, Ware RS, Ranganathan S, Mott LS, et al. Risk factors for bronchiectasis in children with cystic fibrosis. N Engl J Med. 2013;368:1963–70.
61. Henry RL, Mellis CM, Petrovic L. Mucoid Pseudomonas aeruginosa is a marker of poor survival in cystic fibrosis. Pediatr Pulmonol. 1992;12:158–61.
62. McColley SA, Schechter MS, Morgan WJ, Pasta DJ, Craib ML, Konstan MW. Risk factors for mortality before age 18 years in cystic fibrosis. Pediatr Pulmonol. 2017;52:909–15.
63. Sawicki GS, Signorovitch JE, Zhang J, Latremouille-Viau D, von Wartburg M, Wu EQ, et al. Reduced mortality in cystic fibrosis patients treated with tobramycin inhalation solution. Pediatr Pulmonol. 2012;47:44–52.
64. Carmody LA, Zhao J, Schloss PD, Petrosino JF, Murray S, Young VB, et al. Changes in cystic fibrosis airway microbiota at pulmonary exacerbation. Ann Am Thorac Soc. 2013;10:179–87.
65. Carmody LA, Caverly LJ, Foster BK, Rogers MAM, Kalikin LM, Simon RH, et al. Fluctuations in airway bacterial communities associated with clinical states and disease stages in cystic fibrosis. PLoS One. 2018;13:e0194060.
66. O'Brien S, Fothergill JL. The role of multispecies social interactions in shaping Pseudomonas aeruginosa pathogenicity in the cystic fibrosis lung. FEMS Microbiol Lett. 2017;364:15
67. Beaudoin T, Yau YCW, Stapleton PJ, Gong Y, Wang PW, Guttman DS, et al. Staphylococcus aureus interaction with Pseudomonas aeruginosa biofilm enhances tobramycin resistance. NPJ Biofilms Microbi. 2017;3:25.
68. Armbruster CR, Wolter DJ, Mishra M, Hayden HS, Radey MC, Merrihew G, et al. Staphylococcus aureus protein a mediates interspecies interactions at the cell surface of Pseudomonas aeruginosa. MBio. 2016;7:pii: e00538-16.
69. Magalhaes AP, Lopes SP, Pereira MO. Insights into cystic fibrosis Polymicrobial consortia: the role of species interactions in biofilm development, phenotype, and response to in-use antibiotics. Front Microbiol. 2016;7:2146.
70. Limoli DH, Whitfield GB, Kitao T, Ivey ML, Davis MR Jr, Grahl N, et al. Pseudomonas aeruginosa alginate overproduction promotes coexistence with Staphylococcus aureus in a model of cystic fibrosis respiratory infection. MBio. 2017;8:pii: e00186-17.

71. Lipuma JJ. Update on the Burkholderia cepacia complex. Curr Opin Pulm Med. 2005;11:528–33.
72. LiPuma JJ, Spilker T, Coenye T, Gonzalez CF. An epidemic Burkholderia cepacia complex strain identified in soil. Lancet. 2002;359:2002–3.
73. Mahenthiralingam E, Vandamme P, Campbell ME, Henry DA, Gravelle AM, Wong LT, et al. Infection with Burkholderia cepacia complex genomovars in patients with cystic fibrosis: virulent transmissible strains of genomovar III can replace Burkholderia multivorans. Clin Infect Dis. 2001;33:1469–75.
74. Sun L, Jiang RZ, Steinbach S, Holmes A, Campanelli C, Forstner J, et al. The emergence of a highly transmissible lineage of cbl+ Pseudomonas (Burkholderia) cepacia causing CF centre epidemics in North America and Britain. Nat Med. 1995;1:661–6.
75. Zlosnik JE, Speert DP. The role of mucoidy in virulence of bacteria from the Burkholderia cepacia complex: a systematic proteomic and transcriptomic analysis. J Infect Dis. 2010;202:770–81.
76. Huber B, Riedel K, Hentzer M, Heydorn A, Gotschlich A, Givskov M, et al. The cep quorum-sensing system of Burkholderia cepacia H111 controls biofilm formation and swarming motility. Microbiology. 2001;147:2517–28.
77. Loutet SA, Valvano MA. A decade of Burkholderia cenocepacia virulence determinant research. Infect Immun. 2010;78:4088–100.
78. Mahenthiralingam E, Urban TA, Goldberg JB. The multifarious, multireplicon Burkholderia cepacia complex. Nat Rev Microbiol. 2005;3:144–56.
79. Hancock RE. Resistance mechanisms in Pseudomonas aeruginosa and other nonfermentative gram-negative bacteria. Clin Infect Dis. 1998;27(Suppl 1):S93–9.
80. Zlosnik JE, Zhou G, Brant R, Henry DA, Hird TJ, Mahenthiralingam E, et al. Burkholderia species infections in patients with cystic fibrosis in British Columbia, Canada. 30 years' experience. Ann Am Thorac Soc. 2015;12:70–8.
81. Govan JR, Brown PH, Maddison J, Doherty CJ, Nelson JW, Dodd M, et al. Evidence for transmission of Pseudomonas cepacia by social contact in cystic fibrosis. Lancet. 1993;342:15–9.
82. LiPuma JJ, Dasen SE, Nielson DW, Stern RC, Stull TL. Person-to-person transmission of Pseudomonas cepacia between patients with cystic fibrosis. Lancet. 1990;336:1094–6.
83. Campana S, Taccetti G, Ravenni N, Favari F, Cariani L, Sciacca A, et al. Transmission of Burkholderia cepacia complex: evidence for new epidemic clones infecting cystic fibrosis patients in Italy. J Clin Microbiol. 2005;43:5136–42.
84. Corey M, Farewell V. Determinants of mortality from cystic fibrosis in Canada, 1970–1989. Am J Epidemiol. 1996;143:1007–17.
85. Courtney JM, Dunbar KE, McDowell A, Moore JE, Warke TJ, Stevenson M, et al. Clinical outcome of Burkholderia cepacia complex infection in cystic fibrosis adults. J Cyst Fibros. 2004;3:93–8.
86. Jones AM, Dodd ME, Govan JR, Barcus V, Doherty CJ, Morris J, et al. Burkholderia cenocepacia and Burkholderia multivorans: influence on survival in cystic fibrosis. Thorax. 2004;59:948–51.
87. Alexander BD, Petzold EW, Reller LB, Palmer SM, Davis RD, Woods CW, et al. Survival after lung transplantation of cystic fibrosis patients infected with Burkholderia cepacia complex. Am J Transplant. 2008;8:1025–30.
88. Isles A, Maclusky I, Corey M, Gold R, Prober C, Fleming P, et al. Pseudomonas cepacia infection in cystic fibrosis: an emerging problem. J Pediatr. 1984;104:206–10.
89. Kalish LA, Waltz DA, Dovey M, Potter-Bynoe G, McAdam AJ, Lipuma JJ, et al. Impact of Burkholderia dolosa on lung function and survival in cystic fibrosis. Am J Respir Crit Care Med. 2006;173:421–5.
90. Brooke JS. Stenotrophomonas maltophilia: an Emerging Global Opportunistic Pathogen. Clin Microbiol Rev. 2012;25:2–41.
91. Waters VJ, Gomez MI, Soong G, Amin S, Ernst RK, Prince A. Immunostimulatory properties of the emerging pathogen Stenotrophomonas maltophilia. Infect Immun. 2007;75:1698–703.

92. Di Bonaventura G, Spedicato I, D'Antonio D, Robuffo I, Piccolomini R. Biofilm formation by Stenotrophomonas maltophilia: modulation by quinolones, trimethoprim-sulfamethoxazole, and ceftazidime. Antimicrob Agents Chemother. 2004;48:151–60.

93. Pompilio A, Crocetta V, Confalone P, Nicoletti M, Petrucca A, Guarnieri S, et al. Adhesion to and biofilm formation on IB3-1 bronchial cells by Stenotrophomonas maltophilia isolates from cystic fibrosis patients. BMC Microbiol. 2010;10:102.

94. Crossman LC, Gould VC, Dow JM, Vernikos GS, Okazaki A, Sebaihia M, et al. The complete genome, comparative and functional analysis of Stenotrophomonas maltophilia reveals an organism heavily shielded by drug resistance determinants. Genome Biol. 2008;9:R74.

95. Demko CA, Stern RC, Doershuk CF. Stenotrophomonas maltophilia in cystic fibrosis: incidence and prevalence. Pediatr Pulmonol. 1998;25:304–8.

96. Ballestero S, Virseda I, Escobar H, Suarez L, Baquero F. Stenotrophomonas maltophilia in cystic fibrosis patients. Eur J Clin Microbiol Infect Dis. 1995;14:728–9.

97. Talmaciu I, Varlotta L, Mortensen J, Schidlow DV. Risk factors for emergence of Stenotrophomonas maltophilia in cystic fibrosis. Pediatr Pulmonol. 2000;30:10–5.

98. Goss CH, Mayer-Hamblett N, Aitken ML, Rubenfeld GD, Ramsey BW. Association between Stenotrophomonas maltophilia and lung function in cystic fibrosis. Thorax. 2004;59:955–9.

99. Goss CH, Otto K, Aitken ML, Rubenfeld GD. Detecting Stenotrophomonas maltophilia does not reduce survival of patients with cystic fibrosis. Am J Respir Crit Care Med. 2002;166:356–61.

100. Waters V, Atenafu EG, Lu A, Yau Y, Tullis E, Ratjen F. Chronic Stenotrophomonas maltophilia infection and mortality or lung transplantation in cystic fibrosis patients. J Cyst Fibros. 2013;12:482–6.

101. Waters V, Yau Y, Prasad S, Lu A, Atenafu E, Crandall I, et al. Stenotrophomonas maltophilia in cystic fibrosis: serologic response and effect on lung disease. Am J Respir Crit Care Med. 2011;183:635–40.

102. Hadjiliadis D, Steele MP, Chaparro C, Singer LG, Waddell TK, Hutcheon MA, et al. Survival of lung transplant patients with cystic fibrosis harboring panresistant bacteria other than Burkholderia cepacia, compared with patients harboring sensitive bacteria. J Heart Lung Transplant. 2007;26:834–8.

103. Yabuuchi E, Kawamura Y, Kosako Y, Ezaki T. Emendation of genus Achromobacter and Achromobacter xylosoxidans (Yabuuchi and Yano) and proposal of Achromobacter ruhlandii (Packer and Vishniac) comb. nov., Achromobacter piechaudii (Kiredjian et al.) comb. nov., and Achromobacter xylosoxidans subsp. denitrificans (Ruger and Tan) comb. nov. Microbiol Immunol. 1998;42:429–38.

104. Lipuma JJ. The changing microbial epidemiology in cystic fibrosis. Clin Microbiol Rev. 2010;23:299–323.

105. Ridderberg W, Nielsen SM, Norskov-Lauritsen N. Genetic adaptation of achromobacter sp during persistence in the lungs of cystic fibrosis patients. PLoS One. 2015;10:e0136790.

106. Filipic B, Malesevic M, Vasiljevic Z, Lukic J, Novovic K, Kojic M, et al. Uncovering differences in virulence markers associated with Achromobacter species of CF and non-CF origin. Front Cell Infect Microbiol. 2017;7:224.

107. Tom SK, Yau YC, Beaudoin T, LiPuma JJ, Waters V. Effect of high-dose antimicrobials on biofilm growth of Achromobacter species isolated from cystic fibrosis patients. Antimicrob Agents Chemother. 2016;60:650–2.

108. Bador J, Amoureux L, Blanc E, Neuwirth C. Innate aminoglycoside resistance of Achromobacter xylosoxidans is due to AxyXY-OprZ, an RND-type multidrug efflux pump. Antimicrob Agents Chemother. 2013;57:603–5.

109. Decre D, Arlet G, Danglot C, Lucet JC, Fournier G, Bergogne-Berezin E, et al. A beta-lactamase-overproducing strain of Alcaligenes denitrificans subsp. xylosoxydans isolated from a case of meningitis. J Antimicrob Chemother. 1992;30:769–79.

110. De Baets F, Schelstraete P, Van Daele S, Haerynck F, Vaneechoutte M. Achromobacter xylosoxidans in cystic fibrosis: prevalence and clinical relevance. J Cyst Fibros. 2007;6:75–8.

111. Pereira RH, Carvalho-Assef AP, Albano RM, Folescu TW, Jones MC, Leao RS, et al. Achromobacter xylosoxidans: characterization of strains in Brazilian cystic fibrosis patients. J Clin Microbiol. 2011;49:3649–51.
112. Van Daele S, Verhelst R, Claeys G, Verschraegen G, Franckx H, Van Simaey L, et al. Shared genotypes of Achromobacter xylosoxidans strains isolated from patients at a cystic fibrosis rehabilitation center. J Clin Microbiol. 2005;43:2998–3002.
113. Dunne WM Jr, Maisch S. Epidemiological investigation of infections due to Alcaligenes species in children and patients with cystic fibrosis: use of repetitive-element-sequence polymerase chain reaction. Clin Infect Dis. 1995;20:836–41.
114. Kanellopoulou M, Pournaras S, Iglezos H, Skarmoutsou N, Papafrangas E, Maniatis AN. Persistent colonization of nine cystic fibrosis patients with an Achromobacter (Alcaligenes) xylosoxidans clone. Eur J Clin Microbiol Infect Dis. 2004;23:336–9.
115. Ronne Hansen C, Pressler T, Hoiby N, Gormsen M. Chronic infection with Achromobacter xylosoxidans in cystic fibrosis patients; a retrospective case control study. J Cyst Fibros. 2006;5:245–51.
116. Somayaji R, Stanojevic S, Tullis DE, Stephenson AL, Ratjen F, Waters V. Clinical outcomes associated with Achromobacter species infection in patients with cystic fibrosis. Ann Am Thorac Soc. 2017;14:1412–8.
117. Tunney MM, Klem ER, Fodor AA, Gilpin DF, Moriarty TF, McGrath SJ, et al. Use of culture and molecular analysis to determine the effect of antibiotic treatment on microbial community diversity and abundance during exacerbation in patients with cystic fibrosis. Thorax. 2011;66:579–84.
118. Zemanick ET, Harris JK, Wagner BD, Robertson CE, Sagel SD, Stevens MJ, et al. Inflammation and airway microbiota during cystic fibrosis pulmonary exacerbations. PLoS One. 2013;8:e62917.
119. Versalovic J. Manual of clinical microbiology. 10th ed: American Society of Microbiology; Washington, DC: 2011.
120. Hofstad T. Virulence factors in anaerobic bacteria. Euro J Clin Microbiol Infect Dis. 1992;11:1044–8.
121. Brook I. Clinical review: bacteremia caused by anaerobic bacteria in children. Crit Care. 2002;6:205–11.
122. Tunney MM, Field TR, Moriarty TF, Patrick S, Doering G, Muhlebach MS, et al. Detection of anaerobic bacteria in high numbers in sputum from patients with cystic fibrosis. Am J Respir Crit Care Med. 2008;177:995–1001.
123. Worlitzsch D, Rintelen C, Bohm K, Wollschlager B, Merkel N, Borneff-Lipp M, et al. Antibiotic-resistant obligate anaerobes during exacerbations of cystic fibrosis patients. Clin Microbiol Infect. 2009;15:454–60.
124. Muhlebach MS, Hatch JE, Einarsson GG, McGrath SJ, Gilipin DF, Lavelle G, et al. Anaerobic bacteria cultured from cystic fibrosis airways correlate to milder disease: a multisite study. Eur Respir J. 2018;52:pii: 1800242.
125. Harris JK, De Groote MA, Sagel SD, Zemanick ET, Kapsner R, Penvari C, et al. Molecular identification of bacteria in bronchoalveolar lavage fluid from children with cystic fibrosis. Proc Natl Acad Sci U S A. 2007;104:20529–33.
126. Caverly LJ, LiPuma JJ. Good cop, bad cop: anaerobes in cystic fibrosis airways. Eur Respir J. 2018;52:pii: 1801146.
127. Mirkovic B, Murray MA, Lavelle GM, Molloy K, Azim AA, Gunaratnam C, et al. The role of short-chain fatty acids, produced by anaerobic bacteria, in the cystic fibrosis airway. Am J Respir Crit Care Med. 2015;192:1314–24.
128. Ghorbani P, Santhakumar P, Hu Q, Djiadeu P, Wolever TM, Palaniyar N, et al. Short-chain fatty acids affect cystic fibrosis airway inflammation and bacterial growth. Eur Respir J. 2015;46:1033–45.
129. Phan J, Gallagher T, Oliver A, England WE, Whiteson K. Fermentation products in the cystic fibrosis airways induce aggregation and dormancy-associated expression profiles in a CF clinical isolate of Pseudomonas aeruginosa. FEMS Microbiol Lett. 2018;365:10

130. Sherrard LJ, McGrath SJ, McIlreavey L, Hatch J, Wolfgang MC, Muhlebach MS, et al. Production of extended-spectrum beta-lactamases and the potential indirect pathogenic role of Prevotella isolates from the cystic fibrosis respiratory microbiota. Int J Antimicrob Agents. 2016;47:140–5.

131. Zemanick ET, Wagner BD, Robertson CE, Ahrens RC, Chmiel JF, Clancy JP, et al. Airway microbiota across age and disease spectrum in cystic fibrosis. Eur Respir J. 2017;50:pii: 1700832.

132. Zemanick ET, Wagner BD, Robertson CE, Stevens MJ, Szefler SJ, Accurso FJ, et al. Assessment of airway microbiota and inflammation in cystic fibrosis using multiple sampling methods. Ann Am Thorac Soc. 2015;12:221–9.

133. O'Neill K, Bradley JM, Johnston E, McGrath S, McIlreavey L, Rowan S, et al. Reduced bacterial colony count of anaerobic bacteria is associated with a worsening in lung clearance index and inflammation in cystic fibrosis. PLoS One. 2015;10:e0126980.

134. Filkins LM, Hampton TH, Gifford AH, Gross MJ, Hogan DA, Sogin ML, et al. Prevalence of streptococci and increased polymicrobial diversity associated with cystic fibrosis patient stability. J Bacteriol. 2012;194:4709–17.

135. van Ewijk BE, van der Zalm MM, Wolfs TF, van der Ent CK. Viral respiratory infections in cystic fibrosis. J Cyst Fibros. 2005;4(Suppl 2):31–6.

136. Wang EE, Prober CG, Manson B, Corey M, Levison H. Association of respiratory viral infections with pulmonary deterioration in patients with cystic fibrosis. N Engl J Med. 1984;311:1653–8.

137. Scagnolari C, Turriziani O, Monteleone K, Pierangeli A, Antonelli G. Consolidation of molecular testing in clinical virology. Expert Rev Anti-Infect Ther. 2017;15:387–400.

138. Asner S, Waters V, Solomon M, Yau Y, Richardson SE, Grasemann H, et al. Role of respiratory viruses in pulmonary exacerbations in children with cystic fibrosis. J Cyst Fibros. 2012;11:433–9.

139. van Ewijk BE, van der Zalm MM, Wolfs TF, Fleer A, Kimpen JL, Wilbrink B, et al. Prevalence and impact of respiratory viral infections in young children with cystic fibrosis: prospective cohort study. Pediatrics. 2008;122:1171–6.

140. Collinson J, Nicholson KG, Cancio E, Ashman J, Ireland DC, Hammersley V, et al. Effects of upper respiratory tract infections in patients with cystic fibrosis. Thorax. 1996;51:1115–22.

141. Smyth AR, Smyth RL, Tong CY, Hart CA, Heaf DP. Effect of respiratory virus infections including rhinovirus on clinical status in cystic fibrosis. Arch Dis Child. 1995;73:117–20.

142. Wat D, Gelder C, Hibbitts S, Cafferty F, Bowler I, Pierrepoint M, et al. The role of respiratory viruses in cystic fibrosis. J Cyst Fibros. 2008;7:320–8.

143. Scheithauer S, Haase G, Hausler M, Lemmen S, Ritter K, Kleines M. Association between respiratory and herpes viruses on pulmonary exacerbations in cystic fibrosis patients. J Cyst Fibros. 2010;9:234–6.

144. Goffard A, Lambert V, Salleron J, Herwegh S, Engelmann I, Pinel C, et al. Virus and cystic fibrosis: rhinoviruses are associated with exacerbations in adult patients. J Clin Virol. 2014;60:147–53.

145. Hiatt PW, Grace SC, Kozinetz CA, Raboudi SH, Treece DG, Taber LH, et al. Effects of viral lower respiratory tract infection on lung function in infants with cystic fibrosis. Pediatrics. 1999;103:619–26.

146. Ramsey BW, Gore EJ, Smith AL, Cooney MK, Redding GJ, Foy H. The effect of respiratory viral infections on patients with cystic fibrosis. Am J Dis Child. 1989;143:662–8.

147. Flight WG, Bright-Thomas RJ, Tilston P, Mutton KJ, Guiver M, Morris J, et al. Incidence and clinical impact of respiratory viruses in adults with cystic fibrosis. Thorax. 2014;69:247–53.

148. Esther CR Jr, Lin FC, Kerr A, Miller MB, Gilligan PH. Respiratory viruses are associated with common respiratory pathogens in cystic fibrosis. Pediatr Pulmonol. 2014;49:926–31.

149. Etherington C, Naseer R, Conway SP, Whitaker P, Denton M, Peckham DG. The role of respiratory viruses in adult patients with cystic fibrosis receiving intravenous antibiotics for a pulmonary exacerbation. J Cyst Fibros. 2014;13:49–55.
150. Abman SH, Ogle JW, Butler-Simon N, Rumack CM, Accurso FJ. Role of respiratory syncytial virus in early hospitalizations for respiratory distress of young infants with cystic fibrosis. J Pediatr. 1988;113:826–30.
151. de Almeida MB, Zerbinati RM, Tateno AF, Oliveira CM, Romao RM, Rodrigues JC, et al. Rhinovirus C and respiratory exacerbations in children with cystic fibrosis. Emerg Infect Dis. 2010;16:996–9.
152. Ortiz JR, Neuzil KM, Victor JC, Wald A, Aitken ML, Goss CH. Influenza-associated cystic fibrosis pulmonary exacerbations. Chest. 2010;137:852–60.
153. Johansen HK, Hoiby N. Seasonal onset of initial colonisation and chronic infection with Pseudomonas aeruginosa in patients with cystic fibrosis in Denmark. Thorax. 1992;47:109–11.
154. Van Ewijk BE, Wolfs TF, Aerts PC, Van Kessel KP, Fleer A, Kimpen JL, et al. RSV mediates Pseudomonas aeruginosa binding to cystic fibrosis and normal epithelial cells. Pediatr Res. 2007;61:398–403.
155. Hendricks MR, Lashua LP, Fischer DK, Flitter BA, Eichinger KM, Durbin JE, et al. Respiratory syncytial virus infection enhances Pseudomonas aeruginosa biofilm growth through dysregulation of nutritional immunity. Proc Natl Acad Sci U S A. 2016;113:1642–7.

Chapter 6
Fungal Infections and ABPA

Micheál Mac Aogáin, Céline Vidaillac, and Sanjay H. Chotirmall

Patient Perspective

When I was first diagnosed with Scedosporium apiospermum, I did not know what it was or how it would affect my health. Learning that it was a fungal infection, my first reaction was relief. I was relieved because I had been sick for months with increased sputum production, shortness of breath and exhaustion with little to no improvement. It gave me an answer as to why numerous courses of intravenous antibiotics had not worked. I did not realise how complicated or how difficult it could be to treat. Looking back now, I can see that my relief of this diagnosis was a little naïve. My second reaction to this diagnosis was, 'How did I get this?' It was explained to me that soil/dirt was the most likely place I would contract this. If you knew me, you would know that I am probably the least likely person to spend time outside, and I have never even had a house plant. The most likely scenario for someone to get this fungal infection is the least likely place you would find me. No matter how I got it, Scedosporium has been complicated to treat and has affected my life and health.

Additional treatment has included regularly seeing an infectious disease doctor and taking various antifungal medications. The antifungal medication can have drug interactions and affect my liver enzymes, and I must be checked regularly for therapeutic levels. Doctor appointments and blood work are already a part of my life with cystic fibrosis, so these things didn't seem like an extra burden. When I would have a CF exacerbation, the question would be and still is what to treat. Do we treat the bacteria or the fungus? I am usually treated with intravenous antibiotics, and if there is no relief, we switch my long-term antifungal treatment.

There have been a few instances where the Scedosporium apiospermum has had a larger effect on my life. In 2016, after several CF exacerbations in several months

M. Mac Aogáin · C. Vidaillac · S. H. Chotirmall (✉)
Translational Respiratory Research Laboratory, Lee Kong Chian School of Medicine,
Nanyang Technological University, Singapore, Singapore
e-mail: schotirmall@ntu.edu.sg

© Springer Nature Switzerland AG 2020
S. D. Davis et al. (eds.), *Cystic Fibrosis*, Respiratory Medicine,
https://doi.org/10.1007/978-3-030-42382-7_6

and not responding to antibiotics, we switched my antifungal medication from vori-conazole to posaconazole and added micafungin. I was extremely fatigued, and my lung function was declining. Eventually, I was evaluated for a lung transplant. It was a week of tests and appointments that were emotionally and physically exhaust-ing. Part of the evaluation included seeing my infectious disease doctor. I have cultured Scedosporium apiospermum in both my sinuses and my lungs. The risk of this fungus was explained in relation to the transplant and is possibly one of the biggest hurdles of my future transplant. My new lungs are in jeopardy of being infected with this fungus, and other complications and risks were also discussed. I feel like this really changed my perspective on this fungus. It really was more dan-gerous than I had led myself to believe.

As someone with cystic fibrosis, being able to participate in clinical trials has always been important to me. Culturing Scedosporium has impacted my ability to participate in various trials. I had learned of a phase 3 clinical trial of CFTR modu-lators that treat the underlying defect of CF would be conducted at my CF centre. I later learned that I was disqualified from participating due to the fungus that is growing in my lungs and the potential drug interaction with posaconazole.

Something extremely frustrating about having a fungus infection and CF is not fully being able to distinguish whether I am sick from the fungus or another infec-tion. The one thing that I personally have noticed since culturing fungus in my lungs is increased fatigue. Is this fungus the reason why my lungs and health declined so much? Or is this 'normal' CF decline? These are among many questions that I don't have the answers to.

When it comes to this fungus in my lungs, it is nice to know that my doctors are willing to reach out to other physicians to see what has worked for their patients when we feel we have exhausted our options. My antifungal treatment plan has changed several times over the years thanks to physician collaborations.

As I am sitting here doing my inhaled antibiotics and airway clearance vest treatment, I am hoping that better treatment and solutions are in my future. Thank you for taking the time to read about this to learn more about the patient experience.

–Bethany Hawes

Introduction

Chronic lung infection is a key component of cystic fibrosis (CF) pathogenesis, a multi-systemic genetic disorder characterised by mucus hypersecretion and persis-tent airway inflammation [1, 2]. Geographic variation exists in diseases underpinned by genetic and ethnic differences [3, 4]. Reported at lower frequencies in Asian and African settings, CF is most common in Caucasian populations, especially that in Northern Europe (Fig. 6.1) [5, 6]. Recent retrospective analyses suggest that key CF diagnostic pillars, *CFTR* mutations, clinical phenotype and sweat chloride concen-trations, are greatly influenced by Asian genetics and lifestyle differences, support-ing an 'under-diagnosed and more subtle' disease in Asian populations [7]. Gender

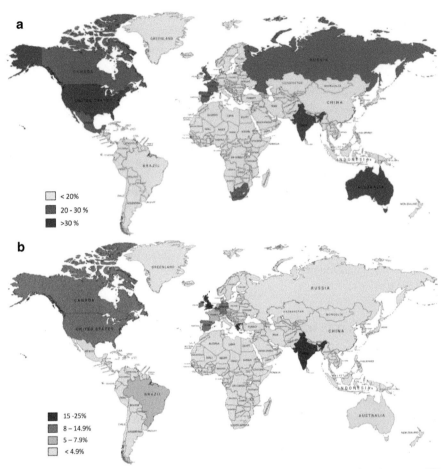

Fig. 6.1 Reported statistics of (**a**) *Aspergillus* sensitisation and (**b**) ABPA based on the current CF literature [13, 14, 16, 239–245]. Country prevalence values are colour coded with regions for which no or limited data is available, indicated by grey colour

and age disparities are also reported in disease prevalence and severity, highlighting some of the key issues faced in the diagnosis and management of CF [8–10]. Critically, the microbial component of disease is dominated by bacterial pathogens, particularly *Pseudomonas aeruginosa* and *Staphylococcus aureus*, both commonly found in stable states and during exacerbations [2, 11]. While the long-standing focus on bacteria remains highly relevant, fungal genera such as *Aspergillus* and *Candida* are now recognised as emerging pathogens playing significant roles in CF pathogenesis, clinical disease trajectory and prognosis [12, 13]. Colonisation with *Aspergillus* species is common and may lead to a range of clinical consequences, largely dependent on the underlying state of host immunity, including allergic bronchopulmonary aspergillosis (ABPA), *Aspergillus* sensitisation and *Aspergillus* bronchitis (immune overactivity), chronic aspergillosis (mild immunodeficiency) and severe invasive pulmonary or haematogenous aspergillosis (severe immunode-ficiency) [14, 15]. The incidence of fungal colonisation and infection varies (Fig. 6.1, Table 6.1), and such variability should be carefully examined as species may har-bour differing antifungal susceptibility profiles that are region-dependent. Importantly, geographic diversity further influences the effect of fungi on lung homeostasis in diverse ways involving a complex and balanced interplay between the host, the environment and their microbiomes. Prevalence of *Aspergillus*-associated sensitisation in CF ranges widely from 20% to 65% globally, with key differences observed between adult and paediatric populations [14, 16]. In contrast, the occurrence of CF-ABPA fluctuates from 3% to 25% and is significantly higher in CF adults when compared to children [14, 16].

In this chapter, we provide an overview of fungal diseases in CF, focusing on the spectrum of species emerging as CF pathogens and evaluating their roles in disease pathogenesis. We detail the CF pulmonary mycobiome and its specific features, including the complex networks that influence lung homeostasis during the stable and exacerbation states. We conclude with the possible treatment options currently used for the management of fungal infection in CF.

Fungal Infections in Cystic Fibrosis

The Aspergilli

Aspergilli represent a ubiquitous genus of saprophytic moulds belonging to the *Ascomycota*, whose airborne conidia are frequently inhaled by mammals [17, 18]. Within this genus, *Aspergillus fumigatus* is a key exemplar and the most significant fungal species implicated in CF-associated disease. Existing across a spectrum of morphological states, including conidia, swollen conidia and hyphal forms, it is encountered by healthy individuals on a daily basis, where it causes little harm due to its control and elimination by working host immune defence mechanisms. Its conidial form, one that reaches the pulmonary alveoli owing to their small size (2–5 um), is removed by innate immune pathways, including mucociliary clearance and macrophage engulfment. Individuals may be exposed to tens of thousands of fungal spores each day during fungal-rich seasons, of which a significant proportion repre-sent spores from Aspergilli [18, 19]. While host defence mechanisms provide pro-tection from invading fungi, dysregulated immunity in the CF lung may explain the observed increased rates of chronic colonisation and allergic complications, which in turn are linked to adverse clinical outcomes in CF, including reduced lung func-tion and increased hospitalisations [20, 21]. If ineffectively cleared from the lung, fungal conidia may germinate forming hyphae, which in turn trigger a cascade of immune responses that drive a wide spectrum of clinical manifestations from colo-nisation and allergic sensitisation to allergic bronchopulmonary aspergillosis (ABPA). Even chronic pulmonary aspergillosis (CPA) and fulminant invasive

Table 6.1 Fungal pathogens in cystic fibrosis: a summary of major clinically relevant species, reported prevalence, clinical roles and risk factors

Genus	Clinically relevant species	Geographic distribution	Reported prevalence	Clinical role	Risk factors in CF	References
Aspergillus	A. fumigatus A. terreus A. niger A. flavus	A. fumigatus is predominant Higher prevalence in Northern Europe	35–40%	1. Coloniser 2. Sensitisation (AS) 3. Allergic response (ABPA) 4. Marker of disease severity 5. Potential role in exacerbations	1. Frequent use of broad-spectrum antibiotics and oral steroids 2. Low BMI 3. Atopy 4. Older age 5. Decreased lung function	[43, 55, 111, 151, 216–220]
Candida	C. albicans C. glabrata C. parapsilosis C. tropicalis C. dubliniensis C. krusei	C. albicans – globally predominant species C. glabrata – second most predominant species in Northern Europe and the USA C. parapsilosis – second most predominant species in Spain and Brazil	Up to 75%	1. Coloniser 2. Localised (thrush) 3. Systemic infection 4. ABPM	1. Low FEV_1 2. Impaired salivary secretion 3. Frequent use of broad-spectrum antibiotics and oral steroids 4. History of diabetes 5. Surgery 6. Medical devices 7. Cancers 8. Organ transplants	[91, 221]
Scedosporium	S. apiospermum S. boydii S. dehoogii S. minutisporum S. prolificans	S. apiospermum is predominant Higher prevalence in Southern Europe	5–10%	1. Coloniser 2. Localised 3. Systemic infections (rare but with high mortality)	1. Pseudomonas 2. Frequent use of β-lactam and steroids 3. Lymphopenia 4. Neutropenia 5. CMV reactivation 6. Low serum albumin level (<3 mg/dl)	[151, 222, 223]

(continued)

Table 6.1 (continued)

Genus	Clinically relevant species	Geographic distribution	Reported prevalence	Clinical role	Risk factors in CF	References
Exophiala	E. dermatitis E. phaeomuriformis E. jeanselmei	Tropical regions	Up to 30%	1. Coloniser 2. Localised	1. Age > 12 2. Colonisation with A. fumigatus 3. Pancreatic failure 4. Advanced disease	[118, 120, 121, 224, 225]
Rasamsonia	R. argillacea R. eburnea R. piperina R. aegroticola	Europe, USA, rare cases in Asia	Emerging	Marker of disease severity	1. Immunodeficiency 2. Organ transplant	[122, 124, 226]
Malassezia	M. restricta M. globosa M. sympodialis		Commensal (skin)		1. Eczema 2. Skin disorders 3. Medical devices	[128, 165]

disease, although rare, have been reported in CF [19, 22]. While several *Aspergillus* species complexes are described in the CF lung, each with their own distinct physiology and associated immune response, *A. fumigatus* remains the predominant species among this genera for reasons yet to be fully understood [23, 24].

Aspergillus *Colonisation*

While precise mechanisms to explain the preferential colonisation and persistence of *A. fumigatus* in the CF lung remain to be determined, some insights may be provided by an analysis of fungal defence mechanisms from a non-CF setting, particularly those known to be dysregulated in the CF patient. These mechanisms include a functional mucociliary system and abundant alveolar macrophages, both of which represent central components of defence against fungi. A key response element of the fungal-host immune interaction is the sentinel pattern recognition receptors (PRR), which recognise fungal pathogen-associated molecular patterns (PAMPs) expressed by fungi that enter the airway. The best described remain the Toll-like receptors (TLRs) and C-type lectin receptors (CLRs), while others include the DC-specific ICAM3-grabbing non-integrin (DC-SIGN), the macrophage-inducible Ca^{2+}-dependent lectin receptor (MINCLE), the mannose receptor, the galectin family of proteins and the receptor for advanced glycation end products (RAGE) [18, 25–27]. Specific TLRs and CLRs activate intracellular pathways upon binding specific fungal PAMPs such as cell wall components, including β-glucans, chitins and mannans (e.g. galactomannan) as well as fungal DNA, present in increasing abundance as conidia convert to hyphae during a prolonged colonisation process (Fig. 6.2a). Bronchial epithelial cells may also phagocytose conidia, although their fungal killing abilities are not as pronounced as those observed in macrophages or neutrophils. Importantly, however, fungi can survive and germinate even within acidic endosomes [28]. Interaction between fungi and host epithelial cells may trigger recognition by membrane-bound TLR and CLR receptors, leading to enhanced T_h1 and T_{reg} responses, which in turn govern defence against and tolerance towards fungi, respectively, while orchestrating an appropriate and holistic host response to fungi at the epithelial interface [29]. This intricate host-fungi dialogue is perturbed at several levels in CF where many of proposed defence mechanisms and tolerance systems are compromised, leading to dysregulated responses that become immunopathogenic when the CF airway is challenged by fungi [30–32]. In the CF lung, the airway surface liquid (ASL), airway epithelium and associated secretions are all notably altered while mucociliary clearance is greatly impaired due to inadequate hydration of the ASL, a further compromise of this key anatomical barrier to fungal colonisation [33]. A general decoupling of protease-antiprotease regulatory systems observed in CF exacerbates the situation, leading unchecked inflammatory cascades to cause disproportionate tissue damage in response to pathogens [34]. Critically, innate immune defences against *A. fumigatus*, such as the expression of the soluble PRR Pentraxin-3 (PTX-3) and the expression of TLR-4 on epithelia, are reduced in

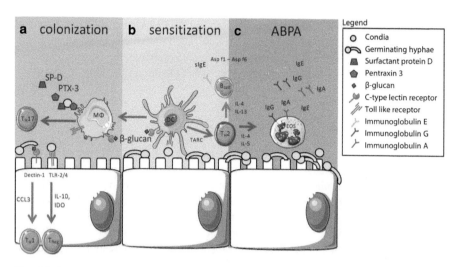

Fig. 6.2 The immunological spectrum of colonisation-sensitisation-ABPA in cystic fibrosis. (**a**) *Aspergillus* colonisation: alveolar macrophages (Mφ) are key components of innate fungal immunity and, together with mucociliary clearance, represent major barriers to fungal infection. Macrophages engulf fungi in a process mediated by soluble recognition factors, including surfactant protein D (SP-D) and pentraxin 3 (PTX-3), that bind to fungal conidia. Cell wall components from actively growing hyphae and germinating spores produce PAMPS such as β-glucans that serve as ligands for membrane-bound PRRs, including Dectin-1. Receptors TLR-2 and Dectin-1 on the macrophage surface cause the production of T_h17-stimulating cytokines that attract neutrophils and other phagocytic cells, while on the epithelial cell surface, these receptors elicit T_h1-driven inflammation and induction of T_{reg} cells that balance fungal tolerance. (**b**) *Aspergillus* sensitisation: if defence systems are compromised, the abundance of *Aspergillus* conidia and hyphae can accumulate, and their recognition by dendritic cells (DC) can orchestrate T_h2-mediated production of specific IgE towards a range of antigens, most notably rAsp f1–f6, which show the strongest association with allergic disease states in CF. (**c**) CF-ABPA: TARC production by dendritic cells causes recruitment of alveolar macrophages, T_h2-driven B-cell (BC) maturation and eosinophil (EOS) recruitment, involving IL-4, IL-5 and IL-13, culminating in an immunological milieu of IgE, IgG and IgA antibodies specific to *A. fumigatus* against a backdrop of increased total IgE production, heightened inflammation and increased fungal burden. Fungal presence can be seen in association with a continuum of clinical manifestations from low fungal burden and tempered immunoregulatory responses in colonised patients to higher fungal burden with Th2-driven hypersensitivity seen in ABPA

CF patients, allowing this inciting fungus to gain the initial foothold [35]. *Aspergillus fumigatus* adopts several immune evasion strategies in the airway, including the production of a hydrophobic rodlet layer and the pigment DHN-melanin, which, respectively, mask the presence of fungal PAMPs and protect the fungus from reactive oxygen species (ROS) by scavenging phagocytic cells [36]. The uptake and destruction of *A. fumigatus* within acidic phagosomes through NADPH oxidase is a primary mechanism of central importance to host fungal defence, and evasion of this permits its airway persistence, colonisation and infection [25]. *Aspergillus fumigatus* produces immunomodulatory toxins, an additional arm of its immunoevasive capabilities. These include (1) gliotoxin, which further disrupts macrophage-related phagocytosis; (2) fumagillin, which inhibits neutrophil function; and (3) galactosaminoglycans (GAGs), a group of compounds that resist neutrophil extracellular traps (NETs) [37–39]. The production of these and other toxic fungal metabolites further impacts airway microbial clearance mechanisms, including ciliary function and antigen presentation, creating an environmental milieu suited to infection [25, 36]. Furthermore, when the fungi's immunoevasive repertoire is coupled to the immunological dysfunction characteristic of CF, including mucosal immunodeficiency and phagocytic dysregulation, it is unsurprising to increasingly observe *Aspergillus* colonisation, persistence and infection become a key clinical issue and research subject in CF over the last years [40, 41]. For instance, *Aspergillus* colonisation is characterised by a gliotoxin-mediated repression of the airway vitamin D receptor (VDR), which is associated to a systemic T_h2 response (IL-5 and IL-13); findings driven by immune evasion, however, are clinically reversible with antifungal (itraconazole) therapy [42]. Collectively, these factors likely explain the high observed rates of fungal, and notably *Aspergillus*, colonisation (6–56%) reported in CF [16, 20, 27]. While fungal colonisation with *Aspergillus* tends to be associated with more severe lung disease, longitudinal analysis has failed to detect any association between colonisation and lung function decline, and the true clinical role of *Aspergillus* colonisation in CF remains controversial [20]. The presence, however, of *Aspergillus* in the CF lung is linked to worse lung disease, including increased exacerbation rates [43, 44]. The treatment of colonised CF patients with itraconazole in a small prospective observational study did reveal radiological and clinical improvement, and well-designed randomised placebo-controlled clinical trials are warranted and ongoing [42, 45]. Early work performed in this space has thus far failed to detect a significant clinical effect of antifungal therapy on clinical outcomes in CF patients chronically colonised by *A. fumigatus*. The only randomised controlled clinical trial performed to date using itraconazole has suffered significant weaknesses, particularly with suboptimal treatment drug levels recorded in approximately half of the enrolled patients [46]. As such, the true role of *A. fumigatus* colonisation in CF pathogenesis remains uncertain, particularly whether colonised patients should be targeted for therapy [47]. Importantly, emerging work focused on early paediatric populations with CF has suggested a non-benign role for *Aspergillus* in the development of structural lung disease including bronchiectasis, outlining its pathogenic potential. Further work is necessary to expound these early observations [48, 49].

Aspergillus *Sensitisation*

An elevated atopic response to an *A. fumigatus*-specific antigen, as confirmed by a skin prick test or elevated serum specific IgE titres, signals Aspergillus sensitisation (AS) [50]. This outcome reflects a Th2-driven response to a fungal antigen that manifests in an increased adaptive response and higher rates of AS observed in CF patients, reflecting the Th1/Th2 imbalance that characterises diseases [51]. A pooled meta-analysis of *Aspergillus* sensitisation in CF reported a high rate of 39.1% compared to 8.9% for confirmed ABPA. Rates were significantly higher in adults compared to children, suggesting that long-term colonisation may represent a harbinger of AS and eventual CF-ABPA in later life across a spectral continuum of *Aspergillus*-associated clinical disease (Fig. 6.2) [16]. Sensitisation manifests along an immunological pathway, whereby antigen presentation by dendritic cells can drive Th2-driven maturation of IgE-producing B cells that recognise specific *Aspergillus* antigens via a process involving thymus- and activation-regulated chemokine (CCL17/TARC), IL-4 and IL-13 (Fig. 6.2b) [52]. Proteases secreted by *A. fumigatus* (some of which are themselves allergenic) are key drivers of the adaptive immune response through desquamation of epithelial cells, causing pro-inflammatory cytokine production and an increased exposure to fungal antigens [53]. Twenty-three allergens of *A. fumigatus* are currently recognised, and specific IgE responses to allergens rAsp f1–rAsp f6 are most widely reported in CF, which exhibit the strongest diagnostic association with CF-ABPA [54]. In contrast to *Aspergillus* colonisation, AS exhibits a much clearer association with clinical manifestations in CF as evidenced by strong correlation to lung function decline [55, 56]. In contrast to CF-ABPA, AS does not exhibit specific anti-*A. fumigatus* IgG production or positive sputum galactomannan and may have variable *Aspergillus* colonisation status, as documented by PCR [55]. This heightened allergic response to allergen reflects the Th2 skew observed in CF patients driven by, among other factors, the direct effect of CFTR mutation on T-cell function and associated expression of *A. fumigatus*-specific IgE, as demonstrated in animal models of diseases [31]. The complex clinical picture and overlapping interrelated immunological status observed with *Aspergillus*-associated disease in CF- and non-CF-related bronchiectasis have prompted novel immunologic classifications to emerge in the literature [55, 57, 58]. Such classification for CF is based on *Aspergillus* PCR status, sputum galactomannan, and specific IgE and anti-*Aspergillus* IgG response classifying patients into non-diseased, colonised, sensitised, with bronchitis and with ABPA.

ABPA

CF-ABPA is associated with significant clinical symptoms and lung function decline and remains a challenging clinical diagnosis to make in practice, owing to its comparability with symptoms of an infective exacerbation. Although several fungal species may lead to allergic bronchopulmonary mycosis (ABPM), the genus *Aspergillus* possesses a high proportion of the predominant organisms causing this pulmonary disorder. While the genus *Aspergillus* has several members, including *A. terreus*, *A. niger* and *A. flavus*, the overwhelming majority of aspergilli cultured from the CF lung is *A. fumigatus* [24]. The diagnosis of CF-ABPA is complicated by overlapping clinical, microbiological, immunological and radiological symptoms to those encountered in exacerbations, including cough, recurrent infection, bronchospasm and the presence of radiological infiltrates against a higher background rate of *Aspergillus* colonisation and sensitisation. This sometimes leads to long delays in reaching a diagnosis, permitting the condition to go untreated for prolonged periods, which in turn causes structural damage and affects lung function, quality of life and disease prognosis [13]. Heightened total and specific IgE antibody counts, combined with elevated specific humoral IgG and eosinophilia, are typical but not always found in CF-ABPA; however they represent central tenants of the established published diagnostic criteria [52, 59]. Several patients who clearly have CF-ABPA that respond well to empirical steroid treatment do not actually meet diagnostic criteria, suggesting that the current CF-ABPA criteria require refinement and inclusion of more objective immunological measures to complement their currently strong emphasis on clinical symptomatology [52, 60]. CF-ABPA patients demonstrate higher fungal burdens suggestive of a sustained failure of typical fungal defence mechanisms, whereby fungal hyphae can be found growing on and between epithelial cells highlighting ineffective immune clearance (Fig. 6.2c) [52, 61]. Higher fungal burden, combined with a Th2 bias, drive IL-4 and IL-13 secretion eliciting differentiation of B cells, IL-5-associated eosinophil recruitment, promotion of local and humoral increases in IgG and IgE production, and immunological and diagnostic hallmarks of CF-ABPA. Basophils are also actively involved in the allergenic process exhibiting hyperresponsiveness to *Aspergillus* antigens in CF where the presence of basophil activation markers, such as CD203c, has been strongly associated with CF-ABPA with potential diagnostic application [62–64].

Given the significant immunological sequelae of CF-ABPA, long-term tapering of oral glucocorticoid treatment has been accepted as a mainstay of CF-ABPA therapy for years. However, the evidence base even for this established choice of therapy is limited, and only recently have controlled trials on dosing regimens suggested that mid-level dosing is comparable to high dosing, mitigating the toxic effects of long-term steroid therapy. Importantly, shorter 'pulsed' doses of steroids, such as methylprednisolone, have shown efficacy and clinical benefit over the long term and are now good alternative treatment choices for CF-ABPA [65, 66]. For individuals who respond poorly to steroid therapy or in whom toxicity is observed, adjunctive antifungal use is an option; this reduces fungal burden and, hence, the deleterious immune response that accompanies CF-ABPA associated with the recognition of PAMPs; however, controlled trials in this area remain scarce [67]. Voriconazole and posaconazole have been employed in the setting of asthma-associated ABPA, while amphotericin B has been used for CF-ABPA and is currently undergoing clinical trials in inhaled formulation for CF-ABPA (NCT02273661). As with any antimicrobial treatment strategy, the emergence of resistance is a concern, and in the case of amphotericin B, the intrinsic resistance of *A. terreus* should also be considered [68]. Immunotherapeutic strategies for CF-ABPA include the use of a humanised anti-IgE monoclonal antibody (omalizumab), which has shown efficacy in treating allergic asthma; however, its usefulness in the setting of CF-ABPA remains to be proven through large controlled studies despite benefits reported through case reports and case series [66, 69–71]. An important emerging concern for CF patients who require antifungal treatment is the drug interaction with CFTR modulators and/or correctors, whose emergence has revolutionised the CF landscape for most but brings added complications for patients suitable for such therapy but with a dependence on antifungals due to severe fungal-associated diseases [72, 73]. The convergence of CFTR potentiators and azole antifungals on the cytochrome P-450 (CYP450) pathway leads to drug interaction when given in combination, with critical implications for fungal therapeutics in CF [73]. Interaction with azoles allows a reduced dosing of ivacaftor with potential cost-saving benefits; however, the 'true' efficacy of lower dose regimens is uncertain and not accompanied by a strong evidence base, presenting a real clinical challenge [74]. The use of ivacaftor reduces fungal burden, further underpinning the importance of CFTR function in immune protection from fungi [75]. Given the predicted increase in the use of first- and second-generation CFTR potentiators, modulators and activators going forwards, this situation requires careful monitoring [76]. Such reconstitution of the immune system may also prompt 'new' implications for CF patients already colonised or infected with A. fumigatus, given that the spectrum of aspergillosis is primarily influenced by host immune function and homeostasis [19].

Chronic and Invasive Aspergillosis

Though considered less common in CF, other Aspergillus-associated conditions should be recognised, particularly in the setting of epidemiological shifts and the evolving CF therapeutic landscape. Classical Aspergillus-associated complications, such as aspergillomas and invasive diseases, are less commonly observed in CF but have been reported with important clinical consequences [77, 78]. Chronic pulmonary aspergillosis (CPA) can manifest as a simple aspergilloma, a chronic cavitary pulmonary aspergillosis (CCPA), a chronic fibrosing pulmonary aspergillosis (CFPA), an Aspergillus nodule, or a sub-acute invasive aspergillosis (SAIA) (Table 6.2) [19, 79]. Simple aspergillomas present as single fungal balls within a pre-existing thoracic cavity. In contrast, CCPA is characterised by multiple cavities containing one or more aspergillomas, while CFPA represents a fibrotic progression of an untreated CCPA with fibrotic destruction of, at least, two lobes [19, 79, 80]. A newer entity has been described recently, and Aspergillus nodules represent an unusual variant of CPA, while SAIA occurs over a shorter time frame with evidence of hyphal invasion into surrounding tissues (Table 6.2). Although CPA is uncommon in CF, improved therapy and longer life expectancies for the disease mean that likely their occurrence rates will increase, particularly at end-stage disease. While invasive pulmonary aspergillosis (IPA) can occur most commonly as a clinical complication of lung transplantation due to immunosuppressive therapy, interestingly, pre-transplant colonisation carries a fourfold higher risk of subsequent invasive disease and should be noted. Overall, however, the occurrence of IPA in CF remains rare despite high rates of Aspergillus-associated airway colonisation [19, 78, 81, 82].

Table 6.2 A summary of the various forms of chronic pulmonary aspergillosis (CPA) based on ESCMID/ERS clinical guidelines [79]

Condition	Description	Timescale
Simple aspergilloma	Single cavitary aspergilloma with diagnostic evidence supporting the presence of *Aspergillus* spp.	>3 months
Chronic cavitary pulmonary aspergillosis (CCPA)	Multiple complicating pulmonary cavities with one or more aspergillomas	
Chronic fibrosing pulmonary aspergillosis (CFPA)	Progression of CCPA with severe fibrotic destruction of at least two lobes	
Aspergillus nodule	One or more non-cavitary nodules	
Sub-acute invasive aspergilloma (SAIA)	Variable radiological features (cavitation, nodules, progressive consolidation) with evidence for hyphal invasion of lung tissue	<3 months

Non-*Aspergillus* Fungi

Candida *spp.*

Candida spp. are ascomycetous moulds found in the oral, lung, genital and intestinal mucosa [83–86]. Reported to colonise the lungs asymptomatically in approximately 50% of the global (healthy) population, *Candida* spp. are present in up to 75% of airways in CF. The genus comprises over 150 species, including some of clinical relevance, which can exist in different morphological forms with variable consequences for human health [84, 87]. *Candida albicans* is the predominant species reported to cause infections in the healthy and CF populations [88–91]. *C. glabrata, C. parapsilosis, C. tropicalis, C. dubliniensis and C. krusei* occasionally cause chronic respiratory infection and have been reported to cause other acute infections in CF [86, 92–94]. Geographic differences in the prevalence of these species are reported. *C. glabrata* dominates in Northern Europe and the USA, whereas *C. parapsilosis* is centred in Brazil and Spain. This bears clinical importance as these species harbour various antifungal susceptibility profiles with implications for therapeutic choice based on region [91].

Candida spp. exist as ovoid yeast cells, in pseudohyphal and hyphal forms exhibiting variable pathogenicity. In *C. albicans*, ovoid yeast cells are predominantly found during commensalism. In contrast, the hyphae cell morphology and the expression of associated genes are required for virulent processes such colonisation, dissemination, tissue adhesion and biofilm formation [95, 96]. Hyphae can breach and damage endothelial cells and induce macrophages and lysis of neutrophils [97]. Morphological transformation of *Candida* spp. is triggered by environmental conditions of high relevance in the CF airway, including limited nutrient availability, changes in temperature and pH, changes in the levels of oxygen and CO_2 and altered cell surface hydrophobicity [87, 98, 99]. In CF, all such conditions are exacerbated, creating an ecological breach in the balance to the benefit of *Candida*. Therefore, the secretion of virulence factors directly modulates inter-species communication in the CF lung, which in turn disrupts ecological homeostasis of pulmonary microbiota, promoting their role in driving diseases [98]. *Pseudomonas aeruginosa*, for example, a major CF pathogen, is capable of establishing biofilms with *Candida* spp. in its hyphal form but not with its yeast cells [100]. The role of *Candida* in CF remains unclear with descriptions ranging from bystander to pathogen [89, 101]. While skin- and genital-related infection by the organism is commonly observed in clinical practice, the previously thought low virulence of *Candida* spp. is now being questioned, with some suggesting that it may have a role in CF morbidity and mortality. Mammalian chitinases target chitin, a major component of the fungal cell wall that has been implicated in the CF response to *Candida*. Higher systemic chitinase activity associates with *C. albicans* colonisation in the CF airway, raising the possibility of its role as a *Candida* biomarker. Importantly, key questions remain on the mechanisms driving this observed systemic response to an airway-associated fungi in CF in the absence of detectable candidaemia [102]. Mutation in the chitotriosidase gene (CHIT1, rs3831317) is linked to an increased fungal colonisation rate, further supporting evidence of the role of chitinases in CF fungal defence strategies [102, 103]. The chitinase-like protein YKL-40 is also elevated in CF, particularly those with the severest lung disease; however, association with a specific inciting fungal pathogen or even whether the observed relationship in CF is primarily fungal-driven remains uncertain [104]. Airway *Candida* has been associated with poorer clinical outcomes, including lung function decline, but this has not translated when inflammatory responses have been examined in vitro against pulmonary cell cultures [105, 106]. Chronic infection with *C. dubliniensis* is associated with a lower FEV_1 and pancreatic insufficiency [94, 107–109]. Impaired salivary secretion observed in CF, frequent use of antibiotics and oral steroids as well as history of diabetes place the CF population at higher risk of developing oral candidiasis [86]. Similarly, CF patients with advanced disease, histories of long-term mechanical ventilation, frequent use of broad-spectrum antimicrobial and anti-inflammatory drugs and chronic infections with mucoid *P. aeruginosa* and diabetes mellitus are at higher risk of developing candidiasis [109]. Patients receiving immunosuppressive treatments after lung transplant are at higher risk for invasive *Candida* infections with systemic dissemination to major organs (kidneys, spleen, skin, eyes, heart and meninges), accompanied by high mortality rates (up to 60%).

Scedosporium *spp.*

The *Scedosporium* genus consists of five clinically relevant species with differing geographic distribution. These include *Scedosporium apiospermum*, *S. boydii*, *S. dehoogii*, *S. minutisporum* and *S. prolificans* [110]. As filamentous ubiquitous moulds, they incite a broad range of clinical consequence, from a transitory colonisation and superficial infection to severe invasive localised or systemic disease, the latter associated with high mortality [110]. These multifaceted and chronic colonisers of the CF airway in select cases are now recognised as emerging pathogens found in other body niches, including the bone, eye, and central nervous system. Now among the top three most prevalent fungal pathogens in CF, its frequency has remained underestimated, owing to challenges to its mycological culture. Technological advances, however, have now led to increased detection rates for this organism, now reported at rates of up to 17% worldwide [111]. Organ transplantation, immunodeficiency, chronic infections with mucoid *Pseudomonas*, frequent use of broad-spectrum lactams and steroids, lymphopenia, neutropenia and low protein levels (serum albumin <3 mg/dl), each with relevance in the setting of CF, have been reported as significant risk factors for the development of scedosporiosis [112–114]. In those immunocompromised, *Scedosporium* has been associated with allergic responses and higher risks of dissemination, but interestingly and dissimilar to *Aspergillus*, its presence does not associate with poorer pulmonary function [115]. Patients colonised with *Scedosporium* are typically colonised by a single strain that illustrates temporal stability. The detection of this pathogen in the CF airway is of clinical significance as *Scedosporium* species harbour high rates of antifungal resistance. Correlations between virulence and metabolic capability have been described, and such early observations encourage further research in the field [116]. Particular amino acids, hexose acids, carboxylic acids, esters and fatty acids have all been found to exhibit growth inhibitory effects on the organism, and these may be considered novel approaches to halt pathogen growth and inhibit spore germination. Close correlation between virulence and metabolism also at least partially explains the variable pathogenicity and patterns of host colonisation in CF. For instance, saline resistance of *S. aurantiacum* has been put forward as a potential reason for its persistence in the salt-rich airway fluid of CF patients [117].

Other Emerging Fungal Threats to the CF Airway

Exophiala, particularly *E. dermatitis*, is a less common but important coloniser of the CF lung. Commonly referred to as the 'black yeast', advances in its detection and physiological characterisation have contributed to the observed increases in CF prevalence. This filamentous and ubiquitous organism, found in moist and warm environments, has the propensity to cause opportunistic and life-threatening infections in immunocompromised patients, including CF patients. While occurrence in Europe has been reported in up to 30% of patients, *E. dermatitis* appears in the main to be a harmless chronic bystander in the lung but importantly can cause invasive and life-threatening mycosis [118, 119]. In people with CF, aged >12 years who have pancreatic insufficiency, co-colonisation with *A. fumigatus* and more advanced disease are at the highest risk of developing systemic *Exophiala* infections [118, 120, 121]. Other clinically apparent and significant moulds described in the airway CF include *Rasamsonia,* an often misidentified genus with underestimated rates of colonisation. Approximately 3% of CF patients are reported to have *Rasamsonia* in their airways [122]. These thermo-tolerant filamentous ascomycete moulds morphologically resemble *Penicillium* and *Paecilomyces* species [123, 124]. Risk factors for colonisation and infection in CF include immune deficiencies and receipt of organ (particularly lung) transplant [124]. *Malassezia* spp. are also frequently described in CF sputum [125]. These fungi are lipid-dependent yeasts of the *Basidiomycota* and commonly occur on the skin and mucosa of mammals. While often associated with skin disorders such as eczema, atopic dermatitis and psoriasis, the use of medical devices has been suggested as a risk factor for systemic infection in immunocompromised patients, for instance, the use of vascular access devices in CF patients [126–128].

Intra/Inter-kingdom Communication in the CF Airway: Roles of the Host, Bacteria and Environmental Cues in CF-Associated Fungal Infection

Recognised as important colonisers of eukaryotes, fungi possess the ability to stimulate and alter host physiology, metabolism and immune response [129, 130]. Changes to holobiont composition are now a recognised powerful mechanism of adaptation to environmental stresses, one far more efficient than genetic mutations or species selection alone [131]. In concert with the coexisting microbiome in the host, fungal communities form a symbiotic holobiome, driven by complex and elaborate networks of dynamic and mutualistic interactions that maintain homeostasis (Fig. 6.3) [132]. Changes to microbiome diversity, particularly characteristic of CF, are associated with greater risks of fungal colonisation, infection and sensitisation (Fig. 6.3) [133–135]. Bacterial and fungal populations may modulate collective behaviour to facilitate access to nutrients and provide collective defences against host and environmental cues employing a myriad of cell-cell communication strategies [136, 137]. Intra- and inter-kingdom signalling occurs by the secretion of extracellular signalling molecules sensed by surrounding cells. Such signalling molecules include the quorum sensing system, lipids, peptides, volatile organic compounds, as well as a wide range of proteases detectable in body fluids, including the ASL, epithelial lining fluid or human plasma [138–140]. More recently, prokaryotic and eukaryotic single-stranded noncoding RNAs secreted and transported by membrane vesicles have been shown to promote communication within and across kingdoms and in turn influence pathogenesis [141–143].

Of great relevance to CF, systemic or localised infection is, in most instances, polymicrobial in nature [144–146]. A dysregulated bacterial diversity likely benefits one or more pathogens in one body niche (such as fungi) and can lead to outgrowth, colonisation and infection at other sites (Fig. 6.3) [145, 146]. In chronic respiratory diseases such as CF, fungal colonisation is thought to exacerbate due to impaired ciliary function or following perturbation of the host microbiome induced by antimicrobial or steroid intake [131]. Therefore, outgrowth of *C. albicans*, for example, is commonly reported following gut dysbiosis and results in an allergic airway response

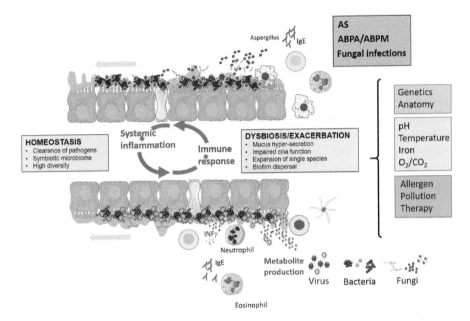

Fig. 6.3 Complex microbial interactions orchestrate intra- and inter-kingdom communications influencing lung holobiont homeostasis in cystic fibrosis. Symbiotic coexistence of virus, bacteria and fungi contributes to host homeostasis. Alterations of microbiome diversity in the gut and/or the lungs lead to the activation of inflammatory and immune responses that trigger allergic responses and pathogen selection. Environmental cues, such as low pH, oxygen levels, temperature, iron concentration and allergens, can exacerbate pathology in CF. Although treatments aim at restoring host homeostasis, they may contribute further infection by species selection, decreasing biodiversity and promoting inflammation. AS *Aspergillus* sensitisation, ABPA/ABPM allergic bronchopulmonary aspergillosis/allergic bronchopulmonary mycoses

to *A. fumigatus* mediated by Th2 cells [147]. To fully appreciate such emerging and clinically complex interactions in CF, it is increasingly clear that a systems biology approach is necessary and that an appreciation of the gut-lung axis, particularly as related to bacterial-fungal communication, must be better understood (Fig. 6.3).

The CF Mycobiome

Diagnostic methodologies targeting fungal pathogens in CF range from mycological culture to molecular techniques and include quantitative polymerase chain reaction (qPCR). Immunoassays are also employed for the detection of specific fungal antigens such as galactomannan [148]. Critically however, detection methodologies for fungi in CF lack standardisation, and variability is consequently observed in reported rates of fungal colonisation and infection even for major pathogens such as *A. fumigatus*, whose reported rates vary between 6% and 60% [149]. Comparing mycological protocols between CF centres is challenging, given the general lack of national mycology guidelines for the processing of respiratory specimens. This has led to the formation of international consortia to propose evidence-based standardised protocols for fungal isolation in CF [150, 151]. Given the inherent challenges of culture-based fungal isolation, a key and emerging complementary approach is the use of culture-independent mycobiome analysis through high-throughput DNA sequencing [152]. The advent of next-generation sequencing has expanded our capacity for culture-independent analysis of the lung microbiome. Though long overlooked due to presuppositions of sterility, the lung has enjoyed a renaissance of renewed focus beginning with the seminal culture independent analysis of the CF airway [153]. As early embracers of these new technologies, the CF field boasts the most advanced respiratory microbiome studies in terms of defined bacterial composition and associated clinical correlates [154–161]. Despite our insight into the bacterial component of the CF lung microbiome, the fungal component– the mycobiome – remains less well studied. This is largely due to the technical challenges in studying mycobiomes. These difficulties range from challenges in extracting adequate DNA from fungi that possess robust cell walls to poorly defined fungal taxonomy and less well-curated comparative databases to that seen with bacteria. Further, a lack of consensus exists in regard to which primer sequences are best to assess the mycobiome by targeted amplicon sequencing relative to more established practices and protocols for analysis of the 16S rRNA gene in bacteria [162, 163]. Whole-genome shotgun metagenomics represents an alternative to targeted amplicon sequencing, but this similarly suffers from deficiencies in reference databases that preclude adequate detection of fungal taxa in CF lung metagenomic data sets [158, 162]. Despite these challenges, a number of studies have now begun to explore culture-independent analysis of fungi in the CF lung [152, 162, 164–169]. These studies demonstrate fungal profiles broadly comparable with fungi detected by routine microbiological culture methods while also revealing the (unculturable) full spectrum of fungal microbiota present in the CF lung [152, 165, 168]. Within these profiles, the presence of stable communities contrasts with more transient fungal species, unstable across serial sampling, which likely represent dynamic trafficking of airborne fungi rather than truly colonising species [167]. Given the limited study population sizes, the composition of the core respiratory mycobiome in CF or indeed non-diseased populations remains speculative at best. However, emerging patterns do include the increased abundance of *Aspergillus* species such as *A. fumigatus*, as well as other filamentous yeasts, including *C. albicans*, *C. parapsilosis* and *Malassezia* species, in CF when compared to non-CF populations [164]. Further evidence supporting the colonisation of the CF lung by specific fungal pathogens comes from observations of genetic adaptation in *Candida* species where mutations in the Nrg1 gene – which causes advantageous constitutive filamentous growth in the lung – are seen to emerge independently among different patients analogous to the adaptive mutations documented in the established bacterial pathogens of the CF lung [168, 170]. While these pioneering studies provide important insight into the CF mycobiome, further work is required before more practical use for such mycobiome analysis in clinical practice can be appreciated and the role of mycobiome assessment in the routine workup of individuals with CF clearly defined [57, 152, 171]. The significance of factors such as ethnicity, geography, gender and therapy – all important variables in determining clinical outcomes in CF – must also be considered in terms of their association on mycobiome profiles [172]. As the field moves forward, many pitfalls, including the underappreciated taxonomic diversity of fungi, the major gaps that still exist in the fungal databases and the emerging interactions between distinct fungal guilds and other microbial kingdoms, must be given due and cautious consideration [173].

Treating Fungi in CF: Existing and Emerging Perspectives

Recurrent infections play a central role in the evolution and pathology of CF [174, 175]. In particular, fungal-associated colonisation and infection often result in atopic sensitisation to mould allergens caused by recurrent lung infections and Th2-driven inflammation (Fig. 6.2) [176]. Consequently, treatments have focused on limiting disease progression and maintaining pulmonary function by targeting both inflammation and infection. Infections are generally polymicrobial in nature and involve pathogens (including fungi) with varying susceptibility profiles and genetic flexibility [145, 146]. Anti-inflammatory agents such as corticosteroids are commonly used in combination with antimicrobial and/or antifungals for the treatment of fungal sensitisation and CF-ABPA [52, 177, 178].

Oral prednisolone (in tapering dose over a prolonged time period) is usually the first-line treatment for CF-ABPA once diagnosed [178–181]. Corticosteroids exerts anti-inflammatory activity through the inhibition of NFκB activation, trafficking and adhesion of cells, mucus secretion, and production and activity of inflammatory mediators [182]. Importantly, and of relevance in CF-ABPA, long-term use substantially alters levels of growth hormone, resulting in a reduction of mineral bone density and associated growth retardation [183–185]. Inhaled corticosteroids have a minimal role in the long-term management of CF-ABPA but remain useful in patients with concurrent reactive airway disease (whether or not related to fungi), and they demonstrate a more favourable side-effect profile to that associated with oral corticosteroids [186–189]. Newer protocols gaining popularity employing pulsed high-dose methylprednisolone (given monthly for nine months) with or without the addition of antifungal treatment permit better symptomatic control, lead to disease resolution in some cases and may achieve greater compliance compared with traditional CF-ABPA protocols while limiting long-term exposure to steroids and their associated side effects [65, 181, 190]. A range of antifungal agents have been employed against fungi in the CF airway, including itraconazole, voriconazole and posaconazole [66, 191–193]. Each has its strengths and limitations. Itraconazole is relatively inexpensive but suffers from poor gastrointestinal absorption and requires close monitoring of therapeutic levels [194]. Voriconazole appears more effective, but photosensitivity has been reported in the CF literature, precluding use in susceptible patients [194, 195]. By far, the greatest emerging challenge and one that requires detailed study is the use of antifungal treatments in patients who are eligible for CFTR modulator or corrector therapy [73]. Most of these new agents cannot be given together, owing to adverse drug reactions or drug-drug interaction with metabolising enzyme systems [73].

Newer and alternative treatment strategies targeting the immune response associated with inflammation and infection in CF and CF-ABPA are emerging [196]. One example is the use of the humanised monoclonal anti-IgE antibody (omalizumab) reported by many and considered an alternative and promising option in the treatment of CF-ABPA [69–71, 197–199]. More recent work, however, has questioned the clinical significance of this agent in CF, and further studies are clearly warranted to evaluate the true value of such an approach [69, 197]. Nonetheless, the broader concept of immunotherapeutic manipulation remains attractive, albeit expensive, and warrants further exploration for fungal infection in CF.

Effective treatments targeting fungal infection directly remain scarce [200]. Only a few classes of antifungal molecules are available, and as antifungal resistance has rapidly emerged and spread globally, the development of new classes of antifungals remains worryingly slow [201, 202]. High levels of resistance to broad-spectrum azole compounds, such as voriconazole or itraconazole, have been reported in *Aspergillus* and *Candida* species and represent one of the greatest global clinical challenges, including those in CF [203–206]. Alternative treatment options include liposomal amphotericin B and newer and safer echinocandin molecules such as caspofungin, micafungin and anidulafungin [206, 207]. Critically, resistance even to these molecules has already been reported in *Candida* and *Aspergillus* species [208–211]. Novel potential targets for antifungal therapy have been identified, and several compounds have accelerated into clinical development pipelines. Immunomodulatory approaches, including anti-IgE therapy (omalizumab), have been reported to illustrate the benefit of the treatment of CF-ABPA in select patients; however, no evidence base or clinical trials have been conducted to attest this. The reported individual cases and case series for omalizumab in CF-ABPA suggest that other developing immunomodulatory agents (used for indications unrelated to CF) may similarly have relevance in select patients as fresh therapeutic approaches against CF-ABPA (Table 6.3) [69–71, 188, 198, 212, 213].

Table 6.3 A summary of antifungal and immunomodulatory and therapies in preclinical and clinical development for pulmonary infection

Compound	Target	Role of the target	Indications	Phase of development	References
Antifungal agents					
Isavuconazole	Ergosterol biosynthesis	Membrane fluidity Trigger of macrophage pyroptosis	Invasive candidiasis	Phase 3	[227–229]
ASP9726	β-glucan synthesis	Cell wall component Inflammasome activation	Invasive pulmonary aspergillosis	Preclinical	[230]
SCY-078			Invasive candidiasis	Phase 2	[231]

Table 6.3 (continued)

Compound	Target	Role of the target	Indications	Phase of development	References
T-2307	Mitochondrial function	Cellular respiration	Candidiasis Aspergillosis	Phase 1	[232]
F901318	Pyrimidine biosynthesis	Amino acid synthesis	Invasive aspergillosis	Phase 1	[233]
APX001	GPI anchor biosynthesis	Lipid anchor with multiple roles Modulation of host immune response	Pulmonary aspergillosis	Phase 1	[234]
OSU-03012	Carbon metabolism	Nutrition and growth	Candida biofilm	Preclinical, granted orphan drug status (EU)	[235]
VL2397	Unknown	Unknown	Invasive aspergillosis	Phase 1	[236]
Immunomodulatory agents					
QGE031 (ligelizumab)	IgE	Antibody	Allergic asthma (potential candidate for ABPA and AS)	Phase 1 (asthma)	[212]
MEDI4212	IgE	Antibody	Allergic asthma (potential candidate for ABPA and AS)	Phase I (asthma)	[237]
Quilizumab	Anti-CεmX	Discrete domain of IgE ε heavy chain	Allergic asthma (potential candidate for ABPA and AS)	Phase II (asthma)	[213, 238]

Conclusion

The interplay that exists between the host, microbiome and mycobiome renders the diagnosis and treatment of fungal infection in CF challenging, especially during concurrent episodes of infective exacerbations. CF-ABPA may be indistinguishable from exacerbations, and guidelines for its diagnosis and treatment require updating. The broad variety of fungi in the CF airway and the complex spectrum of clinical manifestations of fungi in CF make this area of clinical care challenging. Drug regimens, despite lacking strong evidence, must be carefully chosen to ensure fast and optimal eradication of the pathogens while limiting the emergence of drug resistance and further perturbations of the microbiome [2, 165, 214, 215]. Better and more objective diagnostics focused on immune measurements rather than mycological culture and clinical symptoms of CF-ABPA are necessary. Clinical trials for commonly used therapeutic strategies for CF-ABPA are in progress, and this will bolster the weak current evidence base. Novel treatment regimens, immunological classifications that have included the description of *Aspergillus* bronchitis and emerging immunomodulating therapeutic strategies should also be subjected to the full scrutiny of strong longitudinal research and randomised controlled trials so that relevance and efficacy are evaluated. Mechanistic research focused on immunopathogenic pathways and immunoevasive strategies in chronic fungal disease should be pursued, and this will provide a road map to future therapeutic pipelines. Continuing mycobiome studies using systems biology will, with time, reveal microbial interactions relevant to CF, potentially uncovering novel fungal taxa involved in airway pathology, which serves to remind us that we are only at the beginning of understanding the true complexity of the fungal taxonomic landscape as relevant to CF.

Acknowledgements This research is supported by the Singapore Ministry of Health's National Medical Research Council under its Transition Award (NMRC/TA/0048/2016) and the Lee Kong Chian School of Medicine, Nanyang Technological University Start-Up Grant (both S.H.C). The authors would like to acknowledge The Academic Respiratory Initiative for Pulmonary Health (TARIPH) for collaboration support.

References

1. Lyczak JB, Cannon CL, Pier GB. Lung infections associated with cystic fibrosis. Clin Microbiol Rev. 2002;15(2):194–222.
2. Filkins LM, O'Toole GA. Cystic fibrosis lung infections: polymicrobial, complex, and hard to treat. PLoS Pathog. 2015;11(12):e1005258.
3. McIntyre K. Gender and survival in cystic fibrosis. Curr Opin Pulm Med. 2013;19(6):692–7.
4. Goss CH, Burns JL. Exacerbations in cystic fibrosis center dot 1: epidemiology and pathogenesis. Thorax. 2007;62(4):360–7.
5. Corriveau S, Sykes J, Stephenson AL. Cystic fibrosis survival: the changing epidemiology. Curr Opin Pulm Med. 2018;24(6):574–8.
6. Jackson AD, Goss CH. Epidemiology of CF: how registries can be used to advance our understanding of the CF population. J Cyst Fibros. 2018;17(3):297–305.
7. Bosch B, Bilton D, Sosnay P, Raraigh KS, Mak DYF, Ishiguro H, et al. Ethnicity impacts the cystic fibrosis diagnosis: a note of caution. J Cyst Fibros. 2017;16(4):488–91.
8. Taylor-Robinson DC, Schechter MS, Smyth RL. Comparing cystic fibrosis outcomes across the pond. Thorax. 2015;70(3):203–4.
9. Vahedi L, Jabarpoor-Bonyadi M, Ghojazadeh M, Vahedi A, Rafeey M. Gender differences in clinical presentations of cystic fibrosis patients in Azeri Turkish population. Tuberc Respir Dis (Seoul). 2016;79(4):267–73.
10. Harness-Brumley CL, Elliott AC, Rosenbluth DB, Raghavan D, Jain R. Gender differences in outcomes of patients with cystic fibrosis. J Womens Health (Larchmt). 2014;23(12):1012–20.
11. Parkins MD, Floto RA. Emerging bacterial pathogens and changing concepts of bacterial pathogenesis in cystic fibrosis. J Cyst Fibros. 2015;14(3):293–304.
12. Williams C, Ranjendran R, Ramage G. Pathogenesis of fungal infections in cystic fibrosis. Curr Fungal Infect Rep. 2016;10(4):163–9.
13. Janahi IA, Rehman A, Al-Naimi AR. Allergic bronchopulmonary aspergillosis in patients with cystic fibrosis. Ann Thorac Med. 2017;12(2):74–82.

14. Armstead J, Morris J, Denning DW. Multi-country estimate of different manifestations of aspergillosis in cystic fibrosis. PLoS One. 2014;9(6):e98502.
15. Yii AC, Koh MS, Lapperre TS, Tan GL, Chotirmall SH. The emergence of Aspergillus species in chronic respiratory disease. Front Biosci (Schol Ed). 2017;9:127–38.
16. Maturu VN, Agarwal R. Prevalence of Aspergillus sensitization and allergic bronchopulmonary aspergillosis in cystic fibrosis: systematic review and meta-analysis. Clin Exp Allergy. 2015;45(12):1765–78.
17. Latge JP. Aspergillus fumigatus and aspergillosis. Clin Microbiol Rev. 1999;12(2):310–50.
18. van de Veerdonk FL, Gresnigt MS, Romani L, Netea MG, Latge JP. Aspergillus fumigatus morphology and dynamic host interactions. Nat Rev Microbiol. 2017;15(11):661–74.
19. Chotirmall SH, Martin-Gomez MT. Aspergillus species in bronchiectasis: challenges in the cystic fibrosis and non-cystic fibrosis airways. Mycopathologia. 2018;183(1):45–59.
20. de Vrankrijker AM, van der Ent CK, van Berkhout FT, Stellato RK, Willems RJ, Bonten MJ, et al. Aspergillus fumigatus colonization in cystic fibrosis: implications for lung function? Clin Microbiol Infect. 2011;17(9):1381–6.
21. Kraemer R, Delosea N, Ballinari P, Gallati S, Crameri R. Effect of allergic bronchopulmonary aspergillosis on lung function in children with cystic fibrosis. Am J Respir Crit Care Med. 2006;174(11):1211–20.
22. Kosmidis C, Denning DW. The clinical spectrum of pulmonary aspergillosis. Thorax. 2015;70(3):270–7.
23. Slesiona S, Gressler M, Mihlan M, Zaehle C, Schaller M, Barz D, et al. Persistence versus escape: Aspergillus terreus and Aspergillus fumigatus employ different strategies during interactions with macrophages. PLoS One. 2012;7(2):e31223.
24. Sabino R, Ferreira JA, Moss RB, Valente J, Verissimo C, Carolino E, et al. Molecular epidemiology of Aspergillus collected from cystic fibrosis patients. J Cyst Fibros. 2015;14(4): 474–81.
25. Romani L. Immunity to fungal infections. Nat Rev Immunol. 2011;11(4):275–88.
26. Braedel S, Radsak M, Einsele H, Latge JP, Michan A, Loeffler J, et al. Aspergillus fumigatus antigens activate innate immune cells via toll-like receptors 2 and 4. Br J Haematol. 2004;125(3):392–9.
27. Werner JL, Metz AE, Horn D, Schoeb TR, Hewitt MM, Schwiebert LM, et al. Requisite role for the dectin-1 beta-glucan receptor in pulmonary defense against Aspergillus fumigatus. J Immunol. 2009;182(8):4938–46.
28. Wasylnka JA, Moore MM. Aspergillus fumigatus conidia survive and germinate in acidic organelles of A549 epithelial cells. J Cell Sci. 2003;116(Pt 8):1579–87.
29. de Luca A, Bozza S, Zelante T, Zagarella S, D'Angelo C, Perruccio K, et al. Non-hematopoietic cells contribute to protective tolerance to Aspergillus fumigatus via a TRIF pathway converging on IDO. Cell Mol Immunol. 2010;7(6):459–70.
30. Allard JB, Poynter ME, Marr KA, Cohn L, Rincon M, Whittaker LA. Aspergillus fumigatus generates an enhanced Th2-biased immune response in mice with defective cystic fibrosis transmembrane conductance regulator. J Immunol. 2006;177(8):5186–94.
31. Mueller C, Braag SA, Keeler A, Hodges C, Drumm M, Flotte TR. Lack of cystic fibrosis transmembrane conductance regulator in CD3+ lymphocytes leads to aberrant cytokine secretion and hyperinflammatory adaptive immune responses. Am J Respir Cell Mol Biol. 2011;44(6):922–9.
32. Moss RB, Hsu YP, Olds L. Cytokine dysregulation in activated cystic fibrosis (CF) peripheral lymphocytes. Clin Exp Immunol. 2000;120(3):518–25.
33. Boucher RC. Evidence for airway surface dehydration as the initiating event in CF airway disease. J Intern Med. 2007;261(1):5–16.
34. Cosgrove S, Chotirmall SH, Greene CM, McElvaney NG. Pulmonary proteases in the cystic fibrosis lung induce interleukin 8 expression from bronchial epithelial cells via a heme/meprin/epidermal growth factor receptor/Toll-like receptor pathway. J Biol Chem. 2011;286(9):7692–704.

35. Hamon Y, Jaillon S, Person C, Ginies JL, Garo E, Bottazzi B, et al. Proteolytic cleavage of the long pentraxin PTX3 in the airways of cystic fibrosis patients. Innate Immun. 2013;19(6):611–22.
36. Chotirmall SH, Mirkovic B, Lavelle GM, McElvaney NG. Immunoevasive Aspergillus virulence factors. Mycopathologia. 2014;178(5–6):363–70.
37. Schlam D, Canton J, Carreno M, Kopinski H, Freeman SA, Grinstein S, et al. Gliotoxin suppresses macrophage immune function by subverting phosphatidylinositol 3,4,5-trisphosphate homeostasis. MBio. 2016;7(2):e02242.
38. Fallon JP, Reeves EP, Kavanagh K. Inhibition of neutrophil function following exposure to the Aspergillus fumigatus toxin fumagillin. J Med Microbiol. 2010;59(Pt 6):625–33.
39. Lee MJ, Liu H, Barker BM, Snarr BD, Gravelat FN, Al Abdallah Q, et al. The fungal exopolysaccharide galactosaminogalactan mediates virulence by enhancing resistance to neutrophil extracellular traps. PLoS Pathog. 2015;11(10):e1005187.
40. Cohen TS, Prince A. Cystic fibrosis: a mucosal immunodeficiency syndrome. Nat Med. 2012;18(4):509–19.
41. Ratner D, Mueller C. Immune responses in cystic fibrosis: are they intrinsically defective? Am J Respir Cell Mol Biol. 2012;46(6):715–22.
42. Coughlan CA, Chotirmall SH, Renwick J, Hassan T, Low TB, Bergsson G, et al. The effect of Aspergillus fumigatus infection on vitamin D receptor expression in cystic fibrosis. Am J Respir Crit Care Med. 2012;186(10):999–1007.
43. Amin R, Dupuis A, Aaron SD, Ratjen F. The effect of chronic infection with Aspergillus fumigatus on lung function and hospitalization in patients with cystic fibrosis. Chest. 2010;137(1):171–6.
44. McMahon MA, Chotirmall SH, McCullagh B, Branagan P, McElvaney NG, Logan PM. Radiological abnormalities associated with Aspergillus colonization in a cystic fibrosis population. Eur J Radiol. 2012;81(3):e197–202.
45. Liu JC, Modha DE, Gaillard EA. What is the clinical significance of filamentous fungi positive sputum cultures in patients with cystic fibrosis? J Cyst Fibros. 2013;12(3):187–93.
46. Aaron SD, Vandemheen KL, Freitag A, Pedder L, Cameron W, Lavoie A, et al. Treatment of Aspergillus fumigatus in patients with cystic fibrosis: a randomized, placebo-controlled pilot study. PLoS One. 2012;7(4):e36077.
47. Singh A, Ralhan A, Schwarz C, Hartl D, Hector A. Fungal pathogens in CF airways: leave or treat? Mycopathologia. 2018;183(1):119–37.
48. Harun SN, Wainwright CE, Grimwood K, Hennig S, Australasian Cystic Fibrosis Bronchoalveolar Lavage study g. Aspergillus and progression of lung disease in children with cystic fibrosis. Thorax. 2019;74(2):125–31.
49. Engel TGP, Slabbers L, de Jong C, Melchers WJG, Hagen F, Verweij PE, et al. Prevalence and diversity of filamentous fungi in the airways of cystic fibrosis patients – a Dutch, multicentre study. J Cyst Fibros. 2019;18(2):221–6.
50. Agarwal R, Chakrabarti A, Shah A, Gupta D, Meis JF, Guleria R, et al. Allergic bronchopulmonary aspergillosis: review of literature and proposal of new diagnostic and classification criteria. Clin Exp Allergy. 2013;43(8):850–73.
51. Hartl D. Immunological mechanisms behind the cystic fibrosis-ABPA link. Med Mycol. 2009;47(Suppl 1):S183–91.
52. Stevens DA, Moss RB, Kurup VP, Knutsen AP, Greenberger P, Judson MA, et al. Allergic bronchopulmonary aspergillosis in cystic fibrosis – state of the art: Cystic Fibrosis Foundation Consensus Conference. Clin Infect Dis. 2003;37(Suppl 3):S225–64.
53. Svirshchevskaya E, Zubkov D, Mouyna I, Berkova N. Innate immunity and the role of epithelial barrier during Aspergillus fumigatus infection. Curr Immunol Rev. 2012;8(3):254–61.
54. Muthu V, Sehgal IS, Dhooria S, Aggarwal AN, Agarwal R. Utility of recombinant Aspergillus fumigatus antigens in the diagnosis of allergic bronchopulmonary aspergillosis: a systematic review and diagnostic test accuracy meta-analysis. Clin Exp Allergy. 2018;48(9):1107–36.
55. Baxter CG, Dunn G, Jones AM, Webb K, Gore R, Richardson MD, et al. Novel immunologic classification of aspergillosis in adult cystic fibrosis. J Allergy Clin Immunol. 2013;132(3):560–6.e10.

56. Baxter CG, Moore CB, Jones AM, Webb AK, Denning DW. IgE-mediated immune responses and airway detection of Aspergillus and Candida in adult cystic fibrosis. Chest. 2013;143(5):1351–7.
57. Mac Aogain M, Chandrasekaran R, Lim AYH, Low TB, Tan GL, Hassan T, et al. Immunological corollary of the pulmonary mycobiome in bronchiectasis: the CAMEB study. Eur Respir J. 2018;52(1). pii: 1800766.
58. Mac Aogain M, Tiew PY, Lim AYH, Low TB, Tan GL, Hassan T, et al. Distinct 'Immuno-allertypes' of disease and high frequencies of sensitisation in non-cystic-fibrosis bronchiectasis. Am J Respir Crit Care Med. 2019;199(7):842–53.
59. Agarwal R, Khan A, Aggarwal AN, Varma N, Garg M, Saikia B, et al. Clinical relevance of peripheral blood eosinophil count in allergic bronchopulmonary aspergillosis. J Infect Public Health. 2011;4(5–6):235–43.
60. Chotirmall SH, Branagan P, Gunaratnam C, McElvaney NG. Aspergillus/allergic bronchopulmonary aspergillosis in an Irish cystic fibrosis population: a diagnostically challenging entity. Respir Care. 2008;53(8):1035–41.
61. Slavin RG, Bedrossian CW, Hutcheson PS, Pittman S, Salinas-Madrigal L, Tsai CC, et al. A pathologic study of allergic bronchopulmonary aspergillosis. J Allergy Clin Immunol. 1988;81(4):718–25.
62. Gernez Y, Waters J, Mirkovic B, Lavelle GM, Dunn CE, Davies ZA, et al. Blood basophil activation is a reliable biomarker of allergic bronchopulmonary aspergillosis in cystic fibrosis. Eur Respir J. 2016;47(1):177–85.
63. Mirkovic B, Lavelle GM, Azim AA, Helma K, Gargoum FS, Molloy K, et al. The basophil surface marker CD203c identifies Aspergillus species sensitization in patients with cystic fibrosis. J Allergy Clin Immunol. 2016;137(2):436–43.e9.
64. Gernez Y, Dunn CE, Everson C, Mitsunaga E, Gudiputi L, Krasinska K, et al. Blood basophils from cystic fibrosis patients with allergic bronchopulmonary aspergillosis are primed and hyper-responsive to stimulation by aspergillus allergens. J Cyst Fibros. 2012;11(6):502–10.
65. Cohen-Cymberknoh M, Blau H, Shoseyov D, Mei-Zahav M, Efrati O, Armoni S, et al. Intravenous monthly pulse methylprednisolone treatment for ABPA in patients with cystic fibrosis. J Cyst Fibros. 2009;8(4):253–7.
66. Moss RB. Treating allergic bronchopulmonary aspergillosis: the way forward. Eur Respir J. 2016;47(2):385–7.
67. Moreira AS, Silva D, Ferreira AR, Delgado L. Antifungal treatment in allergic bronchopulmonary aspergillosis with and without cystic fibrosis: a systematic review. Clin Exp Allergy. 2014;44(10):1210–27.
68. Dunne K, Prior AR, Murphy K, Wall N, Leen G, Rogers TR, et al. Emergence of persistent Aspergillus terreus colonisation in a child with cystic fibrosis. Med Mycol Case Rep. 2015;9:26–30.
69. Ashkenazi M, Sity S, Sarouk I, Bar Aluma BE, Dagan A, Bezalel Y, et al. Omalizumab in allergic bronchopulmonary aspergillosis in patients with cystic fibrosis. J Asthma Allergy. 2018;11:101–7.
70. Nove-Josserand R, Grard S, Auzou L, Reix P, Murris-Espin M, Bremont F, et al. Case series of omalizumab for allergic bronchopulmonary aspergillosis in cystic fibrosis patients. Pediatr Pulmonol. 2017;52(2):190–7.
71. Perisson C, Destruys L, Grenet D, Bassinet L, Derelle J, Sermet-Gaudelus I, et al. Omalizumab treatment for allergic bronchopulmonary aspergillosis in young patients with cystic fibrosis. Respir Med. 2017;133:12–5.
72. Ramsey BW, Davies J, McElvaney NG, Tullis E, Bell SC, Drevinek P, et al. A CFTR potentiator in patients with cystic fibrosis and the G551D mutation. N Engl J Med. 2011;365(18):1663–72.
73. Jordan CL, Noah TL, Henry MM. Therapeutic challenges posed by critical drug-drug interactions in cystic fibrosis. Pediatr Pulmonol. 2016;51(S44):S61–70.

74. Harrison MJ, Ronan NJ, Khan KA, O'Callaghan G, Murphy DM, Plant BJ. Ivacaftor therapy in siblings with cystic fibrosis-the potential implications of Itraconazole in dosage and efficacy. Pulm Pharmacol Ther. 2015;31:49–50.

75. Heltshe SL, Mayer-Hamblett N, Burns JL, Khan U, Baines A, Ramsey BW, et al. Pseudomonas aeruginosa in cystic fibrosis patients with G551D-CFTR treated with ivacaftor. Clin Infect Dis. 2015;60(5):703–12.

76. Schwarz C, Bouchara JP, Buzina W, Chrenkova V, Dmenska H, de la Pedrosa EGG, et al. Organization of patient management and fungal epidemiology in cystic fibrosis. Mycopathologia. 2018;183(1):7–19.

77. Maguire CP, Hayes JP, Hayes M, Masterson J, FitzGerald MX. Three cases of pulmonary aspergilloma in adult patients with cystic fibrosis. Thorax. 1995;50(7):805–6.

78. Luong ML, Chaparro C, Stephenson A, Rotstein C, Singer LG, Waters V, et al. Pretransplant Aspergillus colonization of cystic fibrosis patients and the incidence of post-lung transplant invasive aspergillosis. Transplantation. 2014;97(3):351–7.

79. Denning DW, Cadranel J, Beigelman-Aubry C, Ader F, Chakrabarti A, Blot S, et al. Chronic pulmonary aspergillosis: rationale and clinical guidelines for diagnosis and management. Eur Respir J. 2016;47(1):45–68.

80. Chotirmall SH, Al-Alawi M, Mirkovic B, Lavelle G, Logan PM, Greene CM, et al. Aspergillus-associated airway disease, inflammation, and the innate immune response. Biomed Res Int. 2013;2013:723129.

81. Mosquera RA, Estrada L, Clements RM, Jon CK. Early diagnosis and treatment of invasive pulmonary aspergillosis in a patient with cystic fibrosis. BMJ Case Rep. 2013;2013. pii: bcr2013201360.

82. Warren TA, Yau Y, Ratjen F, Tullis E, Waters V. Serum galactomannan in cystic fibrosis patients colonized with Aspergillus species. Med Mycol. 2012;50(6):658–60.

83. Kelly MT, MacCallum DM, Clancy SD, Odds FC, Brown AJ, Butler G. The Candida albicans CaACE2 gene affects morphogenesis, adherence and virulence. Mol Microbiol. 2004;53(3):969–83.

84. Odds FC. Morphogenesis in Candida albicans. Crit Rev Microbiol. 1985;12(1):45–93.

85. Blaschke-Hellmessen R. Habitats for Candida in medical and hygienic respects. Mycoses. 1999;42 Suppl 1:22–9.

86. Chotirmall SH, Greene CM, McElvaney NG. Candida species in cystic fibrosis: a road less travelled. Med Mycol. 2010;48(Suppl 1):S114–24.

87. Odds FC. Pathogenesis of Candida infections. J Am Acad Dermatol. 1994;31(3 Pt 2):S2–5.

88. Kleinegger CL, Lockhart SR, Vargas K, Soll DR. Frequency, intensity, species, and strains of oral Candida vary as a function of host age. J Clin Microbiol. 1996;34(9):2246–54.

89. Chotirmall SH, McElvaney NG. Fungi in the cystic fibrosis lung: bystanders or pathogens? Int J Biochem Cell Biol. 2014;52:161–73.

90. Valenza G, Tappe D, Turnwald D, Frosch M, Konig C, Hebestreit H, et al. Prevalence and antimicrobial susceptibility of microorganisms isolated from sputa of patients with cystic fibrosis. J Cyst Fibros. 2008;7(2):123–7.

91. Guinea J. Global trends in the distribution of Candida species causing candidemia. Clin Microbiol Infect. 2014;20(Suppl 6):5–10.

92. Yazici O, Cortuk M, Casim H, Cetinkaya E, Mert A, Benli AR. Candida glabrata pneumonia in a patient with chronic obstructive pulmonary disease. Case Rep Infect Dis. 2016;2016:4737321.

93. Shweihat Y, Perry J 3rd, Shah D. Isolated Candida infection of the lung. Respir Med Case Rep. 2015;16:18–9.

94. Muthig M, Hebestreit A, Ziegler U, Seidler M, Muller FM. Persistence of Candida species in the respiratory tract of cystic fibrosis patients. Med Mycol. 2010;48(1):56–63.

95. Moyes DL, Runglall M, Murciano C, Shen C, Nayar D, Thavaraj S, et al. A biphasic innate immune MAPK response discriminates between the yeast and hyphal forms of Candida albicans in epithelial cells. Cell Host Microbe. 2010;8(3):225–35.

96. Wachtler B, Wilson D, Haedicke K, Dalle F, Hube B. From attachment to damage: defined genes of Candida albicans mediate adhesion, invasion and damage during interaction with oral epithelial cells. PLoS One. 2011;6(2):e17046.
97. Thompson DS, Carlisle PL, Kadosh D. Coevolution of morphology and virulence in Candida species. Eukaryot Cell. 2011;10(9):1173–82.
98. Mayer FL, Wilson D, Hube B. Candida albicans pathogenicity mechanisms. Virulence. 2013;4(2):119–28.
99. Wahab AA, Taj-Aldeen SJ, Kolecka A, ElGindi M, Finkel JS, Boekhout T. High prevalence of Candida dubliniensis in lower respiratory tract secretions from cystic fibrosis patients may be related to increased adherence properties. Int J Infect Dis. 2014;24:14–9.
100. Hogan DA, Kolter R. Pseudomonas-Candida interactions: an ecological role for virulence factors. Science. 2002;296(5576):2229–32.
101. Chotirmall SH. Candida albicans in cystic fibrosis: "opening statements presented, let the trial begin". Pediatr Pulmonol. 2016;51(5):445–6.
102. Hector A, Chotirmall SH, Lavelle GM, Mirkovic B, Horan D, Eichler L, et al. Chitinase activation in patients with fungus-associated cystic fibrosis lung disease. J Allergy Clin Immunol. 2016;138(4):1183–9. e4
103. Seibold MA, Donnelly S, Solon M, Innes A, Woodruff PG, Boot RG, et al. Chitotriosidase is the primary active chitinase in the human lung and is modulated by genotype and smoking habit. J Allergy Clin Immunol. 2008;122(5):944–50. e3
104. Leonardi S, Parisi GF, Capizzi A, Manti S, Cuppari C, Scuderi MG, et al. YKL-40 as marker of severe lung disease in cystic fibrosis patients. J Cyst Fibros. 2016;15(5):583–6.
105. Reihill JA, Moore JE, Elborn JS, Ennis M. Effect of Aspergillus fumigatus and Candida albicans on pro-inflammatory response in cystic fibrosis epithelium. J Cyst Fibros. 2011;10(6):401–6.
106. Chotirmall SH, O'Donoghue E, Bennett K, Gunaratnam C, O'Neill SJ, McElvaney NG. Sputum Candida albicans presages FEV(1) decline and hospital-treated exacerbations in cystic fibrosis. Chest. 2010;138(5):1186–95.
107. AbdulWahab A, Salah H, Chandra P, Taj-Aldeen SJ. Persistence of Candida dubliniensis and lung function in patients with cystic fibrosis. BMC Res Notes. 2017;10(1):326.
108. Gileles-Hillel A, Shoseyov D, Polacheck I, Korem M, Kerem E, Cohen-Cymberknoh M. Association of chronic Candida albicans respiratory infection with a more severe lung disease in patients with cystic fibrosis. Pediatr Pulmonol. 2015;50(11):1082–9.
109. Noni M, Katelari A, Kaditis A, Theochari I, Lympari I, Alexandrou-Athanassoulis H, et al. Candida albicans chronic colonisation in cystic fibrosis may be associated with inhaled antibiotics. Mycoses. 2015;58(7):416–21.
110. Rougeron A, Giraud S, Alastruey-Izquierdo A, Cano-Lira J, Rainer J, Mouhajir A, et al. Ecology of Scedosporium species: present knowledge and future research. Mycopathologia. 2018;183(1):185–200.
111. Tracy MC, Moss RB. The myriad challenges of respiratory fungal infection in cystic fibrosis. Pediatr Pulmonol. 2018;53(S3):S75–85.
112. Schwarz C, Brandt C, Antweiler E, Krannich A, Staab D, Schmitt-Grohe S, et al. Prospective multicenter German study on pulmonary colonization with Scedosporium/Lomentospora species in cystic fibrosis: epidemiology and new association factors. PLoS One. 2017;12(2):e0171485.
113. Sedlacek L, Graf B, Schwarz C, Albert F, Peter S, Wurstl B, et al. Prevalence of Scedosporium species and Lomentospora prolificans in patients with cystic fibrosis in a multicenter trial by use of a selective medium. J Cyst Fibros. 2015;14(2):237–41.
114. Lamaris GA, Chamilos G, Lewis RE, Safdar A, Raad II, Kontoyiannis DP. Scedosporium infection in a tertiary care cancer center: a review of 25 cases from 1989-2006. Clin Infect Dis. 2006;43(12):1580–4.
115. Cimon B, Carrere J, Vinatier JF, Chazalette JP, Chabasse D, Bouchara JP. Clinical significance of Scedosporium apiospermum in patients with cystic fibrosis. Eur J Clin Microbiol Infect Dis. 2000;19(1):53–6.

116. Kaur J, Duan SY, Vaas LA, Penesyan A, Meyer W, Paulsen IT, et al. Phenotypic profiling of Scedosporium aurantiacum, an opportunistic pathogen colonizing human lungs. PLoS One. 2015;10(3):e0122354.
117. Wine JJ. The genesis of cystic fibrosis lung disease. J Clin Invest. 1999;103(3):309–12.
118. Kondori N, Gilljam M, Lindblad A, Jonsson B, Moore ER, Wenneras C. High rate of Exophiala dermatitidis recovery in the airways of patients with cystic fibrosis is associated with pancreatic insufficiency. J Clin Microbiol. 2011;49(3):1004–9.
119. Ziesing S, Suerbaum S, Sedlacek L. Fungal epidemiology and diversity in cystic fibrosis patients over a 5-year period in a national reference center. Med Mycol. 2016;54(8):781–6.
120. Sudhadham M, Prakitsin S, Sivichai S, Chaiyarat R, Dorrestein GM, Menken SB, et al. The neurotropic black yeast Exophiala dermatitidis has a possible origin in the tropical rain forest. Stud Mycol. 2008;61:145–55.
121. Lebecque P, Leonard A, Huang D, Reychler G, Boeras A, Leal T, et al. Exophiala (Wangiella) dermatitidis and cystic fibrosis – prevalence and risk factors. Med Mycol. 2010;48(Suppl 1):S4–9.
122. Steinmann J, Giraud S, Schmidt D, Sedlacek L, Hamprecht A, Houbraken J, et al. Validation of a novel real-time PCR for detecting Rasamsonia argillacea species complex in respiratory secretions from cystic fibrosis patients. New Microbes New Infect. 2014;2(3):72–8.
123. Houbraken J, Spierenburg H, Frisvad JC. Rasamsonia, a new genus comprising thermotolerant and thermophilic Talaromyces and Geosmithia species. Antonie Van Leeuwenhoek. 2012;101(2):403–21.
124. Giraud S, Favennec L, Bougnoux ME, Bouchara JP. Rasamsonia argillacea species complex: taxonomy, pathogenesis and clinical relevance. Future Microbiol. 2013;8(8):967–78.
125. Nagano Y, Elborn JS, Millar BC, Walker JM, Goldsmith CE, Rendall J, et al. Comparison of techniques to examine the diversity of fungi in adult patients with cystic fibrosis. Med Mycol. 2010;48(1):166–76.e1.
126. Leong C, Goh J, Irudayaswamy A, Dawson T. Geographical and ethnic differences in Malassezia species distribution on healthy skin. Med Mycol. 2018;56:S149-S.
127. Prohic A, Sadikovic TJ, Krupalija-Fazlic M, Kuskunovic-Vlahovljak S. Malassezia species in healthy skin and in dermatological conditions. Int J Dermatol. 2016;55(5):494–504.
128. Velegraki A, Cafarchia C, Gaitanis G, Iatta R, Boekhout T. Malassezia infections in humans and animals: pathophysiology, detection, and treatment. PLoS Pathog. 2015;11(1):e1004523.
129. Vylkova S. Environmental pH modulation by pathogenic fungi as a strategy to conquer the host. PLoS Pathog. 2017;13(2).
130. Kale SD, Ayubi T, Chung D, Tubau-Juni N, Leber A, Dang HX, et al. Modulation of immune signaling and metabolism highlights host and fungal transcriptional responses in mouse models of invasive pulmonary aspergillosis. Sci Rep. 2017;7:17096.
131. Goncalves SM, Lagrou K, Duarte-Oliveira C, Maertens JA, Cunha C, Carvalho A. The microbiome-metabolome crosstalk in the pathogenesis of respiratory fungal diseases. Virulence. 2017;8(6):673–84.
132. Kolwijck E, van de Veerdonk FL. The potential impact of the pulmonary microbiome on immunopathogenesis of Aspergillus-related lung disease. Eur J Immunol. 2014;44(11):3156–65.
133. Dickson RP, Erb-Downward JR, Huffnagle GB. The role of the bacterial microbiome in lung disease. Expert Rev Respir Med. 2013;7(3):245–57.
134. Fujimura KE, Lynch SV. Microbiota in allergy and asthma and the emerging relationship with the gut microbiome. Cell Host Microbe. 2015;17(5):592–602.
135. Gensollen T, Blumberg RS. Correlation between early-life regulation of the immune system by microbiota and allergy development. J Allergy Clin Immunol. 2017;139(4):1084–91.
136. Hogan DA. Talking to themselves: autoregulation and quorum sensing in fungi. Eukaryot Cell. 2006;5(4):613–9.
137. Williams P. Quorum sensing, communication and cross-kingdom signalling in the bacterial world. Microbiology. 2007;153(Pt 12):3923–38.

138. Cugini C, Calfee MW, Farrow JM 3rd, Morales DK, Pesci EC, Hogan DA. Farnesol, a common sesquiterpene, inhibits PQS production in Pseudomonas aeruginosa. Mol Microbiol. 2007;65(4):896–906.
139. Hogan DA, Vik A, Kolter R. A Pseudomonas aeruginosa quorum-sensing molecule influences Candida albicans morphology. Mol Microbiol. 2004;54(5):1212–23.
140. Cottier F, Muhlschlegel FA. Communication in fungi. Int J Microbiol. 2012;2012:351832.
141. Tsatsaronis JA, Franch-Arroyo S, Resch U, Charpentier E. Extracellular vesicle RNA: a universal mediator of microbial communication? Trends Microbiol. 2018;26(5):401–10.
142. Peres da Silva R, Puccia R, Rodrigues ML, Oliveira DL, Joffe LS, Cesar GV, et al. Extracellular vesicle-mediated export of fungal RNA. Sci Rep. 2015;5:7763.
143. Sjostrom AE, Sandblad L, Uhlin BE, Wai SN. Membrane vesicle-mediated release of bacterial RNA. Sci Rep. 2015;5:15329.
144. Stacy A, McNally L, Darch SE, Brown SP, Whiteley M. The biogeography of polymicrobial infection. Nat Rev Microbiol. 2016;14(2):93–105.
145. Wolcott R, Costerton JW, Raoult D, Cutler SJ. The polymicrobial nature of biofilm infection. Clin Microbiol Infect. 2013;19(2):107–12.
146. Sibley CD, Parkins MD, Rabin HR, Surette MG. The relevance of the polymicrobial nature of airway infection in the acute and chronic management of patients with cystic fibrosis. Curr Opin Investig Drugs. 2009;10(8):787–94.
147. Kim YG, Udayanga KG, Totsuka N, Weinberg JB, Nunez G, Shibuya A. Gut dysbiosis promotes M2 macrophage polarization and allergic airway inflammation via fungi-induced PGE(2). Cell Host Microbe. 2014;15(1):95–102.
148. Kozel TR, Wickes B. Fungal diagnostics. Cold Spring Harb Perspect Med. 2014;4(4):a019299.
149. Lipuma JJ. The changing microbial epidemiology in cystic fibrosis. Clin Microbiol Rev. 2010;23(2):299–323.
150. Chen SC, Meyer W, Pashley CH. Challenges in laboratory detection of fungal pathogens in the airways of cystic fibrosis patients. Mycopathologia. 2018;183(1):89–100.
151. Delhaes L, Touati K, Faure-Cognet O, Cornet M, Botterel F, Dannaoui E, et al. Prevalence, geographic risk factor, and development of a standardized protocol for fungal isolation in cystic fibrosis: results from the international prospective study "MFIP". J Cyst Fibros. 2019;18(2):212–20.
152. Botterel F, Angebault C, Cabaret O, Stressmann FA, Costa JM, Wallet F, et al. Fungal and bacterial diversity of airway microbiota in adults with cystic fibrosis: concordance between conventional methods and ultra-deep sequencing, and their practical use in the clinical laboratory. Mycopathologia. 2018;183(1):171–83.
153. Rogers GB, Hart CA, Mason JR, Hughes M, Walshaw MJ, Bruce KD. Bacterial diversity in cases of lung infection in cystic fibrosis patients: 16S ribosomal DNA (rDNA) length heterogeneity PCR and 16S rDNA terminal restriction fragment length polymorphism profiling. J Clin Microbiol. 2003;41(8):3548–58.
154. Acosta N, Heirali A, Somayaji R, Surette MG, Workentine ML, Sibley CD, et al. Sputum microbiota is predictive of long-term clinical outcomes in young adults with cystic fibrosis. Thorax. 2018;73(11):1016–25.
155. Heirali AA, Workentine ML, Acosta N, Poonja A, Storey DG, Somayaji R, et al. The effects of inhaled aztreonam on the cystic fibrosis lung microbiome. Microbiome. 2017;5(1):51.
156. Prevaes SM, de Steenhuijsen Piters WA, de Winter-de Groot KM, Janssens HM, Tramper-Stranders GA, Chu ML, et al. Concordance between upper and lower airway microbiota in infants with cystic fibrosis. Eur Respir J. 2017;49(3).
157. Whelan FJ, Heirali AA, Rossi L, Rabin HR, Parkins MD, Surette MG. Longitudinal sampling of the lung microbiota in individuals with cystic fibrosis. PLoS One. 2017;12(3):e0172811.
158. Feigelman R, Kahlert CR, Baty F, Rassouli F, Kleiner RL, Kohler P, et al. Sputum DNA sequencing in cystic fibrosis: non-invasive access to the lung microbiome and to pathogen details. Microbiome. 2017;5(1):20.

159. Carmody LA, Zhao J, Kalikin LM, LeBar W, Simon RH, Venkataraman A, et al. The daily dynamics of cystic fibrosis airway microbiota during clinical stability and at exacerbation. Microbiome. 2015;3:12.

160. Renwick J, McNally P, John B, DeSantis T, Linnane B, Murphy P, et al. The microbial community of the cystic fibrosis airway is disrupted in early life. PLoS One. 2014;9(12):e109798.

161. Zhao J, Schloss PD, Kalikin LM, Carmody LA, Foster BK, Petrosino JF, et al. Decade-long bacterial community dynamics in cystic fibrosis airways. Proc Natl Acad Sci U S A. 2012;109(15):5809–14.

162. Tipton L, Ghedin E, Morris A. The lung mycobiome in the next-generation sequencing era. Virulence. 2017;8(3):334–41.

163. Bokulich NA, Mills DA. Improved selection of internal transcribed spacer-specific primers enables quantitative, ultra-high-throughput profiling of fungal communities. Appl Environ Microbiol. 2013;79(8):2519–26.

164. Nguyen LD, Viscogliosi E, Delhaes L. The lung mycobiome: an emerging field of the human respiratory microbiome. Front Microbiol. 2015;6:89.

165. Delhaes L, Monchy S, Frealle E, Hubans C, Salleron J, Leroy S, et al. The airway microbiota in cystic fibrosis: a complex fungal and bacterial community – implications for therapeutic management. PLoS One. 2012;7(4):e36313.

166. Mounier J, Gouello A, Keravec M, Le Gal S, Pacini G, Debaets S, et al. Use of denaturing high-performance liquid chromatography (DHPLC) to characterize the bacterial and fungal airway microbiota of cystic fibrosis patients. J Microbiol. 2014;52(4):307–14.

167. Willger SD, Grim SL, Dolben EL, Shipunova A, Hampton TH, Morrison HG, et al. Characterization and quantification of the fungal microbiome in serial samples from individuals with cystic fibrosis. Microbiome. 2014;2:40.

168. Kim SH, Clark ST, Surendra A, Copeland JK, Wang PW, Ammar R, et al. Global analysis of the fungal microbiome in cystic fibrosis patients reveals loss of function of the transcriptional repressor Nrg1 as a mechanism of pathogen adaptation. PLoS Pathog. 2015;11(11): e1005308.

169. Kramer R, Sauer-Heilborn A, Welte T, Guzman CA, Abraham WR, Hofle MG. Cohort study of airway mycobiome in adult cystic fibrosis patients: differences in community structure between fungi and bacteria reveal predominance of transient fungal elements. J Clin Microbiol. 2015;53(9):2900–7.

170. Smith EE, Buckley DG, Wu Z, Saenphimmachak C, Hoffman LR, D'Argenio DA, et al. Genetic adaptation by Pseudomonas aeruginosa to the airways of cystic fibrosis patients. Proc Natl Acad Sci U S A. 2006;103(22):8487–92.

171. Chotirmall SH, Gellatly SL, Budden KF, Mac Aogain M, Shukla SD, Wood DL, et al. Microbiomes in respiratory health and disease: an Asia-Pacific perspective. Respirology. 2017;22(2):240–50.

172. Chotirmall SH. The microbiological gender gap in cystic fibrosis. J Womens Health (Larchmt). 2014;23(12):995–6.

173. Nilsson RH, Anslan S, Bahram M, Wurzbacher C, Baldrian P, Tedersoo L. Mycobiome diversity: high-throughput sequencing and identification of fungi. Nat Rev Microbiol. 2019;17(2):95–109.

174. O'Sullivan BP, Freedman SD. Cystic fibrosis. Lancet. 2009;373(9678):1891–904.

175. Schafer J, Griese M, Chandrasekaran R, Chotirmall SH, Hartl D. Pathogenesis, imaging and clinical characteristics of CF and non-CF bronchiectasis. BMC Pulm Med. 2018; 18(1):79.

176. Moss RB. Fungi in cystic fibrosis and non-cystic fibrosis bronchiectasis. Semin Respir Crit Care Med. 2015;36(2):207–16.

177. Khoury O, Barrios C, Ortega V, Atala A, Murphy SV. Immunomodulatory cell therapy to target cystic fibrosis inflammation. Am J Respir Cell Mol Biol. 2018;58(1):12–20.

178. Mahdavinia M, Grammer LC. Management of allergic bronchopulmonary aspergillosis: a review and update. Ther Adv Respir Dis. 2012;6(3):173–87.

179. Vaughan LM. Allergic bronchopulmonary aspergillosis. Clin Pharm. 1993;12(1):24–33.

180. Agarwal R, Dhooria S, Singh Sehgal I, Aggarwal AN, Garg M, Saikia B, et al. A randomized trial of itraconazole vs prednisolone in acute-stage allergic bronchopulmonary aspergillosis complicating asthma. Chest. 2018;153(3):656–64.
181. Singh Sehgal I, Agarwal R. Pulse methylprednisolone in allergic bronchopulmonary aspergillosis exacerbations. Eur Respir Rev. 2014;23(131):149–52.
182. Chmiel JF, Konstan MW, Elborn JS. Antibiotic and anti-inflammatory therapies for cystic fibrosis. Cold Spring Harb Perspect Med. 2013;3(10).
183. Cheng K, Ashby D, Smyth RL. Oral steroids for long-term use in cystic fibrosis. Cochrane Database Syst Rev. 2015;12
184. Dinwiddie R. Anti-inflammatory therapy in cystic fibrosis. J Cyst Fibros. 2005;4(Suppl 2):45–8.
185. Lai HC, FitzSimmons SC, Allen DB, Kosorok MR, Rosenstein BJ, Campbell PW, et al. Risk of persistent growth impairment after alternate-day prednisone treatment in children with cystic fibrosis. N Engl J Med. 2000;342(12):851–9.
186. Balfour-Lynn IM, Welch K. Inhaled corticosteroids for cystic fibrosis. Cochrane Database Syst Rev. 2016;8
187. Agarwal R, Khan A, Aggarwal AN, Saikia B, Gupta D, Chakrabarti A. Role of inhaled corticosteroids in the management of serological allergic bronchopulmonary aspergillosis (ABPA). Intern Med. 2011;50(8):855–60.
188. Moss RB. Treatment options in severe fungal asthma and allergic bronchopulmonary aspergillosis. Eur Respir J. 2014;43(5):1487–500.
189. Katelari A, Petrocheilou A, Doudounakis S. Is the combination of intravenous corticosteroid pulses and inhaled amphotericin a better treatment option than oral corticosteroids and inhaled amphotericin for ABPA? C108 pediatric cystic fibrosis and primary ciliary dyskinesia. American Thoracic Society International Conference Abstracts: American Thoracic Society; 2012. p. A5261-A.
190. Thomson JM, Wesley A, Byrnes CA, Nixon GM. Pulse intravenous methylprednisolone for resistant allergic bronchopulmonary aspergillosis in cystic fibrosis. Pediatr Pulmonol. 2006;41(2):164–70.
191. Wark P. Pathogenesis of allergic bronchopulmonary aspergillosis and an evidence-based review of azoles in treatment. Respir Med. 2004;98(10):915–23.
192. Wark PA, Gibson PG. Allergic bronchopulmonary aspergillosis: new concepts of pathogenesis and treatment. Respirology. 2001;6(1):1–7.
193. Wark P, Wilson AW, Gibson PG. Azoles for allergic bronchopulmonary aspergillosis associated with asthma. Cochrane Database Syst Rev. 2001;4:CD001108.
194. Ashbee HR, Barnes RA, Johnson EM, Richardson MD, Gorton R, Hope WW. Therapeutic drug monitoring (TDM) of antifungal agents: guidelines from the British Society for Medical Mycology. J Antimicrob Chemother. 2014;69(5):1162–76.
195. Markantonis SL, Katelari A, Pappa E, Doudounakis S. Voriconazole pharmacokinetics and photosensitivity in children with cystic fibrosis. J Cyst Fibros. 2012;11(3):246–52.
196. Armstrong-James D, Brown GD, Netea MG, Zelante T, Gresnigt MS, van de Veerdonk FL, et al. Immunotherapeutic approaches to treatment of fungal diseases. Lancet Infect Dis. 2017;17(12):e393–402.
197. Erratum: Omalizumab in allergic bronchopulmonary aspergillosis in patients with cystic fibrosis [Erratum]. J Asthma Allergy. 2018;11:245.
198. Beam KT, Coop CA. Steroid sparing effect of omalizumab in seropositive allergic bronchopulmonary aspergillosis. Allergy Rhinol. 2015;6(2):143–5.
199. Smith S, Rowbotham NJ, Charbek E. Inhaled antibiotics for pulmonary exacerbations in cystic fibrosis. Cochrane Database Syst Rev. 2018;10:CD008319.
200. Campoy S, Adrio JL. Antifungals. Biochem Pharmacol. 2017;133:86–96.
201. Perlin DS, Rautemaa-Richardson R, Alastruey-Izquierdo A. The global problem of antifungal resistance: prevalence, mechanisms, and management. Lancet Infect Dis. 2017;17(12):e383–e92.

202. Denning DW, Bromley MJ. Infectious disease. How to bolster the antifungal pipeline. Science. 2015;347(6229):1414–6.
203. Burgel PR, Baixench MT, Amsellem M, Audureau E, Chapron J, Kanaan R, et al. High prevalence of azole-resistant Aspergillus fumigatus in adults with cystic fibrosis exposed to itraconazole. Antimicrob Agents Chemother. 2012;56(2):869–74.
204. Fischer J, van Koningsbruggen-Rietschel S, Rietschel E, Vehreschild MJ, Wisplinghoff H, Kronke M, et al. Prevalence and molecular characterization of azole resistance in Aspergillus spp. isolates from German cystic fibrosis patients. J Antimicrob Chemother. 2014;69(6):1533–6.
205. Prigitano A, Esposto MC, Biffi A, De Lorenzis G, Favuzzi V, Koncan R, et al. Triazole resistance in Aspergillus fumigatus isolates from patients with cystic fibrosis in Italy. J Cyst Fibros. 2017;16(1):64–9.
206. Hamprecht A, Morio F, Bader O, Le Pape P, Steinmann J, Dannaoui E. Azole resistance in Aspergillus fumigatus in patients with cystic fibrosis: a matter of concern? Mycopathologia. 2018;183(1):151–60.
207. Casciaro R, Naselli A, Cresta F, Ros M, Castagnola E, Minicucci L. Role of nebulized amphotericin B in the management of allergic bronchopulmonary aspergillosis in cystic fibrosis: case report and review of literature. J Chemother. 2015;27(5):307–11.
208. Mesa-Arango AC, Rueda C, Roman E, Quintin J, Terron MC, Luque D, et al. Cell wall changes in amphotericin B-resistant strains from Candida tropicalis and relationship with the immune responses elicited by the host. Antimicrob Agents Chemother. 2016;60(4):2326–35.
209. Garczewska B, Jarzynka S, Kus J, Skorupa W, Augustynowicz-Kopec E. Fungal infection of cystic fibrosis patients – single center experience. Pneumonol Alergol Pol. 2016;84(3):151–9.
210. Mortensen KL, Johansen HK, Fuursted K, Knudsen JD, Gahrn-Hansen B, Jensen RH, et al. A prospective survey of Aspergillus spp. in respiratory tract samples: prevalence, clinical impact and antifungal susceptibility. Eur J Clin Microbiol Infect Dis. 2011;30(11):1355–63.
211. Kordalewska M, Lee A, Park S, Berrio I, Chowdhary A, Zhao Y, et al. Understanding echinocandin resistance in the emerging pathogen Candida auris. Antimicrob Agents Chemother. 2018;62(6).
212. Gauvreau GM, Arm JP, Boulet LP, Leigh R, Cockcroft DW, Davis BE, et al. Efficacy and safety of multiple doses of QGE031 (ligelizumab) versus omalizumab and placebo in inhibiting allergen-induced early asthmatic responses. J Allergy Clin Immunol. 2016;138(4):1051–9.
213. Liour SS, Tom A, Chan YH, Chang TW. Treating IgE-mediated diseases via targeting IgE-expressing B cells using an anti-CepsilonmX antibody. Pediatr Allergy Immunol. 2016;27(5):446–51.
214. Chmiel JF, Aksamit TR, Chotirmall SH, Dasenbrook EC, Elborn JS, LiPuma JJ, et al. Antibiotic management of lung infections in cystic fibrosis. II. Nontuberculous mycobacteria, anaerobic bacteria, and fungi. Ann Am Thorac Soc. 2014;11(8):1298–306.
215. Chmiel JF, Aksamit TR, Chotirmall SH, Dasenbrook EC, Elborn JS, LiPuma JJ, et al. Antibiotic management of lung infections in cystic fibrosis. I. the microbiome, methicillin-resistant Staphylococcus aureus, gram-negative bacteria, and multiple infections. Ann Am Thorac Soc. 2014;11(7):1120–9.
216. Jubin V, Ranque S, Stremler Le Bel N, Sarles J, Dubus JC. Risk factors for Aspergillus colonization and allergic bronchopulmonary aspergillosis in children with cystic fibrosis. Pediatr Pulmonol. 2010;45(8):764–71.
217. Chakrabarti A, Chatterjee SS, Shivaprakash MR. Overview of opportunistic fungal infections in India. Nippon Ishinkin Gakkai Zasshi. 2008;49(3):165–72.
218. Hong G, Psoter KJ, Jennings MT, Merlo CA, Boyle MP, Hadjiliadis D, et al. Risk factors for persistent Aspergillus respiratory isolation in cystic fibrosis. J Cyst Fibros. 2018;17(5):624–30.
219. Bird J, O'Brien C, Moss S. Risk factors for allergic bronchopulmonary aspergillosis in paediatric patients with cystic fibrosis. Arch Dis Child. 2010;95(Suppl 1):A60.

220. Sudfeld CR, Dasenbrook EC, Merz WG, Carroll KC, Boyle MP. Prevalence and risk factors for recovery of filamentous fungi in individuals with cystic fibrosis. J Cyst Fibros. 2010;9(2):110–6.
221. Vardhan V, Mulajker DS. Allergic bronchopulmonary candidiasis. Med J Armed Forces India. 2012;68(4):395–7.
222. Bernhardt A, Sedlacek L, Wagner S, Schwarz C, Wurstl B, Tintelnot K. Multilocus sequence typing of Scedosporium apiospermum and Pseudallescheria boydii isolates from cystic fibrosis patients. J Cyst Fibros. 2013;12(6):592–8.
223. Sahi H, Avery RK, Minai OA, Hall G, Mehta AC, Raina P, et al. Scedosporium apiospermum (Pseudallescheria boydii) infection in lung transplant recipients. J Heart Lung Transplant. 2007;26(4):350–6.
224. Kusenbach G, Skopnik H, Haase G, Friedrichs F, Dohmen H. Exophiala dermatitidis pneumonia in cystic fibrosis. Eur J Pediatr. 1992;151(5):344–6.
225. Diemert D, Kunimoto D, Sand C, Rennie R. Sputum isolation of Wangiella dermatitidis in patients with cystic fibrosis. Scand J Infect Dis. 2001;33(10):777–9.
226. Abdolrasouli A, Bercusson AC, Rhodes JL, Hagen F, Buil JB, Tang AYY, et al. Airway persistence by the emerging multi-azole-resistant Rasamsonia argillacea complex in cystic fibrosis. Mycoses. 2018;61(9):665–73.
227. Maertens JA, Raad II, Marr KA, Patterson TF, Kontoyiannis DP, Cornely OA, et al. Isavuconazole versus voriconazole for primary treatment of invasive mould disease caused by Aspergillus and other filamentous fungi (SECURE): a phase 3, randomised-controlled, non-inferiority trial. Lancet. 2016;387(10020):760–9.
228. Kullberg BJ, Viscoli C, Pappas PG, Vazquez J, Ostrosky-Zeichner L, Rotstein C, et al. Isavuconazole versus caspofungin in the treatment of candidemia and other invasive Candida infections: the ACTIVE trial. Clin Infect Dis. 2019;68(12):1981–89.
229. Katragkou A, McCarthy M, Meletiadis J, Hussain K, Moradi PW, Strauss GE, et al. In vitro combination therapy with isavuconazole against Candida spp. Med Mycol. 2017;55(8):859–68.
230. Wiederhold NP, Najvar LK, Matsumoto S, Bocanegra RA, Herrera ML, Wickes BL, et al. Efficacy of the investigational echinocandin ASP9726 in a guinea pig model of invasive pulmonary aspergillosis. Antimicrob Agents Chemother. 2015;59(5):2875–81.
231. Lamoth F, Alexander BD. Antifungal activities of SCY-078 (MK-3118) and standard antifungal agents against clinical non-Aspergillus mold isolates. Antimicrob Agents Chemother. 2015;59(7):4308–11.
232. Shibata T, Takahashi T, Yamada E, Kimura A, Nishikawa H, Hayakawa H, et al. T-2307 causes collapse of mitochondrial membrane potential in yeast. Antimicrob Agents Chemother. 2012;56(11):5892–7.
233. Oliver JD, Sibley GEM, Beckmann N, Dobb KS, Slater MJ, McEntee L, et al. F901318 represents a novel class of antifungal drug that inhibits dihydroorotate dehydrogenase. Proc Natl Acad Sci U S A. 2016;113(45):12809–14.
234. Gebremariam T, Alkhazraji S, Alqarihi A, Jeon HH, Gu Y, Kapoor M, et al. APX001 is effective in the treatment of murine invasive pulmonary aspergillosis. Antimicrob Agents Chemother. 2018;63:e01713.
235. McCarthy MW, Kontoyiannis DP, Cornely OA, Perfect JR, Walsh TJ. Novel agents and drug targets to meet the challenges of resistant fungi. J Infect Dis. 2017;216(suppl_3): S474–S83.
236. Arendrup MC, Jensen RH, Cuenca-Estrella M. In vitro activity of ASP2397 against Aspergillus isolates with or without acquired azole resistance mechanisms. Antimicrob Agents Chemother. 2016;60(1):532–6.
237. Nyborg AC, Zacco A, Ettinger R, Jack Borrok M, Zhu J, Martin T, et al. Development of an antibody that neutralizes soluble IgE and eliminates IgE expressing B cells. Cell Mol Immunol. 2016;13(3):391–400.

238. Harris JM, Maciuca R, Bradley MS, Cabanski CR, Scheerens H, Lim J, et al. A randomized trial of the efficacy and safety of quilizumab in adults with inadequately controlled allergic asthma. Respir Res. 2016;17:29.
239. Mastella G, Rainisio M, Harms HK, Hodson ME, Koch C, Navarro J, et al. Allergic broncho-pulmonary aspergillosis in cystic fibrosis. A European epidemiological study. Epidemiologic Registry of Cystic Fibrosis. Eur Respir J. 2000;16(3):464–71.
240. Zhao Y, Garnaud C, Brenier-Pinchart MP, Thiebaut-Bertrand A, Saint-Raymond C, Camara B, et al. Direct molecular diagnosis of aspergillosis and CYP51A profiling from respiratory samples of French patients. Front Microbiol. 2016;7:1164.
241. Geller DE, Kaplowitz H, Light MJ, Colin AA. Allergic bronchopulmonary aspergillosis in cystic fibrosis: reported prevalence, regional distribution, and patient characteristics. Scientific Advisory Group, Investigators, and Coordinators of the Epidemiologic Study of Cystic Fibrosis. Chest. 1999;116(3):639–46.
242. Sharma VK, Raj D, Xess I, Lodha R, Kabra SK. Prevalence and risk factors for allergic bronchopulmonary aspergillosis in Indian children with cystic fibrosis. Indian Pediatr. 2014;51(4):295–7.
243. Skov M, McKay K, Koch C, Cooper PJ. Prevalence of allergic bronchopulmonary aspergillosis in cystic fibrosis in an area with a high frequency of atopy. Respir Med. 2005;99(7):887–93.
244. Peetermans M, Goeminne P, De Boeck C, Dupont LJ. IgE sensitization to Aspergillus fumigatus is not a bystander phenomenon in cystic fibrosis lung disease. Chest. 2014;146(3):e99–e100.
245. Fillaux J, Bremont F, Murris M, Cassaing S, Tetu L, Segonds C, et al. Aspergillus sensitization or carriage in cystic fibrosis patients. Pediatr Infect Dis J. 2014;33(7):680–6.

Chapter 7
Nontuberculous Mycobacterium

Thomas Ruffles and Claire Wainwright

Abbreviations

ABPA	Allergic bronchopulmonary aspergillosis
AFB	Acid-fast bacilli
ATS	American thoracic society
BMI	Body mass index
CF	Cystic fibrosis
CFF	Cystic fibrosis foundation
CFRD	Cystic fibrosis related diabetes
CFTR	Cystic fibrosis transmembrane regulator
Cmax	Peak serum concentrations
CT	Computed tomograghy
CYP3A4	Cytochrome P450 3A4
DST	Drug susceptibility testing
ECFS	European cystic fibrosis society
ECG	Electrocardiograph
ELISA	Enzyme-linked immunosorbent assay
erm^{41}	Erythromycin ribosome methyltransferase
FEV_1	Forced expiratory volume in the first second of expiration

T. Ruffles (✉) · C. Wainwright
Queensland Children's Hospital, Department of Respiratory & Sleep Medicine,
South Brisbane, QLD, Australia

Child Health Research Centre, The University of Queensland Brisbane QLD Australia,
Brisbane, QLD, Australia
e-mail: tomruffles@doctors.org.uk

© Springer Nature Switzerland AG 2020
S. D. Davis et al. (eds.), *Cystic Fibrosis*, Respiratory Medicine,
https://doi.org/10.1007/978-3-030-42382-7_7

HRCT	High-resolution computed tomography
IDSA	Infectious Diseases Society of America
IFN-γ	Interferon-gamma
IgG	Immunoglobulin G
ISHLT	International society for heart and lung transplantation
IV	Intravenous
MABS	*Mycobacterium abscessus* species
MABS-PD	*Mycobacterium abscessus* species pulmonary disease
MAC	*Mycobacterium avium* complex
MAC-PD	*Mycobacterium avium* complex pulmonary dusease
NTM	Nontuberculous mycobacteria
NTM-PD	Nontuberculous mycobacteria pulmonary disease
PD	Pharmacodynamic
PK	Pharmacokinetic
PsA	*Pseudomonas aeruginosa*
RCT	Randomised controlled trial
SA	*Staphylococcus aureus*
TDM	Therapeutic drug monitoring
TNF-α	Tumour necrosis factor alpha
WGS	Whole genome sequencing

Patient Perspective

Background

JE is a 16-year-old young man with CF, with a background of homozygous F508 deletion, good nutritional status and nil chronic bacterial colonisation. He presented to the clinic with chronic moist cough, chest pain and fevers along with a decline in lung function. JE's clinical status failed to respond to conventional antibiotic therapy, and CT revealed new nodular changes and tree-in-bud opacification. Two consecutive expectorated sputum cultures grew M. abscessus subspecies abscessus. Our patient was admitted for 1 month of intensive therapy with intravenous amikacin, tigecycline and inhaled amikacin along with oral clofazimine and azithromycin. He found the treatment very challenging and struggled with significant nausea and diarrhoea during the admission. He was discharged on consolidation therapy of oral azithromycin, clofazamine and nebulised amikacin, with clofazimine subsequently being ceased due to suspected clofazimine-induced colitis. JE is mycobacterial culture negative 9 months post completion of intensive therapy. He has no spontaneous cough and his lung function has returned to baseline.

Parents' Perspective

Admission for treatment of Mycobacterium abscessus infection has been the most challenging hospitalisation that we have ever experienced. Given this time again, J says he would prefer to be sedated and woken up when it is over. Getting the nausea under control was one of the most difficult things. Initially J thought that he could manage his admission by himself, but this admission wasn't like any other, *he asked that I just stay in the room with him during the day. Although the medical staff were understanding of the difficulties he faced, many of the other hospital staff thought he was being a difficult teenager, but he was very unwell. People were sometimes unkind to him. He cried, and we were worried he was depressed. This was not a regular CF admission; he vomited every day of the 5 weeks. He struggled with having little control of his life; he was embarrassed, and felt that he had no privacy. I tried hard to get friends to visit him so he could have some timeout. I can't tell you how thankful I am to those kids who did come and visit him. After the admission we thought it would all be over, but then there were withdrawal symptoms from the anti-nausea medicines and more side effects with severe diarrhoea from clofazimine, which was one of his follow-up medications. I thought he didn't want to go to school and got on his back about it when he was actually having more side effects. I couldn't get him to engage with a psychologist, and I was really worried about his mental health. I found that focussing on future goals was really helpful, and we talked about getting fit so he could apply for the air force. He also began to play the guitar. I think this was very therapeutic for him, and he found himself a lovely girlfriend. He still feels annoyed and thinks it is unfair that he has CF and that he has to keep up treatments. As his Mum, I just wish he would do his treatments and clear this infection in the long term.*

Introduction

Nontuberculous mycobacteria (NTM) are increasingly being isolated from the sputum of patients with cystic fibrosis (CF) across a number of countries [1–6]. Over 190 species of *Mycobacteria* have been described, with the genus consisting of a diverse group of obligate aerobes that grow most successfully in oxygen-rich environments, such as the lungs.

NTM are divided into "slow growing" and "rapid growing" species. The slow growing species take 3–6 weeks to culture. *Mycobacterium avium* complex (MAC) are the most common slow growing NTM to cause lung infection and include subspecies *M. avium*, *M. intracellulare* and *M. chimera* amongst many others. MACs are genetically similar to *Mycobacterium tuberculosis* complex and are susceptible to many of the antibiotics used in tuberculosis treatment. The "rapid growing" NTM, *Mycobacterium abscessus* species (MABS), culture within 7–14 days and form a group of three recognised subspecies, *M. abscessus subspecies abscessus*, *M. abscessus subs massiliense* and *M. abscessus subs bolletii*, and are a genetically distinct group.

The proportion of NTM subtypes varies by geographical region, with MAC more common in North America and MABS appearing more commonly in Israel and Europe [2, 5, 7, 8]. Patients with MABS are often of a younger age and with lower baseline lung function [1, 5, 9–11], whilst those with MAC are older and more likely to have residual function Cystic fibrosis transmembrane regulator (CFTR) mutations [4, 10]. MABS is more prone to causing invasive NTM lung disease

(50–80% with culture positive) compared to MAC (<50% with culture positive) [2, 6, 12]. NTM has received a great deal of attention over recent years due to its association with deterioration in lung health in CF [1, 12–14]. The effect of NTM acquisition on CF patients, however, is variable; culture positivity can be transient, and even when persistent, active disease may not follow.

Prevalence and Incidence

NTM pulmonary disease (NTM-PD) is rare in the general population, with an estimated annual prevalence of 40 cases per 100,000 persons in the USA [11]. Rates in the CF population are considerably higher, with impaired mucociliary clearance, nutritional condition and the presence of bronchiectasis as likely important predisposing factors [15].

The best estimates for the prevalence of NTM-positive cultures come from longitudinal reporting through CF data registries [16–19]. In the largest studies (>6000 patients), the NTM positive culture prevalence varies widely from 2% in France [17], 6% in the UK [16] to 13% reported in the USA [18] (Table 7.1). Median age at the first positive culture from the largest data registry report (USA) is 22 years, which is higher than all the other commonly encountered CF pathogens [18].

Estimates for NTM-PD prevalence also vary widely, from 4% to 14% (Table 7.1). Whilst the American Thoracic Society (ATS) definition of NTM-PD is widely accepted [20], clear understanding of the prevalence or comparison between different populations is challenging due to significant differences in environment, frequency of sampling, culture processes and definitions of NTM colonisation, infection and disease. Accurate estimation of NTM prevalence is impeded by the absence of NTM as a notifiable condition in most countries, with Queensland, Australia and some US states as noteworthy exceptions [21].

NTM culture positivity in CF increases with age, from an estimated 10% in children aged 10 years to greater than 30% in adults over 40 years [22].

Table 7.1 Prevalence of NTM positive cultures and NTM-PD in studies since 2000

Country	Year	N	Prevalence of single NTM culture, %	Prevalence of NTM-PD, %	References
Australia	2016	3316	2.6%		[19]
France	2016	6713	1.9%		[17]
France	2004–05	1582	6.6%	3.6%	[4]
Germany	2016	1805	2.4%		[17]
Israel	2016	507	11.2%		[17]
Scandinavia	2000–12	1411	11.1%	8.9%	[6]
UK	2017	9887	6.0%		[16]
USA	2016	14,501	12.7%		[18]
USA	2000–07	829	20.0%	14%	[1]

An Increasing Problem?

The detection of NTM in studies of the general population as well as patients with CF appears to be increasing [1–6, 23, 24]. Prevalence of NTM-positive cultures in CF patients appears to be rising internationally, with longitudinal studies from Israel [5], Europe [4, 6] and the USA [1–3] reporting steady increases. The largest of these studies (16,153 people) reports a significant relative increase of 5% per year from 2010 to 2014 [3].

Improved awareness and greater surveillance and improved diagnostic methods have contributed to the increase in NTM-positive cultures [25, 26]. There is, however, evidence to support a true increase in NTM-positive cultures from studies showing a steady annual increase despite no alteration to laboratory methodology or surveillance frequency during follow-up [23] as well as elevated rates of NTM skin antigen reactivity over time in US-based population studies [24] raising the possibility of increased environmental exposure.

Environmental Exposure

Mycobacteria are ubiquitous in soil and water, forming biofilms [27]. They are found in water pipes, with their innate resistance to disinfectants causing persistence despite processing in water treatment plants [28]. Low temperature hot water systems are also implicated in NTM acquisition with temperatures $\geq 70\ °C$ required for NTM inhibition [29]. The use of showers may be associated with increased exposure with levels of NTM enriched to levels >100-fold above baseline water content [28].

Climate change could also contribute to increased NTM acquisition, with rising temperatures correlating with increased evaporation of water. The observed increase in natural disasters may also be an important factor with a notable spike in NTM-positive cultures in the general population in Louisiana following hurricane Katrina in 2005 [30].

Geographical Variation

There is a wide degree of geographical variability in NTM prevalence, with the factors underlying these observations yet to be fully defined. Multi-centre studies from France [4] and the USA [2, 31] support the concept that NTM is more prevalent in high population density areas.

Studies have shown a correlation of increased rates of NTM culture positivity in areas where humidity is higher [31–33]. A review of data from the US CF patient registry identified higher prevalence (>20%) in predominantly West and Southeast states, with significant spatial clustering of NTM detected in Arizona, Wisconsin, Maryland and Florida. Higher prevalence correlated with increased saturated vapour

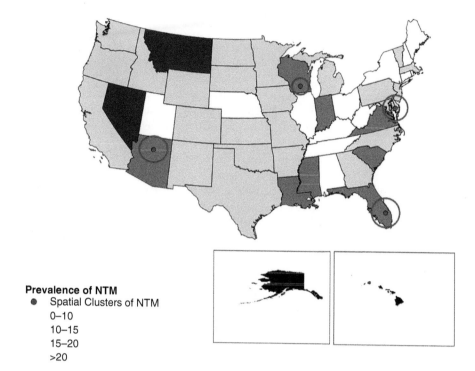

Prevalence of NTM
● Spatial Clusters of NTM
0–10
10–15
15–20
>20

Fig. 7.1 State-level prevalence and significant ($P < 0.05$) clusters of nontuberculous mycobacteria (NTM) among patients with cultured cystic fibrosis, 2010–2011. (Adjemian et al. [33]. Published with permission)

pressure, a measure of atmospheric moisture (Fig. 7.1) [33]. A study from Queensland, Australia, found the odds of NTM acquisition were 2.5-fold higher in CF patients from tropical regions as opposed to subtropical areas [32].

An innovative study combining US Medicare, census and environmental data found an association between high prevalence NTM regions, elevated income levels and raised levels of sodium and copper in the soil [3].

Transmission

It was previously thought that NTM-PD developed exclusively following environmental exposure due to the presence of mycobacterium in soil and water. However, person-to-person transmission has more recently been implicated in clinical outbreaks in CF centres [34–37].

There are a number of reports of nosocomial NTM infection clusters, predominantly from rapid-growing organisms from a variety of surgical procedures, including central venous access devices [29]. A number of outbreaks have been attributed to contaminated hospital tap water, ice machines and showers [38]. In addition, pseudo-outbreaks have been described relating to contaminated bronchoscopes [38].

The first case of possible patient-to-patient NTM spread in CF was reported in 2012 at a lung transplant centre in Seattle, with genetic analysis confirming genetically indistinguishable strains of *M. massiliense* in five patients, with the only link being overlapping clinic visit days [34]. This report has been followed by further studies supporting the concept of cross-infection of MABS in CF [35–37], with whole genome sequencing (WGS) identifying two clustered outbreaks of *M. massiliense* [36]. A subsequent international collaboration found multiple clusters of near-identical MABS isolates from varied locations, suggesting extensive transmission of circulating clones within the worldwide CF community. Estimates from this study have suggested that cross-infection may have a role in as many as 12% of NTM acquisitions [37]. There is conjecture about whether this represents dominant environmental strains that are present globally or international transmission of MABS strains between CF centres.

Prevention

While patient-to-patient spread is possible, environmental contamination through fomites and aerosols is likely to be the more common mechanism of transmission [37]. The ability of NTM to form bio-films on different surfaces could explain the persistence of NTM within the environment and healthcare facilities [39]. Molecular typing of all NTM isolates is essential if there is a possible transmission event [40].

In light of these findings, national infection control policies have been updated [40, 41] with the CF Foundation (CFF) recommending that all healthcare workers adhere to strict contact precautions (e.g. gloves and gown) when caring for patients with CF in all settings [40]. The need for meticulous adherence to robust infection control protocols in both inpatient and outpatient settings is imperative.

Risk Factors

Host Factors

Non-CF analyses have identified a cluster of features associated with NTM-PD, including increased height, low body mass index (BMI) and the presence of skeletal abnormalities, such as scoliosis and pectus excavatum [15, 42]. Malnutrition and low BMI have been associated with NTM acquisition in CF [43], underlining the importance of regular nutritional assessment and good nutritional support in optimal CF care. Prospective analyses of patients with NTM-PD found significantly elevated rates of CFTR mutations (without the diagnosis of CF) compared to population levels [15, 44].

Microbiology

Two recent large retrospective studies from the USA [8] and Europe [9] have attempted to identify potential factors associated with NTM infection. Co-infection with *Stenotrophomonas maltophilia* and *Aspergillus fumigatus* were significantly positively associated with the presence of NTM-positive cultures whilst *Pseudomonas aeruginosa* (PsA) was negatively associated [1, 8]. There is also some evidence of a positive correlation with allergic bronchopulmonary aspergillosis (ABPA) [8].

Immunosuppression

Deficiency of Vitamin D, an innate immune system modulator, has been associated with NTM-PD [45]. However, there are no studies evaluating whether supplementation affects acquisition or outcomes in NTM-PD.

A variety of immunosuppressive medications have been associated with the acquisition of NTM in the general population. Treatment regimens used in solid organ transplant as well as in solid tumour and haematological malignancies have been associated with elevated rates of NTM culture positivity [46]. Biological therapies used in the treatment of autoimmune inflammatory conditions (e.g. rheumatoid arthritis) targeting tumour necrosis factor (TNF)-α, an important cytokine in host immunity to mycobacterium, are also strongly associated with increased risk of NTM acquisition [46].

Interferon-γ (IFN-γ) has been shown to be down-regulated in patients with NTM-PD, with decreased levels correlating with more severe CT changes and reduced lung function [47]. A placebo-controlled randomised controlled trial (RCT) exploring IFN-γ adjuvant therapy in addition to standard antimicrobial treatment for MAC-PD showed encouraging results with improved symptoms, radiology and microbiology [48]. Follow-up studies have not supported these findings [49], and adjuvant IFN-γ therapy is not currently advocated by the CFF/European Cystic Fibrosis Society (ECFS) [26].

Several large CF studies have failed to show a correlation between inhaled or oral corticosteroids and NTM infection [2, 6, 9, 10], in contrast to general population data [50].

Antibiotics

Large retrospective studies have shown a clear association between the use of inhaled antibiotics and NTM-positive cultures, suggesting that targeted suppression of other bacterial species may select for NTM growth within the lung microbiome [9, 10].

The relationship between chronic macrolide therapy and NTM in CF is contentious. The increasing use of long-term azithromycin therapy, which has been shown to reduce pulmonary exacerbation frequency in CF [51, 52], has mirrored increasing NTM prevalence with concern that macrolides may encourage NTM growth. A single centre study found a strong association, supporting the hypothesis, with an in vitro mouse model showing impaired macrophage autophagic killing as a potential mechanism [23]. Whilst this finding has been supported by other reports [9], large retrospective studies have found no such correlation [8, 10, 53] as well as a large case-control analysis that found long-term azithromycin use in the preceding year to be associated with a lower frequency of NTM infections [9]. The CFF/ECFS advises that CF patients who are taking azithromycin as part of their treatment and have a positive NTM culture should discontinue azithromycin whilst further evaluation is undertaken. This recommendation is based on concerns that azithromycin monotherapy could lead to macrolide resistance [26].

Clinical

The diagnosis of NTM-PD is challenging for the CF clinician as there is a significant overlap of clinical and radiological features, with CF pulmonary disease caused by conventional pathogens, such as *Staphylococcus aureus* (SA) and PsA, as well as CF-associated conditions, such as CF-related diabetes (CFRD) and ABPA. The CF clinician should always be suspicious of NTM pulmonary disease in the symptomatic patient who does not respond to conventional therapies.

Symptoms

Symptoms of NTM pulmonary disease are varied, though most patients experience chronic cough and increased sputum production that does not respond to therapy targeting conventional CF pathogens. Other possible features include chest pain, dyspnoea on exertion and haemoptysis [25, 54]. Constitutional symptoms become more apparent with progressive NTM lung disease, including lethargy, anorexia, weight loss, fever and night sweats (Box 7.1) [25, 54].

Box 7.1 Clinical Features Consistent with NTM Infection

1. Respiratory symptoms	Cough, dyspnoea, sputum production, haemoptysis
2. Constitutional symptoms	Lethargy, fever, weight loss
3. Lung function decline	Unexplained
4. HRCT progression	Consolidation with atelectasis, peripheral nodules, cysts or cavities, tree-and-bud opacities not responsive to conventional CF therapies

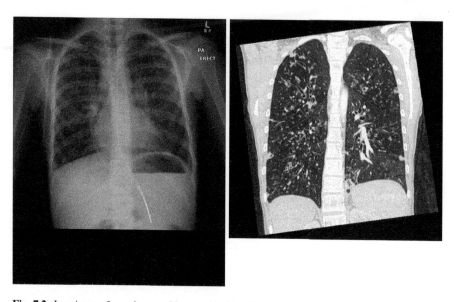

Fig. 7.2 Imaging performed on an 11-year-old girl with *M. abscessus subspecies abscessus*. CXR shows bilateral hyperinflation and extensive bronchiectasis. There is a right-sided central venous access line and nasogastric tube in situ. Multi-detector high-resolution computed tomography (MD-HRCT) shows widespread cylindrical bronchiectasis and mucus plugging. There are several areas of tree-in-bud opacification along with extensive parenchymal nodular changes with areas of cavitation

Imaging

A chest x-ray is advocated in patients suspected of having NTM-PD [55], with a retrospective study finding 77% of patients with MAC having cavitary disease distinguishable on chest x-ray [56]. High-resolution computed tomography (HRCT) is the imaging modality of choice to evaluate possible NTM lung disease [20]. Findings associated with NTM include parenchymal consolidation with atelectasis, peripheral nodules, cysts or cavities as well as tree-and-bud opacities (Fig. 7.2) [57, 58]. Whilst these findings are more frequently seen in CF patients with NTM compared to culture-negative CF controls [58], the radiographic findings are not sufficiently specific to distinguish NTM infection from other possible infective causes [57].

HRCT can assist in the diagnostic challenge of separating indolent infection from NTM disease in the culture-positive patient, with HRCT progression over 15-month follow-up strongly associated with those patients who subsequently fulfilled ATS criteria for NTM-PD [58].

Lung Function

An unexplained fall in forced expiratory volume in the first second of expiration (FEV_1) is associated with NTM-PD in patients with NTM-positive cultures [59, 60]. MABS hastens lung function deterioration when compared to NTM sputum

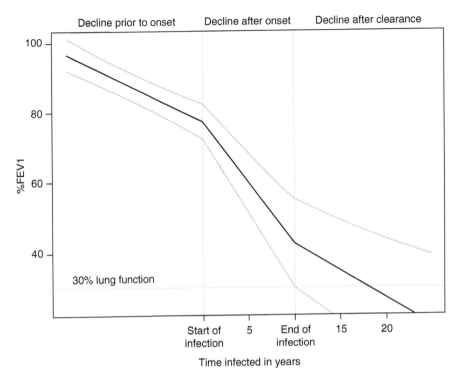

Fig. 7.3 Mean effect on lung function of *Mycobacterium abscessus* complex infection from onset and clearance of the infection in Danish patients with CF. Footnote: Trajectories plotted and held constant for a person born in the 1994–2004 birth cohorts, mutually adjusted for other co-variates in the model and extended beyond the range of the observed data to demonstrate progression to end stage lung disease. (From Qvist et al. [14])

negative controls [1, 12, 14]. A large retrospective study found that FEV$_1$ decline in the preceding 12 months was the strongest predictor of those patients that would go on to develop active NTM disease [13]. The largest study assessing NTM and lung function is a longitudinal Danish registry report that found MABS resulted in a 2.2% annual lung function decline, greater than *Burkholderia cepacia* complex (1.95%) and PsA (0.95%), with MAC infection being found to have no significant effect. Crucially, MABS clearance from sputum resulted in a significant reduction in lung function decline (1.9% improvement) [14] (Fig. 7.3).

Screening

The CFF/ECFS advocate annual NTM cultures in well patients who are able to expectorate to aid diagnosis of NTM-PD given the often insidious and non-specific nature of its presentation [26].

More regular surveillance is advocated in higher risk patients, such as those with advanced lung disease, previous NTM-positive cultures and those living in high prevalence areas [26]. Screening is important prior to consideration of long-term azithromycin therapy to prevent unintentional single agent therapy and encouragement of macrolide resistance in patients with undiagnosed NTM infection [61].

Sputum acid-fast bacilli (AFB) smear and culture is the benchmark screening method advocated [2, 4, 26]. Whilst NTM has been cultured from gastric aspirates and oropharyngeal swabs, there is inadequate data to endorse their use [26]. Serum IgG titre to Mycobacterium antigen A60 has been shown to have a high sensitivity and specificity in NTM lung infection; however, its role in screening has not been proven [62].

Diagnosis of NTM-PD

There are currently no CF-specific diagnostic criteria for NTM-PD. The CFF and ECFS [26] advocate using the American Thoracic Society (ATS)/Infectious Diseases Society of America (IDSA) criteria for the diagnosis of NTM-PD in patients with CF (Box 7.2) [20] and have developed an algorithm for the investigation of CF patients with suspected NTM-PD (Fig. 7.4) [26].

Box 7.2 ATS/IDSA Clinical and Microbiological Criteria for Diagnosis of Nontuberculous Mycobacteria Pulmonary Disease
Clinical criteria (both required)

1. Pulmonary symptoms, nodular or cavitary opacities on chest radiograph or an HRCT scan that shows multi-focal bronchiectasis with multiple small nodules.
2. Appropriate exclusion of other diagnoses

Microbiological criteria (one required)

1. Positive culture results from at least two separate expectorated sputum samples
2. Positive culture results from at least one bronchial wash or lavage
3. Transbronchial or other lung biopsy with mycobacterial histopathological features (granulomatous inflammation or AFB) and positive culture for NTM or biopsy showing mycobacterial histopathological features (granulomatous inflammation or AFB) and one or more sputum or bronchial washings that are culture positive for NTM

Modified with permission from Griffith et al. [20]

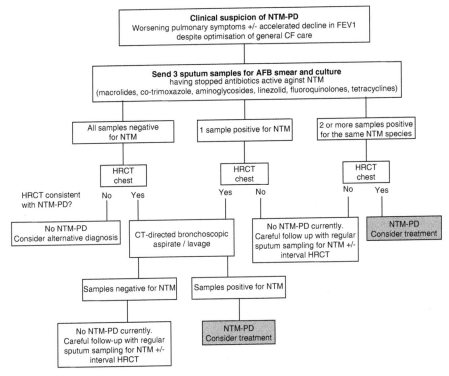

Fig. 7.4 A suggested algorithm for the investigation of individuals with clinical suspicion of NTM-PD (AFB, acid-fast bacilli; CF, cystic fibrosis; FEV$_1$, forced expiratory volume in 1 s; HRCT, high-resolution CT; NTM-PD, nontuberculous mycobacteria pulmonary disease). (From Floto et al. [26])

Clinical Criteria

To make a diagnosis of NTM-PD, a patient must fulfil both clinical and microbiological criteria with appropriate exclusion of other potential diagnoses [20]. The CF team must make a judgement to decide if the observed symptoms and radiological findings are due to NTM [25]. All aspects of a patient's CF management should be appraised and optimised, including nutrition and airway clearance, to help best evaluate the clinical importance of NTM-positive cultures along with consideration of associated conditions, such as CFRD and ABPA [26]. Common CF pathogens (e.g. PsA) should be considered as an explanation for a patient's clinical and radiological findings, and strong consideration should be given to a trial pulmonary optimisation targeting conventional CF pathogens prior to commencing treatment for NTM [26].

Microbiological Criteria

Patients should have two or more NTM-positive sputum cultures of the same species or one positive culture from bronchial wash or lavage [20]. This recommendation is based on non-CF studies that have shown that the risk of developing NTM-PD following only a single positive culture is between 2% and 14% [63–65]. The only CF focused study, a large retrospective study from Colorado, found only 26% of patients re-cultured NTM after initial culture positivity during a 5-year follow-up [13].

Expert consultation should be sought when NTM that are either rarely encountered or usually associated with environmental contamination are obtained from culture [20]. Patients who are believed to have NTM-PD but do not fulfil the diagnostic criteria should be monitored closely with regular samples obtained until the diagnosis is either confirmed or refuted [20]. If repeated sputum samples are NTM culture negative but suspicion of NTM-PD persists, then bronchoscopy with targeted sampling of suggestive areas on HRCT should be contemplated [26].

When to Treat?

Patients fulfilling the ATS/IDSA criteria should be considered for treatment. Making the diagnosis of NTM-PD, however, does not necessitate the instigation of treatment. This is an individualised decision for each patient [20], with consideration and active discussion required with respect to the burden and potential complications of treatment, along with importance of adherence due to the risk of resistance developing with partial treatment. The risks of non-treatment and of potential of treatment failure should also be explained.

It is generally accepted that CF patients with MABS-PD should commence treatment unless contraindicated [25]. However, some have argued that a careful watchful waiting approach may be appropriate for those with MAC-PD with mild clinical features and radiological changes or for those at significant risk of drug interactions or poor tolerance [65].

Treatment

There are no clinical trials evaluating antibiotic treatment combinations for new NTM-PD [66] in patients with CF. Therefore current treatment recommendations are based on the ATS/IDSA guidelines that were developed for the general population based on general experience and considerations [20] as well as the CFF/ECFS guidelines [26]. An example of typical treatment schedules for MABS and MAC is shown in Fig. 7.5.

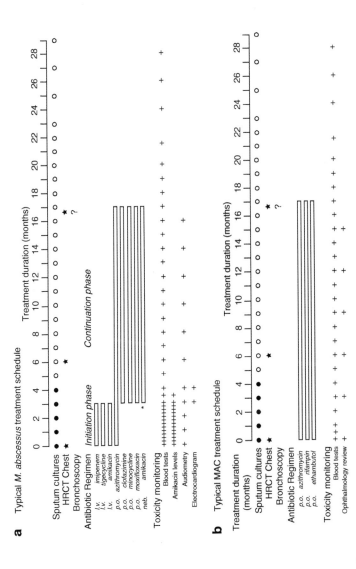

Fig. 7.5 Typical treatment schedules for individuals with CF with *Mycobacterium abscessus* or MAC pulmonary disease. (**a**) *M. abscessus* treatment is divided into an initial intensive phase with an oral macrolide (preferably azithromycin) and intravenous amikacin with one or more additional intravenous antibiotics (tigecycline, imipenem, cefoxitin) for 3–12 weeks (depending on severity of infection, response to treatment and the tolerability of the regimen), followed by a continuation phase of oral macrolide (preferably azithromycin) and inhaled amikacin with 2–3 additional antibiotics (minocycline, clofazimine, moxifloxacin, linezolid). Antibiotic choices should be guided but not dictated by drug susceptibility testing. Baseline and interval testing for drug toxicity is essential (**b**). MAC treatment (for clarithromycin-sensitive disease) should be with a daily oral macrolide (preferably azithromycin), rifampin and ethambutol. An initial course of injectable amikacin or streptomycin should be considered in the presence of (i) AFB smear positive respiratory tract samples, (ii) radiological evidence of lung cavitation or severe infection and (iii) systemic signs of illness. Baseline and interval testing for drug toxicity is essential (AFB, acid-fast bacilli; CF, cystic fibrosis; HRCT, high-resolution CT; MAC, *Mycobacterium avium* complex). (From Floto et al. [26])

Treatment for MABS

MABS are highly resistant to most antibiotics, so combination therapies are required. Conventional MABS treatment is divided into an intensive induction phase, followed by a continuation phase [26]. Given the paucity of trial data, there is wide variation in treatment regimens.

The intensive phase aims to rapidly decrease the bacterial load and usually consists of 3–12 weeks of a daily oral macrolide along with three intravenous antibiotics consisting of amikacin along with one or more from cefoxitin, tigecycline and imipenem [26]. The length of the induction phase is determined by the severity of the MABS-PD along with the response to treatment and the individual's tolerance of the regimen [26].

The continuation phase should include a daily oral macrolide with inhaled amikacin along with two or more oral agents from clofazamine, moxifloxacin, minocycline and linezolid [26]. Ethambutol and co-trimoxazole are less commonly used [20]. Treatment should be continued for at least 12 months post culture conversion [26]. It is advisable for patients to be managed by experts in the treatment of CF and NTM as alterations of therapy are often required on the basis of treatment response, side effects and patient tolerance [26].

MABS consists of the three subspecies: *M. massiliense, M. abscessus* and *M. bolletii*, with the latter two subspecies usually containing the erythromycin ribosome methyltransferase (*erm* [41]) gene, which following macrolide exposure can induce resistance [66]. Most *M. massiliense* contain a non-functional gene and thus do not develop resistance by this mechanism [67]. Inducible macrolide resistance was found to develop in 69% of patients with *M. abscessus* subspecies *abscessus* compared to none with *M. massiliense* in a large non-CF retrospective study [68]. This finding may explain the improved culture conversion observed with *M. massiliense* (88–100%) compared to *M. abscessus* (25–27%) in studies using clarithromycin-based combination regimens [43, 69].

There are a few oral antibiotics with significant in vitro activity against *MABS*, with macrolides being the only ones showing consistent activity [26]. There is debate about whether to include a macrolide in treatment regimens for *M. abscessus* and *M. bolletii* given the presence of a functional *erm* [41] gene. Drug susceptibility testing (DST) is only an adjunct to assist antimicrobial choice and does not dictate drug selection. Azithromycin is advocated for treatment over clarithromycin due to demonstrated lower rates of inducible macrolide resistance [70] as well as improved treatment outcomes in non-CF patients [71].

Challenging MABS Disease

MABS treatment failure (failure of culture conversion) is associated with macrolide resistance, *M. abscessus* and *M. bolletii* infection as well as the presence of four or more positive cultures [6, 72, 73].

Clofazimine has received significant attention, with in vitro reports showing its significant synergistic effect with amikacin [74, 75]. A recent study evaluating clofazimine in combination with other agents in a cohort of both CF and non-CF patients with high rates of refractory NTM-PD showed encouraging results, with 45% exhibiting culture conversion at 12 months [76].

Consideration should be given to trialling the addition of intravenous (IV) tigecycline and/or clofazimine in patients with challenging MABS infection [25, 77, 78]. An in vitro susceptibility study found that tigecycline and clofazimine had synergistic activity in 42% of the isolates tested when multiple drug combinations were evaluated [77].

A recent study in 21 CF patients evaluated IV tigecycline in combination with varying combinations of other IV agents as a salvage treatment for MABS [78]. Encouragingly of those patients with pulmonary disease who were treated for more than a month, 67% were considered to have improved. Unfortunately, there was no data, such as culture conversion rates or lung function, reported to quantify this. Tolerance of tigecycline was also poor, with over half the patients terminating prematurely, primarily due to significant nausea and vomiting [78].

Given the paucity of oral antibiotics with proven activity, inhaled amikacin has been advocated with a recent trial in non-CF patients with refractory MABS-predominant NTM-PD showing symptomatic improvement in 49% along with culture conversion in 18%. However, a significant proportion developed adverse effects, with ototoxicity being the most common (19%) [79]. Subsequent trials, however, have shown less efficacy [80].

Despite arduous multi-agent therapy, sustained MABS culture conversion and clearance rates are low, with less than one third of patients clearing their infection and one quarter undergoing lung transplant or dying during a retrospective Scandinavian study [6]. Treatment for MABS has, however, been shown to slow the decline in lung function with a rate similar to pre-NTM infection [14] Thus, although eradication may not be achievable in a significant proportion of patients, there may be treatment benefits, such as symptom reduction, stabilisation of lung function, radiographic improvement or smear negative status [20].

Treatment for MAC

There are very few randomised controlled trials evaluating the treatment of MAC-PD and none specifically in patients with CF. The CFF/ECFS guidelines advocate that clarithromycin-sensitive MAC-PD should be treated with a daily oral antibiotic regimen containing a macrolide, rifampicin and ethambutol [26]. The recommended treatment length is 12 months following culture conversion, with a positive culture in that time requiring a reset of the treatment duration [20, 26].

Several studies have looked at this combination in treatment of MAC-PD in non-CF bronchiectasis, some in combination with IV amikacin or streptomycin. Approximately 50% attained culture conversion at 6–12 months with mean time to conversion being 3–5 months [81–85]. A comprehensive review of a dozen studies utilising macrolide-based regimens for MAC-PD in the general population reported that despite prolonged therapy, the average clearance rate is 56% [86]. Rates of MAC recurrence are substantial, reaching 40% at 3-year follow-up [20].

A case series of CF patients receiving MAC-PD treatment reported a 91% (10/11 patients) culture conversion rate using ethambutol, rifampicin plus a variety of other agents on the basis of in vitro susceptibility testing [87]. Caution is advised in respect to the significance of these results in light of the small group size and lack of information given with respect to follow-up and recurrence [25].

Azithromycin is preferred to clarithromycin in the treatment of MAC-PD in CF patients due to its improved tolerance and reduced drug interactions. Whilst in vitro models have implicated azithromycin in impaired macrophage autophagic killing of *M. abscessus* [23], this potential disadvantage has not been evaluated in NTM-PD [25].

Challenging MAC Disease

Macrolide resistance testing is advised with all new MAC cultures, when MAC is re-cultured after eradication or following treatment failure, whilst susceptibility testing of other antibiotics has not proved beneficial in the context of new MAC infection [26]. Macrolide-resistant MAC-PD is challenging to treat, with sputum conversion rates as low as 15% [51] and a very poor prognosis, with two non-CF studies reporting 5-year survival between 21% and 53% [51, 52]. Risk factors for resistance include macrolide monotherapy or previous macrolide therapy with a quinolone [52]. Resistance rates of just 4% are recorded using the ATS/IDSA-endorsed combinations [20]. Consequently, it is recommended that macrolide monotherapy should never be used in the management of MAC-PD and that patients with macrolide-resistant MAC-PD should be managed in collaboration with experts in the management of NTM and CF [26].

Liposomal amikacin, which is hypothesised to improve drug delivery into infected macrophages as well as penetrate bio-films, was evaluated in a phase II double blind placebo-controlled randomised study [80]. It was used as additive therapy to multi-drug regimens in 89 CF and non-CF adults with refractory NTM-PD in whom MAC was the most common organism (64%). Culture conversion at 3 months was higher (32% vs 9%) in the amikacin group; however, only 2 of the 17 CF patients (11.8%) achieved culture conversion [80].

Risk factors for MAC treatment failure include macrolide resistance, cavitary disease, AFB smear positivity, poor treatment tolerance and systemic signs of illness [26, 81–83, 85]. Consideration of a 1–3 month course of IV amikacin or streptomycin along with the three drug oral regimen should be given in CF patients with MAC-PD with these risk factors [26]. Whilst there is no CF-specific data, the ATS/IDSA guidelines also recommend considering switching rifampicin to rifabutin and adding either clofazimine and/or moxifloxacin in those with macrolide-resistant MAC [26].

Ongoing treatment should be considered for patients who fail to culture convert despite optimal therapy with the aim of mycobacterial suppression and prevention of disease progression [26].

Monitoring

Clinical

Sputum cultures should be routinely performed every 4–8 weeks throughout the course of treatment to assess microbiological response [26]. HRCT chest should be performed prior to commencing treatment as well as at conclusion to monitor response, with interval HRCT scanning considered if there is a failure of culture conversion or clinical deterioration [26].

Drug Toxicity

A schedule for monitoring for drug toxicity is required prior to initiation of treatment. Regular hearing assessments and renal function screening are advised for patients treated with aminoglycosides (e.g. amikacin), whilst regular ophthalmological review is required for patients receiving ethambutol, rifabutin or linezolid with immediate cessation of therapy advised if visual disturbance occurs. Regular electrocardiograph (ECG) monitoring is recommended with the use of azithromycin, moxifloxacin and clofazimine due to the risk of prolonged QT interval [55]. Monthly full blood count and renal and liver function monitoring is also advocated irrespective of the treatment regimen [26]. A summary of commonly used medications and dosages (Table 7.2) as well as side effects and suggested monitoring regimens (Table 7.3) are endorsed by the CFF/ECFS [26].

Drug Interactions

Careful consideration should be given to potential drug interactions. The rifamycins (e.g. rifampicin and rifabutin) induce cytochrome P450 3A4 (CYP3A4) in the liver potentially reducing the serum concentration of other medications, notably the CFTR modulator ivacaftor. Simultaneous use of the rifamycins and ivacaftor is not advised [88]. In a CF patient receiving ivacaftor or lumacaftor/ivacaftor treatment, possible management options include withholding the modulator during MAC treatment or replacement of rifampicin with a different MAC agent, such as inhaled amikacin or oral clofazimine or moxifloxacin [89]. Consultation with a pharmacist is suggested to help establish potential interactions prior to starting an NTM treatment regimen.

Table 7.2 Antibiotic-dosing regimens used to treat *Mycobacterium avium* complex and *Mycobacterium abscessus* complex pulmonary disease in cystic fibrosis

Antibiotic	Route	Dose suitable for children/adolescents	Dose suitable for adults
Amikacin[a]	Intravenous	Children: 15–30 mg/kg/dose once daily Adolescents: 10–15 mg/kg/dose once daily Maximum dose 1500 mg daily	10–30 mg/kg once daily or 15 mg/kg/day in two divided doses Daily to 3× weekly dosing
Amikacin[a, b, c]	Nebulised	250–500 mg/dose once or twice daily	250–500 mg once or twice daily
Azithromycin	Oral	Children: 10–12 mg/kg/dose once daily Adolescents: adult dosing regimen Maximum dose 500 mg	250–500 mg once daily
Cefoxitin	Intravenous	50 mg/kg/dose thrice daily (maximum dose 12 g/day)	200 mg/kg/day in three divided doses (maximum dose 12 g/day)
Clarithromycin	Oral	7.5 mg/kg/dose twice daily (maximum dose 500 mg)	500 mg twice daily[d]
Clarithromycin	Intravenous	Not recommended	500 mg twice daily[d]
Clofazimine[b, e]	Oral	1–2 mg/kg/dose once daily (maximum dose 100 mg)	50–100 mg once a day
Co-trimoxazole (sulfamethoxazole and trimethoprim)	Oral	10–20 mg/kg/dose twice daily	960 mg twice daily
Co-trimoxazole (sulfamethoxazole and Trimethoprim)	Intravenous	10–20 mg/kg/dose twice daily	1.44 g twice daily
Ethambutol	Oral	Infants and children: 15 mg/kg/dose once daily Adolescents: 15 mg/kg/dose once daily	15 mg/kg once daily
Imipenem	Intravenous	15–20 mg/kg/dose twice daily (maximum dose 1000 mg)	1 g twice daily
Linezolid[f]	Oral	<12 years old: 10 mg/kg/dose thrice daily 12 years and older: 10 mg/kg/dose once or twice daily (maximum dose 600 mg)	600 mg once or twice daily

Table 7.2 (continued)

Antibiotic	Route	Dose suitable for children/adolescents	Dose suitable for adults
Linezolid[f]	Intravenous	<12 years old: 10 mg/kg/dose thrice daily 12 years and older: 10 mg/kg/dose once or twice daily (maximum dose 600 mg)	600 mg once or twice daily
Moxifloxacin	Oral	7.5–10 mg/kg/dose once daily (maximum dose 400 mg daily)	400 mg once daily
Minocycline	Oral	2 mg/kg/dose once daily (maximum dose 200 mg)	100 mg twice daily
Rifampin (Rifampicin)	Oral	10–20 mg/kg/dose once daily (maximum dose 600 mg)	<50 kg 450 mg once daily >50 kg 600 mg once daily
Rifabutin	Oral	5–10 mg/kg/dose once daily (maximum dose 300 mg)	150–300 mg once daily 150 mg if patient taking strong CYP3A4 inhibitor 450–600 mg if patient taking strong CYP3A4 inducer
Streptomycin[a]	Intramuscular/intravenous	20–40 mg/kg/dose once daily (maximum dose 1000 mg)	15 mg/kg once daily (maximum dose 1000 mg)
Tigecycline[b, g]	Intravenous	8–11 years: 1.2 mg/kg/dose twice daily (maximum dose 50 mg) 12 years and older: 100 mg loading dose and then 50 mg once or twice daily	100 mg loading dose and then 50 mg once or twice daily

From Floto et al. [26]

[a]Adjust dose according to levels. Usually, starting dose is 15 mg/kg aiming for a peak level of 20–30 µg/mL and trough levels of <5–10 µg/mL

IND investigational new drug, *FDA* Food and Drug Administration

[b]As tolerated

[c]Mixed with normal saline

[d]For individuals under 55 kg, many practitioners recommend 7.5 mg/kg twice daily

[e]Only available in the USA through an IND application to the FDA

[f]Usually given with high dose (100 mg daily) pyridoxine (vitamin B_6) to reduce risk of cytopaenias

[g]Many practitioners recommend pre-dosing with one or more anti-emetics before dosing and/or gradual dose escalation from 25 mg daily to minimise nausea and vomiting

Table 7.3 Important side effects/toxicities of antibiotics and advisable monitoring procedures for MAC and MABS in CF

Drug	Common side effects/toxicity	Monitoring procedures
Amikacin	Nephrotoxicity	Regular serum amikacin levels[a] Regular serum creatinine levels
	Auditory-vestibular toxicity (tinnitus, high-frequency hearing loss)	Symptoms, baseline and interval audiograms
Azithromycin	Nausea, vomiting, diarrhoea	Symptoms
	Auditory-vestibular toxicity	Symptoms, audiogram
	Prolonged QT	ECG
Clarithromycin	Hepatitis	Liver function tests
	Taste disturbance	Symptoms
	Inhibited hepatic metabolism of rifabutin	Symptoms
Cefoxitin	Fever, rash	Symptoms
	Eosinophilia, anaemia, leucopaenia, thrombocytopaenia	Full blood count
	Interference with common assays to measure serum creatinine	Use alternative assay
Clofazimine	Discoloration of skin[b]	Symptoms
	Enteropathy (sometimes mimicking pancreatic insufficiency)[b]	Symptoms
	Nausea and vomiting	Symptoms
Co-trimoxazole	Nausea, vomiting, diarrhoea	Symptoms
	Anaemia, leucopoenia, thrombocytopaenia	Full blood count
	Fever, rash, Stevens-Johnson syndrome	Symptoms
Ethambutol	Optic neuritis	Symptoms (loss of colour vision/acuity) Baseline and interval testing for colour vision and acuity[c] Ophthalmology opinion if symptoms occur
	Peripheral neuropathy	Symptoms; nerve conduction studies
Imipenem	Hepatitis	Liver function tests
	Nausea, vomiting, diarrhoea	Symptoms
Linezolid	Anaemia, leucopaenia, thrombocytopaenia	Full blood count
	Peripheral neuropathy	Symptoms/clinical evaluation/electrophysiology
	Optic neuritis	Symptoms (loss of colour vision/acuity) Baseline and interval testing for colour vision and acuity Ophthalmology opinion if symptoms occur

Table 7.3 (continued)

Drug	Common side effects/toxicity	Monitoring procedures
Moxifloxacin	Nausea, vomiting, diarrhoea	Symptoms
	Insomnia, agitation, anxiety	Symptoms
	Tendonitis	Symptoms
	Photosensitivity	Symptoms
	Prolonged QT	ECG
Minocycline	Photosensitivity	Symptoms
	Nausea, vomiting, diarrhoea	Symptoms
	Vertigo	Symptoms
	Skin discolouration	Clinical evaluation
Rifampin and rifabutin	Orange discolouration of bodily fluids (can stain contact lenses)	Symptoms
	Hepatitis	Liver function tests
	Nausea, vomiting, diarrhoea	Symptoms
	Fever, chills	Symptoms
	Thrombocytopaenia	Full blood count
	Renal failure (rifampin)	Blood tests
	Increased hepatic metabolism of numerous drugs	Dose adjustment of other medications/serum levels where available
Rifabutin	Leucopaenia,	Full blood count
	Anterior uveitis (when combined with clarithromycin)	Symptoms
	Flu-like symptoms polyarthralgia, polymyalgia	Symptoms
Streptomycin	Nephrotoxicity	Regular serum streptomycin levels Regular serum creatinine levels
	Auditory-vestibular toxicity (tinnitus, high frequency hearing loss)	Symptoms, baseline and interval audiograms
Tigecycline	Nausea, vomiting, diarrhoea	Symptoms
	Pancreatitis	Serum amylase[d]
	Hypoproteinaemia	Serum albumin
	Bilirubinaemia	Serum bilirubin

From Floto et al. [26]

CF cystic fibrosis, *MABS Mycobacterium abscessus* complex, *MAC Mycobacterium avium complex*

[a]Usually aiming for peak levels of 20–30 µg/mL and trough levels of <5–10 µg/mL

[b]It may take up to 3 months for toxicity to resolve following cessation of clofazimine due to its long half-life

[c]Monthly checks if receiving 25 mg/kg/day

[d]In individuals with pancreatic sufficiency

Therapeutic Drug Monitoring (TDM)

Recommended medication doses in NTM treatment are based on pharmacokinetic (PK) and pharmacodynamics data (PD) from healthy individuals. A study of PK and PD for non-CF patients with NTM-PD found peak serum concentrations (Cmax) were frequently below the recommended range for ethambutol (48%), clarithromycin (56%) and azithromycin (35%) [90].

The patient with CF may have very different medication dose responses with potentially impaired absorption and impaired gastric motility along with increased volume of distribution, metabolic rate and elimination [91]. Thus, it is quite possible that patients with CF may need higher doses of anti-mycobacterial agents.

In a single case series of ten CF patients exploring therapeutic drug monitoring (TDM), half the patients had inadequate serum concentrations for one or more commonly used drugs and one patient with persistent MAC became culture negative following dose adjustments that achieved target serum concentrations [92].

The CFF/ECFS guidelines recommend routine TDM in the use of IV amikacin or streptomycin to ensure adequate plasma concentrations as well as to minimise the risk of potential ototoxicity and renal injury [26]. TDM should also be considered in patients who are responding poorly to treatment as well as in those taking medications that can induce liver CYP3A4 enzyme metabolism (e.g. rifampicin) [26].

Non-pharmacological Treatment

Non-pharmacological treatments targeting the underlying CF lung disease, including enhanced attention to airway clearance, are vital for attempted NTM treatment, with evidence showing limitation of achieving bacteriostatic concentrations of antibiotics in mucous plugs in the airway [93]. All NTM treatment plans should involve a multi-disciplinary approach with access to medical, physiotherapy, dietetic, nursing and social care support. There should also be a focus on airway clearance, nutritional optimisation as well as conscientious screening and management of CF co-morbidities such as CFRD [91].

Surgical

Surgical management, including segmentectomy, lobectomy and rarely pneumonectomy, is used as an adjunct to medical therapy in the management of non-CF NTM-PD [72, 73, 94].

The largest study is from Alberta and comprises 69 non-CF patients, 24 of whom underwent adjuvant surgical management (most commonly lobectomy), with indications reported as localised bronchiectasis, cavitary disease and haemoptysis [73].

They report higher culture conversion at follow-up in the dual treatment group (65%) compared to the medical treatment group (39%), with the primary indication for failure to offer surgical management being extensive/multi-lobar disease. An extensive review of indications for thoracic surgery in CF suggested that lobectomy or segmentectomy should be considered with unilateral severe parenchymal localised disease, which has failed to respond to medical therapy and intensive physiotherapy [94]. In patients with CF, however, the disease is invariably diffuse, and given those with NTM are at high risk of acquiring a second NTM [13], surgical resection is very rarely advocated [26].

Failure of Treatment

Treatment failure is defined as the inability to achieve culture conversion within a reasonable period of time [20]. Patients in whom treatment fails require careful evaluation of possible contributing reasons. These include poor adherence, antibiotic resistance, inadequate dosing, poor absorption, inadequate airway clearance, other CF pathogens and co-morbidities such as CFRD [91]. If an appropriate antibiotic combination is being used, serum drug concentration monitoring may also be useful to help ensure there is adequate therapeutic dosing [26].

Transplant

All those being considered for transplant should be screened for NTM-PD and if present commenced on treatment prior to transplant listing [26]. There is understandable concern with respect to disseminated NTM in the immunosuppressed post-transplant patient. There is, however, only sparse literature based on case series with respect to outcomes for CF patients undergoing transplant with previous or on-going NTM-positive cultures [95–97].

A retrospective study from North Carolina of 13 patients who had MABS-PD at some point prior to transplant found four had recurrence of disease with three patients developing post-transplant complications. Complications included MABS wound infection, abscess and empyema. Five-year survival was 50% with no statistical difference compared to the non-NTM cohort [95]. A retrospective Danish study reports on nine CF patients (17% of total) who had NTM-PD prior to transplant, with two patients developing MABS wound infection and two patients dying of non-NTM-related complications [96].

The International Society for Heart and Lung Transplantation (ISHLT) guidelines classifies colonisation with NTM as a relative contraindication for listing as a lung transplant candidate [98], whilst the CFF/ECFS considers persistent infection should not be an absolute contraindication [26]. Progressive disease despite optimal medical therapy is seen as an absolute contra-indication [98]. A recent international survey incorporating 21 transplant centres found current infection with MABS was an absolute contraindication to transplant in 19% of centres. Persisting MABS or MAC infection despite optimal therapy was an absolute contraindication to transplant at 57% of centres [99].

Outcomes

Appropriate treatment has been shown to improve clinical symptoms as well as stabilise lung function in some patients with CF NTM-PD [13, 100]. A recent retrospective paediatric study showed statistically significant improvements in FEV_1 percent predicted trajectory and BMI trajectory in CF patients with MABS-PD that underwent treatment and cleared infection. Completion of the intensive therapy phase appears key for treatment success [100]. The rates of sustained culture conversion following initial treatment in CF patients, however, are disappointing. A retrospective study examining new onset NTM between 2000 and 2010 in an adult and paediatric centre in Colorado reported sustained culture conversion of 45% for MABS and 60% for MAC, although there was no statistically significant difference between the two [13]. In this study, MAC recurred after an average of 1.75 years.

Long-term NTM surveillance is required in CF patients who have had an NTM-positive culture. This is supported by a study that found a second species of NTM was identified in 26% of patients at a 5-year follow-up and 36% of patients at a 10-year follow-up (Fig. 7.6) [13].

The persistent presence of MABS has significant implications on morbidity and mortality in CF. Persistence is associated with a more rapid decline in FEV_1 than with any other commonly cultured organism [14] and elevated rates of transplant and death despite appropriate treatment during long-term follow-up [6]. The imperative for developing more effective treatment strategies has never been greater with encouraging evidence that clearance of MABS results in the rate of lung function decline returning to baseline levels [14].

The Road Ahead

Whole Genome Sequencing

WGS of NTM species has provided valuable insight into understanding NTM transmission as well as global NTM epidemiology [36, 37]. WGS can also be used to recognise the presence or spread of drug resistance mutations. As more NTM isolates are analysed, virulence factors will be identified which can form the basis of new therapeutic targets [89].

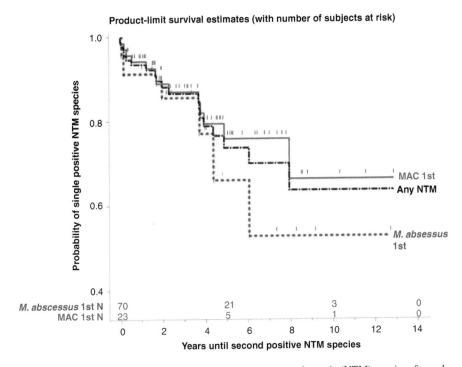

Fig. 7.6 Probability of detecting a second nontuberculous mycobacteria (NTM) species after culturing a first NTM by Kaplan-Meier analysis, separated by initial positive NTM culture species. Twenty-four percent of subjects with *Mycobacterium avium* complex (MAC) initially grew a second NTM species during 5 years of follow-up, whereas 34% of subjects with *M. abscessus* first grew a second NTM species at 5 years. Overall, 26% of subjects grew a second NTM species at 5 years, and 36% grew a second NTM species at 10 years. (From Martiniano et al. [13]. Published with permission)

Serodiagnosis

A serum antibody to MABS (anti-MABSC IgG ELISA) has been shown to be able to discriminate patients with MABS-positive cultures from those with MABS-PD with high sensitivity and specificity. The test was also able to identify infected patients prior to culture results, offering a more reliable and faster indicator of disease [101].

Immune Response

The reason why some CF patients culture NTM from their sputum transiently or persistently without developing NTM-PD while others develop progressive severe disease is not understood, but the impact of the individual host's immune system is likely to be an important factor. A recent study documented anomalies in T cell function in CF patients with past or current MABS infection, showing a marked deficiency in TNF-α production, a finding that may help guide future therapeutic interventions [102].

Therapeutic Targets

New potential treatment targets have been identified with the aim of developing novel treatments. MgtC is a known MABS virulence factor involved in bacterial survival within macrophages. Blocking this factor was protective against aerosolised MABS in the CF mouse model representing a new potential therapeutic target [103]. Gallium-based compounds may represent another potential therapeutic avenue, having been shown to effectively inhibit MABS growth by impairing iron uptake [104].

MABS produces a broad-spectrum β-lactamase $Bla_{Mab,}$ which has been hypothesised to impair the action of and explain the inherent resistance of MABS to cefoxitin and imipenem [105]. Another novel potential future treatment mechanism is through avibactam, a β-lactamase inhibitor that has been shown in vitro in macrophages and in a zebra fish model to inhibit Bla_{Mab} and improve the efficacy of imipenem against MABS [106].

Trials in Progress

Two large Colorado-based studies supported by the CFF are currently in progress. At present, there is a wide degree of variation in practise with respect to interpretation of the guidelines for NTM diagnosis. The PREDICT study will aim to develop a CF-specific, simple, evidence-based, diagnostic protocol [107]. Whilst the PATIENCE trial's goal is to create an evidence-based treatment protocol for new diagnoses of NTM in CF as well as to provide treatment outcome data [108]. The FORMAT trial is a large multinational platform trial that will evaluate outcomes in CF and non-CF patients based on the current treatment guidelines, with new waves evaluating and comparing novel treatment approaches over time [109].

Conclusion

The role of NTM in CF has received growing attention over the last decade, with compelling global evidence of increasing prevalence and a greater understanding of the pathogens' deleterious effects on lung function and survival.

Diagnosis of NTM-PD remains challenging in the CF patient, and there is an urgent need for CF-specific criteria. The management of CF patients with NTM-PD is exceedingly challenging, and treatment protocols are prolonged and burdensome for the patient and often result in a failure to eradicate the organism. International collaboration is required to provide CF-specific clinical trial data to help guide therapeutic management.

References

1. Esther CR Jr, Esserman DA, Gilligan P, Kerr A, Noone PG. Chronic Mycobacterium abscessus infection and lung function decline in cystic fibrosis. J Cyst Fibros. 2010;9(2):117–23.
2. Olivier KN, Weber DJ, Wallace RJ Jr, Faiz AR, Lee JH, Zhang Y, et al. Nontuberculous mycobacteria. I: multicenter prevalence study in cystic fibrosis. Am J Respir Crit Care Med. 2003;167(6):828–34.
3. Adjemian J, Olivier KN, Prevots DR. Epidemiology of pulmonary nontuberculous mycobacterial sputum positivity in patients with cystic fibrosis in the United States, 2010–2014. Ann Am Thorac Soc. 2018;15(7):817–26.
4. Roux AL, Catherinot E, Ripoll F, Soismier N, Macheras E, Ravilly S, et al. Multicenter study of prevalence of nontuberculous mycobacteria in patients with cystic fibrosis in France. J Clin Microbiol. 2009;47(12):4124–8.
5. Bar-On O, Mussaffi H, Mei-Zahav M, Prais D, Steuer G, Stafler P, et al. Increasing nontuberculous mycobacteria infection in cystic fibrosis. J Cyst Fibros. 2015;14(1):53–62.
6. Qvist T, Gilljam M, Jonsson B, Taylor-Robinson D, Jensen-Fangel S, Wang M, et al. Epidemiology of nontuberculous mycobacteria among patients with cystic fibrosis in Scandinavia. J Cyst Fibros. 2015;14(1):46–52.
7. Seddon P, Fidler K, Raman S, Wyatt H, Ruiz G, Elston C, et al. Prevalence of nontuberculous mycobacteria in cystic fibrosis clinics, United Kingdom, 2009. Emerg Infect Dis. 2013;19(7):1128–30.
8. Binder AM, Adjemian J, Olivier KN, Prevots DR. Epidemiology of nontuberculous mycobacterial infections and associated chronic macrolide use among persons with cystic fibrosis. Am J Respir Crit Care Med. 2013;188(7):807–12.
9. Viviani L, Harrison MJ, Zolin A, Haworth CS, Floto RA. Epidemiology of nontuberculous mycobacteria (NTM) amongst individuals with cystic fibrosis (CF). J Cyst Fibros. 2016;15(5):619–23.
10. Catherinot E, Roux AL, Vibet MA, Bellis G, Ravilly S, Lemonnier L, et al. Mycobacterium avium and Mycobacterium abscessus complex target distinct cystic fibrosis patient subpopulations. J Cyst Fibros. 2013;12(1):74–80.
11. Adjemian J, Olivier KN, Seitz AE, Holland SM, Prevots DR. Prevalence of nontuberculous mycobacterial lung disease in U.S. Medicare beneficiaries. Am J Respir Crit Care Med. 2012;185(8):881–6.
12. Esther CR Jr, Henry MM, Molina PL, Leigh MW. Nontuberculous mycobacterial infection in young children with cystic fibrosis. Pediatr Pulmonol. 2005;40(1):39–44.
13. Martiniano SL, Sontag MK, Daley CL, Nick JA, Sagel SD. Clinical significance of a first positive nontuberculous mycobacteria culture in cystic fibrosis. Ann Am Thorac Soc. 2014;11(1):36–44.
14. Qvist T, Taylor-Robinson D, Waldmann E, Olesen HV, Hansen CR, Mathiesen IH, et al. Comparing the harmful effects of nontuberculous mycobacteria and Gram negative bacteria on lung function in patients with cystic fibrosis. J Cyst Fibros. 2016;15(3):380–5.

15. Kim RD, Greenberg DE, Ehrmantraut ME, Guide SV, Ding L, Shea Y, et al. Pulmonary non-tuberculous mycobacterial disease: prospective study of a distinct preexisting syndrome. Am J Respir Crit Care Med. 2008;178(10):1066–74.
16. Trust CF. UK Cystic Fibrosis Registry 2015 annual data report. 2018.
17. Orenti A, Zolin A, Naehrlich L, van Rens J, et al. ECFSPR annual report 2016. 2018.
18. Registry CFFP. 2016 annual data report. Bethesda. 2017.
19. Rasa Ruseckaite SA, Ranger T, Tacey M, Dean J, Gardam M, Bell S, Nettie Burke on behalf of the Australian Cystic Fibrosis Data Registry. The Australian cystic fibrosis data registry annual report, 2016. Monash University, Department of Epidemiology and Preventive Medicine, June 2018, Report No 19.
20. Griffith DE, Aksamit T, Brown-Elliott BA, Catanzaro A, Daley C, Gordin F, et al. An official ATS/IDSA statement: diagnosis, treatment, and prevention of nontuberculous mycobacterial diseases. Am J Respir Crit Care Med. 2007;175(4):367–416.
21. Prevots DR, Loddenkemper R, Sotgiu G, Migliori GB. Nontuberculous mycobacterial pulmonary disease: an increasing burden with substantial costs. Eur Respir J. 2017;49(4).
22. Rodman DM, Polis JM, Heltshe SL, Sontag MK, Chacon C, Rodman RV, et al. Late diagnosis defines a unique population of long-term survivors of cystic fibrosis. Am J Respir Crit Care Med. 2005;171(6):621–6.
23. Renna M, Schaffner C, Brown K, Shang S, Tamayo MH, Hegyi K, et al. Azithromycin blocks autophagy and may predispose cystic fibrosis patients to mycobacterial infection. J Clin Invest. 2011;121(9):3554–63.
24. Khan K, Wang J, Marras TK. Nontuberculous mycobacterial sensitization in the United States: national trends over three decades. Am J Respir Crit Care Med. 2007;176(3):306–13.
25. Skolnik K, Kirkpatrick G, Quon BS. Nontuberculous mycobacteria in cystic fibrosis. Curr Treat Options Infect Dis. 2016;8(4):259–74.
26. Floto RA, Olivier KN, Saiman L, Daley CL, Herrmann JL, Nick JA, et al. US Cystic Fibrosis Foundation and European Cystic Fibrosis Society consensus recommendations for the management of non-tuberculous mycobacteria in individuals with cystic fibrosis: executive summary. Thorax. 2016;71(1):88–90.
27. Halstrom S, Price P, Thomson R. Review: Environmental mycobacteria as a cause of human infection. Int J Mycobacteriol. 2015;4(2):81–91.
28. Feazel LM, Baumgartner LK, Peterson KL, Frank DN, Harris JK, Pace NR. Opportunistic pathogens enriched in showerhead biofilms. Proc Natl Acad Sci U S A. 2009;106(38):16393–9.
29. Phillips MS, von Reyn CF. Nosocomial infections due to nontuberculous mycobacteria. Clin Infect Dis. 2001;33(8):1363–74.
30. Honda JR, Bernhard JN, Chan ED. Natural disasters and nontuberculous mycobacteria: a recipe for increased disease? Chest. 2015;147(2):304–8.
31. Adjemian J, Olivier KN, Seitz AE, Falkinham JO 3rd, Holland SM, Prevots DR. Spatial clusters of nontuberculous mycobacterial lung disease in the United States. Am J Respir Crit Care Med. 2012;186(6):553–8.
32. Sherrard LJ, Tay GT, Butler CA, Wood ME, Yerkovich S, Ramsay KA, et al. Tropical Australia is a potential reservoir of non-tuberculous mycobacteria in cystic fibrosis. Eur Respir J. 2017;49(5).
33. Adjemian J, Olivier KN, Prevots DR. Nontuberculous mycobacteria among patients with cystic fibrosis in the United States: screening practices and environmental risk. Am J Respir Crit Care Med. 2014;190(5):581–6.
34. Aitken ML, Limaye A, Pottinger P, Whimbey E, Goss CH, Tonelli MR, et al. Respiratory outbreak of Mycobacterium abscessus subspecies massiliense in a lung transplant and cystic fibrosis center. Am J Respir Crit Care Med. 2012;185(2):231–2.
35. Johnston DI, Chisty Z, Gross JE, Park SY. Investigation of Mycobacterium abscessus outbreak among cystic fibrosis patients, Hawaii 2012. J Hosp Infect. 2016;94(2):198–200.
36. Bryant JM, Grogono DM, Greaves D, Foweraker J, Roddick I, Inns T, et al. Whole-genome sequencing to identify transmission of Mycobacterium abscessus between patients with

cystic fibrosis: a retrospective cohort study. Lancet (London, England). 2013;381(9877): 1551–60.

37. Bryant JM, Grogono DM, Rodriguez-Rincon D, Everall I, Brown KP, Moreno P, et al. Emergence and spread of a human-transmissible multidrug-resistant nontuberculous mycobacterium. Science (New York, NY). 2016;354(6313):751–7.

38. Wallace RJ Jr, Brown BA, Griffith DE. Nosocomial outbreaks/pseudo-outbreaks caused by nontuberculous mycobacteria. Annu Rev Microbiol. 1998;52:453–90.

39. Sousa S, Bandeira M, Carvalho PA, Duarte A, Jordao L. Nontuberculous mycobacteria pathogenesis and biofilm assembly. Int J Mycobacteriol. 2015;4(1):36–43.

40. Saiman L, Siegel JD, LiPuma JJ, Brown RF, Bryson EA, Chambers MJ, et al. Infection prevention and control guideline for cystic fibrosis: 2013 update. Infect Control Hosp Epidemiol. 2014;35(Suppl 1):S1–s67.

41. Jones A. Mycobacterium abscessus Suggestions for infection prevention and control. Cystic Fibrosis Trust Mycobacterium abscessus Infection Control Working Group. 2013.

42. Kartalija M, Ovrutsky AR, Bryan CL, Pott GB, Fantuzzi G, Thomas J, et al. Patients with nontuberculous mycobacterial lung disease exhibit unique body and immune phenotypes. Am J Respir Crit Care Med. 2013;187(2):197–205.

43. Roux AL, Catherinot E, Soismier N, Heym B, Bellis G, Lemonnier L, et al. Comparing Mycobacterium massiliense and Mycobacterium abscessus lung infections in cystic fibrosis patients. J Cyst Fibros. 2015;14(1):63–9.

44. Ziedalski TM, Kao PN, Henig NR, Jacobs SS, Ruoss SJ. Prospective analysis of cystic fibrosis transmembrane regulator mutations in adults with bronchiectasis or pulmonary nontuberculous mycobacterial infection. Chest. 2006;130(4):995–1002.

45. Jeon K, Kim SY, Jeong BH, Chang B, Shin SJ, Koh WJ. Severe vitamin D deficiency is associated with non-tuberculous mycobacterial lung disease: a case-control study. Respirology. 2013;18(6):983–8.

46. Henkle E, Winthrop KL. Nontuberculous mycobacteria infections in immunosuppressed hosts. Clin Chest Med. 2015;36(1):91–9.

47. Cowman SA, Jacob J, Hansell DM, Kelleher P, Wilson R, Cookson WOC, et al. Whole-blood gene expression in pulmonary nontuberculous mycobacterial infection. Am J Respir Cell Mol Biol. 2018;58(4):510–8.

48. Milanes-Virelles MT, Garcia-Garcia I, Santos-Herrera Y, Valdes-Quintana M, Valenzuela-Silva CM, Jimenez-Madrigal G, et al. Adjuvant interferon gamma in patients with pulmonary atypical Mycobacteriosis: a randomized, double-blind, placebo-controlled study. BMC Infect Dis. 2008;8:17.

49. Lam PK, Griffith DE, Aksamit TR, Ruoss SJ, Garay SM, Daley CL, et al. Factors related to response to intermittent treatment of Mycobacterium avium complex lung disease. Am J Respir Crit Care Med. 2006;173(11):1283–9.

50. Chan ED, Iseman MD. Underlying host risk factors for nontuberculous mycobacterial lung disease. Semin Respir Crit Care Med. 2013;34(1):110–23.

51. Wolter J, Seeney S, Bell S, Bowler S, Masel P, McCormack J. Effect of long term treatment with azithromycin on disease parameters in cystic fibrosis: a randomised trial. Thorax. 2002;57(3):212–6.

52. Clement A, Tamalet A, Leroux E, Ravilly S, Fauroux B, Jais JP. Long term effects of azithromycin in patients with cystic fibrosis: a double blind, placebo controlled trial. Thorax. 2006;61(10):895–902.

53. Radhakrishnan DK, Yau Y, Corey M, Richardson S, Chedore P, Jamieson F, et al. Nontuberculous mycobacteria in children with cystic fibrosis: isolation, prevalence, and predictors. Pediatr Pulmonol. 2009;44(11):1100–6.

54. Griffith DE, Brown-Elliott BA, Langsjoen B, Zhang Y, Pan X, Girard W, et al. Clinical and molecular analysis of macrolide resistance in Mycobacterium avium complex lung disease. Am J Respir Crit Care Med. 2006;174(8):928–34.

55. Haworth CS, Banks J, Capstick T, Fisher AJ, Gorsuch T, Laurenson IF, et al. British Thoracic Society guidelines for the management of non-tuberculous mycobacterial pulmonary disease (NTM-PD). Thorax. 2017;72(Suppl 2):ii1–ii64.

56. Ahn CH, McLarty JW, Ahn SS, Ahn SI, Hurst GA. Diagnostic criteria for pulmonary disease caused by Mycobacterium kansasii and Mycobacterium intracellulare. Am Rev Respir Dis. 1982;125(4):388–91.

57. Martiniano SL, Nick JA. Nontuberculous mycobacterial infections in cystic fibrosis. Clin Chest Med. 2015;36(1):101–15.

58. Olivier KN, Weber DJ, Lee JH, Handler A, Tudor G, Molina PL, et al. Nontuberculous mycobacteria. II: nested-cohort study of impact on cystic fibrosis lung disease. Am J Respir Crit Care Med. 2003;167(6):835–40.

59. Fauroux B, Delaisi B, Clement A, Saizou C, Moissenet D, Truffot-Pernot C, et al. Mycobacterial lung disease in cystic fibrosis: a prospective study. Pediatr Infect Dis J. 1997;16(4):354–8.

60. Leitritz L, Griese M, Roggenkamp A, Geiger AM, Fingerle V, Heesemann J. Prospective study on nontuberculous mycobacteria in patients with and without cystic fibrosis. Med Microbiol Immunol. 2004;193(4):209–17.

61. Mogayzel PJ Jr, Naureckas ET, Robinson KA, Mueller G, Hadjiliadis D, Hoag JB, et al. Cystic fibrosis pulmonary guidelines. Chronic medications for maintenance of lung health. Am J Respir Crit Care Med. 2013;187(7):680–9.

62. Ferroni A, Sermet-Gaudelus I, Le Bourgeois M, Pierre-Audigier C, Offredo C, Rottman M, et al. Measurement of immunoglobulin G against Mycobacterial antigen A60 in patients with cystic fibrosis and lung infection due to Mycobacterium abscessus. Clin Infect Dis. 2005;40(1):58–66.

63. Tsukamura M. Diagnosis of disease caused by Mycobacterium avium complex. Chest. 1991;99(3):667–9.

64. Lee MR, Yang CY, Shu CC, Lin CK, Wen YF, Lee SW, et al. Factors associated with subsequent nontuberculous mycobacterial lung disease in patients with a single sputum isolate on initial examination. Clin Microbiol Infect. 2015;21(3):250.e1–7.

65. Koh WJ, Chang B, Ko Y, Jeong BH, Hong G, Park HY, et al. Clinical significance of a single isolation of pathogenic nontuberculous mycobacteria from sputum specimens. Diagn Microbiol Infect Dis. 2013;75(2):225–6.

66. Leung JM, Olivier KN. Nontuberculous mycobacteria: the changing epidemiology and treatment challenges in cystic fibrosis. Curr Opin Pulm Med. 2013;19(6):662–9.

67. Zelazny AM, Root JM, Shea YR, Colombo RE, Shamputa IC, Stock F, et al. Cohort study of molecular identification and typing of Mycobacterium abscessus, Mycobacterium massiliense, and Mycobacterium bolletii. J Clin Microbiol. 2009;47(7):1985–95.

68. Waters V, Ratjen F. Antibiotic treatment for nontuberculous mycobacteria lung infection in people with cystic fibrosis. Cochrane Database Syst Rev. 2016;12:Cd010004.

69. Koh WJ, Jeon K, Lee NY, Kim BJ, Kook YH, Lee SH, et al. Clinical significance of differentiation of Mycobacterium massiliense from Mycobacterium abscessus. Am J Respir Crit Care Med. 2011;183(3):405–10.

70. Cho EH, Huh HJ, Song DJ, Lee SH, Kim CK, Shin SY, et al. Drug susceptibility patterns of Mycobacterium abscessus and Mycobacterium massiliense isolated from respiratory specimens. Diagn Microbiol Infect Dis. 2019;93(2):107–11.

71. Park J, Cho J, Lee CH, Han SK, Yim JJ. Progression and treatment outcomes of lung disease caused by Mycobacterium abscessus and Mycobacterium massiliense. Clin Infect Dis. 2017;64(3):301–8.

72. Jeon K, Kwon OJ, Lee NY, Kim BJ, Kook YH, Lee SH, et al. Antibiotic treatment of Mycobacterium abscessus lung disease: a retrospective analysis of 65 patients. Am J Respir Crit Care Med. 2009;180(9):896–902.

73. Jarand J, Levin A, Zhang L, Huitt G, Mitchell JD, Daley CL. Clinical and microbiologic outcomes in patients receiving treatment for Mycobacterium abscessus pulmonary disease. Clin Infect Dis. 2011;52(5):565–71.

74. van Ingen J, Totten SE, Helstrom NK, Heifets LB, Boeree MJ, Daley CL. In vitro synergy between clofazimine and amikacin in treatment of nontuberculous mycobacterial disease. Antimicrob Agents Chemother. 2012;56(12):6324–7.

75. Shen GH, Wu BD, Hu ST, Lin CF, Wu KM, Chen JH. High efficacy of clofazimine and its synergistic effect with amikacin against rapidly growing mycobacteria. Int J Antimicrob Agents. 2010;35(4):400–4.

76. Martiniano SL, Wagner BD, Levin A, Nick JA, Sagel SD, Daley CL. Safety and effectiveness of clofazimine for primary and refractory nontuberculous mycobacterial infection. Chest. 2017;152(4):800–9.

77. Singh S, Bouzinbi N, Chaturvedi V, Godreuil S, Kremer L. In vitro evaluation of a new drug combination against clinical isolates belonging to the Mycobacterium abscessus complex. Clin Microbiol Infect. 2014;20(12):O1124–7.

78. Wallace RJ Jr, Dukart G, Brown-Elliott BA, Griffith DE, Scerpella EG, Marshall B. Clinical experience in 52 patients with tigecycline-containing regimens for salvage treatment of Mycobacterium abscessus and Mycobacterium chelonae infections. J Antimicrob Chemother. 2014;69(7):1945–53.

79. Jhun BW, Yang B, Moon SM, Lee H, Park HY, Jeon K, et al. Amikacin inhalation as salvage therapy for refractory nontuberculous mycobacterial lung disease. Antimicrob Agents Chemother. 2018;62(7).

80. Olivier KN, Griffith DE, Eagle G, McGinnis JP 2nd, Micioni L, Liu K, et al. Randomized trial of liposomal amikacin for inhalation in nontuberculous mycobacterial lung disease. Am J Respir Crit Care Med. 2017;195(6):814–23.

81. Wallace RJ Jr, Brown BA, Griffith DE, Girard WM, Murphy DT. Clarithromycin regimens for pulmonary Mycobacterium avium complex. The first 50 patients. Am J Respir Crit Care Med. 1996;153(6 Pt 1):1766–72.

82. Tanaka E, Kimoto T, Tsuyuguchi K, Watanabe I, Matsumoto H, Niimi A, et al. Effect of clarithromycin regimen for Mycobacterium avium complex pulmonary disease. Am J Respir Crit Care Med. 1999;160(3):866–72.

83. Kobashi Y, Matsushima T. The effect of combined therapy according to the guidelines for the treatment of Mycobacterium avium complex pulmonary disease. Intern Med. 2003;42(8):670–5.

84. Griffith DE, Brown BA, Cegielski P, Murphy DT, Wallace RJ Jr. Early results (at 6 months) with intermittent clarithromycin-including regimens for lung disease due to Mycobacterium avium complex. Clin Infect Dis. 2000;30(2):288–92.

85. Griffith DE, Brown BA, Girard WM, Griffith BE, Couch LA, Wallace RJ Jr. Azithromycin-containing regimens for treatment of Mycobacterium avium complex lung disease. Clin Infect Dis. 2001;32(11):1547–53.

86. Field SK, Fisher D, Cowie RL. Mycobacterium avium complex pulmonary disease in patients without HIV infection. Chest. 2004;126(2):566–81.

87. Forslow U, Geborek A, Hjelte L, Petrini B, Heurlin N. Early chemotherapy for non-tuberculous mycobacterial infections in patients with cystic fibrosis. Acta Paediatr. 2003;92(8):910–5.

88. Talamo Guevara M, McColley SA. The safety of lumacaftor and ivacaftor for the treatment of cystic fibrosis. Expert Opin Drug Saf. 2017;16(11):1305–11.

89. Martiniano SL, Davidson RM, Nick JA. Nontuberculous mycobacteria in cystic fibrosis: updates and the path forward. Pediatr Pulmonol. 2017;52(S48):S29–s36.

90. van Ingen J, Egelund EF, Levin A, Totten SE, Boeree MJ, Mouton JW, et al. The pharmacokinetics and pharmacodynamics of pulmonary Mycobacterium avium complex disease treatment. Am J Respir Crit Care Med. 2012;186(6):559–65.

91. Martiniano SL, Nick JA, Daley CL. Nontuberculous mycobacterial infections in cystic fibrosis. Thorac Surg Clin. 2019;29(1):95–108.

92. Gilljam M, Berning SE, Peloquin CA, Strandvik B, Larsson LO. Therapeutic drug monitoring in patients with cystic fibrosis and mycobacterial disease. Eur Respir J. 1999;14(2):347–51.

93. Moriarty TF, McElnay JC, Elborn JS, Tunney MM. Sputum antibiotic concentrations: implications for treatment of cystic fibrosis lung infection. Pediatr Pulmonol. 2007;42(11):1008–17.

94. Rolla M, D'Andrilli A, Rendina EA, Diso D, Venuta F. Cystic fibrosis and the thoracic surgeon. Eur J Cardiothorac Surg. 2011;39(5):716–25.

95. Lobo LJ, Chang LC, Esther CR Jr, Gilligan PH, Tulu Z, Noone PG. Lung transplant outcomes in cystic fibrosis patients with pre-operative Mycobacterium abscessus respiratory infections. Clin Transpl. 2013;27(4):523–9.

96. Qvist T, Pressler T, Thomsen VO, Skov M, Iversen M, Katzenstein TL. Nontuberculous mycobacterial disease is not a contraindication to lung transplantation in patients with cystic fibrosis: a retrospective analysis in a Danish patient population. Transplant Proc. 2013;45(1):342–5.

97. Chalermskulrat W, Sood N, Neuringer IP, Hecker TM, Chang L, Rivera MP, et al. Nontuberculous mycobacteria in end stage cystic fibrosis: implications for lung transplantation. Thorax. 2006;61(6):507–13.

98. Weill D, Benden C, Corris PA, Dark JH, Davis RD, Keshavjee S, et al. A consensus document for the selection of lung transplant candidates: 2014 – an update from the Pulmonary Transplantation Council of the International Society for Heart and Lung Transplantation. J Heart Lung Transplant. 2015;34(1):1–15.

99. Tissot A, Thomas MF, Corris PA, Brodlie M. NonTuberculous Mycobacteria infection and lung transplantation in cystic fibrosis: a worldwide survey of clinical practice. BMC Pulm Med. 2018;18(1):86.

100. Chacko A, Wen SCH, Hartel G, Kapur N, Wainwright CE, Clark JE. Improved clinical outcome after treatment of Mycobacterium abscessus complex pulmonary disease in children with Cystic Fibrosis. Pediatr Infect Dis J. 2019;38(7):660–6.

101. Qvist T, Pressler T, Taylor-Robinson D, Katzenstein TL, Hoiby N. Serodiagnosis of Mycobacterium abscessus complex infection in cystic fibrosis. Eur Respir J. 2015;46(3):707–16.

102. Lutzky VP, Ratnatunga CN, Smith DJ, Kupz A, Doolan DL, Reid DW, et al. Anomalies in T cell function are associated with individuals at risk of Mycobacterium abscessus complex infection. Front Immunol. 2018;9:1319.

103. Le Moigne V, Belon C, Goulard C, Accard G, Bernut A, Pitard B, et al. MgtC as a host-induced factor and vaccine candidate against Mycobacterium abscessus infection. Infect Immun. 2016;84(10):2895–903.

104. Abdalla MY, Switzer BL, Goss CH, Aitken ML, Singh PK, Britigan BE. Gallium compounds exhibit potential as new therapeutic agents against Mycobacterium abscessus. Antimicrob Agents Chemother. 2015;59(8):4826–34.

105. Soroka D, Dubee V, Soulier-Escrihuela O, Cuinet G, Hugonnet JE, Gutmann L, et al. Characterization of broad-spectrum Mycobacterium abscessus class A beta-lactamase. J Antimicrob Chemother. 2014;69(3):691–6.

106. Lefebvre AL, Le Moigne V, Bernut A, Veckerle C, Compain F, Herrmann JL, et al. Inhibition of the beta-Lactamase BlaMab by avibactam improves the in vitro and in vivo efficacy of imipenem against Mycobacterium abscessus. Antimicrob Agents Chemother. 2017;61(4).

107. Martiniano SL, Daley C, Ellington S, Holbrook S, Nick JA. PRospective Evaluation of Nontuberculous Mycobacterial Disease in Cystic Fibrosis (PREDICT) Trial: 298. Pediatric pulmonology. 50:304.

108. Nick JA, SS, Daley C, Ellington S, Holbrook S, Martiniano SL. Prospective algorithm for treatment of nontuberculous mycobacteria in cystic fibrosis (patience) trial: 297. Pediatr Pulmonol 2015;50:303–304.

109. Wainwright CE, Thomson R, Bell S, Grimwood K, Clark J, et al. FORMAT trial. ACTRN12618001831279p. http://www.ANZCTR.org.au/ACTRN12618001831279p.aspx.

Chapter 8
Inflammation in CF: Key Characteristics and Therapeutic Discovery

Deepika Polineni, Dave Nichols, and Alex H. Gifford

Introduction

Inflammation is a critical host response to injury, infection, and noxious environmental insults. In cystic fibrosis (CF), impaired mucociliary clearance and chronic sinopulmonary infection provide ample, sustained inflammatory stimuli. It is widely recognized that airway tissues suffer damage from products of this exuberant, persistent process (e.g. proteases, oxidants), and research has uncovered a variety of involved mechanisms and potential anti-inflammatory targets for therapeutic intervention. As current research continues to investigate whether or not the inflammatory response in CF is inherently abnormal, it is increasingly apparent that inflammation is a central feature of the pathophysiology of this disease and warrants prioritization when working to understand and preserve the health of people with CF.

This chapter focuses on pulmonary inflammation, beginning with a review of several key characteristics and mechanisms of inflammation that have been described (Fig. 8.1). We use that context to discuss a variety of anti-inflammatory strategies that have reached clinical trials in people with CF, with additional emphasis placed on those that subsequently found a place in clinical care. We consider a number of alternative therapeutic interventions that the research community is

D. Polineni
The University of Kansas Health System, Department of Internal Medicine,
Kansas City, KS, USA

D. Nichols
Seattle Children's Hospital, University of Washington School of Medicine,
Department of Pediatrics, Seattle, WA, USA

A. H. Gifford (✉)
Dartmouth Institute for Health Policy and Clinical Practice, Dartmouth-Hitchcock Medical
Center, Department of Pulmonary and Critical Care Medicine, Lebanon, NH, USA
e-mail: alex.h.gifford@hitchcock.org

© Springer Nature Switzerland AG 2020
S. D. Davis et al. (eds.), *Cystic Fibrosis*, Respiratory Medicine,
https://doi.org/10.1007/978-3-030-42382-7_8

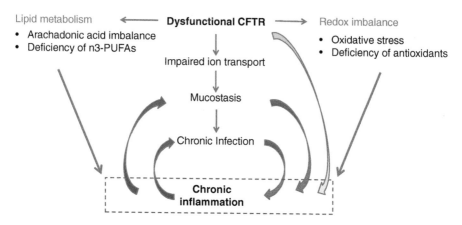

Fig. 8.1 Mechanisms of airway inflammation in CF

already testing or soon will be testing, including drugs that modulate function of CF transmembrane conductance regulator (CFTR), which may reduce inflammation through direct or indirect effects. Such candidates will change over time as new drugs are tested, and our understanding of the role of inflammation in CF continues to improve.

Mechanisms of Inflammation and Injury in the CF Airway

Oxidative stress When we consider the redox milieu of the CF airway, we must first recognize that this chemistry is normally partitioned into the intracellular compartments of bronchial epithelial and recruited phagocytic cells, the mucoid secretions and airway surface liquid (ASL) that overlie and/or contain these cells, and the plasma component of blood circulating through the lung. Multiple lines of evidence suggest that the redox balance of the entire CF lung is injuriously skewed toward oxidative stress due to excess production of oxidant compounds and a relative deficiency of antioxidant substances [1–3].

Dysfunction of Toll-like receptor-4 (TLR-4) and hypoxia-inducible factor-1α (HIF-1α) in human CF bronchial epithelial cells (CFBEs) and the lungs of CFTR knockout mice has been associated with markedly reduced activity of heme oxygenase-1 (HO-1) [4], the linchpin of many intracellular antioxidant pathways [5]. Overexpression of HO-1 in a CF epithelial cell line was shown to protect against damage by *Pseudomonas aeruginosa* [6]. HO-1 overexpression in A549 bronchial epithelial cells induced growth arrest and resistance against oxidative stress [7]. A salient question remains as to whether the antioxidant properties of HO-1 are dependent on the presence of functional CFTR. In CF macrophages, the cellular scaffolding protein caveolin-1 is required for proper membrane localization of HO-1 in order to attenuate TLR-4 signaling, but a physical interaction between CFTR and caveolin-1 was not reported in this study [8] as it was in another investigation [9] which confirmed co-localization of caveolin-1, CFTR, and *Pseudomonas aeruginosa* during bacterial internalization by CFBEs. TLR-4 signaling and internalization of bacteria are arguably distinct processes, but these reports suggest that caveolin-1 might be important to the activity of CFTR as a membrane-associated effector.

Under conditions of hyperoxia-mediated oxidative stress, CFBEs produce large amounts of interleukin-8 (IL-8) and express CXCR1/2 receptors in association with ERK1/2 MAPK and AP-1 activity [10]. This sequence of events promotes neutrophil migration. Neutrophils increase oxidative stress in the CF airway through multiple mechanisms. The first is depletion of extracellular glutathione (GSH) by gamma-glutamyltransferase (GGT) bound to the surfaces of epithelial cells and contained in sputum [11, 12]. Bronchoalveolar lavage fluid (BALF) from children with CF as young as 3 years of age was shown to contain abnormally low concentrations of GSH, and biochemical evidence of GSH consumption in the BALF samples from these children correlated with the presence of bronchiectasis on chest CT [13], both of which suggest that GSH deficiency in the CF lung is harmful. Another neutrophil-derived mediator of oxidative stress, myeloperoxidase (MPO) catalyzes the formation of hypochlorous acid (HOCl) from chloride anion and hydrogen peroxide (H_2O_2) in phagosomes [14]. A considerable body of evidence supports the hypothesis that CF neutrophils are primed to secrete large amounts of MPO and a third promoter of oxidative stress, neutrophil elastase (NE), before they enter the airway [15–17]. Disease longevity does not appear to determine these characteristics of CF airway neutrophils, as they occur in children and adults [16, 18]. The MPO activity of peripheral blood neutrophils from the heterozygous, unaffected parents of children with CF is only slightly reduced by comparison [19], which raises a question of whether the presence of any CFTR mutation informs this neutrophil behavior.

Pro-inflammatory lipid imbalance Abnormal lipid metabolism causes inflammation and injury in the CF airway. A prevailing explanation for this phenomenon is that a quantitative imbalance exists between distinct lipid mediators that precipitate or resolve inflammation [20]. Tracheobronchial secretions from people with CF predominantly contain cholesterol, phospholipids, and glycosphingolipids and are about 30% more lipid-rich than secretions from healthy controls [21]. CFTR dysfunction in human bronchial epithelial cells (HBECs) increases intracellular calcium concentration, which induces phosphorylation of AMP-dependent kinase (AMPK) [22, 23]. AMPK increases the expression and activity of Δ5- and Δ6-desaturase enzymes, which convert the n-6 polyunsaturated linoleic acid (LA) to arachidonic acid (AA) [24]. Levels of LA and another polyunsaturated fatty acid (PUFA), docosahexaenoic acid (DHA), are lower in CFBEs than in wild-type HBECs [25], consistent with CFTR-related derangements in lipid metabolism. Phospholipid-bound AA is more abundant than phospholipid-bound DHA in the tissues of CFTR-deficient mice [26]. Moreover, LA supplementation increases AA content and neutrophil infiltration in the lungs of CFTR knockout but not wild-type mice in association with IL-8, prostaglandin E_2 (PGE$_2$), and prostaglandin $F_{2\alpha}$ (PGF$_{2\alpha}$), all of which come from AA [27]. Taken together, these findings suggest that excess AA metabolites are present in the CF airway and may play an important pro-inflammatory role in this chronic disease.

A relative deficiency of n-3 PUFAs like DHA and eicosapentaenoic acid (EPA) in the CF lung is predicted to restrict the synthesis of specialized pro-resolving mediators (SPMs), which include the D- and E-series resolvins, protectins, and maresins [28]. All three classes of SPMs are derivatives of DHA or EPA [29], although maresins are synthesized by M2 macrophages [28]. Resolvin D1 (RvD1), resolvin D2 (RvD2), and maresin 1 (MaR1) attenuate the production of IL-8, IL-1β, and TNF-α and enhance the production of IL-10 in TLR-4-activated monocytes by increasing phosphorylation of glycogen synthase kinase 3β (GSK 3β) and the CREB transcription factor [30]. Resolvin E1 (RvE1) prevents neutrophils from crossing epithelial cell boundaries by inducing the expression of CD55, an antiadhesive factor, on the epithelial surface [31]. People with CF who have a higher ratio of RvD1 to IL-8 [32] or any RvE1 [33] in their sputum have better lung function than those without these findings, suggesting that SPMs influence the natural history of CF lung disease.

Lipoxin A$_4$ (LXA$_4$) is a molecule with SPM-like effects produced by HBECs and immune effector cells through AA metabolism and the actions of lipoxygenases specific to each cell type [34]. LXA$_4$ facilitates resolution of inflammation by antagonizing NF-κB activity [35], suppressing IL-8 secretion by leukocytes and bronchial epithelial cells [36, 37], inhibiting neutrophil chemotaxis [38], and promoting clearance of apoptotic neutrophils by macrophages [39]. LXA$_4$ concentrations in BALF from individuals with CF are abnormally low relative to those measured in BALF from patients with other inflammatory lung diseases [40], an observation again suggesting that factors specific to CF are responsible.

Local and systemic cytokine excess A panoply of cytokines drive the pulmonary and systemic inflammation observed in CF, and these mediators originate in multiple cell and tissue types. Prominent among the dysregulated cytokines is IL-8, a robust neutrophil chemoattractant [41] produced by bronchial epithelial cells [42] and mononuclear cells [43] and encoded by the *CXCL8* gene. *CXCL8* transcription is potentiated by NF-κB [44], which itself is regulated by complex mechanisms [45]. The contribution of airway infection to IL-8 production cannot be overstated. Pyocyanin from *Pseudomonas aeruginosa* causes wild-type HBECs and CFBEs to produce IL-8 [46]. Lipid A endotoxin from *Burkholderia multivorans* triggers IL-8 release by CFBEs [47]. Interestingly, one or more factors secreted by another CF pathogen, *Staphylococcus aureus*, dampen the IL-8 response triggered in CFBEs by *Pseudomonas aeruginosa* cell-free supernatant [48]. This observation highlights the complexities of immunoregulation in the setting of bacterial co-infection in the CF airway, which is a relatively common occurrence [49].

IL-6 is another cytokine relevant to CF inflammation. Epithelial cells produce IL-6 when pathogen recognition receptors (PRRs) encounter pathogen-associated molecular patterns (PAMPs) in their microenvironment and when dying cells express damage-associated molecular patterns (DAMPs) [50]. In the circulation, IL-6 triggers production of acute phase reactants by the liver, enhances TH17 differentiation of CD4+ T-cells, and induces conversion of B-cells into antibody-producing plasma cells [51]. Increased p38 and ERK MAPK activity in CFBEs after exposure to cell-free *Pseudomonas aeruginosa* filtrates causes excess IL-6 elaboration [52]. Treating CF pulmonary exacerbations with antibiotics reduces serum IL-6 concentrations [53–55], suggesting that lower circulating levels are associated with better health.

However, IL-6 has pleotropic, potentially desirable effects at the tissue level, which might explain why systemic IL-6 antagonism using tocilizumab, a drug approved by the U.S. Food and Drug Administration (FDA), has not found its way into clinical practice in CF. IL-6/STAT-3 signaling promotes regeneration of ciliated bronchial epithelial cells from basal stem cells [56]. LasB, a metalloproteinase produced by *Pseudomonas aeruginosa*, downregulates an IL-6-dependent epithelial repair pathway in HBECs [57]. An absolute deficiency of airway IL-6 also appears to be pro-inflammatory. A study comparing IL-6$^{+/+}$ and IL-6$^{-/-}$ mice showed that the latter population of animals had significantly higher BALF levels of TNF-α, MIP-2, and neutrophils after inhalation of aerosolized endotoxin [58]. There is a need to understand the dualistic nature of IL-6 in the lungs and what roles CFTR might play in regulating IL-6 activity.

There has been considerable recent interest in the contribution of T_H17 inflammation to the pathogenesis of CF lung disease. T_H17 cells develop from naïve T-cells through the engagement of T-cell receptors and co-stimulatory molecules and the influence of IL-1β, IL-6, IL-21, IL-23, and transforming growth factor-β (TGF-β) [59]. T_H17 cells play crucial roles during the earliest phases of infection. The IL-17 produced by T_H17 cells triggers epithelial cells to elaborate the neutrophil chemoattractant CC-chemokine ligand 20 (CCL20) and antimicrobial peptides (β-defensins, lipocalins) and to produce more tight junction proteins like claudin to preserve mucosal integrity [60]. IL-17A concentrations and numbers of T_H17+ effector cells in BALF and airway biopsies from people with CF are uncommonly high [61–63]. The potential problem with T_H17 immunity in CF is that it may operate unchecked. A number of factors, including IL-2, IL-4, IL-27, IFN-γ, the Socs3 inhibitor of STAT signaling, and specific microRNAs, negatively regulate T_H17 cells [64]. Insufficient inhibition of T_H17 immunity in CF could be associated with these factors. Conversely, IL-17 may serve a beneficial role, as it is involved in host-defense and may thus be protective during early life when persons with CF encounter a large number of foreign microbial organisms. The beneficial effect of IL-17 in early life, contrasted with detrimental effects of pro-inflammatory signaling during more advanced disease states, again highlights the complexity of selecting cytokines as therapeutic targets in CF lung disease.

Results of Anti-inflammatory Strategies in CF

Ibuprofen Ibuprofen has been studied in CF for over 3 decades. The immunologic rationale for using ibuprofen in CF is compelling because it interferes with neutrophil chemotaxis. In distinction to naproxen and oxaprozin, and only at a serum concentrations ≥ 50 μM, ibuprofen attenuates *CXCL8*-induced upregulation of the integrin CD11b on human neutrophils [65]. At high concentrations, ibuprofen inhibits activation of the transcription factors NF-κB and AP-1 [66, 67], which govern the expression of genes for numerous inflammatory mediators [68]. Ibuprofen also is an agonist ligand for peroxisome proliferator-activated receptor-γ (PPAR-γ) [69]. In the lung, PPAR-γ modulates leukocyte effector responses and promotes tissue repair [70–72] by blocking DNA sequences targeted by NF-κB and AP-1 [73, 74]. Even though ibuprofen modestly attenuates production of NF-κB in CFBEs after stimulation by TNF-α or IL-1β, it does not reduce stimulated IL-8 mRNA and protein levels [75]. Consistent with this in vitro finding, high-dose ibuprofen did not reduce sputum IL-8 in a 28-day controlled trial [76]. However, this may be more due to the variability of measuring inflammatory markers in sputum and factors related to study design, such as small sample size and short treatment period. Ibuprofen may have intrinsic antimicrobial activity at clinically achievable concentrations, although the mechanism remains conjectural [77], and it corrects F508del-CFTR trafficking in vitro and in vivo by inhibiting cyclooxygenase-1 (COX-1) [78].

The first controlled trial of ibuprofen in CF was published in 1995 by Konstan et al. [79]. In a predominantly adolescent cohort with mildly impaired lung function, these authors observed that subjects who received a daily dose of ibuprofen ($n = 41$) titrated to attain peak plasma concentrations of 50–100 μg/ml experienced a slower annual rate of decline in FEV1 and maintained higher body weight than placebo-treated subjects ($n = 43$) during the 4-year treatment period. Side effects attributable to ibuprofen in the study [79] were epistaxis and conjunctivitis. A subsequent randomized, placebo-controlled trial of ibuprofen in a similar CF population showed that ibuprofen slowed the annual rate of decline of FVC but not FEV1 [80], although this study did not reach its target enrollment. An analysis of CF Foundation Patient Registry (CFFPR) data from 1996 to 2002 revealed that the rate of decline of FEV1 among 6–17-year-old children with baseline FEV1 >60% predicted who were treated with ibuprofen ($n = 1365$) was significantly less rapid than that of 8960 children of similar age and disease severity [81]. The difference in slope of FEV1 decline between the two cohorts was 0.60% predicted per year (95% CI 0.31, 0.89; $p < 0.0001$). The most recent population-level evidence for a favorable effect of ibuprofen on lung function is a propensity score-matched cohort analysis of participants in the Epidemiologic Study of Cystic Fibrosis (ESCF) [82]. On average, FEV1 declined by 1.10% (95% CI 0.51, 1.69) per year in 775 high-dose ibuprofen users and by 1.76% (95% CI 1.48, 2.04) in 3665 nonusers. The rate of decline was 37.5% slower for users compared with nonusers of ibuprofen (95% CI 0.4, 71.3; $p = 0.046$).

Despite the aforementioned molecular and clinical arguments in support of ibuprofen use, uptake into clinical practice has been limited. A case report of renal insufficiency associated with concurrent ibuprofen and parenteral aminoglycoside use [83] and gastrointestinal bleeding exclusively from ibuprofen [81] have been reported, but a single-center study of ibuprofen use did not identify biomarker evidence of occult kidney injury [84]. In addition, there was no significant increase in acute renal failure in people with CF treated with high-dose ibuprofen based upon analyses of the CFFPR [81, 85]. In another study, nearly half of patients prescribed ibuprofen discontinued treatment because of side effects, not preference or nonadherence [86]. So is there a role for ibuprofen or other anti-inflammatory drugs in the CFTR modulator era? The topic is open for debate, but the pulmonary benefits of ibuprofen have been reproducible in multiple studies. Of note, lumacaftor/ivacaftor has been shown to lower peak plasma ibuprofen concentration by 36.4 µg/ml (relative reduction = 41.7%), which appears to reflect a significant drug–drug interaction [87]. We should consider these drug interactions, as increasing numbers of people with CF take CFTR modulators.

Systemic corticosteroids The multifaceted mechanisms and potency with which corticosteroids (GCs) quell inflammation engender them to the management of people with CF [88], but their side effects are myriad and not readily reversible, especially in the context of prolonged use. Binding of GCs to the human glucocorticoid receptor (hGR) triggers phosphorylation of hGR subunits and translocation to the cell nucleus where it not only binds to glucocorticoid-responsive elements (GREs) upstream from numerous genes but also interacts directly with transcription factors like NF-κB and AP-1 [89]. GCs affect multiple cell types in CF, which may explain the scope of their anti-inflammatory effects. The synthetic GC dexamethasone (Dex) reduces TNF-α-stimulated IL-8 secretion by CFBEs in association with reduced NF-κB and AP-1 activity [90]. However, Dex fails to suppress IL-8 production by CFBEs stimulated by NE [91]. This finding highlights the potential for GC responses to be heterogeneous. Dex reduces IL-8 secretion by CF monocyte-derived macrophages [92]. In distinction to other immune cells, neutrophils are protected against apoptosis by GCs [93], which would theoretically promote bacterial clearance in the CF airway, but this has not yet been proved.

The first high-quality evidence supporting the use of a systemic GC (prednisone) in CF was published in 1985 [94]. In this study, 45 children were randomized to 2 mg/kg of prednisone every other day ($n = 21$) or placebo ($n = 24$) for 4 years. At the end of the trial, the prednisone-treated group had better lung function and higher height and weight measurements than the placebo-treated group. Prednisone-treated patients were also admitted less frequently to the hospital for treatment of pulmonary exacerbation during the study period. Ten years later, a multicenter, randomized, placebo-controlled trial was published by Eigen et al. [95]. These investigators randomly assigned children to 1 mg/kg ($n = 95$) or 2 mg/kg of prednisone ($n = 95$) or placebo ($n = 95$) given every other day for 4 years. Lung function was variably better in the 1 mg/kg every other day prednisone-treated group than in the placebo group, but researchers observed linear growth inhibition in both prednisone arms.

Higher-dose prednisone caused abnormal glycemic control. A follow-up analysis of data from this trial [95] and from the CFFPR demonstrated that impaired growth persisted among boys but not girls who received prednisone [96]. GCs are often used as adjuvant therapy during pulmonary exacerbations [97], but this practice is not supported by data from a small controlled trial in which a fixed dose of prednisone given twice daily for 5 days did not improve FEV1 or reduce sputum inflammatory markers [98]. A larger 3-year trial of prednisone during pulmonary exacerbation is now enrolling [99].

Azithromycin Current CF treatment guidelines recommend chronic azithromycin therapy to improve lung function in those with chronic *Pseudomonas aeruginosa* infection and to decrease pulmonary exacerbations in those with and without this infection [100]. A macrolide antibiotic often used to treat acute bacterial infections, azithromycin also exerts beneficial anti-inflammatory effects. A number of studies have shed light on pathways affected by azithromycin. In a study using CFBEs, azithromycin attenuated DNA binding of the pro-inflammatory transcription factors NF-kB and AP-1 by 50–70%, an effect that was associated with reduced IL-8 gene transcription and protein levels [101]. In a murine model of chronic *Pseudomonas aeruginosa* infection, treatment with azithromycin reduced inflammation via inhibition of NLRC4 and NLRC3 inflammasomes [102]. Additional studies in CF mice homozygous for the F508del-*CFTR* mutation showed that exposure to conditioned media collected from *Pseudomonas aeruginosa* strain PAO1 cultures treated with azithromycin attenuated the inflammatory response, as evidenced by lower macrophage chemoattractant protein-1, TNF-α, and IFN-γ concentrations when compared with CF mice treated with untreated PAO1-conditioned media. This difference in response was not observed in the same treatment conditions of wild-type mice. CF versus wild-type mice have been observed to have a 1.7-fold increase in the quantity of alveolar macrophages and tenfold increase in levels of chemokine C-C motif ligand (CCL-2) [103]. Both peritoneal and alveolar macrophages isolated from F508del-*CFTR* homozygous CF versus wild-type mice showed increased M1 and M2 polarization, and treatment with azithromycin following LPS stimulation reduced inflammatory cytokine production, including IL-1β, CCL-2, and TNF-α [103]. Adding to the evidence supporting chronic azithromycin therapy, studies of azithromycin treatment in individuals with CF not infected with *Pseudomonas aeruginosa* demonstrated a reduction in serum amyloid A, calprotectin, and percent of neutrophils in peripheral blood leukocyte counts [104]. A seminal placebo-controlled study in CF which has informed treatment guidelines for azithromycin use showed that after 168 days of azithromycin therapy, FEV1 improved by 94 mL, PEx risk was reduced (HR 0.65, 95% CI 0.44–0.95, $p = 0.007$), and body weight increased by an average of 0.7 kg [105]. A recent randomized controlled trial of azithromycin conducted in a relatively young CF population showed that when it was added to inhaled tobramycin at the time of early *Pseudomonas aeruginosa* identification in respiratory cultures, the onset of subsequent acute pulmonary exacerbation was delayed [106].

Anti-inflammatory Strategies on the Horizon in CF

CFTR modulators Cutting-edge advances in CF treatment include development and FDA approval of CFTR modulators that provide potentiation (ivacaftor; VX-770) or correction (lumacaftor, tezacaftor; VX-809, VX-661, respectively) of mutant CFTR. Use of such therapies is applied singularly or in combination, specific to *CFTR* genotype and its resulting protein defect. While the aim of such therapies is to correct the underlying defect in mutant CFTR, there is current evidence that modulation of CFTR influences inflammation. In vitro studies of CFTR modulators applied to F508del homozygous monocyte-derived macrophages (MDMs) demonstrate mixed effects on inflammatory responses. Although treatment with lumacaftor restored CF MDM bacterial killing and phagocytosis of *Pseudomonas aeruginosa* to nonCF MDM levels, co-treatment with ivacaftor decreased bactericidal and phagocytic effects. Ivacaftor alone, as well as the combination of ivacaftor/lumacaftor, was shown to decrease pro-inflammatory cytokine secretion, including IL-6, IL-8, TNF-α, IFN-γ, and GM-CSF [107]. Early published data of the effects of CFTR modulator on inflammatory signaling in vivo did not show similar reductions in inflammatory cytokines. The GOAL Study was a trial designed to measure clinical effectiveness of ivacaftor in those with G551D. Fourteen participants across five study sites who were part of a substudy focused on inflammatory effects yielded paired induced sputum before and after ivacaftor therapy for analysis. In this cohort (eight males, mean age 27 ± years, mean FEV1 84%pred (± 23%pred) at baseline), induced sputa showed no significant changes in sputum inflammatory markers, including free neutrophil elastase activity, IL-1β, IL-6, IL-8, alpha-1-antitrypsin, and secretory leukocyte protease inhibitory, despite participants maintaining FEV1 improvements and sweat chloride reductions representative of the overall study cohort [108]. In contrast, a single-center study of 12 subjects treated with ivacaftor and followed for 2 years showed that in those participants infected with *Pseudomonas aeruginosa,* spontaneously expectorated sputum showed rapid reductions in NE, IL-8 and IL-1β, with persistent decline (at least tenfold) by day 600, yet high levels of inflammation persisted [109]. The differences in these in vivo studies are several, ranging from baseline characteristics of *Pseudomonas aeruginosa* infection, method of sputum production (induced vs spontaneously expectorated), length of follow-up, and specimen processing (including freeze thaw cycles that may influence some cytokine assays). These differences, and the differing results between studies, emphasize the need for additional work to determine whether and how CFTR modulator drugs affect pulmonary inflammation. While the current evidence for CFTR modulator effects on inflammation remains uncertain, these studies clearly defined that abnormal inflammation persists in CF, even in persons clinically responsive to modulator treatment. The logic of this premise is underscored by the presence of chronic inflammation in non-CF bronchiectasis, wherein CFTR protein remains functional. Thus, clinical trials testing new anti-inflammatory therapies are on the horizon for improving health in CF. Here, we outline studies of anti-inflammatory agents currently under investigation in CF.

Inhaled lactoferrin and hypothiocyanite Lactoferrin (Lf) is a highly conserved glycoprotein which has canonically been discussed with respect to its ability to chelate iron; however, it also mitigates oxidative stress and tissue damage at mucosal boundaries through immunomodulation [110]. In a model of intracellular invasion of human CFBE cells by *Pseudomonas aeruginosa*, bovine lactoferrin (bLf) significantly reduced infection-related production of IL-6, IL-1β, and IL-8, thus implicating Lf as an anti-inflammatory factor in the CF airway [111]. Lf is degraded by proteolysis in the CF airway [112], which is predicted to be deleterious to the host, but no study has associated low sputum Lf with CF disease severity and/or acuity. Hypothiocyanite (OSCN-) is an antimicrobial molecule produced by HBECs from hydrogen peroxide (H_2O_2) and thiocyanate (SCN-) contained in airway surface liquid [113]. This host defense mechanism is defective in CF airway epithelial cells, and preclinical models suggest that SCN- supplementation alone may be beneficial [114–117]. Lower SCN- concentration in upper airway secretions has been correlated with worse lung function in people with CF [118] highlighting the clinical relevance of inadequate OSCN- generation in the airway. Combining Lf with OSCN- for inhalation holds promise as a novel anti-inflammatory strategy in CF. Biofilm formation by laboratory and clinical *Pseudomonas aeruginosa* strains in co-culture with CF bronchial epithelial cells was inhibited by ALX-109, a combination of Lf and OSCN- formulated for inhalation [119]. This evidence suggests a potential anti-infective role for ALX-109 as well. A first-in-human dose-escalation study of inhaled Lf-OSCN- is currently underway [120].

Cannabinoid receptor agonists Ajulemic acid (AJA, JBT-101, anabasum, lenabasum) is a synthetic cannabinoid (CB) similar in structure to Δ^9-THC but sparing psychoactive properties. Lenabasum is a preferential agonist of the CB2 receptor and thus exerts a variety of anti-inflammatory and anti-fibrotic functions, without exerting central nervous system activity [121]. A number of in vitro and animal studies have demonstrated that lenabasum decreases production of IL-1β in synovial fluid monocytes, induces T-cell apoptosis, and increases COX-2 expression and production of LXA_4 by human synovial fibroblasts [122]. In studies focusing on the respiratory system, anabasum reduced TNF-α and IL-6 production from primary lung macrophages stimulated with *Pseudomonas aeruginosa* lipopolysaccharide (LPS) even when the drug was applied concomitantly or after LPS exposure [123]. In persons with CF, a phase 2, double-blind, placebo-controlled trial of lenabasum at various doses for 16 weeks in adults ($n = 85$) demonstrated reductions in not only sputum inflammatory mediator and cell counts but also pulmonary exacerbation frequency [124, 125]. Accordingly, a multicenter phase 2, double-blind, placebo-controlled study assessing the efficacy and safety of lenabasum in patients with CF ≥12 years of age is currently enrolling with a goal of randomizing 415 subjects [126].

Leukotriene antagonism Leukotriene B4 (LTB_4) is produced by the action of leukotriene A_4 hydrolase (LTA_4H) on the arachidonic acid metabolite LTA_4 [127]. LTB_4 secreted by neutrophils in response to formyl peptides from bacteria and necrotic cells is a potent secondary neutrophil chemoattractant and is involved in cell signaling over long distances [128]. In an epithelial monolayer culture model of airway transmigration by neutrophils collected from the peripheral blood of people with CF, inhibition of LTA_4H by acebilustat (CTX 4430) reduced apical (i.e., airway) neutrophil accumulation at 2, 10, and 18 hours after basolateral application; however, acebilustat did not prevent the activation of apical transmigrated neutrophils in response to CF sputum supernatant [17]. A phase I study of acebilustat in 17 subjects with CF with mild to moderate pulmonary disease demonstrated that a daily dose of 100 mg taken for 15 days reduced sputum neutrophil counts by 65% over baseline values [129]. Sputum elastase was also decreased over placebo, and C-reactive protein (CRP) was favorably affected, though not significantly reduced, and the drug was safely tolerated. An early phase II study of 71 persons with CF showed that 49% of people with CF treated with acebilustat were exacerbation free over 48 weeks, compared to 25% of people with CF treated with placebo. This effect accentuated in the portion of participants taking CFTR modulators, wherein 59% of those on modulator therapy were exacerbation free over 48 weeks compared with 22% on placebo. These findings have led to the conduct of ongoing broader phase II studies to determine clinical endpoints, including absolute change in percent-predicted FEV1, reduction in pulmonary exacerbation rates, and time to first pulmonary exacerbation, as well as inflammatory biomarkers [130].

Oral fenretinide At the time of this review, LAU-7B, or oral fenretinide, is the newest anti-inflammatory therapy under clinical trial investigation to determine improvement in inflammatory biomarker and clinical endpoints in adults with CF [131]. LAU-7B works to modify airway lipid metabolism so that epithelial cells produce anti-inflammatory DHA in lieu of pro-inflammatory AA mediators. In CF, DHA-mediated resolution of inflammation may wane, thus contributing to unchecked, exaggerated inflammatory responses that culminate in fibrosis. LAU-7B activates the DHA pathway, thereby triggering endogenous resolution of inflammation, without invoking immunosuppression. Recent in vitro studies of CF airway epithelial cells treated with VX-809 have shown that addition of LAU-7B improves CFTR (WT & F508del) functional responses with improved membrane localization and improved CFTR-dependent current across polarized airway epithelial cells [132]. This stabilization of CFTR depends on membrane lipid composition and emphasizes the relationship between inflammation and CFTR membrane distribution.

We summarize the aforementioned anti-inflammatory therapies in Table 8.1. While these and other anti-inflammatory therapies promise to hasten the resolution of inflammatory responses in CF via manipulation of endogenous anti-inflammatory pathways, additional studies are needed. Importantly, current trials of anti-inflammatory therapies suggest a complementary interplay between CFTR modulation and anti-inflammatory treatment, in which improving the inflammatory milieu may in fact augment the efficacy of CFTR modulators. This indicates a greater rather than a lesser role for anti-inflammatory interventions in the era of improved, but not fully restored, CFTR function.

Table 8.1 Examples of mainstream and investigational anti-inflammatory therapies in cystic fibrosis

Therapy	Availability to patients	Target pathway
Corticosteroids	Approved, not indicated	Activation of glucocorticoid receptors
Ibuprofen	Recommended for 6–17 year old children with CF	Antagonism of NF-κB (at high concentrations)
Azithromycin	FDA approved	Under investigation
CFTR modulator therapies	FDA approved; phase 3 studies; preclinical studies (*dependent upon CFTR mutation*)	Correcting underlying defective CFTR
Lactoferrin	Preclinical studies	Iron sequestration
Hypothiocyanite	Phase 1 studies	Endogenous microbicidal activity
Anabasum/ Lenabasum	Phase 3 studies	Cannabinoid (CB2) receptor agonism
Acebilustat	Phase 3 studies	Leukotriene B4 (LTB4) antagonism
Fenretinide	Phase 2 studies	Docosahexaenoic pathway agonism

Conclusion

The inflammatory host response in CF is complex and not easily manipulated in ways that minimize damage to healthy tissues yet ensure adequate host defense against chronic pathogenic infections. It is challenging in clinical practice to identify individuals with CF whose health is more dramatically undermined by uncontrolled inflammation than that of others. However, recent transcriptomic analyses of airway (i.e., nasal) epithelial cells from individuals with CF have identified associations between heritable patterns of increased inflammatory gene expression and lung disease severity [133]. Despite significant progress in the field of inflammation research in CF, key questions remain, including the nature of the connection between inflammation and CFTR dysfunction, the role of mucociliary impairment and retained airway debris, and the primacy of bacterial or other infectious agents in driving this host response. A few anti-inflammatory drugs are able to reduce inflammation and preserve pulmonary health without worsening infection, and one hopes that novel approaches under development may do so with greater effectiveness, tolerability, and long-term safety.

The current era of CFTR modulation through drug therapy is an exciting opportunity to not only improve outcomes for people with CF but also to better understand inflammation as a central feature of this disease. That said, untangling whether the anti-inflammatory benefits of modulator drugs are direct or indirect may be challenging, and results thus far indicate that a robust inflammatory state dominated by neutrophils may persist in the airways. To what degree longer use or early introduction of these agents may reduce or even eliminate some of the key pathological features of CF lung disease is yet unknown. This is an encouraging prospect to consider, and one hopes that even if CFTR modulators do not normalize the airway environment, they may work in concert with other therapies, including anti-inflammatory drugs, to benefit patients.

References

1. Ziady AG, Hansen J. Redox balance in cystic fibrosis. Int J Biochem Cell Biol. 2014;52: 113–23.
2. Wetmore DR, Joseloff E, Pilewski J, Lee DP, Lawton KA, Mitchell MW, et al. Metabolomic profiling reveals biochemical pathways and biomarkers associated with pathogenesis in cystic fibrosis cells. J Biol Chem. 2010;285(40):30516–22.
3. Roum JH, Buhl R, McElvaney NG, Borok Z, Crystal RG. Systemic deficiency of glutathione in cystic fibrosis. J Appl Physiol (1985). 1993;75(6):2419–24.
4. Chillappagari S, Venkatesan S, Garapati V, Mahavadi P, Munder A, Seubert A, et al. Impaired TLR4 and HIF expression in cystic fibrosis bronchial epithelial cells downregulates heme-oxygenase-1 and alters iron homeostasis in vitro. Am J Physiol Lung Cell Mol Physiol. 2014;307(10):L791–9.
5. Ryter SW, Choi AM. Heme oxygenase-1: redox regulation of a stress protein in lung and cell culture models. Antioxid Redox Signal. 2005;7(1–2):80–91.
6. Zhou H, Lu F, Latham C, Zander DS, Visner GA. Heme oxygenase-1 expression in human lungs with cystic fibrosis and cytoprotective effects against Pseudomonas aeruginosa in vitro. Am J Respir Crit Care Med. 2004;170(6):633–40.
7. Lee PJ, Alam J, Wiegand GW, Choi AM. Overexpression of heme oxygenase-1 in human pulmonary epithelial cells results in cell growth arrest and increased resistance to hyperoxia. Proc Natl Acad Sci U S A. 1996;93(19):10393–8.
8. Zhang PX, Murray TS, Villella VR, Ferrari E, Esposito S, D'Souza A, et al. Reduced caveolin-1 promotes hyperinflammation due to abnormal heme oxygenase-1 localization in lipopolysaccharide-challenged macrophages with dysfunctional cystic fibrosis transmembrane conductance regulator. J Immunol. 2013;190(10):5196–206.
9. Bajmoczi M, Gadjeva M, Alper SL, Pier GB, Golan DE. Cystic fibrosis transmembrane conductance regulator and caveolin-1 regulate epithelial cell internalization of Pseudomonas aeruginosa. Am J Physiol Cell Physiol. 2009;297(2):C263–77.
10. Boncoeur E, Criq VS, Bonvin E, Roque T, Henrion-Caude A, Gruenert DC, et al. Oxidative stress induces extracellular signal-regulated kinase 1/2 mitogen-activated protein kinase in cystic fibrosis lung epithelial cells: potential mechanism for excessive IL-8 expression. Int J Biochem Cell Biol. 2008;40(3):432–46.
11. Corti A, Franzini M, Cianchetti S, Bergamini G, Lorenzini E, Melotti P, et al. Contribution by polymorphonucleate granulocytes to elevated gamma-glutamyltransferase in cystic fibrosis sputum. PLoS One. 2012;7(4):e34772.
12. Hull J, Vervaart P, Grimwood K, Phelan P. Pulmonary oxidative stress response in young children with cystic fibrosis. Thorax. 1997;52(6):557–60.
13. Dickerhof N, Pearson JF, Hoskin TS, Berry LJ, Turner R, Sly PD, et al. Oxidative stress in early cystic fibrosis lung disease is exacerbated by airway glutathione deficiency. Free Radic Biol Med. 2017;113:236–43.
14. Downey DG, Bell SC, Elborn JS. Neutrophils in cystic fibrosis. Thorax. 2009;64(1):81–8.
15. Conese M, Copreni E, Di Gioia S, De Rinaldis P, Fumarulo R. Neutrophil recruitment and airway epithelial cell involvement in chronic cystic fibrosis lung disease. J Cyst Fibros. 2003;2(3):129–35.
16. Tirouvanziam R, Gernez Y, Conrad CK, Moss RB, Schrijver I, Dunn CE, et al. Profound functional and signaling changes in viable inflammatory neutrophils homing to cystic fibrosis airways. Proc Natl Acad Sci U S A. 2008;105(11):4335–9.

17. Forrest OA, Ingersoll SA, Preininger MK, Laval J, Limoli DH, Brown MR, et al. Frontline Science: Pathological conditioning of human neutrophils recruited to the airway milieu in cystic fibrosis. J Leukoc Biol. 2018;104(4):665–75.

18. Kettle AJ, Chan T, Osberg I, Senthilmohan R, Chapman AL, Mocatta TJ, et al. Myeloperoxidase and protein oxidation in the airways of young children with cystic fibrosis. Am J Respir Crit Care Med. 2004;170(12):1317–23.

19. Witko-Sarsat V, Allen RC, Paulais M, Nguyen AT, Bessou G, Lenoir G, et al. Disturbed myeloperoxidase-dependent activity of neutrophils in cystic fibrosis homozygotes and heterozygotes, and its correction by amiloride. J Immunol. 1996;157(6):2728–35.

20. Nichols DP, Chmiel JF. Inflammation and its genesis in cystic fibrosis. Pediatr Pulmonol. 2015;50 Suppl 40:S39–56.

21. Slomiany A, Murty VL, Aono M, Snyder CE, Herp A, Slomiany BL. Lipid composition of tracheobronchial secretions from normal individuals and patients with cystic fibrosis. Biochim Biophys Acta. 1982;710(1):106–11.

22. Kunzelmann K, Mehta A. CFTR: a hub for kinases and crosstalk of cAMP and Ca2+. FEBS J. 2013;280(18):4417–29.

23. Seegmiller AC. Abnormal unsaturated fatty acid metabolism in cystic fibrosis: biochemical mechanisms and clinical implications. Int J Mol Sci. 2014;15(9):16083–99.

24. Umunakwe OC, Seegmiller AC. Abnormal n-6 fatty acid metabolism in cystic fibrosis is caused by activation of AMP-activated protein kinase. J Lipid Res. 2014;55(7):1489–97.

25. Al-Turkmani MR, Andersson C, Alturkmani R, Katrangi W, Cluette-Brown JE, Freedman SD, et al. A mechanism accounting for the low cellular level of linoleic acid in cystic fibrosis and its reversal by DHA. J Lipid Res. 2008;49(9):1946–54.

26. Freedman SD, Katz MH, Parker EM, Laposata M, Urman MY, Alvarez JG. A membrane lipid imbalance plays a role in the phenotypic expression of cystic fibrosis in cftr(-/-) mice. Proc Natl Acad Sci U S A. 1999;96(24):13995–4000.

27. Zaman MM, Martin CR, Andersson C, Bhutta AQ, Cluette-Brown JE, Laposata M, et al. Linoleic acid supplementation results in increased arachidonic acid and eicosanoid production in CF airway cells and in cftr-/- transgenic mice. Am J Physiol Lung Cell Mol Physiol. 2010;299(5):L599–606.

28. Serhan CN. Pro-resolving lipid mediators are leads for resolution physiology. Nature. 2014;510(7503):92–101.

29. Demarquoy J, Le Borgne F. Biosynthesis, metabolism, and function of protectins and resolvins. Clin Lipidol. 2014;9(6):683–93.

30. Gu Z, Lamont GJ, Lamont RJ, Uriarte SM, Wang H, Scott DA. Resolvin D1, resolvin D2 and maresin 1 activate the GSK3beta anti-inflammatory axis in TLR4-engaged human monocytes. Innate Immun. 2016;22(3):186–95.

31. Campbell EL, Louis NA, Tomassetti SE, Canny GO, Arita M, Serhan CN, et al. Resolvin E1 promotes mucosal surface clearance of neutrophils: a new paradigm for inflammatory resolution. FASEB J. 2007;21(12):3162–70.

32. Eickmeier O, Fussbroich D, Mueller K, Serve F, Smaczny C, Zielen S, et al. Pro-resolving lipid mediator Resolvin D1 serves as a marker of lung disease in cystic fibrosis. PLoS One. 2017;12(2):e0171249.

33. Yang J, Eiserich JP, Cross CE, Morrissey BM, Hammock BD. Metabolomic profiling 1of regulatory lipid mediators in sputum from adult cystic fibrosis patients. Free Radic Biol Med. 2012;53(1):160–71.

34. Higgins G, Ringholz F, Buchanan P, McNally P, Urbach V. Physiological impact of abnormal lipoxin A(4) production on cystic fibrosis airway epithelium and therapeutic potential. Biomed Res Int. 2015;2015:781087.

35. Huang YH, Wang HM, Cai ZY, Xu FY, Zhou XY. Lipoxin A4 inhibits NF-kappaB activation and cell cycle progression in RAW264.7 cells. Inflammation. 2014;37(4):1084–90.

36. Jozsef L, Zouki C, Petasis NA, Serhan CN, Filep JG. Lipoxin A4 and aspirin-triggered 15-epi-lipoxin A4 inhibit peroxynitrite formation, NF-kappa B and AP-1 activation, and IL-8 gene expression in human leukocytes. Proc Natl Acad Sci U S A. 2002;99(20):13266–71.

37. Bonnans C, Gras D, Chavis C, Mainprice B, Vachier I, Godard P, et al. Synthesis and anti-inflammatory effect of lipoxins in human airway epithelial cells. Biomed Pharmacother. 2007;61(5):261–7.
38. Weinberger B, Quizon C, Vetrano AM, Archer F, Laskin JD, Laskin DL. Mechanisms mediating reduced responsiveness of neonatal neutrophils to lipoxin A4. Pediatr Res. 2008;64(4):393–8.
39. Godson C, Mitchell S, Harvey K, Petasis NA, Hogg N, Brady HR. Cutting edge: lipoxins rapidly stimulate nonphlogistic phagocytosis of apoptotic neutrophils by monocyte-derived macrophages. J Immunol. 2000;164(4):1663–7.
40. Karp CL, Flick LM, Park KW, Softic S, Greer TM, Keledjian R, et al. Defective lipoxin-mediated anti-inflammatory activity in the cystic fibrosis airway. Nat Immunol. 2004;5(4):388–92.
41. Baggiolini M, Clark-Lewis I. Interleukin-8, a chemotactic and inflammatory cytokine. FEBS Lett. 1992;307(1):97–101.
42. Mizunoe S, Shuto T, Suzuki S, Matsumoto C, Watanabe K, Ueno-Shuto K, et al. Synergism between interleukin (IL)-17 and Toll-like receptor 2 and 4 signals to induce IL-8 expression in cystic fibrosis airway epithelial cells. J Pharmacol Sci. 2012;118(4):512–20.
43. Zaman MM, Gelrud A, Junaidi O, Regan MM, Warny M, Shea JC, et al. Interleukin 8 secretion from monocytes of subjects heterozygous for the deltaF508 cystic fibrosis transmembrane conductance regulator gene mutation is altered. Clin Diagn Lab Immunol. 2004;11(5):819–24.
44. Jundi K, Greene CM. Transcription of Interleukin-8: how altered regulation can affect cystic fibrosis lung disease. Biomol Ther. 2015;5(3):1386–98.
45. Oeckinghaus A, Ghosh S. The NF-kappaB family of transcription factors and its regulation. Cold Spring Harb Perspect Biol. 2009;1(4):a000034.
46. Denning GM, Wollenweber LA, Railsback MA, Cox CD, Stoll LL, Britigan BE. Pseudomonas pyocyanin increases interleukin-8 expression by human airway epithelial cells. Infect Immun. 1998;66(12):5777–84.
47. Ierano T, Cescutti P, Leone MR, Luciani A, Rizzo R, Raia V, et al. The lipid A of Burkholderia multivorans C1576 smooth-type lipopolysaccharide and its pro-inflammatory activity in a cystic fibrosis airways model. Innate Immun. 2010;16(6):354–65.
48. Chekabab SM, Silverman RJ, Lafayette SL, Luo Y, Rousseau S, Nguyen D. Staphylococcus aureus inhibits IL-8 responses induced by Pseudomonas aeruginosa in airway epithelial cells. PLoS One. 2015;10(9):e0137753.
49. Filkins LM, O'Toole GA. Cystic fibrosis lung infections: polymicrobial, complex, and hard to treat. PLoS Pathog. 2015;11(12):e1005258.
50. Chakraborty D, Zenker S, Rossaint J, Holscher A, Pohlen M, Zarbock A, et al. Alarmin S100A8 activates alveolar epithelial cells in the context of acute lung injury in a TLR4-dependent manner. Front Immunol. 2017;8:1493.
51. Tanaka T, Narazaki M, Kishimoto T. IL-6 in inflammation, immunity, and disease. Cold Spring Harb Perspect Biol. 2014;6(10):a016295.
52. Berube J, Roussel L, Nattagh L, Rousseau S. Loss of cystic fibrosis transmembrane conductance regulator function enhances activation of p38 and ERK MAPKs, increasing interleukin-6 synthesis in airway epithelial cells exposed to Pseudomonas aeruginosa. J Biol Chem. 2010;285(29):22299–307.
53. Horsley AR, Davies JC, Gray RD, Macleod KA, Donovan J, Aziz ZA, et al. Changes in physiological, functional and structural markers of cystic fibrosis lung disease with treatment of a pulmonary exacerbation. Thorax. 2013;68(6):532–9.
54. Gifford AH, Moulton LA, Dorman DB, Olbina G, Westerman M, Parker HW, et al. Iron homeostasis during cystic fibrosis pulmonary exacerbation. Clin Transl Sci. 2012;5(4):368–73.
55. Nixon LS, Yung B, Bell SC, Elborn JS, Shale DJ. Circulating immunoreactive interleukin-6 in cystic fibrosis. Am J Respir Crit Care Med. 1998;157(6 Pt 1):1764–9.
56. Tadokoro T, Wang Y, Barak LS, Bai Y, Randell SH, Hogan BL. IL-6/STAT3 promotes regeneration of airway ciliated cells from basal stem cells. Proc Natl Acad Sci U S A. 2014;111(35):E3641–9.

57. Saint-Criq V, Villeret B, Bastaert F, Kheir S, Hatton A, Cazes A, et al. Pseudomonas aeruginosa LasB protease impairs innate immunity in mice and humans by targeting a lung epithelial cystic fibrosis transmembrane regulator-IL-6-antimicrobial-repair pathway. Thorax. 2018;73(1):49–61.

58. Xing Z, Gauldie J, Cox G, Baumann H, Jordana M, Lei XF, et al. IL-6 is an antiinflammatory cytokine required for controlling local or systemic acute inflammatory responses. J Clin Invest. 1998;101(2):311–20.

59. Tsai HC, Velichko S, Hung LY, Wu R. IL-17A and Th17 cells in lung inflammation: an update on the role of Th17 cell differentiation and IL-17R signaling in host defense against infection. Clin Dev Immunol. 2013;2013:267971.

60. Cua DJ, Tato CM. Innate IL-17-producing cells: the sentinels of the immune system. Nat Rev Immunol. 2010;10(7):479–89.

61. Dubin PJ, McAllister F, Kolls JK. Is cystic fibrosis a TH17 disease? Inflamm Res. 2007;56(6):221–7.

62. Tan HL, Regamey N, Brown S, Bush A, Lloyd CM, Davies JC. The Th17 pathway in cystic fibrosis lung disease. Am J Respir Crit Care Med. 2011;184(2):252–8.

63. Brodlie M, McKean MC, Johnson GE, Anderson AE, Hilkens CM, Fisher AJ, et al. Raised interleukin-17 is immunolocalised to neutrophils in cystic fibrosis lung disease. Eur Respir J. 2011;37(6):1378–85.

64. Hirahara K, Ghoreschi K, Laurence A, Yang XP, Kanno Y, O'Shea JJ. Signal transduction pathways and transcriptional regulation in Th17 cell differentiation. Cytokine Growth Factor Rev. 2010;21(6):425–34.

65. Bertolotto M, Contini P, Ottonello L, Pende A, Dallegri F, Montecucco F. Neutrophil migration towards C5a and CXCL8 is prevented by non-steroidal anti-inflammatory drugs via inhibition of different pathways. Br J Pharmacol. 2014;171(14):3376–93.

66. Scheuren N, Bang H, Munster T, Brune K, Pahl A. Modulation of transcription factor NF-kappaB by enantiomers of the nonsteroidal drug ibuprofen. Br J Pharmacol. 1998;123(4):645–52.

67. Tegeder I, Niederberger E, Israr E, Guhring H, Brune K, Euchenhofer C, et al. Inhibition of NF-kappaB and AP-1 activation by R- and S-flurbiprofen. FASEB J. 2001;15(3):595–7.

68. Mitchell S, Vargas J, Hoffmann A. Signaling via the NFkappaB system. Wiley Interdiscip Rev Syst Biol Med. 2016;8(3):227–41.

69. Puhl AC, Milton FA, Cvoro A, Sieglaff DH, Campos JC, Bernardes A, et al. Mechanisms of peroxisome proliferator activated receptor gamma regulation by non-steroidal anti-inflammatory drugs. Nucl Recept Signal. 2015;13:e004.

70. Standiford TJ, Keshamouni VG, Reddy RC. Peroxisome proliferator-activated receptor-{gamma} as a regulator of lung inflammation and repair. Proc Am Thorac Soc. 2005;2(3):226–31.

71. Asada K, Sasaki S, Suda T, Chida K, Nakamura H. Antiinflammatory roles of peroxisome proliferator-activated receptor gamma in human alveolar macrophages. Am J Respir Crit Care Med. 2004;169(2):195–200.

72. Michalik L, Wahli W. Involvement of PPAR nuclear receptors in tissue injury and wound repair. J Clin Invest. 2006;116(3):598–606.

73. Chinetti G, Fruchart JC, Staels B. Peroxisome proliferator-activated receptors (PPARs): nuclear receptors at the crossroads between lipid metabolism and inflammation. Inflamm Res. 2000;49(10):497–505.

74. Perez A, van Heeckeren AM, Nichols D, Gupta S, Eastman JF, Davis PB. Peroxisome proliferator-activated receptor-gamma in cystic fibrosis lung epithelium. Am J Physiol Lung Cell Mol Physiol. 2008;295(2):L303–13.

75. Dauletbaev N, Lam J, Eklove D, Iskandar M, Lands LC. Ibuprofen modulates NF-kB activity but not IL-8 production in cystic fibrosis respiratory epithelial cells. Respiration. 2010;79(3):234–42.

76. Chmiel JF, Konstan MW, Accurso FJ, Lymp J, Mayer-Hamblett N, VanDevanter DR, et al. Use of ibuprofen to assess inflammatory biomarkers in induced sputum: implications for clinical trials in cystic fibrosis. J Cyst Fibros. 2015;14(6):720–6.

77. Shah PN, Marshall-Batty KR, Smolen JA, Tagaev JA, Chen Q, Rodesney CA, et al. Antimicrobial activity of ibuprofen against cystic fibrosis-associated gram-negative pathogens. Antimicrob Agents Chemother. 2018;62(3).
78. Carlile GW, Robert R, Goepp J, Matthes E, Liao J, Kus B, et al. Ibuprofen rescues mutant cystic fibrosis transmembrane conductance regulator trafficking. J Cyst Fibros. 2015;14(1):16–25.
79. Konstan MW, Byard PJ, Hoppel CL, Davis PB. Effect of high-dose ibuprofen in patients with cystic fibrosis. N Engl J Med. 1995;332(13):848–54.
80. Lands LC, Milner R, Cantin AM, Manson D, Corey M. High-dose ibuprofen in cystic fibrosis: Canadian safety and effectiveness trial. J Pediatr. 2007;151(3):249–54.
81. Konstan MW, Schluchter MD, Xue W, Davis PB. Clinical use of ibuprofen is associated with slower FEV1 decline in children with cystic fibrosis. Am J Respir Crit Care Med. 2007;176(11):1084–9.
82. Konstan MW, VanDevanter DR, Sawicki GS, Pasta DJ, Foreman AJ, Neiman EA, et al. Association of high-dose ibuprofen use, lung function decline, and long-term survival in children with cystic fibrosis. Ann Am Thorac Soc. 2018;15(4):485–93.
83. Kovesi TA, Swartz R, MacDonald N. Transient renal failure due to simultaneous ibuprofen and aminoglycoside therapy in children with cystic fibrosis. N Engl J Med. 1998;338(1):65–6.
84. Lahiri T, Guillet A, Diehl S, Ferguson M. High-dose ibuprofen is not associated with increased biomarkers of kidney injury in patients with cystic fibrosis. Pediatr Pulmonol. 2014;49(2):148–53.
85. Konstan MW. Ibuprofen therapy for cystic fibrosis lung disease: revisited. Curr Opin Pulm Med. 2008;14(6):567–73.
86. Fennell PB, Quante J, Wilson K, Boyle M, Strunk R, Ferkol T. Use of high-dose ibuprofen in a pediatric cystic fibrosis center. J Cyst Fibros. 2007;6(2):153–8.
87. Bruch BA, Singh SB, Ramsey LJ, Starner TD. Impact of a cystic fibrosis transmembrane conductance regulator (CFTR) modulator on high-dose ibuprofen therapy in pediatric cystic fibrosis patients. Pediatr Pulmonol. 2018;53:1035.
88. Chmiel JF, Konstan MW, Elborn JS. Antibiotic and anti-inflammatory therapies for cystic fibrosis. Cold Spring Harb Perspect Med. 2013;3(10):a009779.
89. Stahn C, Lowenberg M, Hommes DW, Buttgereit F. Molecular mechanisms of glucocorticoid action and selective glucocorticoid receptor agonists. Mol Cell Endocrinol. 2007;275(1–2):71–8.
90. Rebeyrol C, Saint-Criq V, Guillot L, Riffault L, Corvol H, Chadelat K, et al. Glucocorticoids reduce inflammation in cystic fibrosis bronchial epithelial cells. Cell Signal. 2012;24(5):1093–9.
91. Bedard M, McClure CD, Schiller NL, Francoeur C, Cantin A, Denis M. Release of interleukin-8, interleukin-6, and colony-stimulating factors by upper airway epithelial cells: implications for cystic fibrosis. Am J Respir Cell Mol Biol. 1993;9(4):455–62.
92. Dauletbaev N, Herscovitch K, Das M, Chen H, Bernier J, Matouk E, et al. Down-regulation of IL-8 by high-dose vitamin D is specific to hyperinflammatory macrophages and involves mechanisms beyond up-regulation of DUSP1. Br J Pharmacol. 2015;172(19):4757–71.
93. Belvisi MG. Regulation of inflammatory cell function by corticosteroids. Proc Am Thorac Soc. 2004;1(3):207–14.
94. Auerbach HS, Williams M, Kirkpatrick JA, Colten HR. Alternate-day prednisone reduces morbidity and improves pulmonary function in cystic fibrosis. Lancet. 1985;2(8457):686–8.
95. Eigen H, Rosenstein BJ, FitzSimmons S, Schidlow DV. A multicenter study of alternate-day prednisone therapy in patients with cystic fibrosis. Cystic Fibrosis Foundation Prednisone Trial Group. J Pediatr. 1995;126(4):515–23.
96. Lai HC, FitzSimmons SC, Allen DB, Kosorok MR, Rosenstein BJ, Campbell PW, et al. Risk of persistent growth impairment after alternate-day prednisone treatment in children with cystic fibrosis. N Engl J Med. 2000;342(12):851–9.
97. Hester KL, Powell T, Downey DG, Elborn JS, Jarad NA. Glucocorticoids as an adjuvant treatment to intravenous antibiotics for cystic fibrosis pulmonary exacerbations: a UK Survey. J Cyst Fibros. 2007;6(4):311–3.

98. Dovey M, Aitken ML, Emerson J, McNamara S, Waltz DA, Gibson RL. Oral corticosteroid therapy in cystic fibrosis patients hospitalized for pulmonary exacerbation: a pilot study. Chest. 2007;132(4):1212–8.
99. https://clinicaltrials.gov/ct2/show/NCT03070522. Accession Date: 29 Nov 2018.
100. Mogayzel PJ Jr, Naureckas ET, Robinson KA, Mueller G, Hadjiliadis D, Hoag JB, et al. Cystic fibrosis pulmonary guidelines. Chronic medications for maintenance of lung health. Am J Respir Crit Care Med. 2013;187(7):680–9.
101. Cigana C, Nicolis E, Pasetto M, Assael BM, Melotti P. Anti-inflammatory effects of azithromycin in cystic fibrosis airway epithelial cells. Biochem Biophys Res Commun. 2006;350(4):977–82.
102. Fan LC, Lin JL, Yang JW, Mao B, Lu HW, Ge BX, et al. Macrolides protect against Pseudomonas aeruginosa infection via inhibition of inflammasomes. Am J Physiol Lung Cell Mol Physiol. 2017;313(4):L677–L86.
103. Meyer M, Huaux F, Gavilanes X, van den Brule S, Lebecque P, Lo Re S, et al. Azithromycin reduces exaggerated cytokine production by M1 alveolar macrophages in cystic fibrosis. Am J Respir Cell Mol Biol. 2009;41(5):590–602.
104. Ratjen F, Saiman L, Mayer-Hamblett N, Lands LC, Kloster M, Thompson V, et al. Effect of azithromycin on systemic markers of inflammation in patients with cystic fibrosis uninfected with Pseudomonas aeruginosa. Chest. 2012;142(5):1259–66.
105. Saiman L, Marshall BC, Mayer-Hamblett N, Burns JL, Quittner AL, Cibene DA, et al. Azithromycin in patients with cystic fibrosis chronically infected with Pseudomonas aeruginosa: a randomized controlled trial. JAMA. 2003;290(13):1749–56.
106. Mayer-Hamblett N, Retsch-Bogart G, Kloster M, Accurso F, Rosenfeld M, Albers G, et al. Azithromycin for early pseudomonas infection in cystic fibrosis. The OPTIMIZE Randomized Trial. Am J Respir Crit Care Med. 2018;198(9):1177–87.
107. Barnaby R, Koeppen K, Nymon A, Hampton TH, Berwin B, Ashare A, et al. Lumacaftor (VX-809) restores the ability of CF macrophages to phagocytose and kill Pseudomonas aeruginosa. Am J Physiol Lung Cell Mol Physiol. 2018;314(3):L432–L8.
108. Rowe SM, Heltshe SL, Gonska T, Donaldson SH, Borowitz D, Gelfond D, et al. Clinical mechanism of the cystic fibrosis transmembrane conductance regulator potentiator ivacaftor in G551D-mediated cystic fibrosis. Am J Respir Crit Care Med. 2014;190(2):175–84.
109. Hisert KB, Heltshe SL, Pope C, Jorth P, Wu X, Edwards RM, et al. Restoring cystic fibrosis transmembrane conductance regulator function reduces airway bacteria and inflammation in people with cystic fibrosis and chronic lung infections. Am J Respir Crit Care Med. 2017;195(12):1617–28.
110. Kruzel ML, Zimecki M, Actor JK. Lactoferrin in a context of inflammation-induced pathology. Front Immunol. 2017;8:1438.
111. Frioni A, Conte MP, Cutone A, Longhi C, Musci G, di Patti MC, et al. Lactoferrin differently modulates the inflammatory response in epithelial models mimicking human inflammatory and infectious diseases. Biometals. 2014;27(5):843–56.
112. Rogan MP, Taggart CC, Greene CM, Murphy PG, O'Neill SJ, McElvaney NG. Loss of microbicidal activity and increased formation of biofilm due to decreased lactoferrin activity in patients with cystic fibrosis. J Infect Dis. 2004;190(7):1245–53.
113. Conner GE, Salathe M, Forteza R. Lactoperoxidase and hydrogen peroxide metabolism in the airway. Am J Respir Crit Care Med. 2002;166(12 Pt 2):S57–61.
114. Moskwa P, Lorentzen D, Excoffon KJ, Zabner J, McCray PB Jr, Nauseef WM, et al. A novel host defense system of airways is defective in cystic fibrosis. Am J Respir Crit Care Med. 2007;175(2):174–83.
115. Chandler JD, Min E, Huang J, McElroy CS, Dickerhof N, Mocatta T, et al. Anti-inflammatory and anti-microbial effects of thiocyanate in a cystic fibrosis mouse model. Am J Respir Cell Mol Biol. 2015;53(2):193–205.
116. Chandler JD, Nichols DP, Nick JA, Hondal RJ, Day BJ. Selective metabolism of hypothiocyanous acid by mammalian thioredoxin reductase promotes lung innate immunity and antioxidant defense. J Biol Chem. 2013;288(25):18421–8.

117. Chandler JD, Day BJ. Thiocyanate: a potentially useful therapeutic agent with host defense and antioxidant properties. Biochem Pharmacol. 2012;84(11):1381–7.
118. Lorentzen D, Durairaj L, Pezzulo AA, Nakano Y, Launspach J, Stoltz DA, et al. Concentration of the antibacterial precursor thiocyanate in cystic fibrosis airway secretions. Free Radic Biol Med. 2011;50(9):1144–50.
119. Moreau-Marquis S, Coutermarsh B, Stanton BA. Combination of hypothiocyanite and lactoferrin (ALX-109) enhances the ability of tobramycin and aztreonam to eliminate Pseudomonas aeruginosa biofilms growing on cystic fibrosis airway epithelial cells. J Antimicrob Chemother. 2015;70(1):160–6.
120. https://clinicaltrials.gov/ct2/show/NCT02598999. Accession Date: 29 Nov 2018.
121. Burstein SH. Ajulemic acid: potential treatment for chronic inflammation. Pharmacol Res Perspect. 2018;6(2):e00394.
122. Burstein SH. The cannabinoid acids, analogs and endogenous counterparts. Bioorg Med Chem. 2014;22(10):2830–43.
123. Ribeiro CM, Zhang G, Lubamba BA, Tepper M. Anabasum reduces excessive inflammatory responses in cystic fibrosis patient-derived lung macrophages. Pediatr Pulmonol. 2017;52(S47):251.
124. Martiniano SL, Toprak D, Ong T, Zemanick ET, Daines CL, Muhlebach MS, et al. Highlights from the 2017 north American cystic fibrosis conference. Pediatr Pulmonol. 2018;53(7):979–86.
125. Chmiel J, Elborn S, Constantine S, White B. A double-blind placebo-conrolled phase 2 study in adults with cystic fibrosis of anabasum, a selective cannabinoid receptor type 2 agonist. Pediatr Pulmonol. 2017;52(S47):317.
126. https://clinicaltrials.gov/ct2/show/NCT03451045. Accession Date: 29 Nov 2018.
127. Sadik CD, Luster AD. Lipid-cytokine-chemokine cascades orchestrate leukocyte recruitment in inflammation. J Leukoc Biol. 2012;91(2):207–15.
128. Afonso PV, Janka-Junttila M, Lee YJ, McCann CP, Oliver CM, Aamer KA, et al. LTB4 is a signal-relay molecule during neutrophil chemotaxis. Dev Cell. 2012;22(5):1079–91.
129. Elborn JS, Horsley A, MacGregor G, Bilton D, Grosswald R, Ahuja S, et al. Phase I studies of acebilustat: biomarker response and safety in patients with cystic fibrosis. Clin Transl Sci. 2017;10(1):28–34.
130. Rowe SM, Elborn JS. EMPIRE-CF: a phase 2 trial of a novel anti-inflammatory molecule, acebilustat, in patients with cystic fibrosis. Pediatr Pulmonol. 2018;53(S2):136–7.
131. https://clinicaltrials.gov/ct2/show/NCT03265288. Accession Date: 29 Nov 2018.
132. AbuArish A, Garic D, Pislariu R, Radzioch D, Hanrahan JW. Fenretinide increases CFTR functional expression and recruitment in ceramide microdomains. Pediatr Pulmonol. 2018;53(S2):260.
133. Polineni D, Dang H, Gallins PJ, Jones LC, Pace RG, Stonebraker JR, et al. Airway mucosal host defense is key to genomic regulation of cystic fibrosis lung disease severity. Am J Respir Crit Care Med. 2018;197(1):79–93.

Chapter 9
Pulmonary Exacerbations

Kristina Montemayor, Allison A. Lambert, and Natalie E. West

Abbreviations

CF	Cystic Fibrosis
CFF	Cystic Fibrosis Foundation
CFFPR	Cystic Fibrosis Foundation Patient Registry
CFTR	Cystic Fibrosis Transmembrane Conductance Regulator
ESCF	Epidemiologic Study of Cystic Fibrosis
FEV_1	Forced expiratory volume over 1 second
IV	Intravenous
MRSA	Methicillin-resistant Staphylococcus aureus
PEx	Pulmonary exacerbations
PFTs	Pulmonary Function Tests
PIPE	Prednisone in Cystic Fibrosis Pulmonary Exacerbations
STOP	Standardized Treatment of Pulmonary Exacerbations

Patient Perspective

The hardest part of living with cystic fibrosis is that most of the time you feel like a normal person who has a life to live but CF can creep up at any time. CF has

K. Montemayor · N. E. West (✉)
Johns Hopkins University, Department of Medicine, Division of Pulmonary and Critical Care Medicine, Baltimore, MD, USA
e-mail: kmontem1@jhmi.edu; nwest5@jhmi.edu

A. A. Lambert
University of Washington, Department of Medicine, Division of Pulmonary and Critical Care Medicine, WWAMI Spokane Foundations, UW at Schoenberg Center—Gonzaga, Spokane, WA, USA
e-mail: aalamb@uw.edu

© Springer Nature Switzerland AG 2020
S. D. Davis et al. (eds.), *Cystic Fibrosis*, Respiratory Medicine,
https://doi.org/10.1007/978-3-030-42382-7_9

interrupted so many big moments of my life, but I never let it stop the rest of my life or bring down my positive spirits. I was diagnosed with CF at 6 weeks old with the genes F508del and N1303K, with the second gene being the rarer gene. The problem with the rarer gene is that a lot of the new medications that have come out to alleviate the symptoms of CF will not work for me. This has caused me to be in and out of the hospital more times than I would like within a year.

Over the past few years, my pulmonary function test levels (PFT's) had been steadily declining. Along with my Pulmonary team, we put together many different solutions that may help, even going to the point of doing a bronchoscopy to see if there were any other infections causing my decline. We sent extra tests to see if there were additional IV medicines that were sensitive to my pseudomonas strains. Within the past year I had about seven different CF exacerbations, causing me to miss family gatherings, miss Thanksgiving, quit my job, and eventually reschedule my wedding.

There were times when I felt sick and knew an admission was coming, and I was alright with that. Yet, the hardest admissions were the ones towards the end stage of my lungs. The ones where I was feeling good, but my PFTs were showing otherwise. Those are the ones, the ones that I wasn't expecting, and I had to put off plans that were made weeks ahead of time, or miss family or friend time. All these exacerbations eventually led up to me having a double lung transplant in June of 2018.

To patients who are newly diagnosed with CF, I would say to simply just live your life the way you want. Yes, there are precautions we must take and boundaries we must not cross, but you can't let CF control every aspect of your life. When I was younger, I played baseball all summer long, and my goal was to always stay healthy enough to stay out of the hospital for an exacerbation. There were times during the season that I would get sick and need an admission, but I hated it and wanted to refuse because baseball was my passion. It's what I looked forward to when I woke up, and it was the last thing I thought about before I went to sleep. Baseball was my motivation to stay healthy.

Something I would say to the physicians that care for people with CF is don't just be a doctor. Don't see us as just another patient. Build a relationship, show us that you care and that you have our best interest at heart. The best doctor I've ever had, I trusted my life with. Even when times got dark and my lungs were failing. Without that trust and bond, I don't think that I would have been so confident going into my lung transplant. Be there for our highs and be there to cry with us at our lows, but always make a personal connection with your patient. Luckily, I got to celebrate that my PFTs went to 100% with my CF doctor within a few months of my transplant. I continue to do well and got married to the love of my life in October of 2018.

– Tyler Smith

Introduction

The long-term course of cystic fibrosis (CF) is characterized by chronic progressive loss of lung function with episodes of acute worsening of respiratory symptoms requiring treatment with antibiotics, referred to as a pulmonary exacerbation (PEx).

An objective, measurable, reproducible definition of CF PEx does not exist. Despite the lack of a consensus definition, the prevalence, burden, and multisystem impact of CF PEx is well recognized. This chapter integrates the latest epidemiologic, diagnostic, therapeutic, preventive, and prognostic data in the realm of CF PEx and discusses critical areas for future direction of investigation.

Definition

Interestingly, there is no current agreed-upon definition of a CF PEx, mostly due to lack of robust clinical trial data to define the signs or symptoms and corresponding treatments to impact outcomes and thereby create a definition. Most studies currently define CF PEx by an increase in symptoms and/or a reduction in lung function plus a clinician decision to treat with antibiotics. Calls for a standardized definition of PEx date back to the early 1990s and are supported by the myriad implications of an objective definition, including guiding treatment decisions for individual patients, enhancing the ability of observational studies to consistently identify risk factors and quantify prognosis, and setting standards for clinical trial endpoints [1, 2]. In 2009, the CF Foundation (CFF) convened a working group that was tasked to provide recommendations for the treatment of CF PEx. Although there was insufficient evidence for certain treatment recommendations, Flume and colleagues provided clinical care guidelines for PEx treatment and identified areas for further study [3] (Table 9.1).

A clinician-decision-based definition of a PEx is limited by known variability in clinical practice. Examination of data from the Epidemiologic Study of Cystic Fibrosis (ESCF) has shown variability between clinical sites with regards to frequency of monitoring clinical status, measuring lung function and culturing for respiratory pathogens, which resulted in differences in PEx definition, frequency, and aggressiveness of treatment [4–8]. Using clinical vignettes, Kraynack and colleagues further documented variation by CF clinicians in both the identification and treatment of CF PEx; this variability existed between CF Centers, within each CF Center and at the individual clinician level [9]. Variability extends beyond the definition of a PEx, to how CF PEx are treated, including the route of antibiotic delivery (oral, inhaled, intravenous [IV]), dosing of antibiotics, duration of antibiotics, site of antibiotic delivery (home or hospital), and the addition and timing of steroids [3, 8–13]. Goss and Burns compared the Acute Respiratory Illness Checklist (ARIC), the Respiratory and Systemic Symptoms Questionnaire (RSSQ), and 2 clinical trial definitions and found high variability in symptom profiling, which underscores the need for specificity in a future definition beyond a broad domain, such as "increased respiratory symptoms" [14].

The CFF PEx working group was tasked with designing and conducting robust clinical trials to provide evidence for best practices for treatment of CF PEx. As practice patterns vary widely nationwide and worldwide, optimization through interventional trials could improve outcomes. The Standardized Treatment of

Table 9.1 Summary of cystic fibrosis pulmonary guidelines for treatment of pulmonary exacerbations

Question	Studies	N	Certainty	Magnitude of benefit	Grade of recommendation	Recommendation
Site of treatment[a]	1 RCT(7)	17	Low		I	Insufficient evidence that hospital and home treatment are equivalent
Chronic therapies	[b]	[b]	Moderate	Moderate	B	Continue current practices
Simultaneous use of inhaled and IV antibiotics	0	0	Low		I	Insufficient evidence to recommend for or against simultaneous use
Airway clearance therapies	[b]	[b]	Moderate	Moderate	B	Continue current practices
Number of antibiotics to treat Pseudomonas[a]	17 RCT(25–41) 1 RXO(42) 1 QRT(43)	768	Low		I	Insufficient evidence that a single antibiotic is equivalent to a combination of antibiotics
Aminoglycoside dosing[a]	4 RCT(29, 51–53) 1 RXO(54)	349	Moderate	Small	C	Once-daily dosing is acceptable for treatment Pseudomonas
Continuous infusion beta-lactam antibiotics	1 RXO(54)	5	Low		I	Insufficient evidence to recommend continuous infusion
Duration of antibiotics[a]	0	0	Low		I	Insufficient evidence to define optimal duration of antibiotics
Synergy testing (routine)	1 RCT(24)	132	132	Zero	D	Routine use not recommended
Systemic steroids	2 RCT(63, 64)	44	44		I	Insufficient evidence to recommend use of corticosteroids

Reprinted with permission of the American Thoracic Society. Copyright © 2018 American Thoracic Society

Flume et al. [3]. The *American Journal of Respiratory and Critical Care Medicine* is an official journal of the American Thoracic Society

Definition of abbreviations: *N* number of patients evaluated, *RCT* randomized controlled trial, *RXO* randomized crossover trial, *QRT* quasi-randomized trial, *XO* crossover trial

[a]Cochrane Review exists on this topic

[b]Previous recommendations [26, 67]

Pulmonary Exacerbations (STOP) program conducted the first study in 2014–15, entitled *STOP*, which was designed to "define key clinical endpoints, their magnitude of response, and their variance in order to guide future interventional trials to optimize PEx therapy and outcomes" [15]. This observational study utilized a clinician-decision-based definition of CF PEx and examined 220 patients hospitalized for PEx to collect data on lung function, symptoms, and physician treatment decisions [15, 16]. *STOP* identified highly variable treatments and clinical responses to therapy among patients with CF PEx and served as the foundation for designing the *STOP 2* clinical trial, currently underway, examining three durations of IV antibiotic therapy.

Epidemiology

The CFF Patient Registry (CFFPR) 2017 Annual Report offers insight into the impact of CF PEx upon the general CF patient population [17]. The CFFPR was initiated in 1966 and collects data at each encounter on individuals with CF (lung function, nutritional data, PEx and hospitalizations, microbiology data, amongst numerous other variables). The CFFPR reports provide valuable hypothesis-generating data through the inclusion of patients and practitioners throughout the country and collection of real-world practice patterns, unlike clinical trials which are often centered at urban academic medical centers with predefined interventions and outcomes. In 2017, participants experienced a mean of 0.7 CF PEx requiring IV antibiotics per year, requiring treatment for a median of 13 days (pediatrics) and 14 days (adults) duration for each individual PEx (Fig. 9.1). Participants aged 15–30 were more likely to report CF PEx than those in other age groups, with approximately 45% of adults and 25% of children recorded as having one or more exacerbations requiring IV antibiotics per year [17].

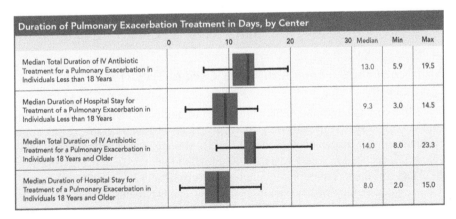

Duration of Pulmonary Exacerbation Treatment in Days, by Center					Median	Min	Max
	0	10	20	30			
Median Total Duration of IV Antibiotic Treatment for a Pulmonary Exacerbation in Individuals Less than 18 Years					13.0	5.9	19.5
Median Duration of Hospital Stay for Treatment of a Pulmonary Exacerbation in Individuals Less than 18 Years					9.3	3.0	14.5
Median Total Duration of IV Antibiotic Treatment for a Pulmonary Exacerbation in Individuals 18 Years and Older					14.0	8.0	23.3
Median Duration of Hospital Stay for Treatment of a Pulmonary Exacerbation in Individuals 18 Years and Older					8.0	2.0	15.0

Fig. 9.1 Duration of pulmonary exacerbation treatment in days, by center. (Reprinted from the Cystic Fibrosis Foundation Patient Registry, 2017 Annual Data Report, with permission from the Cystic Fibrosis Foundation Patient Registry)

Given the prevalence and associated morbidity of CF PEx, identification of risk factors for CF PEx offers both prognostic and preventative value. Consistent with exacerbation risk in other chronic, progressive lung diseases punctuated by episodic increases in symptom burden, frequency of CF PEx and need for IV antibiotics were both independently associated with subsequent CF PEx risk. VanDevanter and colleagues have shown that once a PEx occurs, the risk for subsequent PEx is increased [13]. Thus, it is important to understand what risk factors patients may have that predispose them to a PEx, as well as appropriate maintenance therapies to prevent CF PEx from occurring.

Pulmonary Exacerbation Treatment

In 2009, a systematic review applied the US Preventative Services Task Force grading scheme to provide CF guidelines for the treatment of an acute PEx [3]. Of the 10 CF PEx treatment domains examined, moderate evidence to support recommendations were available among three domains.

Route of Antibiotics to Treat a CF PEx

In addition to chronic therapies, acute PEx require the initiation of antibiotics. The route of antibiotic delivery can include oral, inhaled or IV administration. The decision of which route of therapy to start depends on both subjective and objective data, such as patient-reported symptoms and lung function as measured in forced expiratory volume over 1 second (FEV_1). For milder cases, providers may start oral antibiotics with or without inhaled antibiotics. Alternatively, for individuals with more severe symptoms and a decrease in FEV_1 from baseline, systemic therapy with IV antibiotics will be the preferred choice.

Number of Intravenous Antibiotics Used to Treat a CF PEx

Due to the cost and potential toxicities of systemic antibiotic therapy, there has been considerable research investigating the equivalence of monotherapy versus combined therapy for treatment of an acute PEx [3]. Although the prevalence of *P. aeruginosa* has declined in recent years, 44.6% of individuals captured in the CFFPR in 2017 had a positive respiratory culture for this organism [17]. Therefore, *P. aeruginosa*-targeted therapy with two antipseudomonal agents remains standard of care. A retrospective study utilizing the ESCF database from 2003 to 2005 showed that IV tobramycin was prescribed for 69.6% of CF PEx in conjunction with a second agent [10]. Current treatment regimens typically include an aminoglycoside with concurrent use of an IV cephalosporin, beta-lactam, or carbapenem. In a recent retrospective cross-sectional study, Cogen and colleagues identified the two most commonly utilized antibiotics on hospital admission for an acute PEx in children were tobramycin (58.5%) and ceftazidime (27.3%) [18]. Additionally, if methicillin-resistant *Staphylococcus aureus* (MRSA) is a known respiratory pathogen, IV vancomycin or linezolid is often utilized. Combined therapy remains standard of care, yet, certain circumstances exist in which a single agent is utilized based on an individual's presenting symptoms, medication allergies or intolerances, and case-specific risk/benefit profile.

Duration of Intravenous Therapy

Duration of IV therapy for PEx treatment is variable. Historically, most PEx were treated with a 14-day course of antibiotic therapy [17, 19]. In 2017, the median treatment duration was 13.0 days for individuals less than 18 years of age compared to 14.0 days for individuals greater than 18 years of age, but wide variability in treatment duration exists, ranging from 5 to 20 days in children to 8–23 days in adults [17], Fig. 9.1.

The *STOP* study group first conducted an observational clinical study in 2014–15 of 220 individuals with CF, who were admitted to the hospital for treatment of a PEx with IV antibiotics (*STOP* clinicaltrials.gov: NCT02109822). Physicians were surveyed on treatment decisions, and management practices were observed [15, 16]. Frequent spirometry and daily patient symptom diaries were collected throughout the treatment course. The mean duration of IV antibiotic therapy was 15.9 days (SD 6.0, range 2–51 days). Patients were stratified by age, and there was no statistically significant difference in duration of antibiotics among those less than 18 years of age as compared to those greater than 18 years of age (14.5 days vs 16.2 days, respectively ($p = 0.14$)) [15, 16].

Adjunct Therapies

Optimization of airway clearance and continuation of chronic medications are essential when treating a PEx. Pharmacologic treatments used to aid with airway clearance in the CF population include nebulized 7% hypertonic saline and dornase alpha. Dentice and colleagues conducted a randomized controlled trial ($n = 132$) evaluating the effects of 7% hypertonic saline versus a 0.12% taste-masked control three times daily in the inpatient setting. The hypertonic saline group had significantly higher FEV_1 during the first ten inpatient days compared to the control group (mean FEV_1 difference 172 ml (CI: 42–301 ml)). Additionally, individuals in the hypertonic saline group were 75% more likely to return to their preexacerbation FEV_1 at the time of discharge compared to only 57% of individuals in the control group. Collectively, these results demonstrate that continuation or initiation of hypertonic saline during an acute PEx can help improve patient symptoms and lung function [19, 20]. In addition, dornase alfa is safe, well tolerated, and commonly prescribed during CF PEx either at continued home dosing or more frequently; however, it does not appear to provide significant spirometric benefit beyond antibiotics and physiotherapy [21]. Furthermore, nonpharmacologic airway clearance techniques, such as manual chest percussion, handheld positive expiratory pressure devices and external high-frequency oscillation vests are continued during a PEx [3].

There is insufficient evidence to recommend routine use of oral or inhaled corticosteroids during a PEx [3]. Dovey and colleagues conducted a pilot randomized control trial ($n = 28$) examining the addition of a 5-day course of prednisone (2 mg/kg/day) to standard CF PEx treatment. The primary endpoint, slope of post-bronchodilator FEV_1 between days 1 and 6, was not statistically different between the treatment and placebo groups (52 ml/day vs 51 ml/day, respectively). Furthermore, patient symptom scores were collected and observed to decrease between days 1 and 14, although there was no statistical significance between the group means [22]. Despite lack of robust evidence to support the use of corticosteroids, there are often times when providers prescribe a short course of oral prednisone (typically 40 mg daily or less) if clinical exam suggests underlying bronchospasm. In fact, the *STOP* investigators found that 21% of individuals with a PEx were treated with systemic corticosteroids [16], and Cogen et al. noted a median rate of 23% of systemic corticosteroid use any time during hospital admission for a PEx [18].

Furthermore, the role of continuation or initiation of inhaled antibiotics remains unclear. Scant evidence exists addressing whether continuing chronic inhaled antibiotics or initiating inhaled antibiotics at the onset of a PEx improves patient outcomes [23], and the current CF guidelines report insufficient evidence to recommend for or against the continued use of inhaled antibiotics during an acute PEx [3]. An observational study of 123 CF patients who received IV antibiotics for an acute PEx found that only 10% of individuals were treated with inhaled antibiotics [24]. Additionally, only 10% of patients continued inhaled antibiotics in the *STOP* study, and Cogen and colleagues noted inhaled antibiotic use in 13.1% of PEx, with tobramycin being commonly utilized (87.4%) [16, 18].

Anti-inflammatory pharmacologic treatments have been utilized in the CF population for prevention of acute PEx. Oral ibuprofen and azithromycin have different mechanisms of action, but have both been shown to enhance anti-inflammatory properties. Though there does not appear to be a role for initiation of either of these medications during a PEx, there is little evidence suggesting discontinuation of use during a PEx. There is recent evidence that azithromycin reduces the clinical effectiveness of tobramycin, by inducing adaptive bacterial stress responses in *P. aeruginosa*. This has been shown primarily in retrospective studies, by a secondary analysis of clinical trials involving inhaled tobramycin and aztreonam [25]. Investigators are conducting a prospective clinical trial to evaluate the effect of adding oral azithromycin to inhaled tobramycin among individuals with CF (Clintrials.gov NCT02677701). If an interaction is shown in this prospective trial, it should be considered to stop chronic azithromycin while treating with IV or inhaled tobramycin during a PEx.

Treatment Setting

After the decision is made to initiate IV antibiotics, the provider must decide whether inpatient or outpatient treatment with IV antibiotics is appropriate. Again, insufficient data exist to provide recommendations for treatment location or define patient characteristics to guide location selection. Inpatient admission is warranted in certain circumstances, such as: an individual's first encounter with IV therapy, lack of central venous access, hypoxemia requiring supplemental oxygen therapy, or inability of the patient and/or family to provide consistent medication administration. In 2017, 84% of total PEx treatment occurred in the inpatient setting for individuals less than 18 years compared to 63.2% in individuals 18 years of age and older [17].

Outcomes of home versus hospital IV therapy has previously been examined in both the pediatric and adult populations. Bosworth and colleagues conducted an earlier study comparing 33 cases of inpatient therapy to 27 cases of outpatient therapy and found that outpatient therapy resulted in a longer and more costly treatment course [26]. These findings have not been replicated in a randomized clinical trial, and therefore existing guidelines indicate a lack of certainty regarding preferred location and an insufficient body of evidence to assess the risk versus benefit balance. In another study of the ESCF database, Schechter and colleagues analyzed data to assess whether treatment setting (inpatient or outpatient IV antibiotics) during treatment for a PEx affected outcomes. Approximately 4497 PEx in 2773 individuals with CF were analyzed, who were treated with IV antibiotics between 2002 and 2005. Overall, 75.4% of treated PEx resulted in $FEV_1\%$ predicted returning to $\geq 90\%$ of baseline within 30 days (successful treatment response). The median proportion of IV antibiotic treatment that was spent inpatient was 0.581 (IQR 0.396–0.753), with children spending more time in the inpatient setting (0.664, IQR 0.494–0.770) vs adults (0.471, IQR 0.283–0.636). Overall treatment response was positively correlated with the following: the proportion of inpatient days (Pearson's correlation coefficient $[r] = 0.278$, $p = 0.0.16$); number of days that treatment was administered in the inpatient setting ($r = 0.241$, $p = 0.037$); proportion of treatments that were entirely inpatient regimens ($r = 0.295$, $p = 0.013$). Furthermore, treatment response was negatively correlated with the number of days of home IV therapy ($r = -0.260$, $p = 0.024$). There was an absolute increase of 9.08% in the achievement of return to $\geq 90\%$ of baseline $FEV_1\%$ predicted when comparing complete inpatient treatment to no inpatient treatment ($p = 0.006$) [27].

Additionally, a retrospective study of the CFFPR in 2010–2013 evaluated the effect of treatment setting on the probability of retreatment within 30 days with IV antibiotics. A lower proportion of those individuals who had received at least some part of their IV antibiotic treatment in the hospital were retreated within 30 days compared to those patients who received the entire course of IV antibiotics at home (5.0% vs 8.5%) [12]. Collectively, these studies show that inpatient treatment of PEx may have a significant advantage over outpatient treatment in regards to cost, lung function recovery, and need for retreatment.

Improving PEx Outcomes

Recent quality improvement research has been effective in improving patient outcomes in CF PEx. Researchers have evaluated the implementation of a pulmonary algorithm directed at providing early, consistent care utilizing a multidisciplinary, patient-centered approach. Schechter and colleagues reorganized care at a large academic pediatric care center focusing on chronic maintenance therapies, initiation of antibiotic therapy for a minimum of 5% decrease in FEV_1, with attention to close follow-up in 4–6 weeks. The relative change of $FEV_1\%$ predicted was identified for patients and discussed at weekly multidisciplinary preclinical meetings. Furthermore, after the implementation of the algorithm, the mean of the best $FEV_1\%$ predicted was measured with notable results. The mean of the best $FEV_1\%$ predicted in the previous 12 months rose from 87% predicted to 98% predicted in individuals 6–18 years of age [28]. Implementation of a proactive, multidisciplinary approach across care centers should be considered with the aim to improve patient outcomes worldwide.

Prognosis

PEx are associated with considerable morbidity, loss of lung function (FEV_1), decreased survival, increased healthcare costs, and worsened quality of life [10, 16, 24, 29–42]. A retrospective study evaluating approximately 8500 CF individuals in the CFFPR showed that 25% of individuals did not recover to within 90% of baseline lung function (FEV_1) after treatment with IV antibiotics [32]. A secondary analysis of a randomized clinical trial of IV antibiotic treatment for PEx showed that only 51% of patient's lung function returned to 100% of baseline by day 14 of IV antibiotic treatment [43], and the risk was greater if there was a greater initial decline in FEV_1 and a higher level of inflammatory markers at the end of treatment (C-reactive protein, sputum neutrophil elastase) [43]. The results of the *STOP* prospective study replicated these findings. Only 39% fully recovered lost lung function, and only 65% recovered at least 90% baseline lung function [16], Fig. 9.2.

Individuals with CF who experience more frequent PEx have a more accelerated decline in lung function. A study of almost 8500 individuals in the CFFPR in 2004–2006 showed that in adults, having 3 or more PEx treated with IV antibiotics was associated with a greater decline in lung function over the subsequent 3 years. In children, having *any* number of IV-treated PEx resulted in a greater rate of decline in the next 3 years [31]. A 3-year prospective cohort study in approximately 450 individuals in Canada evaluated lung function decline over the study period and stratified individuals on PEx rates: <1 exacerbation/year, 1–2 exacerbations per year, and >2 exacerbations per year. Individuals with >2 exacerbations/year had an increased risk of having a 5% decline in FEV_1 from baseline FEV_1 compared to individuals with <1 exacerbation/year (adjusted hazard ratio (HR): 1.55 (95% CI:

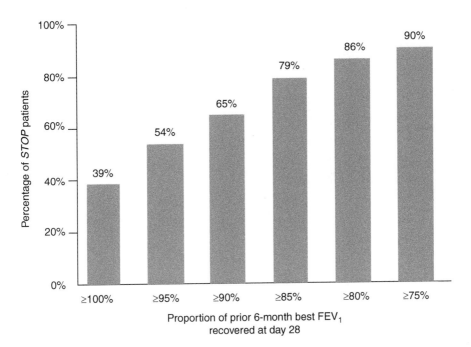

Fig. 9.2 Percentage of *STOP* patients who recovered the specified proportion of their baseline lung function (defined as prior 6-month best FEV_1) at day 28. For example, only 67% of individuals recovered 90% of their baseline lung function. (Reprinted from the West et al. [16], copyright 2017, with permission from Elsevier)

1.10 to 2.18, $p = 0.01$)). In addition, these individuals also had an increased risk of lung transplant or death (HR 4.05 (95% CI: 1.15 to 14.28, $p = 0.03$)) [39]. This accelerated decline in lung function associated with frequent PEx was further demonstrated in a retrospective study of 851 individuals with CF. The annual rate of decline in individuals without a PEx was 1.2% per year compared with 2.5% per year in individuals that did experience a PEx. The proportion of lung function decline that could be attributed to 1 or more PEx was 52% (95% CI 35.0–68.9) [44].

Furthermore, the number of PEx in the previous year is predictive of future PEx. In a retrospective study of the CFFPR, approximately 13,500 individuals with CF were studied to evaluate the number of PEx per year and the associated risk factor for a subsequent PEx. Investigators found that the number of PEx in the previous year was strongly associated with future PEx hazard ratios: 1, 2, 3, ≥4 exacerbations treated with IV antibiotics were 1.8, 2.9, 4.8, and 8.7 more likely to experience a future PEx ($p < 0.0001$) [13]. The number of previous-year PEx was also predictive of time to next PEx (Fig. 9.3). For instance, individuals with zero prior-year PEx had an average time to next PEx of approximately 380 days, while individuals with 1 prior-year PEx had an average of 230 days until next PEx. Alternatively, individuals with ≥4 PEx only had an average of 60 days until next PEx [13]. Therefore, it has been shown that PEx lead to a more accelerated decline in lung

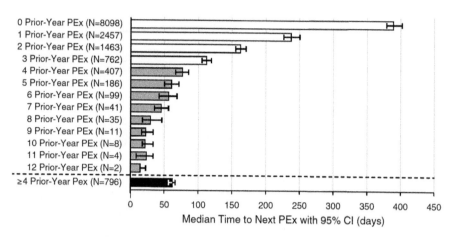

Fig. 9.3 Kaplan–Meier median time-to-PEx by number of Prior-year PEx. White bars highlight Prior-year PEx values where 95% CI for associated median times to next PEx do not overlap with adjacent values. Gray bars show Prior-year PEx values where 95% CI for associated median times to next PEx overlap with adjacent values. The black bar shows the median time to PEx for the group of pooled patients with Prior-year PEx ≥4. CI = confidence interval. (Reprinted from the VanDevanter et al. [13], copyright 2016, with permission from Elsevier)

function and that more frequent PEx lead to subsequent PEx. This vicious cycle highlights the need to both optimize CF PEx treatment but also to prevent initial and recurrent CF PEx.

Route of antibiotic therapy may be contributing to the high proportion of individuals who do not recover baseline lung function after treatment for a PEx. The effect of PEx treated with IV antibiotics has been rigorously studied, yet it is less known about outcomes of PEx treated with oral antibiotics alone. Stanojevic and colleagues evaluated PEx treated with oral antibiotics retrospectively between 2009 and 2014 in Canada in 570 individuals. There was a median of 4 PEx treated with oral antibiotics per patient, (median 0.9/patient/year). At follow-up, 82% were at ≥90% of baseline FEV$_1$, yet only 44% were at ≥100% of baseline FEV$_1$, suggesting loss of baseline lung function. One or more PEx treated with oral antibiotics in the previous 12 months was associated with a decreased FEV$_1$ compared to individuals without a PEx treated with oral antibiotics. In evaluating the cumulative effect, individuals with 6 or more PEx treated with oral antibiotics had the steepest rate of decline in FEV$_1$. This study showed that a large proportion of individuals with a PEx treated with oral antibiotics did not recover baseline lung function, and that an increasing number of PEx treated with oral antibiotics was associated with a more rapid decline in lung function [33]. In a smaller study, 81% of children with CF returned to within 90% of baseline after treatment with oral antibiotics for a PEx [45]. Yet, 19% of children did not experience this return to baseline, echoing previous studies.

Additional research has shown that in individuals aged 6–17, an acute drop in lung function is often not treated with increased antibiotic therapy. Individuals at this age have a high baseline lung function, yet the lack of treatment may explain the increased rate of lung function decline that is seen in this age group. The objective of a retrospective study using the ESCF database, conducted in 1994–2005 in 9875 individuals, was to assess whether a new antibiotic treatment for a PEx was associated with lung function recovery and whether proportion of recovery varied by treatment setting and type of antibiotic therapy. New therapies were classified as: hospitalization with IV antibiotics, home IV antibiotics without hospitalization, inhaled antibiotics, oral quinolone antibiotics, or other oral antibiotics. The results showed that *any* new antibiotic treatment greatly increased the probability of recovery of FEV_1 to 90% of baseline ($p < 0.001$). All four outpatient therapies were also associated with a significantly greater probability of recovery of lung function, compared to no treatment (OR 1.27–1.64). The results of this study accentuate the importance of aggressive antibiotic therapy in the setting of acute lung function decline, and failure to treat acute declines could result in permanent lung function loss [46].

Another retrospective study of the Epidemiologic Study of CF (ESCF) database characterized route of antibiotics and resultant effect on lung function recovery. In 2003–2005, approximately 45,000 PEx were reported in 13,000 individuals; 73% of PEx were treated with oral antibiotics, 39% with IV antibiotics, and 24% with inhaled antibiotics. After treatment with antibiotics, the average improvement for all individuals in FEV_1 was 3.4 ± 12.2% predicted. However, this improvement was higher in those treated with IV antibiotics, 5.1 ± 12.7% predicted, compared to those treated with oral or inhaled antibiotics, 2.0 ± 11.6% predicted [10].

Lastly, in the era of Cystic Fibrosis Transmembrane Conductance Regulator (CFTR) modulators, there has been speculation that these medications may help slow the lung function decline associated with PEx. In the original ivacaftor clinical trial, the rate of PEx in those individuals randomized to ivacaftor was reduced by 55% over the 48-week clinical trial compared to placebo ($p < 0.001$) [47]. In a subsequent study, short-term and long-term lung function recovery data were analyzed from the 161 participants in this clinical trial. While the reduction in rate of PEx was significant, this did not translate into improved recovery of lung function after treatment for a PEx. The proportion of short-term recovery of FEV_1% predicted was similar in ivacaftor versus placebo (57.1% vs 53.7%), as was the proportion of individuals with long-term lung function recovery (46.4% vs 47.7%) [48].

In 2019, the new CFTR modulator elexacaftor/tezacaftor/ivacaftor was approved. In the Phase 3 clinical trials, it reduced exacerbation frequency by 63%. As 90% of the CF population is eligible for elexacaftor/tezacaftor/ivacaftor, the rate of PEx is expected to decline. Hence, the severity of PEx may change over time, and adjustments to our diagnostic and treatment methods may be needed.

Future Directions

The CF Foundation, along with researchers worldwide, are focused on improving patient outcomes related to PEx treatment. Given the strength of evidence of the detrimental effects of PEx, and the poor outcomes after treatment for a PEx, there is a substantial need to improve prevention, detection, and treatment of PEx. There are a number of questions regarding PEx treatment that need robust clinical data to guide development of best practices. This includes antibiotic selection (route, number of antibiotics), dosing of antibiotics, optimal duration of antibiotics, treatment setting (home versus hospital), role of inhaled antibiotics, role of steroids, and role of biomarkers [49].

The *STOP* program first conducted the previously mentioned observational study *STOP*, which was informative in defining potential clinical endpoints and the factors to consider in the design and powering of future clinical trials [50]. *STOP-2* (clinicaltrials.gov NCT02781610) is the first randomized controlled trial to evaluate duration of IV antibiotics. Investigators are categorizing patients as early robust responders (ERR) or nonearly robust responders (NERR) based on patient-reported symptoms and change in lung function response by 7–10 days of treatment. ERR are then being randomized to a 10- or 14-day treatment course, whereas NERR are being randomized to a 14- or 21-day treatment course, with the primary endpoint being change in FEV_1 from the initiation of treatment to 14 days post treatment [51–53]. This trial is expected to complete enrollment at the end of 2019 and should help to establish guidelines in terms of duration of IV antibiotic therapy. The *STOP* investigators will continue to design future clinical trials of PEx with the goal of providing robust clinical data to guide establishment of best practices.

The impact of inhaled antibiotics during treatment for a PEx remains unclear. There is scant evidence of whether continuing chronic inhaled antibiotics or starting a new inhaled antibiotic at the time of initiation of IV antibiotics for treatment of a PEx improves outcomes [23], and CFF guidelines conclude there is insufficient evidence to recommend for or against this practice [3]. Investigators are currently evaluating the role of inhaled antibiotics by retrospectively analyzing several randomized controlled trials of PEx, and a prospective study is planned to begin in 2019.

Waters and colleagues are further addressing the role of oral corticosteroids as an adjunct in PEx treatment with the implementation of a randomized, double-blind, placebo-controlled trial in Canada known as the Prednisone in Cystic Fibrosis Pulmonary Exacerbations (PIPE) study. Investigators are currently enrolling patients and examining the effects of adding oral prednisone at 2 mg/kg/day (max of 60 mg a day) in pediatric and adult patients who do not recover their baseline FEV_1 after 7 days of IV antibiotic treatment [19].

Furthermore, limited data exists regarding sex-based differences in presentation, treatment, and outcomes for a PEx. Multiple studies have shown that while CF is a disease with equal prevalence across sexes, women have worse outcomes, including increased mortality [54–57]. Women with CF have been shown to have reduced survival, more rapid lung function decline, and more frequent CF PEx as compared to men [29, 54, 58–60]. While several mechanisms have been hypothesized to explain this sex disparity (hormone-mediated effects), none can fully account for the difference in outcomes [55, 61, 62]. Puberty and hormonal exposures have been evaluated as a cause, specifically estrogen [58]. Premature acquisition of *Pseudomonas aeruginosa* with conversion to mucoid strains has been hypothesized as the underlying mechanism driving the gender differences in morbidity and mortality [63, 64]. Further supporting this pathway, Chotirmall and colleagues found that mucoid *P. aeruginosa* was selectively grown during periods of high-circulating estradiol and that women receiving oral contraceptives had lower rates of CF PEx [61]. Investigators are currently evaluating sex-based differences in symptom presentation and provider treatment practices for a PEx by retrospectively analyzing several randomized controlled trials of PEx and the CFFPR, as well as collecting data prospectively on sex differences in PEx [65, 66].

Conclusion

While incredible advancements in CF care and survival have been made in the last century, PEx are associated with morbidity, mortality, and reduced quality of life. There is a lack of robust evidence to support guidelines for treatment of PEx. Since the publication of the CF Pulmonary Guidelines in 2009, a working group (*STOP* program) has been established to conduct clinical studies in order to establish best practices for detection and treatment of PEx, in order to improve outcomes for CF PEx. There remain several gaps in knowledge for treatment of PEx, and these interventional studies will guide establishment of best practices for future treatment management of PEx while limiting variability of care across treatment centers.

References

1. Ramsey BW, Boat TF. Outcome measures for clinical trials in cystic fibrosis. Summary of a Cystic Fibrosis Foundation consensus conference. J Pediatr. 1994;124:177–92.
2. Marshall BC. Pulmonary exacerbations in cystic fibrosis: it's time to be explicit! Am J Respir Crit Care Med. 2004;169:781–2.
3. Flume PA, Mogayzel PJ, Robinson KA, Goss CH, Rosenblatt RL, Kuhn RJ, et al. Cystic fibrosis pulmonary guidelines: treatment of pulmonary exacerbations. Am J Respir Crit Care Med. 2009;180:802–8.
4. Morgan WJ, Butler SM, Johnson CA, Colin AA, FitzSimmons SC, Geller DE, et al. Epidemiologic study of cystic fibrosis: design and implementation of a prospective, multicenter, observational study of patients with cystic fibrosis in the U.S. and Canada. Pediatr Pulmonol. 1999;28:231–41.
5. Konstan MW, Butler SM, Schidlow DV, Morgan WJ, Julius JR, Johnson CA. Patterns of medical practice in cystic fibrosis: part I. Evaluation and monitoring of health status of patients. Investigators and Coordinators of the Epidemiologic Study of Cystic Fibrosis. Pediatr Pulmonol. 1999;28:242–7.
6. Konstan MW, Butler SM, Schidlow DV, Morgan WJ, Julius JR, Johnson CA. Patterns of medical practice in cystic fibrosis: part II. Use of therapies. Investigators and Coordinators of the Epidemiologic Study of Cystic Fibrosis. Pediatr Pulmonol. 1999;28:248–54.
7. Johnson C, Butler SM, Konstan MW, Morgan W, Wohl ME. Factors influencing outcomes in cystic fibrosis: a center-based analysis. Chest. 2003;123:20–7.
8. Schechter MS, Regelmann WE, Sawicki GS, Rasouliyan L, VanDevanter DR, Rosenfeld M, et al. Antibiotic treatment of signs and symptoms of pulmonary exacerbations: a comparison by care site. Pediatr Pulmonol. 2015;50:431–40.
9. Kraynack NC, Gothard MD, Falletta LM, McBride JT. Approach to treating cystic fibrosis pulmonary exacerbations varies widely across US CF care centers. Pediatr Pulmonol. 2011;46:870–81.

10. Wagener JS, Rasouliyan L, VanDevanter DR, Pasta DJ, Regelmann WE, Morgan WJ, et al. Oral, inhaled, and intravenous antibiotic choice for treating pulmonary exacerbations in cystic fibrosis. Pediatr Pulmonol. 2013;48:666–73.
11. VanDevanter DR, O'Riordan MA, Blumer JL, Konstan MW. Assessing time to pulmonary function benefit following antibiotic treatment of acute cystic fibrosis exacerbations. Respir Res. 2010;11:137.
12. VanDevanter DR, Flume PA, Morris N, Konstan MW. Probability of IV antibiotic retreatment within thirty days is associated with duration and location of IV antibiotic treatment for pulmonary exacerbation in cystic fibrosis. J Cyst Fibros. 2016;15:783–90.
13. VanDevanter DR, Morris NJ, Konstan MW. IV-treated pulmonary exacerbations in the prior year: an important independent risk factor for future pulmonary exacerbation in cystic fibrosis. J Cyst Fibros. 2016;15:372–9.
14. Goss CH, Burns JL. Exacerbations in cystic fibrosis. 1: epidemiology and pathogenesis. Thorax. 2007;62:360–7.
15. Sanders DB, Solomon GM, Beckett VV, West NE, Daines CL, Heltshe SL, et al. Standardized Treatment of Pulmonary Exacerbations (STOP) study: observations at the initiation of intravenous antibiotics for cystic fibrosis pulmonary exacerbations. J Cyst Fibros. 2017;16:592–9.
16. West NE, Beckett VV, Jain R, Sanders DB, Nick JA, Heltshe SL, et al. Standardized Treatment of Pulmonary Exacerbations (STOP) study: physician treatment practices and outcomes for individuals with cystic fibrosis with pulmonary exacerbations. J Cyst Fibros. 2017;16:600–6.
17. Cystic Fibrosis Foundation. Cystic Fibrosis Foundation Patient Registry, 2017 annual data report. Bethesda. 2018.
18. Cogen JD, Oron AP, Gibson RL, Hoffman LR, Kronman MP, Ong T, et al. Characterization of inpatient cystic fibrosis pulmonary exacerbations. Pediatrics. 2017;139:e20162642.
19. Skolnik K, Quon BS. Recent advances in the understanding and management of cystic fibrosis pulmonary exacerbations. F1000Research. 2018;7:575.
20. Dentice RL, Elkins MR, Middleton PG, Bishop JR, Wark PAB, Dorahy DJ, et al. A randomised trial of hypertonic saline during hospitalisation for exacerbation of cystic fibrosis. Thorax. 2016;71:141–7.
21. Wilmott RW, Amin RS, Colin AA, DeVault A, Dozor AJ, Eigen H, et al. Aerosolized recombinant human DNase in hospitalized cystic fibrosis patients with acute pulmonary exacerbations. Am J Respir Crit Care Med. 1996;153:1914–7.
22. Dovey M, Aitken ML, Emerson J, McNamara S, Waltz DA, Gibson RL. Oral corticosteroid therapy in cystic fibrosis patients hospitalized for pulmonary exacerbation: a pilot study. Chest. 2007;132:1212–8.
23. Hurley MN, Prayle AP, Flume P. Intravenous antibiotics for pulmonary exacerbations in people with cystic fibrosis. Cochrane Database Syst Rev [Internet]. 2015; Available from: https://doi.org/10.1002/14651858.CD009730.pub2.
24. Heltshe SL, Goss CH, Thompson V, Sagel SD, Sanders DB, Marshall BC, et al. Short-term and long-term response to pulmonary exacerbation treatment in cystic fibrosis. Thorax. 2016;71:223–9.
25. Nichols DP, Happoldt CL, Bratcher PE, Caceres SM, Chmiel JF, Malcolm KC, et al. Impact of azithromycin on the clinical and antimicrobial effectiveness of tobramycin in the treatment of cystic fibrosis. J Cyst Fibros. 2017;16:358–66.
26. Bosworth DG, Nielson DW. Effectiveness of home versus hospital care in the routine treatment of cystic fibrosis. Pediatr Pulmonol. 1997;24:42–7.
27. Schechter MS, VanDevanter DR, Pasta DJ, Short SA, Morgan WJ, Konstan MW, et al. Treatment setting and outcomes of cystic fibrosis pulmonary exacerbations. Ann Am Thorac Soc. 2018;15:225–33.
28. Schechter MS, Schmidt HJ, Williams R, Norton R, Taylor D, Molzhon A. Impact of a program ensuring consistent response to acute drops in lung function in children with cystic fibrosis. J Cyst Fibros. 2018;17:769–78.
29. Konstan MW, Wagener JS, VanDevanter DR, Pasta DJ, Yegin A, Rasouliyan L, et al. Risk factors for rate of decline in FEV1 in adults with cystic fibrosis. J Cyst Fibros. 2012;11:405–11.

30. Sanders DB, Hoffman LR, Emerson J, Gibson RL, Rosenfeld M, Redding GJ, et al. Return of FEV1 after pulmonary exacerbation in children with cystic fibrosis. Pediatr Pulmonol. 2010;45:127–34.
31. Sanders DB, Bittner RC, Rosenfeld M, Redding GJ, Goss CH. Pulmonary exacerbations are associated with subsequent FEV1 decline in both adults and children with cystic fibrosis. Pediatr Pulmonol. 2011;46:393–400.
32. Sanders DB, Bittner RC, Rosenfeld M, Hoffman LR, Redding GJ, Goss CH. Failure to recover to baseline pulmonary function after cystic fibrosis pulmonary exacerbation. Am J Respir Crit Care Med. 2010;182:627–32.
33. Stanojevic S, McDonald A, Waters V, MacDonald S, Horton E, Tullis E, et al. Effect of pulmonary exacerbations treated with oral antibiotics on clinical outcomes in cystic fibrosis. Thorax. 2017;72:327.
34. Kerem E, Reisman J, Corey M, Canny GJ, Levison H. Prediction of mortality in patients with cystic fibrosis. N Engl J Med. 1992;326:1187–91.
35. Liou TG, Adler FR, Fitzsimmons SC, Cahill BC, Hibbs JR, Marshall BC. Predictive 5-year survivorship model of cystic fibrosis. Am J Epidemiol. 2001;153:345–52.
36. Mayer-Hamblett N, Rosenfeld M, Emerson J, Goss CH, Aitken ML. Developing cystic fibrosis lung transplant referral criteria using predictors of 2-year mortality. Am J Respir Crit Care Med. 2002;166:1550–5.
37. Emerson J, Rosenfeld M, McNamara S, Ramsey B, Gibson RL. Pseudomonas aeruginosa and other predictors of mortality and morbidity in young children with cystic fibrosis. Pediatr Pulmonol. 2002;34:91–100.
38. Ellaffi M, Vinsonneau C, Coste J, Hubert D, Burgel PR, Dhainaut JF, et al. One-year outcome after severe pulmonary exacerbation in adults with cystic fibrosis. Am J Respir Crit Care Med. 2005;171:158–64.
39. de Boer K, Vandemheen KL, Tullis E, Doucette S, Fergusson D, Freitag A, et al. Exacerbation frequency and clinical outcomes in adult patients with cystic fibrosis. Thorax. 2011;66:680–5.
40. Britto MT, Kotagal UR, Hornung RW, Atherton HD, Tsevat J, Wilmott RW. Impact of recent pulmonary exacerbations on quality of life in patients with cystic fibrosis. Chest. 2002;121:64–72.
41. Konstan MW, Morgan WJ, Butler SM, Pasta DJ, Craib ML, Silva SJ, et al. Risk factors for rate of decline in forced expiratory volume in one second in children and adolescents with cystic fibrosis. J Pediatr. 2007;151:134–9, 139.e1.
42. Lieu TA, Ray GT, Farmer G, Shay GF. The cost of medical care for patients with cystic fibrosis in a health maintenance organization. Pediatrics. 1999;103:e72.
43. Waters VJ, Stanojevic S, Sonneveld N, Klingel M, Grasemann H, Yau YC, et al. Factors associated with response to treatment of pulmonary exacerbations in cystic fibrosis patients. J Cyst Fibros. 2015;14:755–62.
44. Waters V, Stanojevic S, Atenafu EG, Lu A, Yau Y, Tullis E, et al. Effect of pulmonary exacerbations on long-term lung function decline in cystic fibrosis. Eur Respir J. 2012;40:61–6.
45. Hoppe JE, Wagner BD, Accurso FJ, Zemanick ET, Sagel SD. Characteristics and outcomes of oral antibiotic treated pulmonary exacerbations in children with cystic fibrosis. J Cyst Fibros. 2018;17(6):760–8.
46. Morgan WJ, Wagener JS, Pasta DJ, Millar SJ, VanDevanter DR, Konstan MW, et al. Relationship of antibiotic treatment to recovery after acute FEV1 decline in children with cystic fibrosis. Ann Am Thorac Soc. 2017;14:937–42.
47. Ramsey BW, Davies J, McElvaney NG, Tullis E, Bell SC, Dřevínek P, et al. A CFTR potentiator in patients with cystic fibrosis and the G551D mutation. N Engl J Med. 2011;365:1663–72.
48. Flume PA, Wainwright CE, Elizabeth Tullis D, Rodriguez S, Niknian M, Higgins M, et al. Recovery of lung function following a pulmonary exacerbation in patients with cystic fibrosis and the G551D-CFTR mutation treated with ivacaftor. J Cyst Fibros. 2018;17:83–8.
49. West NE, Flume PA. Unmet needs in cystic fibrosis: the next steps in improving outcomes. Expert Rev Respir Med. 2018;12:585–93.

50. VanDevanter DR, Heltshe SL, Spahr J, Beckett VV, Daines CL, Dasenbrook EC, et al. Rationalizing endpoints for prospective studies of pulmonary exacerbation treatment response in cystic fibrosis. J Cyst Fibros. 2017;16:607–15.
51. Heltshe SL, West NE, VanDevanter DR, Sanders DB, Beckett VV, Flume PA, et al. Study design considerations for the Standardized Treatment of Pulmonary Exacerbations 2 (STOP2): a trial to compare intravenous antibiotic treatment durations in CF. Contemp Clin Trials. 2018;64:35–40.
52. Sanders DB, Heltshe S, West NE, VanDevanter DR, Skalland M, Flume PA, et al. Update on the STOP-2 randomized study of IV antibiotic duration in CF pulmonary exacerbations. Pediatr Pulmonol. 2018;52:324.
53. Flume PA, Heltshe SL, West NE, Vandevanter DR, Sanders DB, Skalland M, et al. P094 Design, enrollment, and feasibility of the STOP-2 randomised study of intravenous antibiotic treatment duration in cystic fibrosis pulmonary exacerbations. J Cyst Fibros. 2018;17:S85.
54. Rosenfeld M, Davis R, FitzSimmons S, Pepe M, Ramsey B. Gender gap in cystic fibrosis mortality. Am J Epidemiol. 1997;145:794–803.
55. Harness-Brumley CL, Elliott AC, Rosenbluth DB, Raghavan D, Jain R. Gender differences in outcomes of patients with cystic fibrosis. J Womens Health (Larchmt). 2014;23:1012–20.
56. Warwick WJ, Pogue RE, Gerber HU, Nesbitt CJ. Survival patterns in cyctic fibrosis. J Chronic Dis. 1975;28:609–22.
57. FitzSimmons SC. The changing epidemiology of cystic fibrosis. J Pediatr. 1993;122:1–9.
58. Sutton S, Rosenbluth D, Raghavan D, Zheng J, Jain R. Effects of puberty on cystic fibrosis related pulmonary exacerbations in women versus men. Pediatr Pulmonol. 2014;49:28–35.
59. Dodge J, Lewis P, Stanton M, Wilsher J. Cystic fibrosis mortality and survival in the UK: 1947–2003. Eur Respir J. 2007;29:522–6.
60. Block JK, Vandemheen KL, Tullis E, Fergusson D, Doucette S, Haase D, et al. Predictors of pulmonary exacerbations in patients with cystic fibrosis infected with multi-resistant bacteria. Thorax. 2006;61:969–74.
61. Chotirmall SH, Smith SG, Gunaratnam C, Cosgrove S, Dimitrov BD, O'Neill SJ, et al. Effect of estrogen on pseudomonas mucoidy and exacerbations in cystic fibrosis. N Engl J Med. 2012;366:1978–86.
62. Coakley RD, Sun H, Clunes LA, Rasmussen JE, Stackhouse JR, Okada SF, et al. 17beta-Estradiol inhibits Ca2+-dependent homeostasis of airway surface liquid volume in human cystic fibrosis airway epithelia. J Clin Invest. 2008;118:4025–35.
63. Levy H, Kalish LA, Cannon CL, García KC, Gerard C, Goldmann D, et al. Predictors of mucoid Pseudomonas colonization in cystic fibrosis patients. Pediatr Pulmonol. 2008;43:463–71.
64. Maselli JH, Sontag MK, Norris JM, MacKenzie T, Wagener JS, Accurso FJ. Risk factors for initial acquisition of Pseudomonas aeruginosa in children with cystic fibrosis identified by newborn screening. Pediatr Pulmonol. 2003;35:257–62.
65. Montemayor K, Dezube R, Lechtzin N, Jennings MT, Thaxton AL, Allgood S, et al. Sex differences in pulmonary exacerbations in cystic fibrosis patients. Am J Respir Crit Care Med. 2018;197:A6267.
66. Montemayor K, Dezube R, Lechtzin N, Psoter KJ, Jennings MT, Thaxton AL, et al. Sex differences in pulmonary exacerbations in cystic fibrosis patients. Pediatr Pulmonol. 2018;52:331.
67. Thornton J, Elliott R, Tully MP, Dodd M, Webb AK. Long term clinical outcome and hospital intravenous antibiotic treatment in adults with cystic fibrosis. Thorax. 2004;59:242–6.

Chapter 10
Maintenance of Pulmonary Therapies

Shruti M. Paranjape and Peter J. Mogayzel Jr

Patient Perspective

A Family's Perspective on Chronic Therapies

Diagnosis. Our journey into the world of cystic fibrosis (CF) began very shortly after the birth of our first child. I had a normal pregnancy and Joshua was born early on a winter morning in 1995. The first 30 or so hours were just joyful. Around lunchtime of the second day, Josh began throwing up green bile and was quickly taken for a x-ray. After the x-ray, the doctors came to us and said Josh either had an ileal atresia or meconium ileus, which was indicative of CF. Neither my husband Matt nor I knew of anyone with CF in our extended families, so we were hopeful that it was not CF.

Josh was born at Andrews Air Force Base, which did not have a neonatal intensive care unit (NICU), so he was quickly transferred to Walter Reed Medical Center by ambulance. Late into the night, doctors ran tests and tried various enemas to try and free his blockage without surgery. Shortly after midnight, we were told he would require surgery to clear the blockage. It was extremely devastating, but at this point we were hopeful it was the ileal atresia. I quickly baptized my new baby, in case the worst happened, and they whisked him off to surgery before he was 48 hours old. It was every new parent's worst nightmare.

After surgery, we overheard one of the residents discussing that he was able to assist in the surgery of a baby whose meconium was so thick it was like toothpaste. Josh had not been officially diagnosed with CF, but our hope that it wasn't was quickly waning. Things quickly became a whirlwind. Josh finally underwent a sweat test when he was 8 days old. Throughout the entire day, the doctor and resident kept

S. M. Paranjape (✉)
Johns Hopkins School of Medicine, Eudowood Division of Pediatric Respiratory Sciences, Baltimore, MD, USA
e-mail: sparanj1@jhmi.edu

P. J. Mogayzel Jr
The Johns Hopkins Medical Institutions, Department of Pediatrics, Baltimore, MD, USA

© Springer Nature Switzerland AG 2020
S. D. Davis et al. (eds.), *Cystic Fibrosis*, Respiratory Medicine,
https://doi.org/10.1007/978-3-030-42382-7_10

putting us off and we were certain at this point that no one wanted to break the bad news to us. Late in the day, the resident finally met with us and told us that the sweat test indicated that Josh had CF. Matt and I literally crumbled into each other's arms. I remember the doctor saying that he had a child and if he had to pick a disease for his child to have, it would be CF because he felt there was such hope on the horizon. The gene had been discovered in 1989 and good things were going to come from that. He told us not to read anything published before 1989.

My degree is in rehabilitation counseling and I graduated from college in 1987. All I could think was that life expectancy was 18 to 21 years for those with CF. I had been taught that as a counselor, I would not be working with any clients that had CF because they most likely would either not make it to working age or be well enough to work if they did. It would be their parents that would need our services as they tried to juggle work and manage the care of their sick child. We were terrified of what that meant for both us and Josh.

Of course, I went home and read from my textbooks, all published prior to 1989. The diagnosis consumed us. No one said, "Congratulations on your new baby." Instead everyone said, "I'm sorry." It hurt so badly. We wondered if he would live to graduate high school. All my life, my dream was to be a wife and a mother, more so than having a career. I wanted four children. I wanted a house full of kids and grandchildren like my parents had. I felt what I desired most in life was taken away, along with all the hopes and dreams that I had for my child. So much so, that a few weeks after the diagnosis, I said to Matt, my husband whom I love dearly, "If you don't think you can love me forever, leave me now so we can both have healthy children." That's how raw and unbearable the pain was for me.

I cried every day for 3 months. I was sad and angry. How could our parents have healthy children and give us this gene that didn't allow us to do so? It was horrific. I would hold my beautiful baby and cry and wonder how this could be true. Why him? Why us? Eventually, I saw a counselor and started to deal with what this meant in our lives. Together, Matt and I started to move forward and I was ready to contact the Cystic Fibrosis Foundation and learn more about this disease and what I could do to make things better for my child.

<u>Chronic therapies</u>. As we adjusted to life with a child with CF, it also meant adjusting to the medications and chronic treatments that go hand and hand with it. When our oldest son was born, we had to do manual chest physical therapy (PT). To get a child so young to be still is difficult enough, but finding ways to make it exciting and enjoyable was not easy. In 1999, we had another son, Zachary, who was also diagnosed with CF. Now we had two children who required enzymes and other medications and chest PT.

When the Vest became available to replace manual chest PT, we tried to get it right away but were initially denied it, because our children were too healthy! We were shocked and saddened that something that could keep our children healthy and free up time for us, was denied. Dealing with insurance is an added component that consumes a lot of your time, if you have a child or children with chronic medical needs.

Before Zach turned two, he began nebulized tobramycin. Thirty minute treatments two times a day added to manual chest PT was exceptionally difficult. We tried various ways to entertain him while his treatments were taking place: reading books, watching TV and videos. Eventually, he fell in love with a Disney sing along video and nothing else would do. So for years, and I am not exaggerating, we watched the same video two times a day, 28 days on and 28 days off. He also insisted that whoever was in the room with him at the time wear the fish face nebulizer mask that he wore as he did his treatment as well. Luckily, that only lasted about 6 months!

As the boys grew, they became more and more involved in sports and other activities outside our home and more and more medications and treatments were added. It would not always be easy to fit everything in. They would sometimes need to couple up the vest with a nebulized treatment to get them both in, even though it would be better if one was done before the other.

They were also more inclined to try to get out of treatments that they didn't particularly like. Zach had an aversion to hypertonic saline from the start. "I already cough," he would say. "Why would I do something that makes me cough more?" I would tell him to go do his treatment, he would say he was going to, but when I would check he wasn't. He would put it off until sometimes there wasn't enough time to get it in. It was hard not to become a nag, because as a mom, you are so concerned about your children's health and wanting them to do what they are supposed to be doing. It consumed me and overwhelmed me at times.

Chronic therapy is absolutely necessary for our children with CF to remain healthy. At the same time we would weigh out the benefits versus the time involved. This was especially true with hypertonic saline. Zach felt it made him feel worse and eventually he quit doing it after speaking to one of our CF clinic doctors.

As they grow older, the loss of control over their treatments is extremely stressful. You can no longer force them to do their therapies and letting them do the treatments on their own time wasn't always the best solution. It would force many hard conversations. I think the hardest conversation ever came when both Josh and Zach came to me during their respective senior years in high school. Both told me that they felt the need to live their life to the fullest while they felt well enough to do so. They both felt the pressure of their life expectancy and not knowing when it may be that they would no longer feel healthy enough to do the things they wanted to do. Both felt somewhat overwhelmed with the diagnosis of both CF and CF related diabetes (CFRD).

I would say one of the hardest things through the course of their disease was the diagnosis of CFRD. The burden of measuring multiple blood sugars a day and the introduction of insulin shots twice a day, in addition to an already full plate of treatments did not sit well with either of my sons. Both boys were diagnosed with CFRD at 15 years of age and began regular insulin therapy around the age of 17. Both were angry! Zach took it particularly hard and we really had a rough time the summer he began taking insulin. We probably fought the most about doing his blood sugars and insulin on time than any other treatment introduction. He said he'd rather have CF than diabetes.

The guilt and fear I would feel each time a new therapy was introduced was debilitating at times. This was usually accompanied by worry about what seemed to be progression of the disease. I would always wonder if this would be the turning point where things get exponentially worse and there would be no turning back. Each drop in lung function, each hospitalization, each night the albuterol would not calm the cough takes its toll on you emotionally.

When Orkambi® [lumacaftor/ivacaftor, Vertex Pharmaceuticals, Inc] was approved by the FDA – that was one new therapy we were all on board with and excited to start! The development of a drug targeted to treat the underlying cause of CF and specifically made for our sons' mutations, homozygous F508del, was one of the happier moments of our lives. We now look forward to switching to Symdeko® [tezacaftor/ivacaftor, Vertex Pharmaceuticals, Inc] and future new medications and are hopeful that it will make an even greater difference in our boys' health and longevity.

In time, Josh and Zach each began setting up their medications in the weekly pill organizer and taking control of their treatments. During their senior years in high school, we added ordering medications and dealing with insurance. They became more involved in decisions regarding their treatments. They are both grown now and doing well, but not without the occasional bump in the road.

Josh, now in his early twenties, is in charge of every facet of his care. He transferred all his medications to his new pharmacy and has set up his continued care at the local CF clinic. He attended college at Penn State's main campus for electrical engineering and is now living and working in Colorado – one of the biggest reasons for his move there is to pursue his dream to train and become the first Olympic biathlete with CF.

Zach is in his late teens and attends college full time in the Netherlands. He wants to see the world while he has the time and opportunity and is healthy enough to do so, in his words. This was an extremely hard decision for Matt and me, to let him study so far from home. The healthcare is a bit different there and not all of his medications are readily available. With our older son, we had a 4 hour radius rule when he searched for colleges. He had to be within a reasonable distance that I could pick him up and get him to Johns Hopkins the same day. Our thinking has clearly evolved over the last several years. Although it has taken a while for us to figure everything out about life with CF in the Netherlands, we feel it is important to allow both of our sons to live the lives that they desire.

In the end, as a parent, you know chronic therapy is necessary to manage CF. You are going to make your child do what they need to do to stay healthy. You want to instill in them the importance of doing their therapies every day. You, as a family, have to find a balance that is right for all of you to maintain your sanity in knowing that you are doing everything you can to fight this disease and living your life to the fullest. CF impacts your life in a myriad of ways. It affects how you parent and how you live your life. We have always told our boys that CF is a part of them but it doesn't define them, that they should never let CF hold them back from what they want to do in life. Chronic therapy is the way to ensure they are healthy enough to make their dreams happen.

– Catherine Beeler Berkley

Introduction

Cystic fibrosis (CF) pulmonary disease results from abnormal airway secretions leading to chronic obstruction, infection, inflammation, and eventually bronchiectasis and parenchymal destruction. Treatment is aimed to optimize pulmonary function and prevent disease progression and other complications through (1) management of chronic infection; (2) clearance of mucous secretions; and (3) reduction of airway inflammation [1]. The application of precision medicine [2, 3] and partnered coproduction of care among the individual, family, and clinical care team [4] allow CF pulmonary disease management to be tailored to an individual's respiratory needs and personal preferences. Perhaps the most recognizable precision therapies are cystic fibrosis transmembrane conductance regulator (CFTR) modulators that have been approved by the United States Food and Drug Administration (FDA), for certain *CFTR* genotypes, in adults and children with CF as young as 6 months of age and are described elsewhere in this book.

Whereas most therapeutic interventions in CF, such as selection of antibiotics for specific respiratory infections and modalities for effective airway clearance, are individualized, there is a concurrent need to standardize recommendations for CF pulmonary disease management. Clinical practice guidelines have been developed by the United States Cystic Fibrosis Foundation [5], the European Society of Cystic Fibrosis [6], the CF Trust [7], and others and updated to include the CFTR modulator therapies [8]. How the CFTR modulator therapies might alter the present recommendations for maintenance pulmonary therapies in CF pulmonary disease is a focus for future investigations. Therefore, it is critical for CF care teams to collaborate with individuals and families to develop a therapeutic regimen and optimize individual care [9]. This chapter will review maintenance pulmonary therapies in CF and includes a family's perspectives on chronic daily treatments.

Guidelines for Maintenance Pulmonary Therapies in Cystic Fibrosis

Early diagnosis and intervention are vital to improve and maintain optimal clinical outcomes in CF. Guidelines are available regarding monitoring and chronic therapies for individuals over 6 years of age, preschool age children, and infants. First published in 2007 [10] and updated in 2013 [5], chronic CF treatment guidelines were based on systematic literature review and assessment of the available evidence based on an established grading scale. Guidelines on the use of CFTR modulators were published in 2018 [8]. Because pulmonary disease can progress in early childhood in the absence of overt symptoms, preschool monitoring and management guidelines were published in 2016 [11] that included therapeutics and surveillance. Recommendations for infants with CF were published in 2009 [12] and included disease monitoring and treatment for both nutritional and pulmonary manifestations.

Considerations for infants with CFTR-related metabolic syndrome (CRMS) and CF-screen positive, inconclusive diagnosis (CFSPID) were published separately in 2009 [13] and outlined general guidelines for the implementation of preventive care and subspecialist follow-up.

The major aims of the management of CF pulmonary disease focus on optimizing pulmonary function and preventing disease progression and other disease-associated complications. Treatment is lifelong and generally begins at the time of diagnosis. Individuals with CF in the United States should be cared for in a care center accredited by the CF Foundation, which provides multidisciplinary, patient- and family-centered care. Following diagnosis, frequent clinic visits are recommended to institute and monitor response to therapies and ensure adequate CF teaching. Eventually, visits can be spaced to every 3 months. Similar guidelines are in place in Europe, in accordance with published best practices that were updated in 2018 [6] and include recommendations for CF newborn screening and diagnosis as well as considerations for adult care, transplantation, and end-of-life issues. Chronic pulmonary maintenance therapies include not only prescriptions for various treatments and medications tailored and personalized to an individual's needs and preferences, but also consideration for promoting adherence and improved quality of life. It is important to note that current guidelines are based on available evidence and are subject to change in the modern era of CF therapeutics. Further studies will provide additional insight, given the earlier diagnosis of CF, and help to define the maintenance pulmonary regimen with earlier implementation of the CFTR modulator therapies.

Pulmonary Therapies for Managing Chronic Infection

Airway microbiology is a unique fingerprint for individuals with CF. Several factors have been identified with airway infection including *CFTR* genotype [14], climate, and temperature [15]. Respiratory cultures identify predominant organisms in the CF airway [16]. Bacterial pathogens such as *Pseudomonas aeruginosa,* methicillin-resistant *Staphylococcus aureus* (MRSA), and *Burkholderia cepacia* complex (BCC) are well-known to negatively impact CF pulmonary health. Other organisms, including nontuberculous mycobacteria (NTM) and fungal pathogens, can have significant effects on CF pulmonary disease [17–19]. Non-culture-based detection techniques have demonstrated the presence of additional organisms that may have roles in disease progression and suggest that routine cultures may not fully represent the bacterial communities that populate CF airways. The rich diversity of organisms tends to narrow with antibiotic use and disease progression in older children and adults [20, 21].

Cystic fibrosis infection management includes routine surveillance for acquisition and potential eradication of pathogens and personalizing antimicrobial therapies based on infection severity and chronicity, pulmonary function response, and tolerance of treatments with respect to allergies and modes of delivery [5]. For example, treatment of newly acquired *P. aeruginosa* typically requires treatment with inhaled antibiotics toward the goal of eradication. Individuals with chronic *P. aeruginosa* and other Gram-negative infections can benefit from regular cycled use of inhaled antibiotics, such as tobramycin, aztreonam, or colistimethate. Multiple inhaled antibiotics are available or are in clinical trials for such infections as *P. aeruginosa*, NTM, and MRSA [22].

Tobramycin Tobramycin is an aminoglycoside antibiotic that is bactericidal against Gram-negative bacteria, including *P. aeruginosa*, but notably not against other bacteria seen in CF infections, namely BCC and *Stenotrophomonas maltophilia*. Short-term aerosol administration of inhaled tobramycin has been shown to be both safe and effective in the treatment of *P. aeruginosa*, with improvement in pulmonary function (measured by percent predicted forced expiratory volume in 1 second, FEV_1), decrease in the sputum load of *P. aeruginosa*, and reduction in the risk of hospitalization. The improvement in pulmonary function was most prominent in adolescents with CF between 14 and 17 years of age. In open-label trials, the use of tobramycin inhalation solution in alternating 28-day cycles over 2 years showed that pulmonary function was maintained over baseline with a 25–33% reduction in the number of hospital days in the treatment group compared to placebo [23]. Established guidelines for chronic therapy recommend the use of alternate month inhaled tobramycin for individuals over 6 years of age with moderate to severe pulmonary disease and chronic *P. aeruginosa* in airway cultures [10]. Eradication of early *P. aeruginosa* is the standard of care internationally. In the United States, treatment of first acquisition of *P. aeruginosa*, which consists of a 28-day cycle of inhaled tobramycin, is recommended [24]. The Early Pseudomonas Infection Control (EPIC) trial demonstrated that prophylactic therapy with inhaled tobramycin is not beneficial [25]. Inhaled tobramycin is available in a variety of formulations for nebulization or dry powder for inhalation and is generally well tolerated. Reported side effects include hoarseness of the voice and bronchoconstriction; the emergence of bacterial resistance is uncommon.

Aztreonam Lysine Aztreonam is active against aerobic Gram-negative bacteria by inhibiting bacterial cell wall synthesis. Specifically designed for inhalation therapy, aztreonam lysine for inhalation (AZLI) was well tolerated in phase I clinical trials [26] with sputum concentrations that exceeded the minimum inhibitory concentration (MIC) for *P. aeruginosa*. Phase II clinical trials confirmed optimal dosing at 75 milligrams three times daily and that higher doses were associated with adverse effects such as increased frequency of cough [27]. The use of AZLI also showed increased time to development of the next pulmonary exacerbation as well as an improvement in the respiratory domain using a disease-specific quality of life assessment tool [28]. Secondary endpoints were improvements in pulmonary function and decreased bacterial density in sputum. Additionally, there was no increase in the MIC of *P. aeruginosa* [29].

The traditional approach employs inhaled tobramycin or aztreonam in alternating 28-day cycles on and off therapy but may lead to decline in pulmonary function during the cycle off antibiotic. Therefore, the use of continuously inhaled antibiotics has been proposed as an approach to better suppress *P. aeruginosa* infection and prevent progression of pulmonary disease. A trial of alternating inhaled tobramycin and aztreonam every 28 days was conducted but terminated early because of difficulty in enrolling participants. Individuals receiving three alternating cycles of inhaled tobramycin and aztreonam had fewer exacerbations and hospitalizations than those receiving alternate-month inhaled tobramycin alone, though the measured outcomes did not reach statistical significance [30].

Colistimethate Sodium Colistimethate sodium is a polymyxin derivative that exerts bactericidal activity against Gram-negative bacteria by increasing cell membrane permeability. Inhaled colistimethate sodium has been used for many years for the treatment of chronic *P. aeruginosa* infection, either on alternate month treatment alone or in combination with inhaled tobramycin. Rates of colistimethate resistance to *P. aeruginosa* have remained low. A dry powder formulation has been tested in phase III clinical trials and approved in Europe as a treatment for chronic *P. aeruginosa* infection [22].

Liposomal Amikacin Recently approved by the FDA for treatment of *Mycobacterium avium intracellulare* complex, liposomal amikacin is potent against *P. aeruginosa* as well as nontuberculous mycobacteria. Upon nebulization, the liposomes penetrate CF sputum and are lysed, resulting in prolonged half-life and deposition within the lung. In randomized clinical trials, once daily dosing of liposomal amikacin was safe and well tolerated in individuals with CF with efficacy against *P. aeruginosa* [31].

Inhaled Fluoroquinolones Known for their activity against *P. aeruginosa*, inhaled fluoroquinolones are under study in clinical trials. Inhaled levofloxacin has been approved for use in Europe against chronic *P. aeruginosa* infection. The initial phase I results of inhaled levofloxacin demonstrated tolerability and sputum drug concentrations sufficient for bacterial killing [32]. It has been reported that inhaled levofloxacin leads to a lower rate of hospitalizations for treatment of pulmonary exacerbations and reduced sputum density of *P. aeruginosa* compared to inhaled tobramycin. Phase III clinical trials demonstrated favorable safety and efficacy with improvement in pulmonary function and quality of life [33]. Also in development are liposomal and dry powder formulations of inhaled ciprofloxacin for treatment of chronic *P. aeruginosa* infection.

Inhaled Vancomycin There is presently no consensus recommendation for the management of MRSA infection in individuals with CF. Inhaled vancomycin has been used for both eradication and decolonization of MRSA infection. Prior work [34] has demonstrated MRSA eradication, defined by negative cultures over a minimum 6-month period, but had small sample sizes. Because MRSA is present in over 25% of the CF population, a recent double-blind, randomized, placebo-controlled study utilized an MRSA eradication protocol that included topical decontamination, environmental cleaning, and oral antibiotics with randomized treatment with either inhaled vancomycin or placebo. This study showed no difference in MRSA eradication rates one and three months after completion of treatment and concluded that persistent MRSA infection is difficult to eradicate with a single course of treatment with inhaled vancomycin [35].

Antifungal Therapy The use of antifungal agents is not presently part of chronic CF management [18]. Colonization or chronic infection with *Aspergillus* species has been treated with antifungal agents. Treatment of allergic bronchopulmonary aspergillosis (ABPA) consists of extended corticosteroid therapy, sometimes given in combination with antifungal agents. More randomized, controlled clinical trials are needed to guide recommendations for treatment. While bacterial pathogens such as *P. aeruginosa* and MRSA remain a primary research and treatment focus in CF pulmonary disease, there is an increasing body of evidence regarding the role of fungal pathogens. It remains unclear as to whether fungi are actively involved in CF infections or are merely bystanders in a dysregulated microenvironment, as discussed elsewhere in this book.

Pulmonary Therapies for Clearing Mucous Secretions

Airway clearance therapy (ACT) in the management of CF pulmonary disease serves to remove airway secretions and lessen the burden of infection through the removal of bacteria and other irritants and thus improve gas exchange, reduce airway resistance, correct ventilation-perfusion mismatch, and decrease proteolytic activity. There are established consensus guidelines for airway clearance, including exercise, in CF [36]. Airway clearance therapies are typically performed twice daily as maintenance therapy and increased in frequency for treatment of acute pulmonary disease exacerbations [36]. Frequently, airway clearance therapies are used in conjunction with inhaled mucus modulating therapies to facilitate mucus removal. Exercise is an adjunct to regular airway clearance modalities. As with other CF therapies, airway clearance should be personalized to maximize efficacy through adherence.

Commonly used airway clearance techniques include postural drainage and percussion, active cycle of breathing, autogenic drainage, positive expiratory pressure (high pressure or oscillating), high-frequency chest wall oscillation, and exercise. Airway clearance maneuvers are typically used in conjunction with inhaled mucus altering therapies designed to thin viscous secretions and facilitate their removal from the airways. Inhaled mucus altering agents include: recombinant human DNase (dornase alfa, rhDNase) N-acetylcysteine, mannitol, and hypertonic saline.

Recommended exclusively in the chronic management of CF pulmonary disease, dornase alfa is an enzyme that cleaves DNA polymers released from neutrophils in the characteristically purulent airway secretions [10]. Dornase alfa has been shown to improve pulmonary function and decrease exacerbations in individuals with CF, and is thus part of the recommended chronic maintenance treatment regimen. N-acetylcysteine has free sulfhydryl groups that hydrolyze disulfide bonds in mucins and thus lower mucus viscosity and elasticity. Although N-acetylcysteine has been used for decades as a mucolytic agent in CF, there are no data that conclusively demonstrate a beneficial effect in CF [37]. Approved for use in Europe and Australia in the treatment of both CF and non-CF bronchiectasis, inhaled mannitol acts as an expectorant by drawing water and mucus secretions into the airway [38, 39].

Aerosolized hypertonic saline (typically used and prescribed as a 3% or 7% solution) causes expectoration by inducing water and mucus secretion into the airway, primarily based on studies from Australia that demonstrated improvement in pulmonary function and decreased exacerbations [40]. Long-term use of inhaled hypertonic saline is recommended to improve pulmonary function and reduce the frequency of exacerbations in adults and children over 6 years of age [10]. Data regarding the effectiveness of hypertonic saline in younger children are mixed. In infants and children with CF younger than 6 years of age, treatment with 7% hypertonic saline did not reduce the rate of pulmonary exacerbations over the course of 48 weeks of treatment [41]. However, a recent study demonstrated improvements in lung clearance index and weight gain in infants less than 4 months of age with CF with preventive inhalation of 6% hypertonic saline [42]. Therefore, CF Foundation guidelines recommend selective use of inhaled hypertonic saline in children 2–5 years of age for either chronic treatment or during an acute pulmonary exacerbation [11].

Pulmonary Therapies for Reducing Airway Inflammation

Cystic fibrosis pulmonary disease is caused in part by chronic airway inflammation. Currently used anti-inflammatory therapies include high-dose ibuprofen and oral azithromycin [5, 10]. The routine use of oral or inhaled corticosteroids as chronic maintenance therapy is not recommended for individuals with CF unless the treatment is for co-existing inflammatory conditions, such as asthma or allergic bronchopulmonary aspergillosis (ABPA). High-dose ibuprofen has been shown to decrease neutrophil migration in CF individuals between 6 and 17 years of age when serum ibuprofen levels are between 50 and 100 μg/mL. Although clear benefit of this anti-inflammatory therapy has been demonstrated in clinical trials, treatment with high-dose ibuprofen is not widely used in clinical practice because of the small increased risk of gastrointestinal bleeding and need for drug level monitoring [43].

Oral azithromycin, typically dosed three times a week, has been shown to improve pulmonary function and reduce the frequency of pulmonary exacerbations in patients with and without evidence of chronic *P. aeruginosa* infection [44, 45]. The use of azithromycin as anti-inflammatory therapy has been used for decades and is included in guidelines for chronic medication therapy in CF, but at the present time, is somewhat controversial [5]. A 2014 retrospective study reported a significant decrease in lung function in a cohort reporting regular azithromycin use and randomized to inhaled tobramycin use compared to a cohort not reporting azithromycin use and concluded that oral azithromycin may antagonize the therapeutic benefits of inhaled tobramycin in individuals with chronic *P. aeruginosa* infection [46]. A 2017 study reported improvements in pulmonary function and respiratory domain quality of life scores in participants treated with azithromycin and concomitant use of inhaled tobramycin and inhaled aztreonam compared to participants who did not use azithromycin [47]. Data obtained using clinical *P. aeruginosa* strains in vitro showed selective reduction of the bactericidal effects of tobramycin and upregulation of an efflux antibiotic resistance mechanism. Taken together, these studies suggest that the concomitant use of oral azithromycin may lessen the effectiveness of inhaled tobramycin for chronic *P. aeruginosa* infection. Recently, the OPTIMIZE (Optimizing Treatment for Early *Pseudomonas aeruginosa* Infection in Cystic Fibrosis) trial demonstrated that 18 months of azithromycin therapy, three times weekly, significantly reduced pulmonary exacerbations and improved weight gain without impacting *P. aeruginosa* infections in young children with CF [48]. These reports further emphasize the need for confirmatory, prospective studies to not only delineate mechanisms of bacterial resistance, but also identify which individuals may be more vulnerable to potential drug interactions; thereby improving safety and tolerability of chronic pulmonary anti-infective therapies.

There is concern that chronic azithromycin use in individuals who have occult nontuberculous mycobacterial infection will lead specifically to antibiotic resistance and further complicate treatment. Individuals with CF should be screened for nontuberculous mycobacterial infection before starting oral azithromycin and at least annually. Additionally, azithromycin should be discontinued with newly acquired nontuberculous mycobacterial infection until comprehensive therapy is started. Interestingly, recent data suggest that chronic azithromycin therapy may in fact decrease the risk of acquiring nontuberculous mycobacterial infection [49].

Although inflammation leads to pulmonary damage in CF, it also plays a role in controlling infection [50]. While current anti-inflammatory therapies, including oral azithromycin and high-dose ibuprofen, have broad effects on immune function, newer drugs, such as acebilustat and lenabasum, target inflammatory pathways and can also play a role in controlling infection. Acebilustat is a leukotriene A_4 (LTA_4) hydrolase inhibitor that targets excessive neutrophil influx [51, 52] and is presently in phase II clinical trials assessing change in pulmonary function, frequency of pulmonary exacerbations, time to first pulmonary exacerbation, and effects on pulmonary and systemic inflammatory biomarkers [53]. Lenabasum, a selective cannabinoid receptor type 2 (CB2) agonist, reduced lipopolysaccharide inflammation in an in vitro airway macrophage model. In phase II clinical trials, lenabasum showed a decrease in pulmonary exacerbations and reduced synthesis of key airway proinflammatory cytokines in adults with CF [54]. The increase in pulmonary exacerbations observed in subjects receiving the leukotriene B_4 (LTB_4) receptor antagonist BIIL 284 BS in a 2014 phase II trial demonstrated that maintaining an appropriate inflammatory response is vitally important [55]. Studies have demonstrated the influence of inflammatory genes as CF pulmonary disease modifiers [56–58]. Effects of inflammatory genes can be greatly altered by environmental factors. For example, the effect of secondhand cigarette smoke exposure is influenced by TGF-β polymorphisms [59, 60].

Personalizing Chronic Pulmonary Therapies in the Era of CFTR Modulator Treatment

Understanding disease pathogenesis in CF has led to the continued development of novel and effective therapies as well as treatment guidelines to further personalize CF care and treatment regimens beyond the use of chronic medications. While one goal is to standardize treatment for all affected individuals, CF treatment must still be personalized and include input from individuals, their families and caregivers, and CF care teams, in line with the concept of family and provider coproduction in clinical care [4]. The design of a long-term, daily pulmonary treatment regimen is not simply choosing from available options of inhaled or oral medications, airway clearance modalities, and regular exercise. Customizing CF care should be based on multiple factors, such as genotype, associated systemic manifestations, microbiology profile, and individual preference to improve not only clinical outcomes but also adherence to a complex treatment regimen.

With availability of CFTR modulator treatment, it is now possible to speculate that there may be fewer disease-associated complications once effective medication combinations are available for all affected CF individuals and treatment is initiated as early as possible in the course of disease. Future studies will be needed to determine the long-term impact of CFTR modulators on acquisition or establishment of chronic infection. This raises the question of how chronic therapies, sometimes referred to as the "legacy" therapies, will be utilized in future CF management. For the foreseeable future, there will remain major challenges with respect to treatment of respiratory bacterial infections and other extrapulmonary manifestations of CF, which will define how chronic therapies are prescribed and recommended and how they should be used, for example, in the setting of pulmonary exacerbations. The full impact on health care costs has yet to be realized. Nevertheless, a major advantage of CFTR modulator therapy is the promise it holds for dramatically slowing disease progression, reducing daily treatment burden and aggressive pulmonary disease management, and improving quality of health, quality of life, and overall survival.

References

1. Davis PB. Cystic fibrosis since 1938. Am J Respir Crit Care Med. 2006;173(5):475–82.
2. Paranjape SM, Mogayzel PJ Jr. Cystic fibrosis in the era of precision medicine. Paediatr Respir Rev. 2018;25:64–72.
3. Spielberg DR, Clancy JP. Cystic fibrosis and its management through established and emerging therapies. Annu Rev Genomics Hum Genet. 2016;22:22.
4. Sabadosa KA, Batalden PB. The interdependent roles of patients, families and professionals in cystic fibrosis: a system for the coproduction of healthcare and its improvement. BMJ Qual Saf. 2014;23(Suppl 1):i90–4.
5. Mogayzel PJ Jr, Naureckas ET, Robinson KA, Mueller G, Hadjiliadis D, Hoag JB, et al. Cystic fibrosis pulmonary guidelines. Chronic medications for maintenance of lung health. Am J Respir Crit Care Med. 2013;187(7):680–9.

6. Castellani C, Duff AJA, Bell SC, Heijerman HGM, Munck A, Ratjen F, et al. ECFS best practice guidelines: the 2018 revision. J Cyst Fibros. 2018;17(2):153–78.

7. Robinson KA, Saldanha IJ, McKoy NA. Management of infants with cystic fibrosis: a summary of the evidence for the cystic fibrosis foundation working group on care of infants with cystic fibrosis. J Pediatr. 2009;155(6 Suppl):S94–s105.

8. Ren CL, Morgan RL, Oermann C, Resnick HE, Brady C, Campbell A, et al. Cystic Fibrosis Foundation pulmonary guidelines. Use of cystic fibrosis transmembrane conductance regulator modulator therapy in patients with cystic fibrosis. Ann Am Thorac Soc. 2018;15(3):271–80.

9. Riekert KA, Eakin MN, Bilderback A, Ridge AK, Marshall BC. Opportunities for cystic fibrosis care teams to support treatment adherence. J Cyst Fibros. 2015;14(1):142–8. https://doi.org/10.1016/j.jcf.2014.10.003. Epub Oct 24

10. Flume PA, O'Sullivan BP, Robinson KA, Goss CH, Mogayzel PJ Jr, Willey-Courand DB, et al. Cystic fibrosis pulmonary guidelines: chronic medications for maintenance of lung health. Am J Respir Crit Care Med. 2007;176(10):957–69.

11. Lahiri T, Hempstead SE, Brady C, Cannon CL, Clark K, Condren ME, et al. Clinical practice guidelines from the Cystic Fibrosis Foundation for preschoolers with cystic fibrosis. Pediatrics. 2016;137(4):pii: e20151784.

12. Borowitz D, Robinson KA, Rosenfeld M, Davis SD, Sabadosa KA, Spear SL, et al. Cystic Fibrosis Foundation evidence-based guidelines for management of infants with cystic fibrosis. J Pediatr. 2009;155(6 Suppl):S73–93.

13. Borowitz D, Parad RB, Sharp JK, Sabadosa KA, Robinson KA, Rock MJ, et al. Cystic Fibrosis Foundation practice guidelines for the management of infants with cystic fibrosis transmembrane conductance regulator-related metabolic syndrome during the first two years of life and beyond. J Pediatr. 2009;155(6 Suppl):S106–16.

14. Corvol H, Blackman SM, Boelle PY, Gallins PJ, Pace RG, Stonebraker JR, et al. Genome-wide association meta-analysis identifies five modifier loci of lung disease severity in cystic fibrosis. Nat Commun. 2015;6:8382. https://doi.org/10.1038/ncomms9382.

15. Collaco JM, Raraigh KS, Appel LJ, Cutting GR. Respiratory pathogens mediate the association between lung function and temperature in cystic fibrosis. J Cyst Fibros. 2016;15(6):794–801. https://doi.org/10.1016/j.jcf.2016.05.012. Epub Jun 11

16. 2017 Annual data report. Bethesda, MD: Cystic Fibrosis Foundation Patient Registry 2018.

17. Chotirmall SH, McElvaney NG. Fungi in the cystic fibrosis lung: bystanders or pathogens? Int J Biochem Cell Biol. 2014;52:161–73. https://doi.org/10.1016/j.biocel.2014.03.001. Epub Mar 10

18. Moss RB. Fungi in cystic fibrosis and non-cystic fibrosis bronchiectasis. Semin Respir Crit Care Med. 2015;36(2):207–16. https://doi.org/10.1055/s-0035-1546750. Epub 2015 Mar 31

19. Prevots DR, Adjemian J, Fernandez AG, Knowles MR, Olivier KN. Environmental risks for nontuberculous mycobacteria. Individual exposures and climatic factors in the cystic fibrosis population. Ann Am Thorac Soc. 2014;11(7):1032–8. https://doi.org/10.1513/AnnalsATS.201404-184OC.

20. Springman AC, Jacobs JL, Somvanshi VS, Sundin GW, Mulks MH, Whittam TS, et al. Genetic diversity and multihost pathogenicity of clinical and environmental strains of Burkholderia cenocepacia. Appl Environ Microbiol. 2009;75(16):5250–60. https://doi.org/10.1128/AEM.00877-09. Epub 2009 Jun 19

21. Zhao J, Schloss PD, Kalikin LM, Carmody LA, Foster BK, Petrosino JF, et al. Decade-long bacterial community dynamics in cystic fibrosis airways. Proc Natl Acad Sci U S A. 2012;109(15):5809–14. https://doi.org/10.1073/pnas.1120577109. Epub 2012 Mar 26

22. Tay GT, Reid DW, Bell SC. Inhaled antibiotics in Cystic Fibrosis (CF) and non-CF bronchiectasis. Semin Respir Crit Care Med. 2015;36(2):267–86.

23. Moss RB. Long-term benefits of inhaled tobramycin in adolescent patients with cystic fibrosis. Chest. 2002;121(1):55–63.

24. Mogayzel PJ Jr, Naureckas ET, Robinson KA, Brady C, Guill M, Lahiri T, et al. Cystic Fibrosis Foundation pulmonary guideline. Pharmacologic approaches to prevention and eradication of initial Pseudomonas aeruginosa infection. Ann Am Thorac Soc. 2014;11(10):1640–50.

25. Treggiari MM, Retsch-Bogart G, Mayer-Hamblett N, Khan U, Kulich M, Kronmal R, et al. Comparative efficacy and safety of 4 randomized regimens to treat early Pseudomonas aeruginosa infection in children with cystic fibrosis. Arch Pediatr Adolesc Med. 2011;165(9):847–56.
26. Gibson RL, Retsch-Bogart GZ, Oermann C, Milla C, Pilewski J, Daines C, et al. Microbiology, safety, and pharmacokinetics of aztreonam lysinate for inhalation in patients with cystic fibrosis. Pediatr Pulmonol. 2006;41(7):656–65.
27. Retsch-Bogart GZ, Burns JL, Otto KL, Liou TG, McCoy K, Oermann C, et al. A phase 2 study of aztreonam lysine for inhalation to treat patients with cystic fibrosis and Pseudomonas aeruginosa infection. Pediatr Pulmonol. 2008;43(1):47–58.
28. Retsch-Bogart GZ, Quittner AL, Gibson RL, Oermann CM, McCoy KS, Montgomery AB, et al. Efficacy and safety of inhaled aztreonam lysine for airway pseudomonas in cystic fibrosis. Chest. 2009;135(5):1223–32.
29. Oermann CM, McCoy KS, Retsch-Bogart GZ, Gibson RL, McKevitt M, Montgomery AB. Pseudomonas aeruginosa antibiotic susceptibility during long-term use of aztreonam for inhalation solution (AZLI). J Antimicrob Chemother. 2011;66(10):2398–404.
30. Flume PA, Clancy JP, Retsch-Bogart GZ, Tullis DE, Bresnik M, Derchak PA, et al. Continuous alternating inhaled antibiotics for chronic pseudomonal infection in cystic fibrosis. J Cyst Fibros. 2016;15(6):809–15.
31. Clancy JP, Dupont L, Konstan MW, Billings J, Fustik S, Goss CH, et al. Phase II studies of nebulised Arikace in CF patients with Pseudomonas aeruginosa infection. Thorax. 2013;68(9):818–25.
32. Elborn JS, Flume PA, Cohen F, Loutit J, VanDevanter DR. Safety and efficacy of prolonged levofloxacin inhalation solution (APT-1026) treatment for cystic fibrosis and chronic Pseudomonas aeruginosa airway infection. J Cyst Fibros. 2016;15(5):634–40.
33. Flume PA, VanDevanter DR, Morgan EE, Dudley MN, Loutit JS, Bell SC, et al. A phase 3, multi-center, multinational, randomized, double-blind, placebo-controlled study to evaluate the efficacy and safety of levofloxacin inhalation solution (APT-1026) in stable cystic fibrosis patients. J Cyst Fibros. 2016;15(4):495–502.
34. Lo DK, Muhlebach MS, Smyth AR. Interventions for the eradication of meticillin-resistant Staphylococcus aureus (MRSA) in people with cystic fibrosis. Cochrane Database Syst Rev. 2018;7:CD009650.
35. Dezube R, Jennings MT, Rykiel M, Diener-West M, Boyle MP, Chmiel JF, et al. Eradication of persistent methicillin-resistant Staphylococcus aureus infection in cystic fibrosis. J Cyst Fibros. 2018;8(3):357–63.
36. Flume PA, Robinson KA, O'Sullivan BP, Finder JD, Vender RL, Willey-Courand DB, et al. Cystic fibrosis pulmonary guidelines: airway clearance therapies. Respir Care. 2009;54(4):522–37.
37. Rubin BK. Aerosol medications for treatment of mucus clearance disorders. Respir Care. 2015;60(6):825–9. discussion 30–2
38. Tildy BE, Rogers DF. Therapeutic options for hydrating airway mucus in cystic fibrosis. Pharmacology. 2015;95(3–4):117–32.
39. Hurt K, Bilton D. Inhaled mannitol for the treatment of cystic fibrosis. Expert Rev Respir Med. 2012;6(1):19–26.
40. Elkins MR, Robinson M, Rose BR, Harbour C, Moriarty CP, Marks GB, et al. A controlled trial of long-term inhaled hypertonic saline in patients with cystic fibrosis. N Engl J Med. 2006;354(3):229–40.
41. Rosenfeld M, Ratjen F, Brumback L, Daniel S, Rowbotham R, McNamara S, et al. Inhaled hypertonic saline in infants and children younger than 6 years with cystic fibrosis: the ISIS randomized controlled trial. JAMA. 2012;307(21):2269–77.
42. Stahl M, Wielputz MO, Ricklefs I, Dopfer C, Barth S, Schlegtendal A, et al. Preventive Inhalation of Hypertonic Saline in Infants with Cystic Fibrosis (PRESIS): a randomized, double-blind, controlled study. Am J Respir Crit Care Med. 2018;199(10):1238–48.
43. Konstan MW, Davis PB. Pharmacological approaches for the discovery and development of new anti-inflammatory agents for the treatment of cystic fibrosis. Adv Drug Deliv Rev. 2002;54(11):1409–23.

44. Saiman L, Anstead M, Mayer-Hamblett N, Lands LC, Kloster M, Hocevar-Trnka J, et al. Effect of azithromycin on pulmonary function in patients with cystic fibrosis uninfected with Pseudomonas aeruginosa: a randomized controlled trial. JAMA. 2010;303(17):1707–15.

45. Saiman L, Marshall BC, Mayer-Hamblett N, Burns JL, Quittner AL, Cibene DA, et al. Azithromycin in patients with cystic fibrosis chronically infected with Pseudomonas aeruginosa: a randomized controlled trial. JAMA. 2003;290(13):1749–56.

46. Nick JA, Moskowitz SM, Chmiel JF, Forssen AV, Kim SH, Saavedra MT, et al. Azithromycin may antagonize inhaled tobramycin when targeting Pseudomonas aeruginosa in cystic fibrosis. Ann Am Thorac Soc. 2014;11(3):342–50.

47. Nichols DP, Happoldt CL, Bratcher PE, Caceres SM, Chmiel JF, Malcolm KC, et al. Impact of azithromycin on the clinical and antimicrobial effectiveness of tobramycin in the treatment of cystic fibrosis. J Cyst Fibros. 2017;16(3):358–66.

48. Mayer-Hamblett N, Retsch-Bogart G, Kloster M, Accurso F, Rosenfeld M, Albers G, et al. Azithromycin for early pseudomonas infection in cystic fibrosis. The OPTIMIZE randomized trial. Am J Respir Crit Care Med. 2018;198(9):1177–87.

49. Binder AM, Adjemian J, Olivier KN, Prevots DR. Epidemiology of nontuberculous mycobacterial infections and associated chronic macrolide use among persons with cystic fibrosis. Am J Respir Crit Care Med. 2013;188(7):807–12.

50. Cantin AM, Hartl D, Konstan MW, Chmiel JF. Inflammation in cystic fibrosis lung disease: pathogenesis and therapy. J Cyst Fibros. 2015;14(4):419–30. https://doi.org/10.1016/j.jcf.2015.03.003. Epub Mar 23

51. Elborn JS, Bhatt L, Grosswald R, Ahuja S, Springman EB. Phase I studies of Acebilustat: pharmacokinetics, pharmacodynamics, food effect, and CYP3A induction. Clin Transl Sci. 2017;10(1):20–7. https://doi.org/10.1111/cts.12426. Epub 2016 Oct 28

52. Elborn JS, Horsley A, MacGregor G, Bilton D, Grosswald R, Ahuja S, et al. Phase I studies of Acebilustat: biomarker response and safety in patients with cystic fibrosis. Clin Transl Sci. 2017;10(1):28–34. https://doi.org/10.1111/cts.12428. Epub 2016 Nov 2

53. Elborn JS, Ahuja S, Springman E, Mershon J, Grosswald R, Rowe SM. EMPIRE-CF: a phase II randomized placebo-controlled trial of once-daily, oral acebilustat in adult patients with cystic fibrosis – study design and patient demographics. Contemp Clin Trials. 2018;72:86–94.

54. Lubamba B, Zhang G, Tepper M, Ribeiro C. Lenabasum reduces LPS-induced inflammation in airway macrophages from human cystic fibrosis lungs. Pediatr Pulmonol. 2018;53(Supplement 2):S242.

55. Konstan MW, Doring G, Heltshe SL, Lands LC, Hilliard KA, Koker P, et al. A randomized double blind, placebo controlled phase 2 trial of BIIL 284 BS (an LTB4 receptor antagonist) for the treatment of lung disease in children and adults with cystic fibrosis. J Cyst Fibros. 2014;13(2):148–55. https://doi.org/10.1016/j.jcf.2013.12.009. Epub 4 Jan 17

56. Cutting GR. Modifier genes in Mendelian disorders: the example of cystic fibrosis. Ann N Y Acad Sci. 2010;1214:57–69. https://doi.org/10.1111/j.749-6632.2010.05879.x.

57. Knowles MR. Gene modifiers of lung disease. Curr Opin Pulm Med. 2006;12(6):416–21.

58. Merlo CA, Boyle MP. Modifier genes in cystic fibrosis lung disease. J Lab Clin Med. 2003;141(4):237–41.

59. Collaco JM, Vanscoy L, Bremer L, McDougal K, Blackman SM, Bowers A, et al. Interactions between secondhand smoke and genes that affect cystic fibrosis lung disease. JAMA. 2008;299(4):417–24. https://doi.org/10.1001/jama.299.4.417.

60. Drumm ML, Konstan MW, Schluchter MD, Handler A, Pace R, Zou F, et al. Genetic modifiers of lung disease in cystic fibrosis. N Engl J Med. 2005;353(14):1443–53.

Chapter 11
Advanced Stage Lung Disease

Bryan Garcia, Jessica Mattson, and Patrick A. Flume

The pathogenesis of cystic fibrosis (CF) lung disease is the downstream result of multiple factors including chronic airways infection and unabated pulmonary and systemic inflammation resulting in progressive loss of lung function. Therapeutic advancements including airway clearance therapies, antibiotics, and highly effective CFTR modulators have resulted in improved health outcomes and improved survival; however, the predicted life expectancy for CF patients remains well below that of the rest of the population, and respiratory failure is the most common cause of death [1–3]. As such, the patients, their families, and CF care providers must be prepared to manage the challenges of advanced stage lung disease. The focus of this chapter is the care of CF patients with advanced stage lung disease and includes defining advanced CF lung disease, risk factors associated with the development of advanced lung disease, the pulmonary complications associated with advanced CF lung disease and their corresponding management, and, finally, referral for transplantation and palliative care.

B. Garcia (✉)
Department of Medicine, Medical University of South Carolina, Charleston, SC, USA
e-mail: garciab@musc.edu

J. Mattson
Person with CF2, Bluffton, SC, USA

P. A. Flume
Department of Medicine, Medical University of South Carolina, Charleston, SC, USA

Department of Pediatrics, Medical University of South Carolina, Charleston, SC, USA

© Springer Nature Switzerland AG 2020
S. D. Davis et al. (eds.), *Cystic Fibrosis*, Respiratory Medicine,
https://doi.org/10.1007/978-3-030-42382-7_11

Advanced Stage Lung Disease in Cystic Fibrosis

Advanced stage lung disease is defined as a severity of lung impairment such that the end of life is predicted to be near and for which additional planning should be performed. Objective measurement of lung function using spirometry is the primary indicator of disease severity with forced expiratory volume in 1 second (FEV_1) used to define severity of airway obstruction. Because all patients with advanced CF lung disease have low FEV_1, the forced vital capacity (FVC) is used by transplant pulmonologists for the purpose of risk stratification pertaining to the risk of the transplantation as well as to further subcategorize disease severity among CF patients with end-stage disease awaiting transplantation as it pertains to lung allocation score [4]. Lung function measures are normalized and reported as a percent of predicted. Since the percent of predicted is normalized for age, a 15-year-old with an FEV_1 of 50% predicted should be considered at a more advanced stage of disease compared to a 30-year-old with the same lung function [5].

Patients with advanced stage lung disease based on pulmonary function alone commonly request prognostic timelines, and this information is relevant for the purpose of transplantation timing. As will be described in greater detail later in this chapter, broad heterogeneity in disease progression makes prognostication complex. Additionally, the rapid growth of therapeutics available to CF patients means that prognostication is evolving as additional therapeutics altering disease course become available. For example, the median transplant-free survival for CF patients with $FEV_1 < 30\%$ predicted in 1998 was 3.9 years and has increased to 6.6 years in 2013 [6, 7]. Importantly, these data reflect the time period prior to the broad utilization of CFTR modulators, and their effect on survival in advanced stage disease remains uncertain [8].

FEV_1 as a percent of predicted has been associated with survival on a population basis, but for the individual patient, it is a poor independent predictor of mortality risk [4, 7]. Given the broad heterogeneity in disease progression at advanced stages, alternative markers of disease progression, beyond lung function alone, have been proposed such as rate of lung function decline and exacerbation frequency [9]. Recent formulas have sought to address this further by including a range of clinically relevant variables including gender, CFTR genotype, age, pulmonary function, nutritional status, presence of CF-related diabetes, and presence of specific airway pathogens [10–12]. Despite increased predicted survival in advanced CF, such models remain limited in their predictive capacity at an individual level.

Risk Factors for Disease Progression

Clinically relevant variables that have been identified as risk factors associated with disease progression include CFTR genotype, female gender, exacerbation frequency (>1 per year), presence of specific respiratory pathogens (including but not limited to *Staphylococcus aureus*, *Pseudomonas aeruginosa*, and *Burkholderia cepacia*), pancreatic insufficiency, cystic fibrosis-related diabetes (CFRD), low body mass index (BMI), uncontrolled mental health disorders including depression, and poor medication compliance [13–15]. Furthermore, given the complex nature of disease management and high disease treatment burden, socioeconomic status, low medical literacy, concomitant mental health issues, substance abuse, and lack of access to care have also previously been associated with both compliance and disease progression [16, 17].

The underlying assessment and management of patients with advanced stage CF lung disease is not inherently different from that of a patient with preserved lung function, but the identification of disease progression or development of other complications should prompt further evaluation to identify the precipitating etiology. Medications approved for the treatment of CF lung disease (e.g., dornase alfa, hypertonic saline, inhaled antibiotics, CFTR modulators) have demonstrated improvement in lung function, and adherence to the use of these medications is associated with improved clinical outcomes [2, 16, 18, 19]. Therefore, failure to optimize a treatment regimen on the part of the clinician and failure to adhere to the use of these therapies are primary risk factors for the development of progression of CF lung disease and the pulmonary complications associated with it. Risk factors associated with poor adherence are similar to those for disease progression and include clinical depression, substance abuse, low socioeconomic status, lack of access to medical care, high treatment burden, and low medical literacy [17, 20–23]. To address these issues, consensus guidelines recommend annual screening for depression and anxiety in the CF population [24]. Additionally, a trained medical social worker should be employed to help identify and assess any unmet psychosocial needs [25].

Pulmonary exacerbations, defined as acute worsening of respiratory symptoms and drop in lung function, occur throughout the course of CF disease, and patients with advanced disease experience an increase in exacerbation frequency and severity, a key complication of advanced disease. Additional key pulmonary complications associated with advanced stage CF lung disease include pneumothorax and hemoptysis. Diagnosis and management of pneumothorax and hemoptysis are discussed in greater detail later in this chapter; however, it is important to note that these events are associated with acute drops in lung function that often are not fully recovered. Furthermore, despite aggressive treatment, less than 50% of pulmonary exacerbations result in a return to pre-exacerbation baseline FEV_1 [26, 27]. Thus, exacerbation frequency is a predictor of increased risk for rapid loss of lung function.

Extrapulmonary manifestations of CF disease can also result in progressive lung function decline, and key extrapulmonary manifestations include the presence of pancreatic insufficiency, CFRD, and poor caloric intake [13]. CF treatment guidelines recommend annual screening for unrecognized CFRD [28]. Progressive loss of lung function with associated decline in BMI should prompt evaluation for development of CFRD and late-onset pancreatic insufficiency resulting in caloric malabsorption and nutritional deficiencies. Pancreatic sufficient patients should be screened annually for development of pancreatic insufficiency, and when present enzyme supplementation can result in improved nutrient absorption and BMI, a key predictor of lung function [29]. Similarly, uncontrolled hyperglycemia will result in loss of lean body mass, and improved glucose control may improve BMI and lung function [30].

Pulmonary Complications of Advanced Stage Lung Disease

Pneumothorax

Spontaneous pneumothorax is a well-recognized complication of CF lung disease with an average annual incidence of 0.64% or 1 in 167 patients per year, and approximately 3.4% of all CF patients will suffer a pneumothorax during their lifetime [31]. These events most commonly occur in older patients and those with more advanced lung impairment. A prior analysis demonstrated a median age of 21 years and demonstrated that 72.4% of all pneumothoraces occurred in patients over the age of 18 years. The primary risk factor for the occurrence of a pneumothorax in this analysis was the presence of severe obstructive airway disease with 75% of all pneumothoraces occurring in patients with an FEV_1 less than 40% predicted [31].

Pneumothoraces in CF are hypothesized to be the result of air trapping distal to bronchioles impacted by mucus plugs. This can result in alveolar pressure exceeding interstitial pressure and escape of air into the pleural space [32]. Patients typically present with acute-onset chest pain, but acute worsening dyspnea may also be a prominent symptom. Diagnosis is made by chest radiograph demonstrating the presence of free air within the thorax (however small); anterior pneumothoraces may require chest CT for visualization. Two-year mortality among CF patients with pneumothorax is high (48.6%); thus referral for lung transplant evaluation upon first event is appropriate [33, 34].

Previously, an expert panel utilized the Delphi technique to formalize consensus recommendations toward the management of both pneumothorax and hemoptysis in CF patients [34]. Recommendations from this panel included initial outpatient observation of small pneumothoraces (<3 cm) if the patient is clinically stable, while larger pneumothoraces (>3 cm) should be monitored in the hospital. Patients exhibiting signs of clinical instability or those with large pneumothoraces require evacuation of the pleural space via tube thoracostomy [34]. Patients should be maintained on airway clearance therapies, although the use of positive airway pressure in the form of BiPAP and intrapulmonary percussive ventilation may complicate resolution of the pneumothorax; many clinicians will add antibiotics and manage pneumothoraces as they would a typical pulmonary exacerbation.

In many cases, the pneumothorax will resolve, and the chest tube can be removed. However, cases of persistent air leak will require pleurodesis. A surgical approach to management of a non-resolving pneumothorax in CF patients was previously considered the preferred method, but it is recognized that CF patients are at increased risk for perioperative complications related to thoracic surgery. No prior random-ized control trial has described the results of either medical or surgical pleurodesis for this patient subset [35].

Recurrence rates of pneumothorax are high with estimates up to 50–90% [33]. There is risk for a subsequent contralateral pneumothorax, indicative of the underly-ing advanced lung disease and associated structural lung abnormalities such as severe bronchiectasis [32]. Utilization of early pleurodesis, given the high rate of ipsilateral recurrence, is controversial in this population due to lack of evidence sup-porting its use and because pleurodesis creates potential issues related to lung trans-plantation due to increased intraoperative bleeding during native lung dissection as a result of the development of pleural adhesions, potentially impacting the patient's transplant candidacy [34].

Hemoptysis

The prevalence of hemoptysis in the CF population is not known, and a prior retro-spective study reported a rate of 9.1% over a 5-year period; however this may be an underestimation as [36] analysis of placebo groups from prior clinical trials has demonstrated rates of hemoptysis of 21–31% over periods as short as 6 months [37–39]. A retrospective cohort study using data from eight prospective, longitudi-nal randomized trials found 8% of patients in the placebo groups reported hemopty-sis during an average period of 8 months [40]. These events occur more commonly in patients who are older, have *Pseudomonas* in sputum cultures, and have greater impairment in lung function.

CF clinicians define hemoptysis as scant (blood-streaked sputum), mild (>5 mL), or massive (>240 mL in 1 day or 2 days of greater than 100 mL), and management is dependent on severity [34, 41]. Massive hemoptysis occurs when bronchial arter-ies rupture, resulting in arterial blood flow into the airway, while scant or mild hemoptysis is likely the result of chronic inflammation causing localized destruc-tion of the airway epithelium. Increased presence of angiogenic mediators as a result of chronic airway inflammation leads to bronchial artery hypertrophy and enlarged, tortuous, and dilated vessels that are at increased risk of rupture.

The impact of hemoptysis on progression of lung disease is unknown, but mas-sive hemoptysis can be life-threatening. There is an average annual rate of massive hemoptysis of 0.87% or 1 in 115 patients per year, and 4.1% of all patients will suffer this complication in their lifetime [42]. Similar to pneumothorax, massive hemoptysis is more common in patients with severe obstructive lung disease; how-ever 22% of patients will have normal or mild obstruction on pulmonary function testing. The median age for this complication is 23 years, and 75% of patients will be greater than 18 years of age [42, 43]. Furthermore, massive hemoptysis has a high expected mortality, with an attributable risk for mortality between 5.8% and 16.1%; thus patients with massive hemoptysis warrant consideration for lung trans-plantation evaluation [41].

Most clinicians will treat hemoptysis as if it were a manifestation of a pulmonary exacerbation [34]. Therapeutic management includes systemic antibiotics; however the role for airway clearance and inhaled therapies are dependent upon the amount of bleeding. For those with mild bleeding, it is recommended to continue the full armamentarium of inhaled airway clearance therapies, but patients with evidence of massive hemoptysis may require withholding airway clearance therapies so as to not cause cough clearance of a formed clot [34]. Airway clearance therapies can be reinstituted once the bleeding has resolved, but guidelines regarding the precise timing and order of reinstitution do not exist. Additional assessment to identify and correct any underlying coagulopathy is also appropriate [34, 42].

For patients who fail to respond to conservative therapy, are unstable, or are experiencing massive hemoptysis, bronchial artery embolization (BAE) can be life-saving and is the preferred method of achieving resolution of the airway bleed. Although the source of bleeding could be identified by CT scan of the chest or by direct visualization by bronchoscopy, these diagnostic procedures are not recommended due to low clinical yield and increased delay in definitive management [34]. Despite successful initial embolization, recurrence is not uncommon, and utilization of BAE is associated with increased risk for respiratory failure, death, and requirement for lung transplantation, likely indicative of the presence of severe underlying lung disease [34, 44, 45]. Furthermore, complications of embolization range from mild including headache and chest pain to severe including the development of pulmonary hypertension, stroke, and permanent paralysis from spinal artery infarction.

Respiratory Failure and Pulmonary Hypertension

Chronic airway infection and inflammation results in progressive bronchiectasis, airflow obstruction, and airway remodeling. As a result of worsening bronchiectasis, ventilation-perfusion mismatching occurs leading to the development of chronic respiratory failure marked by both hypoxemia and hypercapnia. At present, there are no guidelines regarding the screening for hypercapnia; however, symptoms including morning headaches, fatigue, and poor sleep quality should prompt a clinician to assess for hypercapnia with blood gas sampling, and, if present, patients may be candidates for nocturnal noninvasive positive pressure ventilation (NIPPV) [46]. Recently, physicians have identified increased sleep disturbances among healthy CF patients, including the pediatric population. Routine screening with polysomnography has not been recommended, and, at present, the initiation of NIPPV for hypercapnia related to worsening lung disease is based on expert opinion [47, 48]. Furthermore, studies have not demonstrated survival benefit with the use of either nocturnal oxygen supplementation or NIPPV, but improvements in quality of life and functional status have been reported [49–51].

As lung function worsens and FEV_1 decreases below 40%, there is an increased risk for development of pulmonary hypertension, and patients should be assessed for exercise-induced hypoxemia [42]. Supplemental oxygen is indicated for anyone with resting hypoxemia or desaturation below 88% during exercise testing. The development of hypoxemic-induced pulmonary hypertension in CF is complex and a result of the interplay of hypoxemic vasoconstriction and vascular endothelial dysfunction, with resultant remodeling of pulmonary vasculature via subintimal fibrosis and muscularization of pulmonary arterioles [52, 53]. The prevalence of pulmonary hypertension remains unclear in the CF population with a recent study identifying a 57% rate of pulmonary hypertension in patients undergoing lung transplant evaluation [54]. Pulmonary hypertension is likely an under-recognized complication in CF patients due to symptomatic overlap with other aspects of CF lung disease; however, identification is important as the presence of pulmonary hypertension is associated with significantly increased risk of mortality without lung transplantation [54]. Transthoracic echocardiography can estimate the presence of elevated pulmonary pressures by utilizing tricuspid regurgitation jet velocity, but this method tends to underestimate pressures in patients, and right heart catheterization is the gold standard for measurement of arterial pressures; however this requires an invasive procedure [55].

Treatment modalities for pulmonary hypertension in CF patients are limited with the exception of supplemental oxygen in those with hypoxemia. Utilization of phosphodiesterase inhibitors and inhaled prostacyclins including sildenafil and iloprost has been described with success in case reports; however high-quality clinical trial data are lacking [56, 57].

Mechanical Ventilation and Extracorporeal Life Support

CF patients with acute respiratory failure may require mechanical ventilation for survival. Previously, the outcomes of CF patients treated with mechanical ventilation were so poor that its use was considered futile. More recent data reported a 40% mortality among CF patients on mechanical ventilation, demonstrating that many patients will successfully be weaned from ventilatory support [58, 59]. The patient's baseline lung function at the time of hospital admission is informative in predicting the likelihood of successful liberation from the ventilator [60]. Among patients with FEV_1 less than 25% of predicted or severe malnutrition, the prognosis is exceedingly poor, and mechanical ventilation is discouraged if imminent lung transplantation is not an option; for those patients currently listed for lung transplant, mechanical ventilation could be used as a bridge to transplant and does not adversely affect posttransplant survival [61].

In patients who suffer intractable respiratory failure despite mechanical ventilation, extracorporeal membrane oxygenation (ECMO) has been utilized with mixed success as a bridge to transplant. ECMO is a form of life support in which blood is removed through a dual-lumen catheter typically placed in the right internal jugular vein. Blood is pumped through an external membrane where it is oxygenated and carbon dioxide is removed, and subsequently blood is returned via the catheter to the right atrium. Ambulatory veno-venous ECMO (VV-ECMO) has been utilized as a bridge to lung transplant in an attempt to improve nutritional status and physical rehabilitation in patients with end-stage respiratory failure [62]. In patients with pre-existing severe disease who are not lung transplant candidates, use of ECMO is not recommended.

Transplant Referral Timing and Palliative Care

Lung transplantation is a therapeutic option for CF patients with advanced lung disease whose predicted 3-year survival is less than 50% [63]. CF is the indication for approximately 25% of all lung transplants performed worldwide [52, 64]. Historically transplant referral was indicated for patients with FEV_1 less than 30%; however this recommendation stems from single-center data demonstrating a 2-year survival of <50% for patients with $FEV_1 < 30\%$ predicted [65].

As previously described, due to the heterogenous disease course of CF and the recent success with CFTR modulator therapies, indications for timing of lung transplantation referral and lung transplant surgery require frequent reassessment. As evidence of the difficulty with mortality prediction, recently proposed models predicting mortality related to CF lung disease failed to produce significant improvement in prediction over FEV_1 less than 30% predicted alone [10, 66]. A recent study suggests patient-reported physical function and quality of life scores may significantly add to the identification of mortality risk related to CF lung disease and which patients are suitable for lung transplant referral [64].

Despite therapeutic advancements, improved management of complications of advanced CF lung disease, and lung transplantation, a majority of CF patients will ultimately succumb to respiratory failure that is typically preceded by recurrent pulmonary exacerbations, worsened lung function, increased healthcare utilization, and frequent hospitalization over a period of several months or years [67]. Therefore, providing high-quality care throughout the lifespan on the part of the CF providers includes helping navigate and manage end-of-life healthcare-related decisions. In addition to referral for transplant evaluation, inclusion of palliative care is necessary [68, 69]. Palliative therapies are intended to reduce symptoms of dyspnea and pain. For most CF patients, conventional therapies, including intravenous and inhaled antibiotics, and airway clearance therapies may be continued late into the disease course if the patient reports perceived symptomatic relief in response to therapy. Noninvasive ventilation may provide relief of dyspnea, reduced nocturnal headaches, and improved vitality when the patients have significant hypercarbia. Pain and dyspnea regimens will often include opiates, but they should be used judiciously as they may exacerbate other CF-related health issues such as constipation, and they should not be used as a substitute therapy for mental health problems such as depression.

It is imperative that providers address patient preferences regarding care planning via a process of structured discussion to ensure a patient's wishes are identified. This discussion should ensure the patient and the family understand that aggressive care can be continued per their wishes while also increasing focus on the alleviation of distressing symptoms including intractable dyspnea, nausea, anxiety, and constipation [67]. Additionally patient preference regarding place of death should be frankly discussed [70]. Interestingly, although few CF patients (<5%) report discussing advanced care planning with their CF team, they do report a desire to implement an early approach to advanced care planning, to address this topic during periods of clinical stability, and to receive insight from their primary pulmonologist in decision-making [71]. Thus, it is essential for CF clinicians to consider early discussion regarding advanced care planning as this may help identify long-term treatment goals and rationale for therapeutic decision-making as disease state progresses.

Summary

Therapeutic advancements including the identification of highly effective CFTR modulators, improved nutritional support modalities, and improved management of airways infections have resulted in improved life expectancy for CF patients. Despite these improvements, a subset of patients continue to experience progression of lung disease and respiratory complications associated with advanced stage disease including pneumothorax, hemoptysis, and hypoxic and hypercapnic respiratory failure. The effect of therapeutic advancements has demonstrated improvement in mortality even among patients with advanced stage disease, and CF clinicians must be astute in the management of these complex patients.

References

1. Keogh RH, Szczesniak R, Taylor-Robinson D, Bilton D. Up-to-date and projected estimates of survival for people with cystic fibrosis using baseline characteristics: a longitudinal study using UK patient registry data. J Cyst Fibros. 2018;17:218–27.
2. Taylor-Cousar JL, Munck A, McKone EF, van der Ent CK, Moeller A, Simard C, Wang LT, Ingenito EP, McKee C, Lu Y, Lekstrom-Himes J, Elborn JS. Tezacaftor-ivacaftor in patients with cystic fibrosis homozygous for phe508del. N Engl J Med. 2017;377:2013–23.
3. Cystic Fibrosis Foundation. 2016 annual data report to the center directors. Bethesda; 2017.
4. Hayes D Jr, Kirkby S, Whitson BA, Black SM, Sheikh SI, Tobias JD, Mansour HM, Kopp BT. Mortality risk and pulmonary function in adults with cystic fibrosis at time of wait listing for lung transplantation. Ann Thorac Surg. 2015;100:474–9.
5. Konstan MW, Wagener JS, VanDevanter DR. Characterizing aggressiveness and predicting future progression of cf lung disease. J Cyst Fibros. 2009;8(Suppl 1):S15–9.
6. George PM, Banya W, Pareek N, Bilton D, Cullinan P, Hodson ME, Simmonds NJ. Improved survival at low lung function in cystic fibrosis: cohort study from 1990 to 2007. BMJ. 2011;342:d1008.
7. Ramos KJ, Quon BS, Heltshe SL, Mayer-Hamblett N, Lease ED, Aitken ML, Weiss NS, Goss CH. Heterogeneity in survival in adult patients with cystic fibrosis with fev1 < 30% of predicted in the United States. Chest. 2017;151:1320–8.

8. Taylor-Cousar J, Niknian M, Gilmartin G, Pilewski JM, VX11-770-901 investigators. Effect of ivacaftor in patients with advanced cystic fibrosis and a g551d-cftr mutation: safety and efficacy in an expanded access program in the United States. J Cyst Fibros. 2016;15:116–22.
9. Flume PA. Cystic fibrosis: when to consider lung transplantation? Chest. 1998;113:1159–61.
10. Liou TG, Adler FR, Fitzsimmons SC, Cahill BC, Hibbs JR, Marshall BC. Predictive 5-year survivorship model of cystic fibrosis. Am J Epidemiol. 2001;153:345–52.
11. Aaron SD, Stephenson AL, Cameron DW, Whitmore GA. A statistical model to predict one-year risk of death in patients with cystic fibrosis. J Clin Epidemiol. 2015;68:1336–45.
12. Augarten A, Akons H, Aviram M, Bentur L, Blau H, Picard E, Rivlin J, Miller MS, Katznelson D, Szeinberg A, Shmilovich H, Paret G, Laufer J, Yahav Y. Prediction of mortality and timing of referral for lung transplantation in cystic fibrosis patients. Pediatr Transplant. 2001;5:339–42.
13. Kerem E, Viviani L, Zolin A, MacNeill S, Hatziagorou E, Ellemunter H, Drevinek P, Gulmans V, Krivec U, Olesen H, Group EPRS. Factors associated with FEV1 decline in cystic fibrosis: analysis of the ECFS patient registry. Eur Respir J. 2014;43:125–33.
14. Cogen J, Emerson J, Sanders DB, Ren C, Schechter MS, Gibson RL, Morgan W, Rosenfeld M, EPIC Study Group. Risk factors for lung function decline in a large cohort of young cystic fibrosis patients. Pediatr Pulmonol. 2015;50:763–70.
15. Konstan MW, Wagener JS, Vandevanter DR, Pasta DJ, Yegin A, Rasouliyan L, Morgan WJ. Risk factors for rate of decline in fev1 in adults with cystic fibrosis. J Cyst Fibros. 2012;11:405–11.
16. Quittner AL, Zhang J, Marynchenko M, Chopra PA, Signorovitch J, Yushkina Y, Riekert KA. Pulmonary medication adherence and health-care use in cystic fibrosis. Chest. 2014;146:142–51.
17. Lin AH, Kendrick JG, Wilcox PG, Quon BS. Patient knowledge and pulmonary medication adherence in adult patients with cystic fibrosis. Patient Prefer Adherence. 2017;11:691–8.
18. Donaldson SH, Bennett WD, Zeman KL, Knowles MR, Tarran R, Boucher RC. Mucus clearance and lung function in cystic fibrosis with hypertonic saline. N Engl J Med. 2006;354:241–50.
19. Wainwright CE, Elborn JS, Ramsey BW, Marigowda G, Huang X, Cipolli M, Colombo C, Davies JC, De Boeck K, Flume PA, Konstan MW, McColley SA, McCoy K, McKone EF, Munck A, Ratjen F, Rowe SM, Waltz D, Boyle MP, Group TS. Lumacaftor-ivacaftor in patients with cystic fibrosis homozygous for Phe508del CFTR. N Engl J Med. 2015;373:220–31.
20. Sawicki GS, Sellers DE, Robinson WM. High treatment burden in adults with cystic fibrosis: challenges to disease self-management. J Cyst Fibros. 2009;8:91–6.
21. Modi AC, Quittner AL. Barriers to treatment adherence for children with cystic fibrosis and asthma: what gets in the way? J Pediatr Psychol. 2006;31:846–58.
22. Snell C, Fernandes S, Bujoreanu IS, Garcia G. Depression, illness severity, and healthcare utilization in cystic fibrosis. Pediatr Pulmonol. 2014;49:1177–81.
23. Ploessl C, Pettit RS, Donaldson J. Prevalence of depression and antidepressant therapy use in a pediatric cystic fibrosis population. Ann Pharmacother. 2014;48:488–93.
24. Quittner AL, Abbott J, Georgiopoulos AM, Goldbeck L, Smith B, Hempstead SE, Marshall B, Sabadosa KA, Elborn S, International Committee on Mental Health; EPOS Trial Study Group. International Committee on Mental Health in Cystic Fibrosis: Cystic Fibrosis Foundation and European Cystic Fibrosis Society consensus statements for screening and treating depression and anxiety. Thorax. 2016;71:26–34.
25. Conway S, Balfour-Lynn IM, De Rijcke K, Drevinek P, Foweraker J, Havermans T, Heijerman H, Lannefors L, Lindblad A, Macek M, Madge S, Moran M, Morrison L, Morton A, Noordhoek J, Sands D, Vertommen A, Peckham D. European cystic fibrosis society standards of care: framework for the cystic fibrosis Centre. J Cyst Fibros. 2014;13(Suppl 1):S3–22.
26. West NE, Beckett VV, Jain R, Sanders DB, Nick JA, Heltshe SL, Dasenbrook EC, VanDevanter DR, Solomon GM, Goss CH, Flume PA, STOP investigators. Standardized Treatment of Pulmonary Exacerbations (STOP) study: physician treatment practices and outcomes for individuals with cystic fibrosis with pulmonary exacerbations. J Cyst Fibros. 2017;16:600–6.
27. Flume PA, Wainwright CE, Elizabeth Tullis D, Rodriguez S, Niknian M, Higgins M, Davies JC, Wagener JS. Recovery of lung function following a pulmonary exacerbation in patients with cystic fibrosis and the G551D-CFTR mutation treated with ivacaftor. J Cyst Fibros. 2018;17:83–8.

28. Moran A, Brunzell C, Cohen RC, Katz M, Marshall BC, Onady G, Robinson KA, Sabadosa KA, Stecenko A, Slovis B, Committee CG. Clinical care guidelines for cystic fibrosis-related diabetes: a position statement of the American Diabetes Association and a clinical practice guideline of the Cystic Fibrosis Foundation, endorsed by the Pediatric Endocrine Society. Diabetes Care. 2010;33:2697–708.

29. Turck D, Braegger CP, Colombo C, Declercq D, Morton A, Pancheva R, Robberecht E, Stern M, Strandvik B, Wolfe S, Schneider SM, Wilschanski M. ESPEN-ESPGHAN-ECFS guidelines on nutrition care for infants, children, and adults with cystic fibrosis. Clin Nutr. 2016;35:557–77.

30. Chan CL, Vigers T, Pyle L, Zeitler PS, Sagel SD, Nadeau KJ. Continuous glucose monitoring abnormalities in cystic fibrosis youth correlate with pulmonary function decline. J Cyst Fibros. 2018;17:783–90.

31. Flume PA. Pneumothorax in cystic fibrosis. Curr Opin Pulm Med. 2011;17:220–5.

32. Flume PA. Pneumothorax in cystic fibrosis. Chest. 2003;123:217–21.

33. Flume PA, Strange C, Ye X, Ebeling M, Hulsey T, Clark LL. Pneumothorax in cystic fibrosis. Chest. 2005;128:720–8.

34. Flume PA, Mogayzel PJ Jr, Robinson KA, Rosenblatt RL, Quittell L, Marshall BC, Clinical Practice Guidelines for Pulmonary Therapies Committee, Cystic Fibrosis Foundation Pulmonary Therapies Committee. Cystic fibrosis pulmonary guidelines: pulmonary complications: hemoptysis and pneumothorax. Am J Respir Crit Care Med. 2010;182:298–306.

35. Amin R, Noone PG, Ratjen F. Chemical pleurodesis versus surgical intervention for persistent and recurrent pneumothoraces in cystic fibrosis. Cochrane Database Syst Rev. 2012;12:CD007481.

36. Efrati O, Harash O, Rivlin J, Bibi H, Meir MZ, Blau H, Mussaffi H, Barak A, Levy I, Vilozni D, Kerem E, Modan-Moses D. Hemoptysis in Israeli CF patients – prevalence, treatment, and clinical characteristics. J Cyst Fibros. 2008;7:301–6.

37. Fuchs HJ, Borowitz DS, Christiansen DH, Morris EM, Nash ML, Ramsey BW, Rosenstein BJ, Smith AL, Wohl ME. Effect of aerosolized recombinant human DNase on exacerbations of respiratory symptoms and on pulmonary function in patients with cystic fibrosis. The Pulmozyme Study Group. N Engl J Med. 1994;331:637–42.

38. Ramsey BW, Davies J, McElvaney NG, Tullis E, Bell SC, Drevinek P, Griese M, McKone EF, Wainwright CE, Konstan MW, Moss R, Ratjen F, Sermet-Gaudelus I, Rowe SM, Dong Q, Rodriguez S, Yen K, Ordonez C, Elborn JS, Group VXS. A CFTR potentiator in patients with cystic fibrosis and the G551D mutation. N Engl J Med. 2011;365:1663–72.

39. Ramsey BW, Pepe MS, Quan JM, Otto KL, Montgomery AB, Williams-Warren J, Vasiljev KM, Borowitz D, Bowman CM, Marshall BC, Marshall S, Smith AL. Intermittent administration of inhaled tobramycin in patients with cystic fibrosis. Cystic fibrosis inhaled tobramycin study group. N Engl J Med. 1999;340:23–30.

40. Thompson V, Mayer-Hamblett N, Kloster M, Bilton D, Flume PA. Risk of hemoptysis in cystic fibrosis clinical trials: a retrospective cohort study. J Cyst Fibros. 2015;14:632–8.

41. Flume PA, Yankaskas JR, Ebeling M, Hulsey T, Clark LL. Massive hemoptysis in cystic fibrosis. Chest. 2005;128:729–38.

42. Flume PA. Pulmonary complications of cystic fibrosis. Respir Care. 2009;54:618–27.

43. Stenbit A, Flume PA. Pulmonary complications in adult patients with cystic fibrosis. Am J Med Sci. 2008;335:55–9.

44. Vidal V, Therasse E, Berthiaume Y, Bommart S, Giroux MF, Oliva VL, Abrahamowicz M, du Berger R, Jeanneret A, Soulez G. Bronchial artery embolization in adults with cystic fibrosis: impact on the clinical course and survival. J Vasc Interv Radiol. 2006;17:953–8.

45. Barben J, Robertson D, Olinsky A, Ditchfield M. Bronchial artery embolization for hemoptysis in young patients with cystic fibrosis. Radiology. 2002;224:124–30.

46. Noone PG. Non-invasive ventilation for the treatment of hypercapnic respiratory failure in cystic fibrosis. Thorax. 2008;63:5–7.

47. Shakkottai A, O'Brien LM, Nasr SZ, Chervin RD. Sleep disturbances and their impact in pediatric cystic fibrosis. Sleep Med Rev. 2018;42:100–10.

48. Vandeleur M, Walter LM, Armstrong DS, Robinson P, Nixon GM, Horne RSC. What keeps children with cystic fibrosis awake at night? J Cyst Fibros. 2017;16:719–26.
49. Young AC, Wilson JW, Kotsimbos TC, Naughton MT. Randomised placebo controlled trial of non-invasive ventilation for hypercapnia in cystic fibrosis. Thorax. 2008;63:72–7.
50. Elphick HE, Mallory G. Oxygen therapy for cystic fibrosis. Cochrane Database Syst Rev. 2013;(7):CD003884.
51. Archangelidi O, Carr SB, Simmonds NJ, Bilton D, Banya W, Cullinan P, CF-EpiNet. Non-invasive ventilation and clinical outcomes in cystic fibrosis: findings from the UK CF registry. J Cyst Fibros. 2019;18(5):665–70.
52. Tonelli AR. Pulmonary hypertension survival effects and treatment options in cystic fibrosis. Curr Opin Pulm Med. 2013;19:652–61.
53. Poore S, Berry B, Eidson D, McKie KT, Harris RA. Evidence of vascular endothelial dysfunction in young patients with cystic fibrosis. Chest. 2013;143:939–45.
54. Hayes D Jr, Tobias JD, Mansour HM, Kirkby S, McCoy KS, Daniels CJ, Whitson BA. Pulmonary hypertension in cystic fibrosis with advanced lung disease. Am J Respir Crit Care Med. 2014;190:898–905.
55. Arcasoy SM, Christie JD, Ferrari VA, Sutton MS, Zisman DA, Blumenthal NP, Pochettino A, Kotloff RM. Echocardiographic assessment of pulmonary hypertension in patients with advanced lung disease. Am J Respir Crit Care Med. 2003;167:735–40.
56. Montgomery GS, Sagel SD, Taylor AL, Abman SH. Effects of sildenafil on pulmonary hypertension and exercise tolerance in severe cystic fibrosis-related lung disease. Pediatr Pulmonol. 2006;41:383–5.
57. Tissieres P, Nicod L, Barazzone-Argiroffo C, Rimensberger PC, Beghetti M. Aerosolized iloprost as a bridge to lung transplantation in a patient with cystic fibrosis and pulmonary hypertension. Ann Thorac Surg. 2004;78:e48–50.
58. Sood N, Paradowski LJ, Yankaskas JR. Outcomes of intensive care unit care in adults with cystic fibrosis. Am J Respir Crit Care Med. 2001;163:335–8.
59. Oud L. Critical illness among adults with cystic fibrosis in Texas, 2004-2013: patterns of ICU utilization, characteristics, and outcomes. PLoS One. 2017;12:e0186770.
60. King CS, Brown AW, Aryal S, Ahmad K, Donaldson S. Critical care of the adult patient with cystic fibrosis. Chest. 2019;155(1):202–14.
61. Bartz RR, Love RB, Leverson GE, Will LR, Welter DL, Meyer KC. Pre-transplant mechanical ventilation and outcome in patients with cystic fibrosis. J Heart Lung Transplant. 2003;22:433–8.
62. Hayes D Jr, Kukreja J, Tobias JD, Ballard HO, Hoopes CW. Ambulatory venovenous extracorporeal respiratory support as a bridge for cystic fibrosis patients to emergent lung transplantation. J Cyst Fibros. 2012;11:40–5.
63. Morrell MR, Pilewski JM. Lung transplantation for cystic fibrosis. Clin Chest Med. 2016;37:127–38.
64. Sole A, Perez I, Vazquez I, Pastor A, Escriva J, Sales G, Hervas D, Glanville AR, Quittner AL. Patient-reported symptoms and functioning as indicators of mortality in advanced cystic fibrosis: a new tool for referral and selection for lung transplantation. J Heart Lung Transplant. 2016;35:789–94.
65. Kerem E, Reisman J, Corey M, Canny GJ, Levison H. Prediction of mortality in patients with cystic fibrosis. N Engl J Med. 1992;326:1187–91.
66. Mayer-Hamblett N, Rosenfeld M, Emerson J, Goss CH, Aitken ML. Developing cystic fibrosis lung transplant referral criteria using predictors of 2-year mortality. Am J Respir Crit Care Med. 2002;166:1550–5.
67. Sands D, Repetto T, Dupont LJ, Korzeniewska-Eksterowicz A, Catastini P, Madge S. End of life care for patients with cystic fibrosis. J Cyst Fibros. 2011;10(Suppl 2):S37–44.
68. Bourke SJ, Booth Z, Doe S, Anderson A, Rice S, Gascoigne A, Quibell R. A service evaluation of an integrated model of palliative care of cystic fibrosis. Palliat Med. 2016;30:698–702.

69. Robinson WM, Ravilly S, Berde C, Wohl ME. End-of-life care in cystic fibrosis. Pediatrics. 1997;100:205–9.
70. Ford D, Flume PA. Impact of lung transplantation on site of death in cystic fibrosis. J Cyst Fibros. 2007;6:391–5.
71. Linnemann RW, Friedman D, Altstein LL, Islam S, Bach KT, Georgiopoulos AM, Moskowitz SM, Yonker LM. Advance care planning experiences and preferences among people with cystic fibrosis. J Palliat Med. 2019;22(2):138–44.

Chapter 12
Lung Transplantation for Cystic Fibrosis

Joseph M. Pilewski

Patient Perspective

I am a 45-year-old mother with cystic fibrosis who had a double-lung transplant 10 years ago. As my disease progressed, I hoped that transplant would be an option, especially with all of the resistant bacteria I had battled for many years. I knew there would be a chance it might not happen for me.

I had a lot of preconceived notions prior to transplant because my brother had a transplant in 1991. It was many years before mine, but his recovery, medicines, and in the end, his death 18 months later made my mind wonder whether it would be right for me. Looking back, I wish I would have been more open to discussion about transplant in the earlier stages of my disease. I feel like it could have helped alleviate fears I had about having a successful procedure. Having the discussions closer to when transplant was actually going to happen didn't really give me time to prepare myself mentally because at the time, I was dealing with the end stages of my disease and trying to prepare my family. Patients need to feel comfortable bringing the topic up and so do physicians. If it is gradual and more casual at regular care appointments than an emergent issue, it would seem like it is a part of the plan rather than a last resort and put patients, like myself, at ease.

When discussions have been initiated between you and your physician, you will be tempted to hit the web, like I was. Do not over-research things online and in forums. I have found that people tend to discuss negative symptoms more than positive ones. So, you really aren't seeing the big picture. There are many positive stories like my own, but you do not always have access to them. Currently, I am a part

J. M. Pilewski (✉)
University of Pittsburgh, Pittsburgh, PA, USA

Pulmonary, Allergy, and Critical Care Medicine Division, University of Pittsburgh Medical Center, Pittsburgh, PA, USA

Cystic Fibrosis Center, UPMC Children's Hospital of Pittsburgh, Pittsburgh, PA, USA
e-mail: pilewskijm@upmc.edu

© Springer Nature Switzerland AG 2020
S. D. Davis et al. (eds.), *Cystic Fibrosis*, Respiratory Medicine,
https://doi.org/10.1007/978-3-030-42382-7_12

of a few support groups, and it is helpful to discuss symptoms or new things that pop up after transplant and see if there is anyone out there who is feeling the same. I looked at some of the groups prior to transplant, and I found them overwhelming at times. Be cautious what information you allow yourself to obtain.

Once you have had the discussions, and you are at the point to be listed, I highly encourage you to keep your body moving! Exercise is difficult when you feel so poorly but keeping your muscles strong and endurance high will help you on the flip side. It doesn't have to be a marathon; it can be at a slow crawl but try and keep going. Utilize your team and physical therapy specialist at your facility. Mine were extremely encouraging and did whatever they could to support me.

Speaking of support, make sure you plan on keeping your network informed and by your side before and after transplant. Having a good support system can help keep you on track and keep you focused on getting better. I felt like having friends and family around both before and after transplant kept everyone fresh and positive. A positive outlook helped healing and encouraged me to push through. Use the people around you. Talk with them. Don't keep everything to yourself. They want to help in a helpless situation.

When you make it to transplant, stay positive! I asked many questions before transplant, but honestly, I did not know what I should be asking because everything was going to be new. The best advice given to me was by one of my doctors. They said to take it one day at a time. Do not get ahead of myself. They will let me know if there is anything I need to worry about and that I should just focus on healing. Sometimes it is one day at a time, and sometimes it will be minutes at a time. You are basically trading a disease you know everything about and starting from scratch with another. Trust in your team to teach you what you need to know, but at the same point, advocate for yourself and make sure you keep a line of communication open for questions and explanations of how you are feeling both physically and mentally.

After transplant, it took a little time to get into a new routine with medications, blood work, and follow-up appointments, but it has all been worth it. I still have hospital stays and viral/bacterial infections, but keeping close contact with my care teams helps prevent a downward spiral. Having a transplant has not been a cure, but it has enabled me to be alive for 10 more years and enjoy my family. I will forever be grateful I took the chance and, in turn, a facility took the chance on me. I could not have asked for a better result.

–Mindy Ladd

Introduction

Lung transplantation is an attractive treatment option for many patients with end-stage lung disease, particularly individuals with cystic fibrosis (CF). Since inception in the 1980s, over 65,000 adult lung transplantations have been performed worldwide, and more than 4000 are performed annually in recent years, according to the most recent International Society of Heart and Lung Transplantation registry report

[1]. Despite the development of newer CF therapies and improved delivery of care, which has resulted in improved median survival for patients with CF [2], most individuals with CF succumb to respiratory failure. For those who progress to advanced lung disease, lung transplantation provides an opportunity for better quality of life and prolonged survival. In 1983, the first lung transplant for CF was performed, and CF now accounts for approximately 15% of all pretransplant diagnoses [1]. Despite the changes in lung allocation policies, 10–20% of individuals with CF die while waiting for lung transplantation [3].

Among the challenges for transplant as a treatment option, inability to predict survival has made it difficult to identify the optimal time for individuals to pursue transplant. Historically, the fraction of expiratory volume in 1 second (FEV_1) has been the most often used functional variable to predict prognosis, with early reports of $FEV_1 < 30\%$ predicted being associated with a 2-year mortality of 50% [4]. A more recent analysis of the Cystic Fibrosis Foundation Patient Registry determined that the median survival of individuals with CF and $FEV_1 < 30\%$ predicted has improved in recent decades, to 6.6 years [5], and the development of highly effective CFTR modulators is likely to extend survival further [6, 7]. In addition to FEV_1, other variables associated with a high risk of death from CF are hypoxia, hypercapnia, pulmonary hypertension, reduced 6-minute walk distance, and female gender [4]. From these variables, a few predictive models of survival in patients with CF have been developed; however predicting survival for patients with CF is imprecise at best [5, 8, 9]. The goal of lung transplantation in patients with CF is to not only extend survival but also to improve quality of life. In comparison to other patients with end-stage lung disease, individuals with CF face unique challenges when considering lung transplantation, yet the median survival for individuals with CF after transplant exceeds those of individuals transplanted for other end-stage lung diseases [1].

Overview of the Journey to Lung Transplant

Due to complexities in patient selection, comorbidities, and availability of suitable organ donors, the journey to lung transplant typically requires significant time – rarely weeks and more typically months to years. The journey can be broken into phases and transitions to highlight the processes and requirements (see Fig. 12.1). The initial phase is discussion with the individual with CF and her or his psychosocial support system regarding the risk of death from lung disease, trajectory of disease, and difficulties predicting survival with CF. Ideally, lung transplant is presented in the context of other CF treatment options, from routine airway clearance and exercise to inhaled mucolytics, inhaled and systemic antibiotics, CFTR modulators, and respiratory support with oxygen and noninvasive ventilation. Because transplant is a complex intervention, introduction of transplant as a treatment is best done well before the onset of respiratory failure to allow for education and timely referral to a transplant program. Initial discussions are often most effective over the course

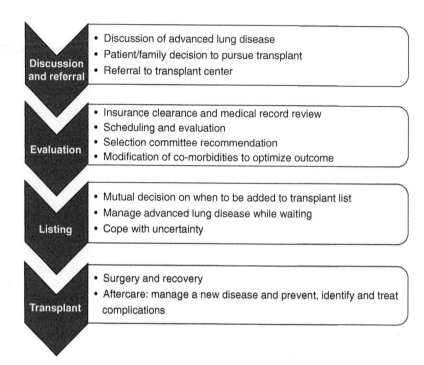

Fig. 12.1 Phases of the lung transplant journey

of several clinic visits and incorporate discussions of survival and quality of life with and without a lung transplant, as well as educational materials from sources such as the United Network for Organ Sharing (https://transplantliving.org/) and the Cystic Fibrosis Foundation in the USA (https://www.cff.org/Life-With-CF/Treatments-and-Therapies/Lung-Transplantation/) or the country of residence (https://www.cysticfibrosis.ca/; https://www.ecfs.eu/). The goal of these discussions is to assess the individual with CF or their parents' interest in the second phase of the journey – referral for consideration of lung transplant as a future treatment option. Referral to a transplant center involves identification of a specific lung transplant program and sending pertinent demographic and medical records to the transplant center. Referral is the beginning of a transition of care, as the CF team engages with the transplant team to share information and allow the transplant team to make an educated decision of when a transplant evaluation should be scheduled.

Guidelines for Referral and Evaluation

To date, there are no prospective, randomized, well-powered studies that define the optimal timing of transplant referral and listing, particularly for CF. Contributing to the challenge of when to refer is the limited data regarding survival with advanced CF lung disease. For many years, CF clinicians relied on data published in the early

1990s that reported median survival for individuals with CF and $FEV_1 < 30\%$ predicted while clinically stable was 2 years [4]. A subsequent attempt to develop a multivariable model identified variables associated with 2-year mortality but had no better positive or negative predictive value for survival than FEV1 alone [8]. Analysis of a more contemporary dataset provides important insight to survival with advanced CF lung disease. Ramos et al., using the US CF Foundation Patient Registry, reported that for individuals with CF and $FEV_1 < 30\%$ predicted during periods of clinical stability, median survival is 6.6 years, markedly improved compared to the earlier study. However, 10% of those with $FEV_1 < 30\%$ predicted died each year [5]. In the USA, a significant percentage – approximately one-third of individuals with CF and $FEV_1 < 30\%$ predicted between 2003 and 2013 – died without a lung transplant [3], due to patient preference, failure of the CF provider to refer prior to the development of respiratory failure, and misperceptions regarding transplant criteria, particularly with respect to resistant pathogens [10]. Due to significant variability in transplant recipient criteria among transplant centers, CF providers are encouraged to defer decisions on transplant candidacy to transplant programs. Early referral to a lung transplant center, prior to the anticipated need for listing, is highly encouraged to initiate patient and family education and to identify and correct potential barriers to lung transplantation (e.g., malnutrition, substance abuse, poor psychosocial support).

Expert consensus recommendations for CF lung transplant referral were published in 2019 [11] and highlight several key areas: (1) the need to discuss lung transplant as a treatment option early in the course of CF lung disease; (2) approaches to identify modifiable risk factors that can be addressed prior to transplant to maximize transplant benefit and reduce morbidity; (3) the variability in criteria among transplant programs and need to consult multiple programs if an initial center declines the individual as a transplant candidate; and (4) the benefit of frequent communication between CF and transplant centers from time of initial referral through listing, transplant, and postoperative care.

Discussing Lung Transplant as a Treatment Option for CF

The consensus guidelines recommended introduction of lung transplant as a routine part of CF care and formal referral for transplant based on variables that predict shortened survival. As death without lung transplant occurs for significant numbers of individuals with CF, and as lung transplant has become more available with improved posttransplant survival, the guidelines recommend general discussion of lung transplant as a treatment option as part of an annual assessment of disease trajectory and no later than when the FEV_1 falls below 50% predicted; formal transplant referral should occur no later than when the FEV_1 is <30% predicted. For individuals with FEV_1 30–40% predicted, and for selected individuals with $FEV_1 > 40\%$ predicted, referral is encouraged for individuals with risk factors that have been shown to increase mortality, including hypoxemia, hypercapnia, life-threatening hemoptysis, frequent infectious exacerbations, and pulmonary

Table 12.1 Information for CF providers to discuss with individuals with CF and advanced lung disease

Despite significant advances in treatments for CF, lung disease in CF is generally progressive and leads to premature death
Predicting survival for individuals with advanced CF lung disease, defined as $FEV_1 < 40\%$ predicted, is difficult, so discussion of all treatment options is critical
Lung transplant is a treatment option for many individuals with CF who suffer from severe lung disease, with median survival after transplant now approaching 10 years
Determination of who is an acceptable lung transplant candidate varies among transplant centers, and decisions on candidacy are best deferred to transplant centers rather than determined by CF care teams
Early referral for transplant is critical to optimize the chance of having a successful transplant before dying of CF lung disease; early referral allows time to address modifiable barriers and risks for transplant, particularly adherence, narcotic use, and malnutrition
Concerns about surgical recovery and pain management should not preclude lung transplant referral and evaluation
Referral for lung transplant does not mean listing for lung transplant, as the decision to list for transplant requires both patient and transplant team to agree on timing; no one is ever forced to undergo transplant and patients decide on listing in collaboration with transplant and CF providers
Lung transplant is a complex procedure and requires significant commitment and resources; routine care after transplant is critical to a good outcome, but daily treatments after transplant are less time-consuming than CF care before transplant
Approximately 90% of individuals with CF who undergo transplant enjoy marked improvements in functional capacity and quality of life, in addition to longer survival than if they had not undergone transplant; ~10% of transplant recipients have a poor outcome with complications that lead to survival of less than a year; transplant physicians are often unable to predict which patients are certain to have a poor outcome
Infections and acute rejection are common complications after lung transplant but typically respond to treatment; chronic rejection is the major cause of mortality after transplant
Monthly monitoring of laboratory and pulmonary function tests can often allow for early, successful treatment of complications
Optimal care of individuals with CF after lung transplant is achieved through collaboration between a transplant team and CF team

hypertension [9]. Discussion of transplant should focus on general principles and not include preconceived ideas based on CF clinician experiences because lung transplant outcomes are improving and determination of which patients are suitable lung transplant candidates should be deferred to the transplant program. Facts that are helpful for discussion regarding lung transplant are summarized in Table 12.1.

Selection of Candidates for Lung Transplantation

Lung transplantation should be considered for patients whose clinical status has progressively declined despite maximal medical therapy. Candidates should have a high risk of death from lung disease (>50%) within 2 years without lung

Table 12.2 Studies performed during lung transplant evaluation for CF

Chest X-ray	Complete blood count
Computed tomography of the chest	Renal function panel
Complete pulmonary function tests	Hepatic function panel
Six minute walk	Arterial blood gas
Quantitative ventilation/perfusion scan	Sputum culture
Barium swallow	24 hour urine for creatinine clearance
Electrocardiogram	Thrombosis risk panel
Transthoracic echocardiogram	HLA molecular typing
Right +/− left heart catheterization	HLA antibody screen
Bone densitometry	Blood group type
Age-appropriate health maintenance exams	Hemoglobin A1C
	Urinalysis
	PPD/QuantiFERON-TB Gold test
	Serologies
	HIV
	Hepatitis B
	Hepatitis C
	Syphilis
	Herpes simplex virus
	Varicella zoster virus
	Cytomegalovirus
	Epstein-Barr virus
	Toxoplasmosis

transplantation and a high likelihood of 5-year posttransplant survival in the setting of acceptable graft function [12]. To determine the severity of disease and appropriateness for lung transplantation, several studies are performed during the evaluation process (Table 12.2). The ideal candidate should be free of significant extrapulmonary comorbidities; however, the other systemic manifestations of CF rarely preclude lung transplantation. The absolute and relative contraindications for lung transplantation are constantly in flux as surgical techniques and management of complications have improved over the past decade. In general, patients with CF should be free from malignancy within the past 2 years; however decisions regarding cancer-free interval prior to transplant are increasingly based on tumor biology and prognosis rather than absolute timelines. Ideally, suitable lung transplant candidates are free of significant heart, renal, or hepatic dysfunction, but coronary interventions, a viable plan for renal replacement, liver disease with preserved synthetic function, or combined heart-lung or liver-lung transplant may overcome seemingly unsurmountable extrapulmonary disease in younger individuals. Other challenges may also be acceptable at some transplant programs, such as significant chest wall deformity or bleeding disorders. In contrast, uncontrolled psychiatric, psychosocial, or financial issues may not be remedied and preclude adherence to a complex posttransplant medical regimen and compliance with follow-up care. Candidates should demonstrate an ability to partner with healthcare providers and be compliant with medical therapies, have good insight and a reliable social support system, have potential for physical rehabilitation, and be free of any recent substance abuse or dependence [12]. Practices on use of cannabinoids and chronic opioids, in the absence of abuse, vary among transplant programs, so they should be addressed proactively. As some barriers to transplant are modifiable prior to the development of respiratory failure, early referral is important to allow sufficient time to address barriers and optimize the opportunity for a successful transplant.

Type of Transplantation

While the initial approach to lung transplant for CF was a combined heart and lung transplantation, bilateral sequential lung transplantation became the preferred procedure in the early 1990s [13, 14]. This procedure originally involved transection of the sternum in a "clamshell procedure" to fully expose the chest cavity. However, bilateral anterior thoracotomies are now performed at some centers, as a sternal-sparing procedure to avoid surgical complications such as non-union of the sternum and sternal osteomyelitis [15, 16]. However, for cases in which surgical challenges with recipient pneumonectomy are anticipated, the "clamshell procedure" remains ideal to fully expose all intrathoracic structures.

To combat the high mortality among patients with CF awaiting lung transplantation, and limited donor lung availability, living donor lobar lung transplantation was implemented as an alternative to conventional cadaveric lung transplantation [17]. With this procedure, single lobes are removed from one or more living donors and implanted in the recipient. Despite reports of comparable short- and long-term outcomes compared to conventional lung transplantation, this procedure is rarely performed now due to occasional donor complications and to the recent changes in the urgency/benefit allocation system for cadaveric lung transplantation in the USA [18, 19]. Cadaveric lobar lung transplantation carries the benefit of reducing waitlist mortality for patients with small stature without imposing any risk to a living donor. In this procedure, individual lobes from deceased donors with larger chest cavities are implanted in recipients with smaller chest cavities. In this decade, cadaveric lobar lung transplantation has been safely performed in individuals with CF with encouraging short- and long-term outcomes [20, 21].

Comorbidities in CF and Impact on Transplant Candidacy and Outcomes

An important consideration for lung transplantation is the impact of pretransplant comorbidities on outcomes. Several reports of single-center outcomes for patients with CF have been published and identify risk factors for worse transplant outcome;

Table 12.3 Controversial comorbidities in CF and their impact on transplant outcomes

Comorbidity	Impact on outcomes
Multiple drug-resistant *Pseudomonas aeruginosa*	None
Gram-negative CF pathogens other than *Burkholderia gladioli* and *B. cenocepacia*	None
Burkholderia cenocepacia	Approximately 40% decrease in 1-year survival; minimal effect on 5-year survival
Mycobacterium abscessus	Increase in perioperative morbidity; no appreciable effect on mortality
Aspergillus fumigatus	None
Cirrhosis	None with Child-Pugh A and perhaps B
Malnutrition	Debated but worst case estimate 10% lower survival at 3 and 5 years with BMI < 18
Mechanical support with invasive ventilation or ECMO	Increase morbidity; no appreciable decrease in short-term survival and unknown impact on long-term survival
HIV and hepatitis C	Unknown but likely none if viral infection cleared prior to transplant

however, to date there are no predictive models that allow estimation of risk associated with multiple comorbidities. CF-specific comorbidities and their individual impact on survival are listed in Table 12.3. Candidacy for lung transplant is based largely on center experience and level of risk aversion, which varies widely among transplant programs. Typically, higher-volume transplant centers will often offer transplant to patients previously declined at less experienced centers. For this reason, it is imperative that CF clinicians be familiar with the criteria at their regional transplant centers and, to maximize opportunity for motivated individuals with CF, explore referral to multiple transplant centers when necessary to overcome barriers to transplant.

Prior Thoracic Procedures

Historically, prior thoracic procedures were a major contraindication to lung transplantation. Pneumothoraces are a risk factor for mortality in CF patients [22], and for the transplant surgeon, less aggressive measures are preferred over chemical or surgical pleurodesis. Many patients can be managed with prolonged chest tube drainage, often with a PleurX catheter and valve, to minimize the short- and long-term risk of pleurodesis. Nevertheless, while few studies have detailed the impact of pleural procedures on transplant outcomes, many centers have found that prior pleural procedures increase the complexity of recipient pneumonectomy and increase pleural bleeding. In one large single-center report, Meachery et al. reported on outcomes for 176 individuals with CF who underwent lung or heart-lung transplantation from 1989 to 2007. For the 12% who had prior pneumothorax (including six patients with medical or surgical pleurodesis), outcomes were no worse in individuals with prior pneumothoraces and pleurodesis compared to the larger cohort [23]. Thus, individuals with prior pneumothoraces, including those treated by pleurodesis, can, in the care of an experienced transplant team, have comparable outcomes. Similarly, prior lobectomy or pneumonectomy is not a contraindication to lung transplant at some programs.

CF Bacterial Pathogens

Some transplant centers consider pretransplant colonization with pan-resistant strains of *Pseudomonas aeruginosa* or *Burkholderia cepacia* as predictive of poor posttransplant outcomes and, therefore, a contraindication to transplantation. Beginning with studies in 1997, there has been some controversy over the impact of pan-resistant bacteria other than *Burkholderia cepacia* on outcomes from lung transplantation for CF. In one of the larger reviews, Hadjiliadis and colleagues retrospectively reviewed the experience at two transplant centers with 99 patients transplanted between 1988 and 2001 [24]. Pan-resistant *Pseudomonas* was defined as those isolates having resistant or intermediate susceptibility to one antibiotic from each class of antibiotics against these bacteria (e.g., antipseudomonal penicillins, cephalosporins, carbapenems, quinolones, and aminoglycosides). Individuals in the group with pan-resistant *Pseudomonas* ($n = 45$) had worse outcomes by overall comparison of survival to those with sensitive organisms ($n = 58$). The difference in survival was appreciable up until 2 years after transplant, after which the survival curves were comparable. In addition, patients in the pan-resistant *Pseudomonas* group tended to have infection as a more common cause of death than the sensitive *Pseudomonas* group; however, pan-resistant *Pseudomonas* was directly responsible for death in only 3 of the 45 patients in this group. Individuals in the pan-resistant group comprised almost half the study population, highlighting the frequency of highly resistant *Pseudomonas* in the CF population with end-stage lung disease. While the authors' conclusion that patients with pan-resistant *Pseudomonas* have a statistically worse outcome than those with sensitive *Pseudomonas* appears substantiated, outcomes in the pan-resistant group were comparable to those in the UNOS registry. Thus, a corollary point is that patients with sensitive *Pseudomonas* appear to have better outcomes than other transplant recipients. Nevertheless, as the authors propose, both groups had very good outcomes, leading to the conclusion that patients with more resistant *Pseudomonas* species should not be excluded from consideration for transplantation. A more recent registry analysis confirmed this conclusion [25].

There remains considerable debate regarding whether patients infected with *Burkholderia* species are appropriate candidates for lung transplantation. Studies in the 1990s indicated that individuals infected with *B. cepacia* had a high risk of posttransplant mortality, and over time, fewer and fewer transplant centers have offered transplant evaluation and listing for patients infected with *B. cepacia* [26]. Over the last decade or more, LiPuma and colleagues have contributed immensely to understanding the microbiology of *Burkholderia*, first by distinguishing this group of pathogens from *Pseudomonas* and then more recently by identifying genotypically distinct species that appear to impact differently on transplant outcomes. Using two large databases [the CF Foundation Patient Registry and the Scientific Registry of Transplant Recipients (SRTR)] to identify cohorts of over 1000 transplant candidates and over 500 recipients, and the data available from the *Burkholderia* Research Laboratory and Repository, Murray et al. were able to assess the mortality risk of different *Burkholderia* species [27]. *Burkholderia* infection significantly impacted posttransplant survival in several ways:

1. Patients infected with *B. gladioli* had a significantly higher posttransplant mortality than uninfected recipients and recipients infected with *B. multivorans*.
2. Recipients infected with *B. multivorans* prior to transplant had no appreciable difference in mortality compared to uninfected patients.
3. Overall, transplant recipients infected with *B. cenocepacia* ($n = 31$) prior to transplant did not have an overall worse 1- and 5-year survival compared to uninfected patients.
4. In contrast, subgroup analysis revealed that patients infected with non-epidemic *B. cenocepacia* strains (e.g., strains other than the two epidemic strains in this dataset – the Midwest clone and PHDC) prior to transplant had a significantly higher risk of mortality compared to uninfected recipients or recipients infected with *B. multivorans*.

Notably, the excess mortality associated with *B. gladioli* and non-epidemic strains of *B. cenocepacia* occurred in the first 6 months after transplant and was typically attributable to recurrent infection. Similar observations were reported in individuals with CF infected prior to transplant with *B. dolosa* [28].

Other investigators have reported comparative analyses of transplant outcomes for individuals infected with *Burkholderia cepacia* complex (Bcc) transplanted between 1990 and 2006. Survival rates for patients infected with *B. cenocepacia* were significantly lower than for those infected with other species, and patients with *B. cenocepacia* were six times more likely to die in the first year after transplantation (1-year survival: 89–92% for non-*Burkholderia* and Bcc species other than *cenocepacia* versus 29% for *B. cenocepacia* infected) [29]. Similarly, in a study from France, individuals infected with *B. cenocepacia* prior to transplant had higher mortality rates than those infected with other *Burkholderia* species, while patients infected with strains other than *cenocepacia* did not have a statistically higher mortality risk compared to those not infected with Bcc species. Three of the six deaths in *cenocepacia* patients occurred in the postoperative period and were directly attributable to *cenocepacia* infection [30]. A recent meta-analysis of risk factors for posttransplant mortality confirmed risk associated with cenocepacia [31]. These cumulative data suggest that more aggressive, or alternative, antibiotic regimens targeted at preventing early infection will be necessary to improve outcomes for individuals with *B. cenocepacia*. In addition, further correlation of molecularly characterized species with outcomes are needed to fully resolve subtype differences and to determine definitively whether it is ethically appropriate to exclude all patients with *B. cenocepacia* from lung transplantation. Reasonable outcomes in at least one transplant center [32] support a recommendation to refer individuals with CF and *Burkholderia* spp. and allow the transplant program to determine candidacy, rather than a common practice to not refer [10] and deny the individual an opportunity to be considered.

The impact of other less frequent Gram-negative CF pathogens is not well defined. *Stenotrophomonas* and *Achromobacter* species do not appear to pose an increased risk for early mortality [33]. Several studies have demonstrated a negative impact of infection with methicillin-resistant *Staphylococcus aureus* (MRSA) on survival with CF [34], but the impact of pretransplant MRSA on posttransplant outcomes is unclear.

Fungal Pathogens

Aspergillus and other fungi are found in respiratory cultures from a significant fraction of adults with CF but, with few exceptions, do not appear to adversely impact transplant outcomes. Up to 70% of adults with CF harbor *Aspergillus fumigatus*, and allergic bronchopulmonary aspergillosis may occur in up to 10% of patients over the course of their disease. Mycetomas are much less common, and true invasive aspergillosis has rarely been reported. In one recent single-center study, 70% of patients transplanted for CF had *Aspergillus* prior to transplant, and almost 40% had fungus in explanted lung cultures. The risk of invasive aspergillus after transplant was high (22%) and often temporally related to treatment for acute cellular rejection; however, preoperative aspergillus did not appreciably increase the risk for early mortality after transplant [35]. Particularly with the availability of newer azole antifungals and experience with inhaled amphotericin [36], *Aspergillus* spp. are not considered a contraindication to lung transplant. Other fungal pathogens such as *Scedosporium* spp. are seen much less frequently and should be considered carefully given case reports of early mortality attributable to these fungi [37].

Non-tuberculous Mycobacteria

Non-tuberculous mycobacteria (NTM) appear to be an increasing challenge in CF and significantly impact lung transplant candidacy. Prevalence studies at a large number of US CF Centers over a decade ago demonstrated that approximately 13% over the age of 10 had respiratory cultures with NTM, with 72% being *M. avium* and 16% *M. abscessus* [38]. While decline in lung function was not appreciably different between those with and without NTM, a subset with multiple positive cultures had serial CT changes suggestive of progressive disease [39]. Differentiating colonization from infection is often difficult; however, what is clear is that individuals with *M. abscessus* who undergo transplantation are at risk for dissemi-nated or, more frequently, localized infections (e.g., at wounds or in pleural space). Consequently, potential transplant candidates with CF and NTM colonization or infection are often deemed to be unsuitable for transplant due to infectious compli-cations. However, data to support any NTM as an absolute contraindication for transplant are lacking, and data for the more virulent and antibiotic-resistant *M. abscessus* are generally poor, but most single-center and small case series sup-port lung transplantation in this CF population.

In one study, almost 20% of transplant referrals with CF had a history of NTM, and of the 18 patients who had NTM prior to transplant, 7 were culture positive after transplant [40]. However, only four of these had NTM disease, including two wound infections among eight patients who had *M. abscessus* prior to transplant. Six of eight patients with pretransplant *M. abscessus* had negative airway cultures after transplant. There were no deaths attributable to NTM, and median survival among the NTM positive and negative cohorts was not appreciably different. An update reported six patients with *M. abscessus* disease prior to transplant, with three post-transplant mycobacterial infections, all of which were controlled with therapy and were not associated with worse survival [41]. Similar conclusions resulted from a review of four individuals with pretransplant *M. abscessus*; three developed wound infections or cutaneous abscesses, and all resolved with debridement and prolonged mycobacterial therapy [42]. A similarly high frequency of postoperative infections in recipients with pretransplant *M. abscessus* was reported by others, supporting the notion that pretransplant *M. abscessus* increases posttransplant infectious risk and morbidity, without excess mortality [43]. Most recently, two centers reported acceptable outcomes in individuals with pretransplant *M. abscessus*, including those with positive cultures at time of transplant [44, 45]. With the emergence of alternative agents for NTM, including clofazimine [46] and bedaquiline and bacte-riophages [47], most transplant centers and infectious disease clinicians currently take a conservative approach that potentially pathogenic NTM, particularly *M. abscessus*, be controlled with a tolerable NTM regimen prior to transplantation to minimize the posttransplant risk. Infection with NTM should not preclude trans-plant referral; however, during the transplant evaluation, individuals with CF should be educated in detail about the risk and burden of prolonged posttransplant NTM therapy when NTM are isolated within the year prior to transplant.

Gastrointestinal Comorbidities

A number of GI manifestations of CF potentially impact transplant candidacy and outcomes, including liver dysfunction, exocrine pancreatic insufficiency, and mal-nutrition. Early autopsy studies reported almost uniform focal biliary cirrhosis among adults with CF, while more recent reviews report cholestasis by laboratory testing in over a quarter of adults with CF. A very small proportion of individuals with CF (<5%) manifest cirrhosis and portal hypertension, with the majority recognized prior to adulthood. While the natural history of cirrhosis in CF appears to be relatively indolent, perhaps due to aggressive use of ursodeoxycholic acid for cholestasis in CF, most individuals with cirrhosis complicating CF can be managed medically and/or endoscopically and do not require liver transplantation [48–50]. A number of adults with CF are known to have cirrhosis and/or portal hypertension prior to referral for lung transplantation or are found to have varying degrees of liver dysfunction during the evaluation process. Patients with liver disease limited to cholestasis are generally deemed low risk for perioperative liver decompensation. However, patients with cirrhosis are more controversial, as many are prematurely deemed unsuitable for isolated lung transplantation.

Data on the impact of cirrhosis are limited to small case series, making evidence-based decisions regarding lung transplantation with CF liver disease difficult. A recent case control series strongly suggested that selected patients with CF and advanced liver disease can undergo uneventful lung transplantation without concomitant liver transplantation. Six patients with CF and liver cirrhosis, defined as esophageal varices, imaging evidence of cirrhosis, and/or splenomegaly or diagnostic histology, underwent isolated lung transplantation, with no appreciable difference in perioperative complications or survival compared to a matched control group [50]. Notably, none of the six patients with cirrhosis, with Model for End-Stage Liver Disease (MELD) scores ranging from 27 to 34 and Child-Pugh scores of 5–8, exhibited decompensation of liver disease in the first 4 years after lung transplantation [50]. This single-center experience at a high-volume lung transplant program demonstrates the feasibility of isolated lung transplant with CF and cirrhosis. Experience at the authors' institution is similar. For over 16 patients with CF and Child's A or B cirrhosis who underwent isolated lung transplantation, there was no perioperative mortality. The published and anecdotal experiences at high-volume transplant centers indicate that concomitant lung-liver transplant is likely only necessary when there is hepatocellular dysfunction and uncontrolled complications of CF liver disease. Therefore, most individuals with CF and mild cirrhosis should not be declined for lung transplant due to liver disease. Because it is often challenging to obtain lung and liver en bloc in the USA, it is critical to better define the severity of CF liver disease that precludes isolated lung transplantation. For the few individuals who require combined lung liver transplant, survival appears comparable to lung-only transplant recipients [51].

Pancreatic insufficiency and malnutrition are more common GI complications of CF. Pancreatic insufficiency affects >85% of adults with CF; thus lung transplantation in individuals with CF who are pancreatic sufficient is relatively uncommon. Surprisingly, one recent review demonstrated that pancreatic sufficient transplant recipients have a higher risk of mortality than those who are pancreatic insufficient, and malnutrition (BMI <18.5) was not associated with worse outcomes [32]. The latter contradicts the conclusion of an earlier study using a larger registry cohort which demonstrated an approximately 10% lower 5-year survival for patients with CF who had a BMI <18.5 compared to a cohort with normal pretransplant BMI [52]. However, even individuals with a BMI <17 were recently demonstrated to have comparable survival to recipients with pulmonary fibrosis [53], suggesting that mild malnutrition in itself should not preclude lung transplant referral and listing. Further studies that examine nutritional status as assessed both by BMI and by markers of protein and fat-soluble vitamin deficiency are necessary, as are studies of vitamin D deficiency and transplant outcomes [54]. While many US transplant centers will not offer lung transplant to patients with BMI <18, most view this as at most a relative contraindication and example of an often modifiable risk factor for poorer outcomes after lung transplantation.

Sinus Disease

Sinus disease, manifesting as chronic sinusitis with or without nasal polyposis, is nearly ubiquitous in CF, particularly those with advanced lung disease. Very few studies have attempted to determine the impact of CF sinus disease on transplant outcomes. It is assumed that the sinuses in CF patients provide a reservoir for bacterial pathogens that predisposes patients to lower airway colonization or infection and may contribute to allograft dysfunction and worse posttransplant outcomes. In a recent study, cultures of the sinuses of lung recipients with CF after transplantation were compared to lower airway cultures; there was significant concordance in isolates from sinus aspirates and bronchoscopic cultures [55, 56], which is consistent with the reservoir hypothesis. Moreover, patients who underwent sinus surgery followed by routine nasal douches had a higher incidence of negative sinus and lower airway *Pseudomonas* colonization after transplantation and improved survival and freedom from higher-grade bronchiolitis obliterans syndrome/chronic rejection. These findings corroborate earlier reports that lung recipients with CF and *Pseudomonas* colonization after transplantation had worse outcomes compared to a *Pseudomonas*-negative cohort [57, 58]. This suggests that outcomes after transplant in patients with CF may be improved by preventive measures against lower airway infection, particularly with management of sinus disease, and perhaps routine mucosal antibiotics to prevent lower airway colonization and infection, and judicious endoscopic sinus surgery [58–62].

Osteoporosis

Osteoporosis is common in advanced lung disease, and osteoporosis with fractures has long been considered a relative contraindication to lung transplantation. In adults with CF, osteoporosis is very common, with mean average bone mineral densities two standard deviations below an age-matched control population [63]. Individuals with CF had increased fracture rates, particularly vertebral-compression and rib fractures, and a surprisingly high incidence of kyphosis associated with loss of height. While the possible mechanisms for this high rate of severe bone disease in a young population are not fully defined, vitamin D deficiency, malnutrition, early puberty, glucocorticoid exposure, and chronic inflammation are favored mechanisms. The implication of this for transplantation is that the fracture risk is often high prior to transplant and may increase further with the required immunosuppressive regimen following transplantation. Some studies have demonstrated safety and efficacy for bisphosphonates in conjunction with vitamin D and calcium supplementation to improve bone mineral density in adults with CF. [64, 65] Thus, for most transplant centers, osteoporosis is perceived as a remediable comorbidity, and only uncontrolled pain related to fractures is considered a contraindication to lung transplantation.

Diabetes

Cystic fibrosis-related diabetes (CFRD) is the most common comorbidity in patients with CF, occurring in approximately 20% of adolescents and 40–50% of adults [66]. CFRD is associated with worse lung function, more chest infections, overall poorer nutrition, and increased mortality irrespective of lung transplantation [67]. New-onset diabetes occurs in approximately 38% of patients without preexisting CFRD following lung transplantation. Potential candidates with CF should be counseled about the risk of developing diabetes following transplantation. In one study, both de novo and preexisting diabetes were associated with an increased risk of death following transplantation [68]. However, a more recent analysis did not demonstrate an impact of diabetes on transplant outcomes for recipients with CF. [32] Poorly controlled diabetes is considered by many to be a relative contraindication for lung transplantation, as this may be a surrogate for adherence with medical therapies. Aggressive treatment of diabetes is strongly recommended prior to, and following, lung transplantation. However, further studies evaluating the impact that tight glycemic control has on overall survival after transplant are warranted.

Listing for Lung Transplantation

From the provider perspective, the decision to recommend that an individual with CF and advanced lung disease be listed for transplant is complex and should consider the rate of decline in pulmonary function, frequency of exacerbations, complications such as pneumothorax and hemoptysis, troublesome pathogens, and the development of awake hypercapnia, hypoxemia, and/or pulmonary hypertension. Current recommendations from the International Society of Heart and Lung Transplantation are based upon small studies and expert opinion consensus (Table 12.4).

Listing for lung transplantation should be considered when survival from respiratory-related complications from CF is anticipated to be less than survival after lung transplantation. The decision on when to list is best a mutual one based

Table 12.4 Criteria
for listing for lung
transplantation
for cystic fibrosis

FEV$_1$ < 30% predicted or rapidly declining lung function
Frequent exacerbations requiring antimicrobial therapy
Recent exacerbation requiring mechanical ventilation
Increasing oxygen requirements
Recurrent hemoptysis despite embolization procedures
Refractory or recurrent pneumothorax
Baseline hypercapnia (pCO$_2$ > 50 mmHg)
Pulmonary hypertension
Ongoing weight loss despite aggressive nutritional supplementation

on informed and detailed discussion between the individual with CF, the CF physician, and the transplant team. Limitations in predicting 1-year survival without a transplant preclude data-driven decision-making to identify the time point at which survival with a transplant exceeds survival with CF. Compounding this problem is the unpredictability of waiting time once placed on the lung transplant list. Wait times vary from days to months to years, and while the Lung Allocation System in the USA attempts to prioritize organs to individuals with the highest risk of 1-year mortality, up to 15% of individuals with CF die while waiting for transplant. Ideally, transplant should occur prior to the onset of respiratory failure and need for mechanical ventilation or extracorporeal support, to reduce morbidity and maximize transplant survival. Lastly, the decision of when to list is challenged by the increasing experience of individuals with CF and advanced lung disease suffering rapid decline to respiratory failure when seemingly stable clinically. In some instances, there is a clear precipitant to the acute decline, such as an infectious exacerbation or pneumonia, hemoptysis, pneumothorax or viral infection, and pulmonary embolism; however, in others a clear precipitant cannot be identified. Ultimately, the decision to list and proceed with transplant must be mutual and consider anticipated survival, quality of life, patient preferences, and transplant program experience with transplanting individuals with respiratory failure.

Transplant Waitlist and Lung Allocation

The time from transplant listing to transplant is highly variable; however, changes to the allocation of lungs since 2005 have attempted to minimize waiting time for the sickest transplant candidates to reduce the chances of death while awaiting transplant. Prior to 2005, donor lungs were distributed based on blood group, size, and time on the transplant waiting list. As such, donor lungs were first distributed to individuals with the longest waitlist time, and many listed patients waited many months to a few years before undergoing transplant. For individuals with progressive lung diseases, like CF, many who were most in need of transplant due to respiratory failure died while waiting. To address this problem, allocation based on waitlist time was replaced by the Lung Allocation Score (LAS) in 2005 to distribute donor lungs based on parameters that predicted waitlist mortality, balanced twofold relative to factors that predicted 1-year survival [69]. Since implementation, the LAS has undergone revisions as additional data provided clinical parameters predictive of waitlist mortality and/or 1-year posttransplant survival, and overall waitlist mortality has improved [70]. Moreover, a lawsuit in 2017 led to removal of some geographic constraints to organ allocation and prompted evaluation of geographic sharing that has potential to reduce waitlist mortality [71, 72]. Despite these efforts, the LAS remains limited in its ability to identify patients most likely to benefit from transplantation. Waitlist time currently varies from days to 1–2 years, with lung candidates with smaller chest cavities waiting longer and those with severe hypoxemia and acute respiratory failure waiting shorter times. Most individuals with CF require supplemental oxygen and have advanced pulmonary impairment prior to achieving a sufficiently high LAS to receive donor lungs, and based on practices at most transplant centers, individuals with CF undergo transplant in the several weeks to months after listing.

Given the variable waiting, after addition to the UNOS lung transplant waitlist, transplant candidates are assessed regularly by the lung transplant program and undergo updated testing approximately every 3 months, in parallel with maximizing conditioning and medical therapy for their underlying medical problems. Most transplant programs require regular exercise or pulmonary rehabilitation. Also, maintenance of optimal nutrition and good control of extrapulmonary manifestations of CF, including sinusitis and diabetes, is important to transplant candidates achieving optimal transplant outcomes with low morbidity. Communication between the CF team and transplant team, on a regular basis and more acutely with changes in clinical status, is critical to ensuring that lung transplant candidates remain candidates for transplant and enjoy good outcomes.

Mechanical Support as a Bridge to Lung Transplantation

Historically, the requirement of mechanical ventilation had been considered to be a relative contraindication to lung transplantation as mechanical ventilation prior to lung transplantation was associated with an increased risk of mortality in the first year after lung transplantation [1]. However, in individuals with CF, the risk attributed to mechanical ventilation has been controversial, with some reports suggesting that mechanical ventilation may be associated with a longer intensive care unit stay and longer need for mechanical ventilation post-lung transplantation without a significant change in overall survival [73, 74]. Noninvasive ventilation is useful to control respiratory acidosis and has been helpful to support patients with advanced lung disease while waiting for lung transplantation. Noninvasive ventilation in patients with CF prior to lung transplantation is not associated with any adverse outcomes post-lung transplant [75, 76]. In recent years, accumulating experience indicates that extracorporeal membrane oxygenation (ECMO) is useful as a bridge to lung transplantation with comparable post-lung transplantation short- and mid-term outcomes, as well as low mortality [77, 78]. Newer ECMO strategies, including the use of a dual-lumen single cannula which allows for ambulatory veno-venous ECMO, can be done in awake, spontaneously breathing patients and allow for oral intake and participation in physical therapy [79]. In general, mechanical support can be efficacious as a bridge to lung transplantation, and perhaps as a bridge to recovery, in experienced centers with adequate resources.

Survival and Quality of Life Concerns

The median survival from lung transplantation in the international registry for patients with CF is approaching 10 years, which is significantly better than patients who were transplanted in earlier eras or for patients with other diseases such as chronic obstructive pulmonary disease and pulmonary fibrosis [1]. Patients with CF who survive beyond the first year have a median survival of well over 10 years [1]. This may reflect the overall younger age and less cardiac and renal comorbidity of CF recipients, in comparison to other lung transplant recipients. The major causes of death within the first year following lung transplantation, irrespective of pretransplant lung disease, involve technical problems; primary graft dysfunction resulting, ultimately, in graft failure; and acute infections. Infections account for approximately 35% of deaths between 1 month and 1 year following lung transplantation [1]. After the first year, bronchiolitis obliterans syndrome, the major form of chronic lung allograft dysfunction (CLAD), and non-cytomegalovirus infections account for the majority of deaths [1].

The overall survival benefit from lung transplantation in patients with CF has been controversial. In 2005, an analysis involving data from the United Network for Organ Sharing (UNOS) and the CF Foundation Patient Registry found that youth, the presence of *Burkholderia cepacia*, and CF-related arthropathy were associated with a higher hazard of death [80]. Adult patients with CF with a 5-year predicted survival of <50%, without *B. cepacia* or arthropathy, had improved survival compared to control CF patients who did not undergo lung transplantation [80]. As pediatric lung transplantation is now uncommon for CF, some have questioned whether the prior studies associating younger age with poor survival are valid. Liou and colleagues subsequently performed proportional hazards analysis on a cohort of CF patients to identify variables that were associated with change in survival [81]. In addition to transplantation, four variables were identified that impacted survival: *Burkholderia cepacia* infection, diabetes, infection with *Staphylococcus aureus*, and age. *B. cepacia* infection was associated with shortened survival with or without transplantation, whereas diabetes was associated with shorter pretransplant survival. Age and *S. aureus* infection were also associated with shorter posttransplant survival. Using these variables as covariates, the authors estimated the benefit or harm of transplant, and of the 514 children on the waiting list during the analysis period of 1992–2002, the analysis estimated clear survival advantage for only 5 patients, risk of harm for 315 patients, and neither benefit nor harm for 194 patients. The authors concluded that benefit from lung transplantation cannot be assumed for children with CF. [81]

Several critiques of these findings included the author's utilization of covariates obtained more than 2 years prior to transplantation, thus leading to a potential bias against transplantation. In addition, many covariates that are known to predict survival in patients with CF, such as the need for mechanical ventilation, use of supplemental oxygen, and change in pulmonary function over time, were neglected from the study. Furthermore, the study was performed in an era prior to initiation of the US Lung Allocation Score (LAS) and may not be applicable to current practice [82]. Thus, only an analysis of outcomes with LAS will determine the relative benefit of lung transplantation for children.

A strong association between LAS and lung transplantation was identified, in that the higher the LAS at the time of transplantation, the greater the survival benefit of lung transplantation [83]. Overall, survival in cystic fibrosis is determined by multiple interactive factors involving the respiratory system, and lung transplantation is widely accepted as an appropriate option for many individuals with CF who have a high risk of short-term mortality.

Prior studies have documented worsening health-related quality of life in patients with CF as lung function declines [84, 85]. Patients with CF are younger, spend more days on the waiting list, and are more likely to be working or going to school in comparison to other patients on the lung transplant waiting list [86]. However, in comparison to other patients with other end-stage lung diseases, patients with CF waiting for lung transplantation have lower levels of anxiety, higher levels of social support, and use more functional coping strategies [87]. Following lung transplantation, patients with CF report better quality of life, including physical and social functioning, treatment burden, and chest symptoms [88, 89]. In addition, energy level and sleep quality are also significantly improved following lung transplantation [86]. In general, patients with CF have the same improvements in overall quality of life in comparison to patients with other solid organ transplants [90].

Complications of Lung Transplant

Most individuals who undergo transplant have one or more complications, ranging from the time of transplant to many years later. Figure 12.2 provides a high-level overview of the more common complications and their relative timeline. Surgical complications from the transplant itself include bleeding from pleural adhesions and coagulopathy from platelet and coagulation factor consumption that may require significant transfusions, distributive shock from release of endotoxin during manipulation of the recipient lungs, acute kidney injury, and primary graft dysfunction (PGD). Progress in surgical techniques and use of extracorporeal membrane oxygenation (ECMO) in lieu of cardiopulmonary bypass has potential to reduce these early complications. With improved techniques to identify recipient

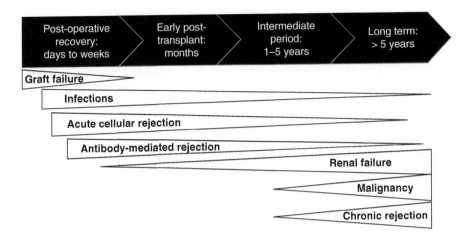

Fig. 12.2 Complications of lung transplant

antibodies against HLA antigens and avoidance of these antigens (referred to as a "virtual crossmatch"), hyperacute rejection caused by antibody deposition and complement-mediated lung injury is exceedingly rare. In contrast, PGD, defined as hypoxemia related to capillary leak and inflammatory changes [91–94], occurs in over 50% of lung transplants, but severe PGD is uncommon. With supportive measures that may include postoperative ECMO, PGD typically resolves over a period of days to weeks, and many transplant recipients who had significant PGD at time of transplant recover to long-term survival [95]. Airway ischemia reperfusion injury (IRI) occurs to varying degrees [96] and results from poor perfusion of the airway associated with loss of the bronchial circulation. The airway wall and mucosa typically heal; however, airway IRI may lead to bronchial stenosis that requires balloon dilatation and/or endobronchial stents. Given these potential complications, the duration of mechanical ventilation and need for tracheostomy varies widely, but most lung transplant recipients require <3–5 days of ventilator support, and <10% require posttransplant tracheostomy to provide support as PGD resolves [97].

Infections are a common complication after lung transplant and may occur at any time. Donor-derived and early postoperative pneumonia and empyema are uncommon with antibiotics prophylaxis, despite many recipients with CF having multidrug or pan-resistant bacterial pathogens in the native airways. Avoiding early bacterial infections with inhaled antibiotics and typically a several-week course of intravenous antibiotics has made early posttransplant pneumonia very uncommon. After the initial transplant, the lung allograft is susceptible to a broad range of infections, including viral (opportunistic such as CMV to community-acquired viruses such as influenza, parainfluenza, and respiratory syncytial virus), bacterial (in CF, often typical CF pathogens that are likely related to residual bacteria in the sinuses), mycobacterial (*Mycobacterium avium-intracellulare* and *M. abscessus* in particular), and opportunistic (fungi such as *Aspergillus fumigatus* and *Scedosporium* spp., *Nocardia* spp., *Pneumocystis jiroveci*, and others). Extrapulmonary infections may be more frequent after lung transplant, particularly in CF, and acute and chronic sinusitis that may prove difficult to manage. A variety of systemic viral infections may occur after transplant, including reactivation or primary infection with Epstein-Barr virus that may lead to posttransplant lymphoproliferative disorder (PTLD) and CMV in the retina or GI tract with or without pneumonitis. Thus, infection remains a significant cause of morbidity and mortality after lung transplant.

Acute cellular rejection (ACR) is a relatively common complication of lung transplant, as ~40% of recipients require augmented immunosuppression to resolve cellular rejection and potentially reduce the risk of more chronic rejection. The standard for preventing ACR is maintenance immunosuppression that typically consists of a calcineurin inhibitor (tacrolimus or cyclosporine), an antimetabolite (mycophenolate or azathioprine), and a corticosteroid (prednisone). Less commonly, a mTOR inhibitor such as everolimus or sirolimus is a component of maintenance immunosuppression. Despite broad immunosuppression, ACR is common in the first few years after transplant. ACR may manifest as respiratory or systemic symptoms, such as cough, fever, malaise, shortness of breath, and decline in lung function, or ACR may be asymptomatic. Consequently, most lung transplant programs perform surveillance transbronchial biopsy at defined intervals after transplant to detect ACR. Antibody-mediated rejection, caused by recipient antibodies against donor HLA or other antigens, occurs less commonly than cellular rejection and may require antibody depletion with plasmapheresis and therapies such as rituximab, bortezomib, or carfilzomib to deplete antibody-producing B and plasma cells. As donor-specific antibodies increase the risk of chronic rejection and are associated with shortened survival, techniques to detect and deplete donor-directed antibodies may improve posttransplant survival.

The primary cause of longer-term death after lung transplant is chronic rejection, recently recategorized within the broad term, chronic lung allograft dysfunction (CLAD). Based on current consensus among lung transplant experts, CLAD consists of chronic fibrosis involving either or both compartments of the lung: (1) fibrosis of the airways, bronchiolitis obliterans syndrome (BOS), known pathologically as obliterative bronchiolitis and physiologically as progressive airway obstruction, and (2) fibrosis involving the lung parenchyma, restrictive allograft syndrome (RAS), causing restrictive physiology and manifest as subpleural fibrotic changes on imaging. The pathophysiology of CLAD remains to be defined; however, the current paradigm is that CLAD results from recipient immune cells or antibodies injuring the allograft airway or alveolar compartments to cause loss of lung function. While new techniques to identify early CLAD with blood or bronchoalveolar lavage biomarkers or imaging, such as parametric response monitoring (PRM), are in progress [98], much work remains to define pathogenesis and optimal treatments. Azithromycin [99] and perhaps Montelukast [100] appear to be useful adjuncts to maintenance immunosuppression; however, augmenting immunosuppression often leads to infections, and the role of steroids and other immunosuppressive agents in treatment of CLAD is unclear. New therapies for treatment of CLAD are in clinical trials, including inhaled cyclosporine and extracorporeal photopheresis. Survival after the development of CLAD remains highly variable, from a few months to many years with a median of 3–4 years for double-lung recipients [101], and many individuals with CLAD after transplant for CF succumb to respiratory failure or require re-transplantation.

Opportunities for Improved Transplant Outcomes

Despite improvements in surgical techniques that have reduced early mortality after lung transplantation, long-term survival remains poor relative to other solid organ transplants, with 5- and 10-year survivals estimated at 65% and 50%, respectively, based on registries [1, 32]. Improvements in 1-year survival have not translated to improved long-term survival due to the high frequency of CLAD that most commonly manifests as bronchiolitis obliterans pathologically and progressive obstructive lung disease physiologically. Potential explanations for the lack of progress in preventing this common complication are infrequent patient follow-up with physicians trained in transplantation, resulting in late recognition of chronic rejection; lack of available biomarkers for early allograft dysfunction; wide variability in transplant center experience with transplant for CF; poor insight to the pathophysiology of chronic rejection; and lack of a defined optimal immunosuppressive regimens to prevent chronic rejection. The observation that there are differences in transplant outcomes between US centers[1] and across national boundaries [32, 102] suggests that benchmarking to identify best practices for posttransplant monitoring and care and co-management of the individual with CF after lung transplantation may be productive. Also, creation of a detailed registry of transplant outcomes, akin to the CF patient registry that has facilitated comparative effectiveness research and helped transform routine CF care, may provide critical observations that could improve the quality of posttransplant care, establish standard therapies that will facilitate multicenter clinical trials of new interventions, and ultimately improve the long-term survival for lung transplant recipients with CF.

Routine Care of the Posttransplant Patient by the CF Team

After lung transplant, longitudinal care of the individual with CF who has undergone transplant is optimal when the transplant and CF teams collaborate. Unless the lung transplant physician is also a CF provider, routine visits to both transplant and CF centers are encouraged to capitalize on the complementary areas of expertise. Establishing mutual expectations and maintaining regular communication are important to seamless posttransplant care. The transplant team should make all decisions regarding pulmonary care, including immunosuppression management, prophylactic antibiotics, and treatment of acute infections. Typically, the CF team manages non-pulmonary manifestations of CF, including sinus disease, nutrition, bone disease, and, in the absence of an endocrinologist with experience in CF, diabetes. CF lung transplant recipients monitor lung function at home and/or in the pulmonary function laboratory at regular intervals to assess allograft function and typically are assigned a lung transplant coordinator for all communications on transplant-related issues and hospitalizations. The lung recipient or CF team should inform the transplant team of any acute illnesses, hospitalizations, and medication changes to avoid unwanted drug interactions and decide whether transfer to the transplant hospital is appropriate in lieu of local care; the transplant team should provide regular communication to the CF team on recipient progress and complications. Lastly, other members of the CF and transplant teams, such as social workers, mental health providers, and dieticians, often benefit from communication with one another on problems to optimize care plans.

Conclusion

Lung transplantation is an attractive option for individuals with CF and end-stage lung disease. Despite comorbidities including infections with multidrug-resistant organisms, diabetes, and gastrointestinal complications, adults with CF clearly benefit from lung transplantation in terms of quantity and quality of life. Further studies are needed to optimize referral, candidate selection, lung allocation [103], and post-transplant management to further improve outcomes following lung transplantation. Additional opportunities for research and discussion include mechanisms to prevent allograft colonization with CF pathogens, immune responses of transplant recipients with CF, and the effect that socioeconomic status and healthcare systems influence access to lung transplantation and outcomes [32, 102, 104].

References

1. Chambers DC, Cherikh WS, Harhay MO, Hayes D Jr, Hsich E, Khush KK, Meiser B, Potena L, Rossano JW, Toll AE, Singh TP, Sadavarte A, Zuckermann A, Stehlik J, International Society for Heart and Lung Transplantation. The International Thoracic Organ Transplant Registry of the International Society for Heart and Lung Transplantation: thirty-sixth adult lung and heart-lung transplantation Report-2019; focus theme: donor and recipient size match. J Heart Lung Transplant. 2019;38(10):1042–55.
2. MacKenzie T, Gifford AH, Sabadosa KA, et al. Longevity of patients with cystic fibrosis in 2000 to 2010 and beyond: survival analysis of the Cystic Fibrosis Foundation patient registry. Ann Intern Med. 2014;161:233–41.
3. Valapour M, Lehr CJ, Skeans MA, Smith JM, Uccellini K, Lehman R, Robinson A, Israni AK, Snyder JJ, Kasiske BL. OPTN/SRTR 2017 annual data report: lung. Am J Transplant. 2019;19(Suppl 2):404–84. https://doi.org/10.1111/ajt.15279.
4. Kerem E, Reisman J, Corey M, Canny GJ, Levison H. Prediction of mortality in patients with cystic fibrosis. N Engl J Med. 1992;326:1187–91.
5. Ramos KJ, Quon BS, Heltshe SL, Mayer-Hamblett N, Lease ED, Aitken ML, Weiss NS, Goss CH. Heterogeneity in survival in adult patients with cystic fibrosis with $FEV_1 < 30\%$

of predicted in the United States. Chest. 2017 Jun;151(6):1320–8. https://doi.org/10.1016/j.chest.2017.01.019.

6. Middleton PG, Mall MA, Dřevínek P, Lands LC, McKone EF, Polineni D, Ramsey BW, Taylor-Cousar JL, Tullis E, Vermeulen F, Marigowda G, McKee CM, Moskowitz SM, Nair N, Savage J, Simard C, Tian S, Waltz D, Xuan F, Rowe SM, Jain R, VX17-445-102 Study Group. Elexacaftor-Tezacaftor-Ivacaftor for cystic fibrosis with a single Phe508del allele. N Engl J Med. 2019;381(19):1809–19.

7. Heijerman HGM, McKone EF, Downey DG, Van Braeckel E, Rowe SM, Tullis E, Mall MA, Welter JJ, Ramsey BW, McKee CM, Marigowda G, Moskowitz SM, Waltz D, Sosnay PR, Simard C, Ahluwalia N, Xuan F, Zhang Y, Taylor-Cousar JL, McCoy KS, VX17-445-103 Trial Group. Efficacy and safety of the elexacaftor plus tezacaftor plus ivacaftor combination regimen in people with cystic fibrosis homozygous for the F508del mutation: a double-blind, randomised, phase 3 trial. Lancet. 2019. pii: S0140–6736(19)32597–8.

8. Mayer-Hamblett N, Rosenfeld M, Emerson J, Goss CH, Aitken ML. Developing cystic fibrosis lung transplant referral criteria using predictors of 2-year mortality. Am J Respir Crit Care Med. 2002;166:1550–5.

9. Augarten A, Akons H, Aviram M, et al. Prediction of mortality and timing of referral for lung transplantation in cystic fibrosis patients. Pediatr Transplant. 2001;5:339–42.

10. Ramos KJ, Somayaji R, Lease ED, Goss CH, Aitken ML. Cystic fibrosis physicians' perspectives on the timing of referral for lung transplant evaluation: a survey of physicians in the United States. BMC Pulm Med. 2017;17(1):21. https://doi.org/10.1186/s12890-017-0367-9.

11. Ramos KJ, Smith PJ, McKone EF, Pilewski JM, Lucy A, Hempstead SE, Tallarico E, Faro A, Rosenbluth DB, Gray AL, Dunitz JM, CF Lung Transplant Referral Guidelines Committee. Lung transplant referral for individuals with cystic fibrosis: Cystic Fibrosis Foundation consensus guidelines. J Cyst Fibros. 2019;18(3):321–33. https://doi.org/10.1016/j.jcf.2019.03.002.

12. Weill D, Benden C, Corris PA, et al. A consensus document for the selection of lung transplant candidates: 2014--an update from the Pulmonary Transplantation Council of the International Society for Heart and Lung Transplantation. J Heart Lung Transplant. 2015;34:1–15.

13. Mendeloff EN, Huddleston CB, Mallory GB, et al. Pediatric and adult lung transplantation for cystic fibrosis. J Thorac Cardiovasc Surg. 1998;115:404–13; discussion 13–4.

14. Shennib H, Noirclerc M, Ernst P, et al. Double-lung transplantation for cystic fibrosis. The Cystic Fibrosis Transplant Study Group. Ann Thorac Surg. 1992;54:27–31; discussion −2.

15. Venuta F, Diso D, Anile M, et al. Evolving techniques and perspectives in lung transplantation. Transplant Proc. 2005;37:2682–3.

16. Meyers BF, Sundaresan RS, Guthrie T, Cooper JD, Patterson GA. Bilateral sequential lung transplantation without sternal division eliminates posttransplantation sternal complications. J Thorac Cardiovasc Surg. 1999;117:358–64.

17. Cohen RG, Barr ML, Schenkel FA, DeMeester TR, Wells WJ, Starnes VA. Living-related donor lobectomy for bilateral lobar transplantation in patients with cystic fibrosis. Ann Thorac Surg. 1994;57:1423–7; discussion 8.

18. Date H, Sato M, Aoyama A, et al. Living-donor lobar lung transplantation provides similar survival to cadaveric lung transplantation even for very ill patients. Eur J Cardiothorac Surg. 2015;47:967–73.

19. Battafarano RJ, Anderson RC, Meyers BF, et al. Perioperative complications after living donor lobectomy. J Thorac Cardiovasc Surg. 2000;120:909–15.

20. Shigemura N, D'Cunha J, Bhama JK, et al. Lobar lung transplantation: a relevant surgical option in the current era of lung allocation score. Ann Thorac Surg. 2013;96:451–6.

21. Stanzi A, Decaluwe H, Coosemans W, et al. Lobar lung transplantation from deceased donors: a valid option for small-sized patients with cystic fibrosis. Transplant Proc. 2014;46:3154–9.

22. Flume PA, Strange C, Ye X, Ebeling M, Hulsey T, Clark LL. Pneumothorax in cystic fibrosis. Chest. 2005;128:720–8.

23. Meachery G, De Soyza A, Nicholson A, et al. Outcomes of lung transplantation for cystic fibrosis in a large UK cohort. Thorax. 2008;63:725–31.

24. Hadjiliadis D, Steele MP, Chaparro C, et al. Survival of lung transplant patients with cystic fibrosis harboring panresistant bacteria other than Burkholderia cepacia, compared with patients harboring sensitive bacteria. J Heart Lung Transplant. 2007;26:834–8.
25. Lay C, Law N, Holm AM, Benden C, Aslam S. Outcomes in cystic fibrosis lung transplant recipients infected with organisms labeled as pan-resistant: an ISHLT Registry–based analysis. J Heart Lung Transplant. 2019;38(5):545–52.
26. Aris RM, Gilligan PH, Neuringer IP, Gott KK, Rea J, Yankaskas JR. The effects of panresistant bacteria in cystic fibrosis patients on lung transplant outcome. Am J Respir Crit Care Med. 1997;155:1699–704.
27. Murray S, Charbeneau J, Marshall BC, LiPuma JJ. Impact of burkholderia infection on lung transplantation in cystic fibrosis. Am J Respir Crit Care Med. 2008;178:363–71.
28. Wang R, Welsh SK, Budev M, Goldberg H, Noone PG, Gray A, Zaas D, Boyer D. Survival after lung transplantation of cystic fibrosis patients infected with Burkholderia dolosa (genomovar VI). Clin Transpl. 2018 May;32(5):e13236.
29. Alexander BD, Petzold EW, Reller LB, et al. Survival after lung transplantation of cystic fibrosis patients infected with Burkholderia cepacia complex. Am J Transplant. 2008;8:1025–30.
30. Boussaud V, Guillemain R, Grenet D, et al. Clinical outcome following lung transplantation in patients with cystic fibrosis colonised with Burkholderia cepacia complex: results from two French centres. Thorax. 2008;63:732–7.
31. Koutsokera A, Varughese RA, Sykes J, Orchanian-Cheff A, Shah PS, Chaparro C, Tullis E, Singer LG, Stephenson AL. Pre-transplant factors associated with mortality after lung transplantation in cystic fibrosis: a systematic review and meta-analysis. J Cyst Fibros. 2019;18(3):407–15.
32. Stephenson AL, Sykes J, Berthiaume Y, Singer LG, Aaron SD, Whitmore GA, Stanojevic S. Clinical and demographic factors associated with post-lung transplantation survival in individuals with cystic fibrosis. J Heart Lung Transplant. 2015;34(9):1139–45.
33. Lobo LJ, Tulu Z, Aris RM, Noone PG. Pan-resistant Achromobacter xylosoxidans and Stenotrophomonas maltophilia infection in cystic fibrosis does not reduce survival after lung transplantation. Transplantation. 2015;99(10):2196–202.
34. Dasenbrook EC, Checkley W, Merlo CA, Konstan MW, Lechtzin N, Boyle MP. Association between respiratory tract methicillin-resistant Staphylococcus aureus and survival in cystic fibrosis. JAMA. 2010;303:2386–92.
35. Luong ML, Chaparro C, Stephenson A, et al. Pretransplant Aspergillus colonization of cystic fibrosis patients and the incidence of post-lung transplant invasive aspergillosis. Transplantation. 2014;97:351–7.
36. Peghin M, Monforte V, Martin-Gomez MT, Ruiz-Camps I, Berastegui C, Saez B, Riera J, Ussetti P, Solé J, Gavaldá J, Roman A. 10 years of prophylaxis with nebulized liposomal amphotericin B and the changing epidemiology of Aspergillus spp. infection in lung transplantation. Transpl Int. 2016;29(1):51–62.
37. Symoens F, Knoop C, Schrooyen M, et al. Disseminated Scedosporium apiospermum infection in a cystic fibrosis patient after double-lung transplantation. J Heart Lung Transplant. 2006;25:603–7.
38. Olivier KN, Weber DJ, Wallace RJ Jr, et al. Nontuberculous mycobacteria. I: multicenter prevalence study in cystic fibrosis. Am J Respir Crit Care Med. 2003;167:828–34.
39. Olivier KN, Weber DJ, Lee JH, et al. Nontuberculous mycobacteria. II: nested-cohort study of impact on cystic fibrosis lung disease. Am J Respir Crit Care Med. 2003;167:835–40.
40. Chalermskulrat W, Sood N, Neuringer IP, et al. Non-tuberculous mycobacteria in end stage cystic fibrosis: implications for lung transplantation. Thorax. 2006;61:507–13.
41. Lobo LJ, Chang LC, Esther CR Jr, Gilligan PH, Tulu Z, Noone PG. Lung transplant outcomes in cystic fibrosis patients with pre-operative Mycobacterium abscessus respiratory infections. Clin Transpl. 2013;27:523–9.
42. Gilljam M, Schersten H, Silverborn M, Jonsson B, Ericsson HA. Lung transplantation in patients with cystic fibrosis and Mycobacterium abscessus infection. J Cyst Fibros. 2010;9:272–6.

43. Qvist T, Pressler T, Thomsen VO, Skov M, Iversen M, Katzenstein TL. Nontuberculous myco-bacterial disease is not a contraindication to lung transplantation in patients with cystic fibro-sis: a retrospective analysis in a Danish patient population. Transplant Proc. 2013;45:342–5.
44. Perez AA, Singer JP, Schwartz BS, Chin-Hong P, Shah RJ, Kleinhenz ME, Gao Y, Venado A, Leard LE, Golden JA, Kukreja J, Greenland JR, Hays SR. Management and clinical outcomes after lung transplantation in patients with pre-transplant Mycobacterium abscessus infection: a single center experience. Transpl Infect Dis. 2019;21(3):e13084.
45. Raats D, Lorent N, Saegeman V, Vos R, van Ingen J, Verleden G, Van Raemdonck D, Dupont L. Successful lung transplantation for chronic Mycobacterium abscessus infection in advanced cystic fibrosis, a case series. Transpl Infect Dis. 2019;21(2):e13046.
46. Hamad Y, Pilewski JM, Morrell M, D'Cunha J, Kwak EJ. Outcomes in lung transplant recipi-ents with Mycobacterium abscessus infection: a 15-year experience from a large tertiary care center. Transplant Proc. 2019;51(6):2035–42.
47. Dedrick RM, Guerrero-Bustamante CA, Garlena RA, Russell DA, Ford K, Harris K, Gilmour KC, Soothill J, Jacobs-Sera D, Schooley RT, Hatfull GF, Spencer H. Engineered bacterio-phages for treatment of a patient with a disseminated drug-resistant Mycobacterium abscessus. Nat Med. 2019;25(5):730–3.
48. Nash KL, Allison ME, McKeon D, et al. A single Centre experience of liver disease in adults with cystic fibrosis 1995-2006. J Cyst Fibros. 2008;7:252–7.
49. Rowland M, Gallagher CG, O'Laoide R, et al. Outcome in cystic fibrosis liver disease. Am J Gastroenterol. 2011;106:104–9.
50. Nash EF, Volling C, Gutierrez CA, et al. Outcomes of patients with cystic fibrosis undergoing lung transplantation with and without cystic fibrosis-associated liver cirrhosis. Clin Transpl. 2012;26:34–41.
51. Salman J, Grannas G, Ius F, Sommer W, Siemeni T, Avsar M, Kuehn C, Boethig D, Fleissner F, Bobylev D, Gottlieb J, Klempnauer J, Welte T, Haverich A, Tudorache I, Warnecke G, Lehner F. The liver-first approach for combined lung and liver transplantation. Eur J Cardiothorac Surg. 2018;54(6):1122–7.
52. Lederer DJ, Wilt JS, D'Ovidio F, et al. Obesity and underweight are associated with an increased risk of death after lung transplantation. Am J Respir Crit Care Med. 2009;180:887–95.
53. Ramos KJ, Kapnadak SG, Bradford MC, Somayaji R, Pilewski JM, Lease ED, Mulligan MS, Aitken ML, Gries CJ, Goss CH. Underweight patients with cystic fibrosis are suitable candi-dates for lung transplantation. Chest. 2020 Jan 17. pii: S0012-3692(20)30019-2. https://doi.org/10.1016/j.chest.2019.11.043. [Epub ahead of print] PMID: 31958441.
54. Lowery EM, Bemiss B, Cascino T, et al. Low vitamin D levels are associated with increased rejection and infections after lung transplantation. J Heart Lung Transplant. 2012;31:700–7.
55. Vital D, Hofer M, Benden C, Holzmann D, Boehler A. Impact of sinus surgery on pseudo-monal airway colonization, bronchiolitis obliterans syndrome and survival in cystic fibrosis lung transplant recipients. Respiration. 2013;86:25–31.
56. Vos R, Vanaudenaerde BM, Geudens N, Dupont LJ, Van Raemdonck DE, Verleden GM. Pseudomonal airway colonisation: risk factor for bronchiolitis obliterans syndrome after lung transplantation? Eur Respir J. 2008;31:1037–45.
57. Botha P, Archer L, Anderson RL, et al. Pseudomonas aeruginosa colonization of the allograft after lung transplantation and the risk of bronchiolitis obliterans syndrome. Transplantation. 2008;85:771–4.
58. Vital D, Hofer M, Boehler A, Holzmann D. Posttransplant sinus surgery in lung transplant recipients with cystic fibrosis: a single institutional experience. Eur Arch Otorhinolaryngol. 2013;270:135–9. https://doi.org/10.1007/s00405-012-2002-y.
59. Aanaes K, von Buchwald C, Hjuler T, Skov M, Alanin M, Johansen HK. The effect of sinus surgery with intensive follow-up on pathogenic sinus bacteria in patients with cystic fibrosis. Am J Rhinol Allergy. 2013;27:e1–4. https://doi.org/10.2500/ajra.2013.27.3829.
60. Virgin FW, Rowe SM, Wade MB, Gaggar A, Leon KJ, Young KR, Woodworth BA. Extensive surgical and comprehensive postoperative medical management for cystic fibrosis chronic rhi-nosinusitis. Am J Rhinol Allergy. 2012;26:70–5. https://doi.org/10.2500/ajra.2012.26.3705.

61. Liang J, Higgins T, Ishman SL, Boss EF, Benke JR, Lin SY. Medical management of chronic rhinosinusitis in cystic fibrosis: a systematic review. Laryngoscope. 2014;124:1308–13. https://doi.org/10.1002/lary.24503.
62. Alanin MC, Aanaes K, Høiby N, Pressler T, Skov M, Nielsen KG, Taylor-Robinson D, Waldmann E, Krogh Johansen H, von Buchwald C. Sinus surgery postpones chronic Gram-negative lung infection: cohort study of 106 patients with cystic fibrosis. Rhinology. 2016;54:206–13. https://doi.org/10.4193/Rhin15.347.
63. Aris RM, Renner JB, Winders AD, et al. Increased rate of fractures and severe kyphosis: sequelae of living into adulthood with cystic fibrosis. Ann Intern Med. 1998;128:186–93.
64. Aris RM, Lester GE, Renner JB, et al. Efficacy of pamidronate for osteoporosis in patients with cystic fibrosis following lung transplantation. Am J Respir Crit Care Med. 2000;162:941–6.
65. Aris RM, Lester GE, Caminiti M, et al. Efficacy of alendronate in adults with cystic fibrosis with low bone density. Am J Respir Crit Care Med. 2004;169:77–82.
66. Moran A, Dunitz J, Nathan B, Saeed A, Holme B, Thomas W. Cystic fibrosis-related diabetes: current trends in prevalence, incidence, and mortality. Diabetes Care. 2009;32:1626–31.
67. Brennan AL, Geddes DM, Gyi KM, Baker EH. Clinical importance of cystic fibrosis-related diabetes. J Cyst Fibros. 2004;3:209–22.
68. Hackman KL, Bailey MJ, Snell GI, Bach LA. Diabetes is a major risk factor for mortality after lung transplantation. Am J Transplant. 2014;14:438–45.
69. Egan TM, Murray S, Bustami RT, Shearon TH, McCullough KP, Edwards LB, et al. Development of the new lung allocation system in the United States. Am J Transplant. 2006;6(5 Pt 2):1212–27.
70. Egan TM, Edwards LB. Effect of the lung allocation score on lung transplantation in the United States. J Heart Lung Transplant. 2016;35(4):433–9.
71. Glazier A. The lung lawsuit: a case study in organ allocation policy and administrative law. J Health Biomedical. 2018;XIV:139–48.
72. Mooney JJ, Bhattacharya J, Dhillon GS. Effect of broader geographic sharing of donor lungs on lung transplant waitlist outcomes. J Heart Lung Transplant. 2019;38:136–44.
73. Bartz RR, Love RB, Leverson GE, Will LR, Welter DL, Meyer KC. Pre-transplant mechanical ventilation and outcome in patients with cystic fibrosis. J Heart Lung Transplant. 2003;22:433–8.
74. Vermeijden JW, Zijlstra JG, Erasmus ME, van der Bij W, Verschuuren EA. Lung transplantation for ventilator-dependent respiratory failure. J Heart Lung Transplant. 2009;28:347–51.
75. Spahr JE, Love RB, Francois M, Radford K, Meyer KC. Lung transplantation for cystic fibrosis: current concepts and one center's experience. J Cyst Fibros. 2007;6:334–50.
76. Moran F, Bradley JM, Piper AJ. Non-invasive ventilation for cystic fibrosis. Cochrane Database Syst Rev. 2013;4:CD002769.
77. Bermudez CA, Rocha RV, Zaldonis D, et al. Extracorporeal membrane oxygenation as a bridge to lung transplant: midterm outcomes. Ann Thorac Surg. 2011;92:1226–31; discussion 31–2.
78. Toyoda Y, Bhama JK, Shigemura N, et al. Efficacy of extracorporeal membrane oxygenation as a bridge to lung transplantation. J Thorac Cardiovasc Surg. 2013;145:1065–70; discussion 70–1.
79. Hayes D Jr, Kukreja J, Tobias JD, Ballard HO, Hoopes CW. Ambulatory venovenous extracorporeal respiratory support as a bridge for cystic fibrosis patients to emergent lung transplantation. J Cyst Fibros. 2012;11:40–5.
80. Liou TG, Adler FR, Huang D. Use of lung transplantation survival models to refine patient selection in cystic fibrosis. Am J Respir Crit Care Med. 2005;171:1053–9.
81. Liou TG, Adler FR, Cox DR, Cahill BC. Lung transplantation and survival in children with cystic fibrosis. N Engl J Med. 2007;357:2143–52.
82. Sweet SC, Aurora P, Benden C, et al. Lung transplantation and survival in children with cystic fibrosis: solid statistics – flawed interpretation. Pediatr Transplant. 2008;12:129–36.
83. Thabut G, Christie JD, Mal H, et al. Survival benefit of lung transplant for cystic fibrosis since lung allocation score implementation. Am J Respir Crit Care Med. 2013;187:1335–40.

84. Gee L, Abbott J, Conway SP, Etherington C, Webb AK. Validation of the SF-36 for the assessment of quality of life in adolescents and adults with cystic fibrosis. J Cyst Fibros. 2002;1:137–45.
85. Gee L, Abbott J, Conway SP, Etherington C, Webb AK. Quality of life in cystic fibrosis: the impact of gender, general health perceptions and disease severity. J Cyst Fibros. 2003;2:206–13.
86. Vermeulen KM, van der Bij W, Erasmus ME, Duiverman EJ, Koeter GH, TenVergert EM. Improved quality of life after lung transplantation in individuals with cystic fibrosis. Pediatr Pulmonol. 2004;37:419–26.
87. Burker EJ, Carels RA, Thompson LF, Rodgers L, Egan T. Quality of life in patients awaiting lung transplant: cystic fibrosis versus other end-stage lung diseases. Pediatr Pulmonol. 2000;30:453–60.
88. Gee L, Abbott J, Hart A, Conway SP, Etherington C, Webb AK. Associations between clinical variables and quality of life in adults with cystic fibrosis. J Cyst Fibros. 2005;4:59–66.
89. Singer LG, Chowdhury NA, Faughnan ME, et al. Effects of recipient age and diagnosis on health-related quality of life benefit of lung transplantation. Am J Respir Crit Care Med. 2015;192:965–73. https://doi.org/10.1164/rccm.201501-0126OC.
90. Busschbach JJ, Horikx PE, van den Bosch JM, Brutel de la Riviere A, de Charro FT. Measuring the quality of life before and after bilateral lung transplantation in patients with cystic fibrosis. Chest. 1994;105:911–7.
91. Snell GI, Yusen RD, Weill D, Strueber M, Garrity E, Reed A, Pelaez A, Whelan TP, Perch M, Bag R, Budev M, Corris PA, Crespo MM, Witt C, Cantu E, Christie JD. Report of the ISHLT Working Group on Primary Lung Graft Dysfunction, part I: definition and grading-A 2016 Consensus Group statement of the International Society for Heart and Lung Transplantation. J Heart Lung Transplant. 2017;36:1097–103. https://doi.org/10.1016/j.healun.2017.07.021.
92. Diamond JM, Arcasoy S, Kennedy CC, Eberlein M, Singer JP, Patterson GM, Edelman JD, Dhillon G, Pena T, Kawut SM, Lee JC, Girgis R, Dark J, Thabut G. Report of the International Society for Heart and Lung Transplantation Working Group on Primary Lung Graft Dysfunction, part II: epidemiology, risk factors, and outcomes-A 2016 Consensus Group statement of the International Society for Heart and Lung Transplantation. J Heart Lung Transplant. 2017;36:1104–13. https://doi.org/10.1016/j.healun.2017.07.020.
93. Gelman AE, Fisher AJ, Huang HJ, Baz MA, Shaver CM, Egan TM, Mulligan MS. Report of the ISHLT Working Group on primary lung graft dysfunction part III: mechanisms: a 2016 consensus group statement of the International Society for Heart and Lung Transplantation. J Heart Lung Transplant. 2017;36:1114–20. https://doi.org/10.1016/j.healun.2017.07.014.
94. Van Raemdonck D, Hartwig MG, Hertz MI, Davis RD, Cypel M, Hayes D Jr, Ivulich S, Kukreja J, Lease ED, Loor G, Mercier O, Paoletti L, Parmar J, Rampolla R, Wille K, Walia R, Keshavjee S. Report of the ISHLT Working Group on primary lung graft dysfunction part IV: prevention and treatment: a 2016 consensus group statement of the International Society for Heart and Lung Transplantation. J Heart Lung Transplant. 2017;36:1121–36. https://doi.org/10.1016/j.healun.2017.07.013.
95. Cantu E, Diamond JM, Suzuki Y, Lasky J, Schaufler C, Lim B, Shah R, Porteous M, Lederer DJ, Kawut SM, Palmer SM, Snyder LD, Hartwig MG, Lama VN, Bhorade S, Bermudez C, Crespo M, McDyer J, Wille K, Orens J, Shah PD, Weinacker A, Weill D, Wilkes D, Roe D, Hage C, Ware LB, Bellamy SL, Christie JD, Lung Transplant Outcomes Group. Quantitative evidence for revising the definition of primary graft dysfunction after lung transplant. Am J Respir Crit Care Med. 2018;197:235–43. https://doi.org/10.1164/rccm.201706-1140OC.
96. Crespo MM, McCarthy DP, Hopkins PM, Clark SC, Budev M, Bermudez CA, Benden C, Eghtesady P, Lease ED, Leard L, D'Cunha J, Wigfield CH, Cypel M, Diamond JM, Yun JJ, Yarmus L, Machuzak M, Klepetko W, Verleden G, Hoetzenecker K, Dellgren G, Mulligan M. ISHLT Consensus Statement on adult and pediatric airway complications after lung transplantation: definitions, grading system, and therapeutics. J Heart Lung Transplant. 2018;37:548–63. https://doi.org/10.1016/j.healun.2018.01.1309.

97. Eberlein M, Arnaoutakis GJ, Yarmus L, Feller-Kopman D, Dezube R, Chahla MF, Bolukbas S, Reed RM, Klesney-Tait J, Parekh KR, Merlo CA, Shah AS, Orens JB, Brower RG. The effect of lung size mismatch on complications and resource utilization after bilateral lung transplantation. J Heart Lung Transplant. 2012;31:492–500. https://doi.org/10.1016/j.healun.2011.12.009.

98. Belloli EA, Degtiar I, Wang X, Yanik GA, Stuckey LJ, Verleden SE, Kazerooni EA, Ross BD, Murray S, Galbán CJ, Lama VN. Parametric response mapping as an imaging biomarker in lung transplant recipients. Am J Respir Crit Care Med. 2017;195:942–52. https://doi.org/10.1164/rccm.201604-0732OC.

99. Ruttens D, Verleden SE, Vandermeulen E, Bellon H, Vanaudenaerde BM, Somers J, Schoonis A, Schaevers V, Van Raemdonck DE, Neyrinck A, Dupont LJ, Yserbyt J, Verleden GM, Vos R. Prophylactic azithromycin therapy after lung transplantation: post hoc analysis of a randomized controlled trial. Am J Transplant. 2016;16:254–61. https://doi.org/10.1111/ajt.13417.

100. Vos R, Eynde RV, Ruttens D, Verleden SE, Vanaudenaerde BM, Dupont LJ, Yserbyt J, Verbeken EK, Neyrinck AP, Van Raemdonck DE, Verleden GM, Leuven Lung Transplant Group. Montelukast in chronic lung allograft dysfunction after lung transplantation. J Heart Lung Transplant. 2019;38:516–27. https://doi.org/10.1016/j.healun.2018.11.014.

101. Kulkarni HS, Cherikh WS, Chambers DC, Garcia VC, Hachem RR, Kreisel D, Puri V, Kozower BD, Byers DE, Witt CA, Alexander-Brett J, Aguilar PR, Tague LK, Furuya Y, Patterson GA, Trulock EP 3rd, Yusen RD. Bronchiolitis obliterans syndrome-free survival after lung transplantation: an International Society for Heart and Lung Transplantation Thoracic Transplant Registry analysis. J Heart Lung Transplant. 2019;38:5–16. https://doi.org/10.1016/j.healun.2018.09.016.

102. Quon BS, Psoter K, Mayer-Hamblett N, Aitken ML, Li CI, Goss CH. Disparities in access to lung transplantation for patients with cystic fibrosis by socioeconomic status. Am J Respir Crit Care Med. 2012;186:1008–13.

103. Lehr CJ, Skeans M, Dasenbrook EC, Fink A, Fernandez G, Faro A, Valapour M. Effect of including important clinical variables on accuracy of the lung allocation score for cystic fibrosis and chronic obstructive pulmonary disease. Am J Respir Crit Care Med. 2019;200:1013–21. https://doi.org/10.1164/rccm.201902-0252OC.

104. Merlo CA, Clark SC, Arnaoutakis GJ, et al. National healthcare delivery systems influence lung transplant outcomes for cystic fibrosis. Am J Transplant. 2015;15:1948–57.

Part III
Gastrointestinal Manifestations

Chapter 13
Exocrine Pancreatic Insufficiency and Nutritional Complications

Amar Mandalia and Matthew J. DiMagno

Abbreviations

AUC	Area under the (receiver operating) curve
BMD	Bone mineral density
CCK	Cholecystokinin
CF	Cystic fibrosis
CFF	Cystic Fibrosis Foundation
CFTR	Cystic fibrosis transmembrane conductance regulator
CP	Chronic pancreatitis
CT	Computed tomography
DEXA	Dual-energy X-ray absorptiometry
DHA	Docosahexaenoic acid
ELISA	Enzyme-linked immunosorbent assay
ERCP	Endoscopic retrograde cholangiopancreatography
EUS	Endoscopic ultrasonography
FE	Fecal elastase
MRCP	Magnetic resonance cholangiopancreatography
NPV	Negative predictive value
PERT	Pancreatic enzyme replacement therapy
PFT	Pancreatic function test
PI	Pancreatic insufficiency
PPI	Proton pump inhibitor
PPV	Positive predictive value

A. Mandalia
University of Michigan Hospital and Health Systems, Department of Internal Medicine,
Division of Gastroenterology and Hepatology,
Ann Arbor, MI, USA
e-mail: amandali@med.umich.edu

M. J. DiMagno (✉)
University of Michigan School of Medicine, Department of Internal Medicine,
Division of Gastroenterology and Hepatology, Ann Arbor, MI, USA
e-mail: mdimagno@umich.edu

© Springer Nature Switzerland AG 2020
S. D. Davis et al. (eds.), *Cystic Fibrosis*, Respiratory Medicine,
https://doi.org/10.1007/978-3-030-42382-7_13

PS   Pancreatic sufficiency
PTH   Parathyroid hormone
USP   United States Pharmacopeia

Patient Perspective

I was born with Cystic Fibrosis in 1989, a year that would result in the discovery of the CF gene. My parents were told that they needed to prepare themselves for their child to have a difficult and hard life ahead of her. That statement was followed-up with that if by a miracle your child survives her toddler years she will never see thirteen. In the years that followed I would learn my true strengths, I would learn my true desire to survive, and I would learn to have courage when facing unsurmountable odds. One diagnose would lead to another and that would lead to another. Today, I have a medical chart that reads more like a medical dictionary. When it comes to my gastrointestinal issues, they have resulted in having to have three intestinal surgeries with the possibility of more in the future. My first surgery was when I was only 23 hours old. I was born with meconium ileus. From the three intestinal surgeries, I have had 70 cms removed from my small intestines.

There are many diagnoses that I remember receiving. I remember that feeling of being told you have a new diagnosis. I remember how those moments would stand still, and I remember all the emotions that you go through. After a while, you learn to adapt and expect there will be more things that you will just have to overcome. Then, there are some that I do not remember. Most of my stomach issues, including the diagnosis of Exocrine Pancreatic Insufficiency (PI), fall into that category of diagnoses that I do not remember. Being born with Cystic Fibrosis, there has never been a time in my life where I did not have stomach issues of one kind or another. I have taken enzymes with meals for 29 years. My parents tell me stories about the looks they got when they had to cut open my pills and add the powder. I myself remembering mixing enzyme in applesauce, and I can still taste the little beads that were in the big capsules that we used to break open so we could swallow them. Then, advancing to the whole capsule one at a time. There has always been a variety of additional intestinal medications that have been taken to ensure that everything stays working as it should.

There are times that it does not bother me that I have PI, and there are other times where I feel the true burden of the disease. Knowing that I cannot eat if I happen to forget the enzymes and knowing that there are foods I must avoid or limit to ensure my stomach is okay can be difficult. As I have aged, the side effects of having stomach issues seem to be increasing. For example, I get stomach aches that last for days, I have pelvic floor muscles strained resulting in over tightening, and I suffer from bleeding issues. My regimen to maintain my stomach health is becoming more demanding. On a regular basis, I must take three or more medications, depending on the symptoms. I average 32 enzymes a day. I have had to do pelvic floor therapy. I have found that even though it is demanding, if I can keep up with all that is required of me to maintain my health that I have fewer stomach issues. However, they do not ever go away completely.

Talking about one's intestine is sensitive. It can be embarrassing at times. I know personally, there are many things that I kept to myself for years. I suffered in silence, embarrassed to talk about my symptoms. Then, when I got to my breaking point and finally mentioned it, it has lead to three medical diagnoses that required me to change up my medication routine. It also resulted in me having long-term damage that may never be undone. As a young child and teenager, I wish I would have mentioned my issues sooner so that I would not have to be doing things like pelvic floor therapy, anal botox shots, and possible surgery. I would encourage all to speak up and remember that there is no shame in saying that you have this new health problem that is concerning. I also feel that medical professionals need to ask better questions than just how many times a patient is going and what it looks like. Those questions will not always get to the root of the problem. I recommend asking more thorough questions like, "Is there pain?", "Is there blood?", "When you go, how does it feel?". Patients should also be educated about what we should be experiencing. With more specific knowledge, we will be less likely to chalk it up to more CF stuff. We will know that there is help out there to manage our symptoms and that we are not alone in what we are going through.

– Kayleen Flanery

Objectives
- Review the historical observations of exocrine pancreatic insufficiency (PI) in cystic fibrosis (CF).
- Understand the pathophysiology of PI in CF.
- Define severe PI.
- Describe the clinical manifestations and differential diagnosis of PI and vitamin deficiencies.
- Recognize tests for PI, including tubeless testing and tests that use a gastroduodenal tube.
- Select appropriate treatment of PI and vitamin deficiencies.
- Assess the effectiveness of therapy.

Introduction

Exocrine pancreatic insufficiency (PI) is a common manifestation of cystic fibrosis (CF), contributing to nutritional and vitamin deficiencies and the inability of a patient to thrive. A minority of patients have pancreatic sufficiency (PS) for a portion or entirety of their life. This chapter on PI and nutrition in CF reviews historical observations, pathophysiology, prevalence, definitions, clinical manifestations, and differential diagnosis of the disease. The chapter also highlights direct and indirect tests of pancreatic function and treatment of PI, including correctors and potentiators of the CF transmembrane conductance regulator (*CFTR*) protein and the mainstay of treatment, pancreatic enzyme replacement therapy (PERT). Finally, the chapter provides an overview of the screening and management of nutritional and vitamin deficiencies, a summary of key points for the treatment of PI, and a discussion of future directions.

Historical Observations

In 1595, Pieter Pauw identified a link between pancreatic pathology and CF by describing the pancreas in an autopsy of a "bewitched" 11-year-old girl as "swollen, hardened, gleaming white" [1, 2]. Additionally, from the mid-1600s, there were descriptions of symptoms synonymous with steatorrhea, likely in those with exocrine pancreatic insufficiency (PI) [1]. Reports in the nineteenth and early twentieth centuries associated pancreatic lesions, steatorrhea, and meconium ileus [1]. Pancreatic lesions and steatorrhea were initially thought to be a variant of celiac disease, but bronchopulmonary complications were also noted. In 1938, Dorothy Andersen and her colleagues introduced the term "cystic fibrosis of the pancreas," based on histological findings of "fibrocystic" lesions in the pancreas [3]. In 1946, Andersen and Hedges presented compelling evidence that CF was an autosomal recessive genetic disease [3]. During the 1948 heat wave in New York, Dr. Paul di Sant'Agnese noticed that many infants with heat prostration had CF. He then demonstrated that CF patients had a fivefold excess of sodium and chloride in their sweat, which persisted even after the heat wave subsided. This observation led to development of the "sweat test" [4]. It was not until 1983 when Paul Quinton identified chloride transport as the basic defect in CF [1], which was followed by the discovery of the *CFTR* gene [5–7]. Since bicarbonate transport is coupled to severity of disease in CF [8], pancreatic function can be correlated with mutations in this gene. This relationship between genotype and phenotype is the basis for predicting exocrine pancreatic insufficiency (PI) and sufficiency (PS) among patients.

Pathophysiology

Normal Function of the Pancreas

The pancreas is a retroperitoneal organ consisting of a head, body, tail, and uncinate process and has endocrine and exocrine functions. The former comprises islets of Langerhans, which constitute 1–2% of the pancreas of about one million cell clusters. Subtypes of islet cells secrete insulin, glucagon, pancreatic polypeptide, amylin, or somatostatin. Insulin positively regulates and somatostatin negatively regulates exocrine function [9].

The exocrine pancreas constitutes 98–99% of pancreatic mass, composed of acinar-, ductal-, and centro-acinar cells that synthesize and secrete digestive enzymes, bicarbonate, electrolytes, and fluid. The acinar cells synthesize digestive enzymes, which are stored in zymogen granules. The digestive enzymes are 90% proteases, packaged as proenzymes (e.g., trypsinogen), and 10% active enzymes (amylase, lipase, and nucleases) [10]. When acinar cells are stimulated, through neurohormonal regulatory mechanisms [11], the zymogen granules fuse with the apical plasma membrane and release their contents into the central acinar lumen, transported to the duodenum through a series of ducts [12]. Within the duodenum, trypsinogen is proteolytically cleaved to its active trypsin by the small bowel brush border enzyme enterokinase. Subsequently, trypsin recognizes lysine and arginine sites, thus activating more trypsinogen and other proenzymes [13]. Cuboidal cells that line the smaller pancreatic side-branching ducts secrete a bicarbonate-rich fluid. Bicarbonate buffers pancreatic fluid and neutralizes gastric acid to provide an optimal pH for digestive enzymes, particularly lipase, which is inactivated below pH 4.5 [14, 15]. The proximal duct columnar cells express the CFTR protein in humans [16, 17].

CFTR Gene Mutations and the Pancreas

There are seven classes of CFTR gene mutations (Table 13.1). Each class induces an effect at the molecular level (Figure? in another chapter). More than >2000 CFTR gene mutations have been identified, but not all are pathogenic [18, 19]. As

Table 13.1 CF phenotype and CFTR gene mutations

Class	Genotype (examples)	CFTR protein disturbance	Exocrine pancreatic function	Corrective therapy
Severe genotypes (classes I–III, VII)				
I	Nonsense G542X	No protein produced	Insufficient	Rescue synthesis
II	Missense deletion F508	*Trafficking defect*: protein formed but fails to reach apical membrane	Insufficient	Rescue trafficking
III	Missense G551D	*Regulation defect*: channel opening unresponsive to cAMP	Insufficient	Restore channel function
VII[a]	Splice junction 1717-1G->A	No mRNA produced	Insufficient	Not rescuable
Milder genotypes (classes IV–VI)				
IV	Missense R117H	*Channel defect*: responds to cAMP with attenuated chloride conductance	Sufficient	Restore channel activity
V	Missense A455E Alternative splicing 3849 + 10kbc->T	*Synthesis defect*: decreased synthesis or partially defective protein processing	Sufficient	Correct splicing
VI	Rescued F508 c. 120del123	*Decreased stability and regulation defect*: degrades quickly, not enough protein present, inadequate channel opening	Sufficient	Stabilizers

CFTR mutations are classified as I to VII according to type and severity of genotype, the aberrant pattern of intracellular CFTR protein handling, severity of phenotype, impact on exocrine pancreatic function, and corrective therapy [20, 274]. Approximately 80% of patients with CF have a severe phenotype, suffer from PI, have either of two severe mutations (F508) or compound heterozygosity [22], and have class I–III defects, corresponding to the loss of chloride channel functioning [275]. 20% of CF patients exhibit a milder phenotype with PS and have one or two "mild" CFTR mutations associated with class IV–VI defects or associated with a responsive but functionally impaired chloride channel or a functional but unstable channel [275]

PI pancreatic insufficiency, *PS* pancreatic sufficiency

[a]Class VII formerly grouped with class I

of August 31, 2018, a total of 400 variants are annotated on the Clinical and Functional Translation of CFTR website: 336 cause CF, 35 have varying clinical consequences, 20 are not CF-causing, and 9 are of unknown significance [19]. CFTR function is virtually absent with class I–III and VII mutations, while class IV–VI mutations allow for some residual CFTR function [20]. Pancreatic function is the most predictable measure of CFTR function based on genotype [21–23]. PI is seen almost exclusively in patients who are homozygous for severe CFTR mutations (class I–III and VII mutations). Patients who are homozygous for mild CFTR mutations (classes IV–VI) or heterozygous for a mild and severe mutation typically have PS. Patients with PS, however, can progress to PI in late childhood or adulthood.

The Pancreas in CF

The severity of pancreatic damage in CF variably correlates with age [3]. Early pancreatic histology may appear relatively normal, but somewhat subtle morphological changes are often present, including increases in the ratio of connective tissue to acini [24]. With advanced disease, the pancreas may appear small, hard, and nodular and may have cystic features associated with obstruction of small ducts [3, 25, 26]. Pancreatic damage appears to begin in utero, interfering with normal maturation of the pancreas, and to continue during infancy and early childhood [27, 28]. Imrie and colleagues identified pancreatic damage at autopsy of 60 patients with CF less than 4 months of age at death [28]. Evidence of inflammation is rarely present [24, 29].

Prevalence of PI in CF

In the United States, the overall prevalence of PI in CF is estimated to be 85–88% based on PERT prescriptions [30] and pancreatic fecal elastase 1 test <200 ug/g stool [31]. At birth, the prevalence of PI ranges between 50 and 65% [27], but 30% of patients with PS rapidly develop PI within the first 36 months of life [32]. Couper reported in CF with eventual PI a greatly elevated trypsinogen value during infancy, followed by a rapid decline over several years [27]. By contrast, those with PS maintain normal range serum trypsinogen and as a group have wide-ranging exocrine pancreatic functions owing to highly variable colipase and lipase secretion [27]. Hence, repeat testing, particularly with pancreatic fecal elastase and/or fecal fat testing (see diagnosis), may be required to correctly classify patients as having PS or PI in need of PERT. Although impaired bicarbonate secretion is the earliest sign of abnormal exocrine pancreatic function [33–42], its association with pancreatic enzyme secretion is highly variable [35–38, 40–44], at least initially (Table 13.2).

Table 13.2 Pancreatic bicarbonate secretion reduced more than enzymes in CF

Author	Year	# patients	Comments (diagnosis/testing)
Secretin (i.v.) evoked pancreatic secretion			
Gibbs [276]	1950	11	Secretin juice output and concentrations[A, F, T] in 11 CF (age 1–132 mos) and 12 controls (age 2–100 mos). Those with CF had reduced fluid and trypsin outputs/concentrations compared to controls
di Sant'Agnese [43]	1955	9	Secretin juice concentrations[T] and fecal balance studies in 9 CF children. Pancreatic function was normal in 3, partially reduced in 3, and declining from normal to low in the remaining 3
Short, endoscopic, secretin (i.v.) evoked pancreatic secretion			
Engjom [277]	2015	31	Secretin juice concentrations[A, B, Ch, E, L] in 31 CF patients and 25 controls. Patients were classified as PS ($n = 13$) or PI ($n = 18$) based on a pancreatic fecal elastase cutoff value of 100 µg/g. Mean (range) values were 560 (169–703) for PS and 0 (0–17) for PI. Duodenal bicarbonate and enzyme concentrations (obtained 30–45 min post secretin) discriminated between PS and PI
CCK (i.v.) evoked pancreatic secretion			
Rick [278]	1963	NA	Secretin and pancreozymin stimulation in CF. No data provided. The degree of pancreatic ductal and acinar cell dysfunction may be discordant in CF patients
Hadorn [37]	1968	10	Secretin and pancreozymin juice outputs[A, B, L, T] in 10 CF children and young adults (age 4–23) with PS ($n = 5$) or PI ($n = 5$) and 27 controls (age 6 weeks to 13 years). In CF, outputs of bicarbonate were more severely reduced than enzymes, particularly in the group with CF and PI
Hadorn [36]	1968	10	Secretin and pancreozymin juice outputs[A, B, L, Ca, Ch, T] in 10 CF children and young adults (age 4–23) with PS and 27 controls. 10 of 10 had low bicarbonate secretion (<10% lowest normal), more severely reduced than enzyme secretion, for which there was great variability. Enzyme concentrations were greater than controls
Shwachman [41]	1975	10	Secretin and pancreozymin juice concentrations[A, B, Ch, T] in 10 adolescent and young adults with CF and PI. 100% had low bicarbonate but near normal enzyme secretions
Wong [42]	1982	14	Secretin and pancreozymin juice outputs[A, B, Ch, L, T] in 14 CF patients and 38 controls. In CF, outputs were lower for bicarbonate in 13 of 13 and for enzymes in 9 of 13
Gaskin [35]	1984	55	Secretin and pancreozymin juice outputs[Co, L, T]. Enzyme outputs were reduced in all patients. Steatorrhea (fecal fat excretion >7%) did not occur until lipase output was <4% lowest normal values (based on 14 healthy controls)
Kopelman [39]	1985	28	Secretin and pancreozymin juice outputs[T, F, P] in 28 CF patients and 21 controls. 24 of 28 CF patients had fecal balance studies. All CF patients had hyperconcentration of protein. 11 of 15 CF patients with low trypsin output (≤50 U/kg body weight/hour) had steatorrhea

(continued)

Table 13.2 (continued)

Author	Year	# patients	Comments (diagnosis/testing)
Davidson [34]	1986	65	Secretin and cholecystokinin juice outputs[B,F,L,T] in 65 CF and 11 control children. 55 of 65 CF patients had fecal balance studies. In CF, outputs were reduced for bicarbonate in 96.5% and for trypsin (but also lipase) in 79% (but near normal or normal in 21%)
Kopelman [38]	1988	56	Secretin and cholecystokinin juice outputs[B,F,T] in 56 CF patients and 56 controls. Decreased fluid secretion correlated with bicarbonate and chloride secretion. Fluid and trypsin outputs correlated
Kopelman [40]	1989	40	Secretin and cholecystokinin juice outputs[B,F,T] in 40 CF patients without steatorrhea and 69 controls. In CF, outputs were lower for bicarbonate but not trypsin.

CD celiac disease, *CCK* cholecystokinin, *CFA* coefficient of fat absorption, *PI* pancreatic insufficiency, *GFD* gluten free diet, *i.v.* intravenous, *PERT* pancreatic enzyme replacement therapy, *PFT* pancreatic function testing

Pancreatic juice content: [A]amylase, [B]bicarbonate, [Ca]carboxypeptidase, [Ch]chymotrypsin, [Co]colipase, [E]elastase, [F]fluid volume, [L]lipase, [P]protein, [Ph]phospholipase A2, [T]trypsin

Pathogenesis of PI in CF

Four mechanisms have been postulated to cause PI:

- Obstruction of pancreatic ducts by inspissated mucus plugs [24]
- Inhibition of endocytosis in acinar cells [45–47]
- Inflammation
- Imbalance of membrane lipids

As acinar secretion traverses the pancreatic ducts, its composition is altered by fluid and bicarbonate secretion into the lumen, a function regulated mainly by CFTR in ductal epithelial cells. In CF, there is low volume flow, acidic conditions, and increased mucus production, resulting in precipitation of proteins and mucus plugs, causing ductal obstruction, damage, and pancreatic atrophy [3, 24, 33–39, 42, 45, 48]. Luminal acidification decreases solubilization of luminal proteins, resulting in the formation of lamellar plugs, and also impairs acinar function through defective pH-sensitive apical endocytosis (and retrieval) of zymogen granule membranes, blocking the recycling of the membranes and reducing intracellular packaging of newly synthesized digestive enzymes [45, 46, 49].

Recurrent acute and chronic pancreatitis (CP) are complications of CF that can play a role in the development and progression of PI [50]. The development of pancreatitis, however, is uncommon in PI and typically reflects an underlying PS (10.3% with PS develop pancreatitis vs 0.5% with PI). The onset of pancreatitis requires some preserved acinar function [41, 51, 52]. As an extension of this observation, up to 50% of patients with early-onset idiopathic (CP) have CFTR gene mutations and PS

[53–56]. Some CP patients have evidence supporting the diagnoses of CF, a CFTR-related disorder, or a CFTR-related metabolic syndrome (CRMS) based on further testing [57]. Mild CFTR genotypes carry the greatest risk of pancreatitis [58, 59].

CFTR mutations appear responsible for alterations in fatty acid metabolism, resulting in essential fatty acid deficiency [60, 61], even in the absence of nutritional deficiencies [62, 63]. Linoleic and docosahexaenoic acid (DHA) levels are generally low, while arachidonic acid levels are high in CF [60–63]. These fatty acids are important regulators of membrane fluidity and transport systems. The imbalance between DHA and arachidonic acids may explain mucin hypersecretion, alterations in the acinar cell endocytosis, and pancreatic inflammation in CF [62]. In an experimental murine model of CF, dietary supplementation with DHA partially reverses abnormal pancreatic, lung, and intestinal phenotypes [64]. Clinical trials suggest that dietary DHA supplementation may reduce inflammatory markers in the lung, intestine, and blood [65, 66]. Whether dietary DHA supplementation leads to clinical improvement requires further investigation.

Defining Severity of Exocrine Pancreatic Insufficiency (PI)

Severe PI is defined as impaired pancreatic enzyme output that causes steatorrhea [67–69]. Mild and moderate PI occurs with abnormal enzyme output and bicarbonate secretion without the presence of steatorrhea. Using direct pancreatic function testing (PFT), DiMagno and colleagues defined that steatorrhea and creatorrhea may develop when lipase and trypsin thresholds fall below 10% of normal, respectively [67]. Complementary studies of patients with PI due to CP [67] and to CF [35] observed a similar absolute threshold for all to develop steatorrhea, specifically when lipase output falls below 2–4% of lowest normal. Although reduced bicarbonate secretion precedes impaired enzyme output, it does not necessarily mean severe PI (steatorrhea) [33, 36, 37, 41, 42].

Clinical Manifestations and Differential Diagnosis

The major consequence of PI is fat malabsorption and less commonly creatorrhea. Hallmarks include weight loss or failure to gain weight, malnutrition, micronutrient deficiencies, and metabolic bone disease [70, 71], but there are multiple possible clues to PI in CF upon taking a history and performing a physical examination (Table 13.3). The calorie and protein losses are usually associated with oily stools and lead to a decrease in fat stores with loss of subcutaneous fat, decreased muscle mass, and failure to thrive within the first few months of life. Fat malabsorption can also cause deficiencies of fat-soluble vitamins A, D, E, and K, which can lead to various clinical manifestations (Table 13.4). Less common micronutrient deficiencies include deficiency in zinc, selenium, and copper (Table 13.4).

Table 13.3 Clinical manifestations of PI in CF

History	Physical exam
Failure to thrive	Loss of subcutaneous fat
Short stature	Decreased muscle mass
Poor weight gain	Digital clubbing
Weight loss	Edema
Edema	Abdominal tenderness
Steatorrhea	Acrodermatitis
Diarrhea	Neuropathy
Bloating	
Flatulence	
Abdominal pain	
Bleeding tendencies	
Bone fractures	
Night blindness	
Constipation*	
Distal intestinal obstruction syndrome (DIOS)*	
Rectal prolapse*	
Meconium ileus*	

CF cystic fibrosis, *PI* pancreatic insufficiency
*gastrointestinal condition associated with PI in CF

Table 13.4 Clinical manifestation of fat-soluble vitamin and select mineral deficiencies

Micronutrient	Clinical manifestations of deficiency
Vitamin A	Xerophthalmia
	Night blindness
	Bitot's spots
	Follicular hyperkeratosis
	Immune dysfunction
Vitamin D	Rickets
	Bowed legs
	Osteomalacia
Vitamin E	Peripheral neuropathy
	Spinocerebellar ataxia
	Skeletal muscle atrophy
	Retinopathy
	Anemia
Vitamin K	Elevated prothrombin time
	Coagulopathy
	Decreased bone health
Zinc	Dermatitis
	Alopecia
	Diarrhea
	Weight loss
	Infection
	Hypogonadism
Copper	Neutropenia
	Impaired bone calcification
	Myelopathy
	Neuropathy
	Anemia

Malnutrition and poor growth in the pediatric population are driven by PI. Infants at diagnosis are more malnourished, as evidenced by poor weight gain, depressed fat stores, low serum albumin, and blood urea nitrogen [72]. Rectal prolapse and digital clubbing are common in children with CF and PI [73, 74].

Differential Diagnosis

Differential diagnosis of PI includes primary (including CF) and secondary causes (Table 13.5). Diagnostic testing (see below) serves to avoid pitfalls of defining exocrine pancreatic function on the basis of PERT prescriptions [30], which incorrectly classifies 5% (57 of 1131) as PI and 29% (24 of 84) as PS, the latter defined by pancreatic fecal elastase >200 ug/g stool [75]. It is also important to consider non-pancreatic causes of malabsorption in CF to avoid misclassifying patients as having PI and to troubleshoot the management of patients with PI but persistent steatorrhea despite PERT (Table 13.6).

Diagnosis

Pancreatic function tests (PFT) measure pancreatic secretion and are useful to differentiate pancreatic and nonpancreatic causes of malabsorption [76–78]. There are two categories of PFTs, those requiring a gastroduodenal tube and tubeless tests. The gold standard PFT is the direct pancreatic stimulation test, but they are performed far less commonly than tubeless tests due to the arduous and time-consuming nature of the test and need for specially trained personnel to perform and analyze the results.

Table 13.5 Malabsorption from causes of luminal pancreatic enzyme deficiency

Primary PI	Secondary PI
Reduced secretory capacity	*Preserved secretory capacity*
Agenesis of the pancreas	Obstruction: pancreatic and ampullary neoplasm
Congenital pancreatic	Decreased CCK release: small bowel disease (e.g., celiac,
hypoplasia	Crohn's)
Shwachman-Diamond	Intraluminal lipase inactivation (gastrinoma, lipase inhibitor)
syndrome	Postcibal asynchrony (poor mixing, decreased CCK release,
Johanson-Blizzard syndrome	decreased contact time): gastrointestinal surgery, dysmotility
Adult pancreatic lipomatosis or	Enterokinase deficiency: reduced luminal activation of
atrophy	pancreatic proteases
Cystic fibrosis	Reduced synthesis: protein calorie malnutrition (marasmus,
Isolated lipase deficiency	kwashiorkor), reversible with repletion of essential amino
Chronic pancreatitis	acids
Pancreatic resection	

CCK cholecystokinin, *PI* pancreatic insufficiency

Table 13.6 Evaluation of persistent steatorrhea despite PERT for PI

Factors	Details
PERT	Dose and adherence
Acid inhibition	pH <4.5 degrades uncoated PERT Low pH delays release of coated PERT (until the jejunum) Low pH precipitates bile acids, decreasing micellar solubilization of lipids
Bile acid deficiency	Bacterial overgrowth (deconjugation) Biliary obstruction and ileal disease
Duodenal disease	Celiac disease, tropical sprue, plus others Infection (e.g., giardia)
Mixing disorder (asynchrony)	Timing of PERT Gastroparesis Intestinal surgery

Adapted from DiMagno et al. [171] with permission
PERT pancreatic enzyme replacement therapy, *PI* pancreatic insufficiency

PFT Requiring a Gastroduodenal Tube

These PFTs collect pancreatic fluid from the duodenum through a gastroduodenal tube. These PFTs are classified as direct or indirect. The direct test requires intravenous secretagogues (secretin, CCK or its analogues, or both) to stimulate pancreatic secretion and fluoroscopic placement of a double-lumen tube. The gastric aspiration port, positioned in the distal stomach, continuously aspirates gastric juice to prevent the contamination of pancreatic juice aspirated from the duodenal port. Duodenal fluid is collected at specific time intervals pre- and post-administration of secretagogue(s) and subsequently analyzed for juice volume and concentrations of bicarbonate and enzymes (e.g., lipase, trypsin, etc.). A peak bicarbonate fluid concentration of less than 80 milliequivalents/liter (mEq/L), lipase output <77,000 IU/h, and trypsin output <25,000 U/h indicates impaired pancreatic secretory function [76]. Direct PFTs are accurate, sensitive (67–97%), and specific (78–100%) for detecting PI [67, 79–87].

The indirect Lundh PFT employs a single- rather than double-lumen gastroduodenal tube for pancreatic juice collection and a test meal to stimulate pancreatic secretion [88]. The test meal comprises a standardized 300 milliliters (mL) of dried milk, vegetable oil, and dextrose. Duodenal concentrations of chymotrypsin below 12.6 international units (IU)/L suggest PI, with a sensitivity ranging from 66% to 94% [89–91].

Tubeless Testing

Noninvasive tubeless PFTs indirectly measure pancreatic function by relying on two bioassay principles. First, the maldigestion and malabsorption of fat, protein, and carbohydrate may be measured in stool. Alternatively, oral administration of a synthetic compound that is acted upon by a specific pancreatic digestive enzyme will generate a product that may be measured in stool, blood, breath, or urine. Overall, these tests have limited utility as a positive test is typically present only with severe PI [78]. These tests include oral PFTs, fecal pancreatic enzyme output, and fecal fat quantitation.

Oral PFTs

Pancreolauryl and bentiromide tests are oral indirect tests of pancreatic exocrine function but are rarely used in clinical practice due to lack of availability and relatively low sensitivity [37–100%] and specificity [39–100%] [69, 77, 92–100]. The accuracy of these tests is affected by previous gastrointestinal surgery, nonpancreatic malabsorption syndromes, liver disease, and alterations to gut microbiome.

The ^{13}C mixed triglyceride breath test involves orally administered ^{13}C-labeled fat, which releases free fatty acids or monoglycerides when digested in the proximal gut by pancreatic lipolytic activity. These products are absorbed in the gut and oxidized in the liver to $^{13}CO_2$, which is exhaled in breath [101–103]. The sensitivity and specificity of these tests (in non-CF populations) are 92–93% and 86–92%, respectively [104, 105]. Factors that may affect the accuracy and precision of these tests include diabetes mellitus, celiac disease, small intestinal bacterial overgrowth, or previous small bowel surgery.

Fecal Pancreatic Enzyme (Elastase, Chymotrypsin) Measurements

Human pancreatic elastase 1 is an endoprotease and sterol-binding protein that is present in both human pancreatic secretion and feces [100]. Fecal elastase (FE) is not degraded during intestinal transit and correlates with duodenal lipase, amylase, trypsin, and bicarbonate concentration [106–108]. Monoclonal FE testing via enzyme-linked immunosorbent assay (ELISA) is more sensitive than polyclonal ELISA [109, 110] and is unaffected by PERT.

FE is recommended for all infants with CF age < 2 years [111] and at least annually in patients with PS. FE-1 < 100 ug/g stool (see below) suggests conversion to PI [112] and warrants PERT therapy.

FE-1 < 200 ug/g stool has too low sensitivity as a screen for mild PI (without steatorrhea) [108] but a high sensitivity and specificity for severe PI [108, 113, 114]. Importantly, FE-1 value >100 ug/g stool has a 99% negative predictive value for severe PI due to CF. FE-1 testing is inaccurate in children less than 2 weeks [115], and false positive tests occur in patients with diarrhea [116].

In non-CF populations, FE-1 testing is less useful for the diagnosis of PI with a 40% sensitivity for mild-moderate PI and 83% sensitivity for severe PI [117]. In CP with PI, the optimal cut-off is 84 ug/g stool (87.5% sensitivity, 81.6% specificity, 66.7% PPV, 93.9% NPV, and AUC 0.861) [118]. FE-1 false positive tests, however, occur in 25–30% of patients with small bowel conditions [113, 117, 119–121] and also are common in diabetes mellitus. In type 1 diabetes mellitus, FE-1 has a low specificity and positive predictive value compared with direct PFTs [122].

Fecal chymotrypsin may be performed on random stool samples [123, 124] and is 45–100% sensitive and 49–90% specific for PI in CF [123, 125–127]. It, however, is more useful for identifying severe rather than mild-to-moderate PI [128, 129] but is inferior to fecal elastase to screen for PI in CF and of limited use [130].

Tests for Fecal Fat Determination

The 72-h quantitative fecal fat determination is the gold standard to detect steatorrhea [131] but does not discriminate between pancreatic and nonpancreatic causes of fat malabsorption. Quantitative fecal fat testing requires consuming a high-fat diet (100 grams of fat daily) starting at least 3 days prior to the 72-h stool collection. Research protocols include methods too cumbersome for clinical use, namely, ingestion of colored stool markers (e.g., carmine) at the beginning of test meals and collecting stool for 72 h following passage of the marker.

There is a linear correlation between ingestion and excretion of fat [132]. Upon ingesting 100 grams of fat/day, steatorrhea is present if more than 7 grams of fat is excreted in stool/24 h in children and adults [76] but more than 15 gram/day in infants [111]. In clinical studies, the quantitative fecal fat test results are expressed as the coefficient of fat absorption (CFA). The coefficient of nitrogen absorption (CNA) [133] is a related but less sensitive marker of PI; reductions in pancreatic juice lipase output (and decreases in CFA) typically occur prior to reductions in trypsin (and decreases in CNA) [81, 134, 135]. Both CFA and CNA are used, however, as clinical trial endpoints for PERT effectiveness.

CFA is defined by the following equation:

$$\mathrm{CFA}\,(\%) = 100 \times \left[\left(\text{mean daily fat intake} - \text{mean daily stool fat} \right) / \text{mean daily fat intake} \right]$$

Steatocrit, a rapid gravimetric method for measuring stool fat, is not an effective method to determine steatorrhea [136, 137].

Comparison of PFT and Imaging in Cystic Fibrosis

In CF, common pancreatic imaging abnormalities are fatty replacement of the pancreas with atrophy or enlargement (less common), pancreatic atrophy without fatty replacement, pancreatic cystosis, and less commonly ductal abnormalities [138]. Abnormal pancreatic imaging in CF may suggest PI, but PI may be present with normal pancreatic imaging in 25–33% of patients [139, 140]. Functional imaging, namely, secretin-stimulated ultrasound (US) [141, 142] and MRI [142], which measure peak duodenal area and fluid filling, respectively, may better discriminate between PS and PI. However, in CF, impaired fluid and bicarbonate secretion have a highly variable association with pancreatic enzyme secretion [35–38, 40–44], at least initially.

Treatment

Targeting the CFTR Defect

CFTR modulators are a mainstay of therapy to improve CFTR protein function. Potentiators, such as ivacaftor (KALYDECO®), improve the gating of chloride and bicarbonate on the luminal epithelial surface. Correctors, such as lumacaftor and tezacaftor, stabilize misfolded CFTR and increase protein trafficking to the luminal epithelial surface. Combination potentiator/corrector drugs include lumacaftor/ivacaftor (ORKAMBI®) and tezacaftor/ivacaftor (SYMDECO®).

Conceivably, CFTR modulators should improve pancreatic exocrine function by augmenting ductal secretion of fluid and bicarbonate, solubilizing inspissated proteins, restoring acinar recycling, and flushing and restoring patency of the ducts. Ivacaftor improves exocrine pancreatic function (based on fecal elastase) in children ages 12 to <24 months [143] and 2–5 years [144]. Up to 67% of 2–5-year-old children transitioned from PI (FE-1 < 50 ug/g stool) to PS (FE-1 > 200 ug/g stool) [143]. In case reports, improvement in exocrine pancreatic function may also occur [145]. Both ivacaftor and combination treatment with lumacaftor/ivacaftor increase body mass index, but it is uncertain if body weight also increases [143, 144, 146–151]. Ivacaftor also improves bone mineralization [152].

CFTR modulators may also increase exocrine function by improving islet cell function. CFTR plays a crucial role in the insulin secretion of pancreatic beta cells [153], and insulin potentiates postprandial and secretagogue-evoked exocrine pancreatic secretion [154–161]. Ivacaftor treatment of CF patients increases insulin secretion [162, 163].

Pancreatic Enzyme Replacement Therapy (PERT)

PERT is the primary treatment of PI secondary to CF, CP, surgery, and other causes (Table 13.5). Dosing and timing of PERT administration can be confusing because treatment recommendations for patients with CF and PI differ by patient age and CF society/organization. In addition, there are different PERT recommendations for CP, which are included to highlight possible research and future updates in guidelines.

PERT Formulations

Five commercial products are approved by the Food and Drug Administration (FDA) (Table 13.7) [164]. All contain pancrelipase, a mixture of porcine-derived lipases, amylases, and proteases. Four products are enteric-coated, delayed-release formulations. Based on package insert information, each product releases at pH

Table 13.7 Currently available enzyme products for treating PI

Product	Formulation		Lipase units/dose	Manufacturer
Immediate release (nonenteric coated)				
Viokace®	Porcine, oral, tablet		10,440, 20,880	Aptalis Pharmaceutical Technologies, Birmingham, AL
[a]*Delayed release (enteric coated)*				
Zenpep®	Porcine, oral, bead		3000, 5000, 10,000, 15,000, 20,000, 25,000, 40,000	Aptalis Pharmaceutical Technologies, Birmingham, AL
	[b]*Size (mm)*	*Dose (KU)*		
	1.8–1.9	3–5		
	2.2–2.5	10–40		
Creon®	Porcine, oral, microsphere		3000, 6000, 12,000, 24,000, 36,000	Abbott Laboratories, Abbott Park, IL
	[b]*Size (mm)*	*Dose (KU)*		
	0.7–1.6	All		
Pancreaze®	Porcine, oral, microtablet		4200, 10,500, 16,800, 21,000	Johnson and Johnson, New Brunswick, NJ
	[b]*Size (mm)*	*Dose (KU)*		
	~2	All		
Pertzye®	Porcine, oral, microsphere with bicarbonate		4000, 8000, 16,000	Digestive Care, Inc., Bethlehem, PA
	[b]*Size (mm) Dose (KU)*			
	0.8–1.4	4–8		
	0.8–2.2	16		

PI pancreatic insufficiency

[a]According to package insert information, each enteric-coated product releases enzyme contents at pH >5.5

[b]Enteric-coated particles >2 mm diameter may have delayed prandial gastric emptying [165–167], which would reduce duodenal mixing with the meal

>5.5 and has enteric-coated particles close to the critical 2 mm diameter (Table 13.7), above which particles have delayed prandial gastric emptying [165–167], which would reduce duodenal mixing with the meal. One product, Pertzye, is buffered with bicarbonate. Viokace is an uncoated, immediate-release formulation approved for use with a proton pump inhibitor to reduce acid denaturation of lipase. In CF patients receiving enteral feeding, a new lipase delivery system [RELiZORB] has been developed, but studies of clinical efficacy are limited; it is a disposable cartridge containing lipase immobilized onto polymeric carrier beads, which is connected to gastrostomy tubing for hydrolyzing lipid in enteral nutrition [168].

PERT Dosing and Timing for PI due to CF

PERT dosing is based on lipase content, owing to greater reduction in lipase than other digestive enzymes in PI [134]. The practice guidelines for PERT from the CF Foundation (CFF) [70, 111] is consensus rather than evidence-based [75, 169, 170] and is calculated by either dietary fat intake or body weight (which can be used at any age) (Table 13.8). Diet-based dosing is useful in infants who receive a known amount of fat in their formula or in patients receiving enteral feeding. The consensus dosing approach was developed in response to safety concerns about dose-dependent complications (discussed below) [111] and not by physiologic measurements to ascertain the amount of intraduodenal lipolytic activity necessary to adequately hydrolyze fat, as are recommendations for PERT in CP with PI (see recent review [171]).

The recommended PERT timing (before, during, or after meals and snacks) in CF patients with PI appears settled in children but is less clear in adults. In a randomized, crossover study of two schedules of PERT (before vs during meals) for CF patients [172], children <10 years old had a significantly greater CFA by taking PERT before meals, and children >10 years old had a nonsignificant trend toward a greater CFA by taking PERT during meals [172]. According to CF guidelines of North America

Table 13.8 PERT dosing strategies in CF

Age	USP units of lipase (in PERT)
Dietary fat-based dosing [70, 111]	
[a]Infants	2000–5000/120 mL formula (~1600/g fat injested)
	2000–5000/ breastfeeding (~1600/g fat injested)
[a]Children/adults	<4000 units lipase per gram of dietary fat per day
Weight-based dosing [70, 111, 223]	
[a]Age < 4 years	1000–2500/kg/meal
[a]Age > 4 years	500–2500/kg/meal, fewer with snacks (e.g., 250/kg)

[a]Max PERT dose is 2500 USP units of lipase/kg/meal and 10,000 USP units of lipase/kg/day [111] or < 4000 USP units of lipase/g dietary fat/day [70, 223]

(CFF) [173] and Australia [174], children and adolescents should take PERT immediately *before* meals and snacks. In adults, recommendations for PERT timing are conflicting: *before* meals (CFF) [173], *during* meals (Australia) [174], and no specific recommendations (European CF societies) [112, 175] except to reference the Cochrane analysis conclusion that information is lacking on the timing of PERT dosing [176]. Clinically, we recommend that adults take PERT during meals and refer readers to the CF study discussed above [172] and the CP studies discussed below.

Contrasting PERT Dosing and Timing in PI due to CP

PERT dosing in CP is derived from physiologic studies in PI patients with CP. In these patients, normal fat absorption requires more than 5–10% of lowest normal lipase output per meal, equivalent to 45,000–90,000 United States Pharmacopeia (USP) units of lipase [67, 177]. Steatorrhea is abolished if this dose results in more than 5% of maximal postprandial duodenal lipase concentration [178] (Table 13.9). This range of PERT dosing for PI in CP is recommended by authors of CP book chapters [179–181], guidelines [182–185], and expert reviews [171, 184–188].

PERT timing recommendations in CP (for PI) are derived from several observations. First, prandial ingestion of PERT compared to hourly ingestion (the historical standard) resulted in similar delivery of lipase to the duodenum and reductions in steatorrhea [14, 171], corroborating and extending earlier observations [189]. More recently, it was found that fat digestion was significantly greater when PERT was distributed with meals or just after meals [190]. Currently, authors of book chapters [179–181], guidelines [182–185], and expert reviews [171, 184–188] recommend taking PERT during or after meals, the former by taking one quarter of the dose with the first few bites of the meal, one half during the meal, and one quarter with the last bites of the meal.

Table 13.9 Lipase units (IU vs USP) in health and PI

	IU[a]	USP
Mean *normal* postprandial lipase output [14, 67]	140,000/h × 4 h = 560,000/ meal	420,00/h × 4 h = 1,680,000/ meal
Lowest *normal* lipase output (2 SD below mean) [14, 67]	75,000/h × 4 h = 300,000/ meal	225,000/h × 4 h = 900,000/ meal
~10% normal lipase output = steatorrhea (>7 g/24 h) [67]	7500/h × 4 = 30,000/meal[b]	22,500/h × 4 = 90,000/meal[b]

Adapted from DiMagno et al. [171] with permission
IU international units, *USP* United States Pharmacopeia
Lipolytic units based on hydrolysis of substrate. [a]Based on hydrolysis of triolein, sometimes called triolein units. [b]In chronic pancreatitis with fat malabsorption, when gastric acid secretion is blocked, ~ 30,000 IU (3833 IU/tablet × 8, ~90,000 USP units) given with meals abolishes steatorrhea [178]

Applying Conflicting PERT Recommendations

Clinical decisions regarding PERT for PI in CF should follow the current CF guidelines. When PERT is ineffective, alternate PERT dosing and timing that are used in CP and other potential causes of a suboptimal clinical response should be considered, as discussed in the next section.

Monitoring PERT Effectiveness

In patients with CF, gastrointestinal symptoms correlate poorly with PERT dosing and are poor indicators of undertreated malabsorption [191]. Nevertheless, monitoring the effectiveness of therapy includes tracking weight, body mass index, micronutrient status (discussed below), symptoms (less reliable), and measurement of CFA. According to multiple systematic reviews, PERT therapy may abolish, but usually only reduces, steatorrhea, regardless of PI etiology [192–195]. Treatment options for patients with features of ineffective PERT treatment (Table 13.6) include assessing adherence with PERT, possibly by measuring fecal chymotrypsin (low values indicate inadequate PERT) [186]; encouraging PERT ingestion throughout meals (see timing); increasing PERT dose; and adding inhibitors of acid secretion.

Postprandial duodenal acidity occurs in PI due to CP [14] and CF [196] and irreversibly denatures lipase [14, 15, 178], delays pH-dependent (pH > 5.0) release of enteric-coated PERT [197, 198] until jejunal or ileal segments [199–202], and precipitates (inactivates) bile acids [203, 204], thereby impairing mixed micelle formation [203, 204] and fat absorption, which occurs predominantly in the duodenum during normal human physiology [205].

According to the 2016 Cochrane systematic review of 17 trials (6 of children or adults, 7 of children only, 4 of adults only), the suppression of gastric acid generally augments PERT-evoked increases in CFA in patients with PI and only partial responses to PERT [206]. Early studies of nonenteric-coated PERT for PI in CP observed that coadministration of H2 blockers increased luminal lipase activity [178, 207], micellar bile acid concentrations [203], and CFA [178, 207]. Similar findings were observed during the treatment of PI with enteric-coated PERT, both in CP, by coadministering H2 blockers or proton pump inhibitors (PPIs) [208], and in CF populations, by coadministering H2 blockers [204, 209, 210] or PPIs [211, 212]. Even though potential side effects of long-term PPI use may be overstated, it is advisable to create specific treatment goals for beginning, tapering, and stopping PPI therapy [213]. Another promising approach in CF patients with PI is to raise luminal pH using CFTR correctors [201].

Persistent steatorrhea in PI may involve causes other than acid denaturation of lipase, commonly small intestinal bacterial overgrowth (SIBO) [214, 215], but other factors may need attention (Table 13.6). If addressing these factors fails to abolish steatorrhea, other primary and secondary causes of luminal pancreatic enzyme deficiency leading to maldigestion of fat need consideration [179] (Table 13.5).

PERT Complications

Fibrosing Colonopathy In the 1990s, microencapsulated PERT were introduced without a recommendation for max dosing and were temporarily withdrawn after reports of a dose-dependent association with colonic strictures, termed fibrosing colonopathy [216–218]. To address this drug safety concern, attendees of a consensus conference generated weight-based (as opposed to symptom-based) PERT dosing guidelines [75, 219]. The etiology of this complication is thought to be iatrogenic due to high doses of pancreatic enzymes (specifically due to protease), unrelated to a specific formulation, and also possibly due to a local immune response to porcine enzymes. A discredited concept is that fibrosing colonopathy is due to Eudragit, a polymer used in PERT preparations to delay release of enzymes until a higher, optimal intraluminal pH is present [220]. Potential risk factors for fibrosing colonopathy include high PERT dose >6000 lipase units/kg/meal, duration of PERT >6 months, prior GI surgery, H2 blocker use, Pulmozyme (DNAse) use, and distal intestinal obstructive syndrome [216, 218]. Currently there is an active 10-year prospective study registered on clinicaltrials.gov (NCT01652157) to assess the occurrence and risk factors for this disorder.

Other Complications Common reactions (≥10%), according to a representative PERT package insert for Pertzye (https://resources.chiesiusa.com/Pertzye/PERTZYE_PI.pdf), include diarrhea, dyspepsia, and cough. Hyperglycemia can occur with abrupt dose changes [221]. Additional adverse events include hyperuricemia [222], allergic reactions (including anaphylaxis, asthma, hives, and pruritus), and oral mucosal ulcerations, which may develop with prolonged contact to PERT, particularly when microspheres are administered with food in infants'/toddlers' mouth [223].

Fat-Soluble Vitamins: Monitoring and Treatment

Fat-soluble vitamins (A, D, E, K) are essential for health. The prevalence of deficiencies is variable in CF patients, for which screening tests, treatment, and monitoring are recommended (see Table 13.10 for vitamin D). The same applies for bone health (see Table 13.11), discussed in conjunction with vitamin D.

Vitamin A

Vitamin A is essential for eye health, cellular integrity, growth, immune function, and bone and tooth development. Important cautions are that excessive vitamin A intake leading to above normal blood levels (hypervitaminosis A) may be harmful, causing changes in bone health, dermatitis, liver damage, and rarely pseudotumor

Table 13.10 Summary of CF guideline recommendations for vitamin D deficiency

Assessment
Annual serum vitamin D 25(OH) (preferably end of winter)
Goal: > = 30 ng/ml (75 nmol/liter)
During vitamin D replacement
Recheck level in 3 months after changing dose
Confirm adherence to treatment if repeat levels low
Avoid indirect markers of vitamin D: PTH, osteocalcin, alkaline phosphatase

Management
All individuals
Maintain serum vitamin D 25(OH) level ≥ 30 ng/ml (75 nmol/liter)
Infants < 12 months old
Initial vitamin D3 dose: 400–500 IU
Level 20–30 ng/mL (50–75 nmol/L): increase to 800–1000 IU/day
Level 20–30 ng/mL despite above increase: increase to max 2000 IU/day
Level ≤ 20 ng/mL (50 nmol/L): maximum 2000 IU/day
Referral to specialist
Level < 10 ng/mL (<25 nmol/L): – also assess for rickets
Level < 30 ng/mL (75 nmol/L) after treatment
Children 1–10 years old
Initial vitamin D3 dose: 800–1000 IU
Level 20–30 ng/mL (50–75 nmol/L): increase to 1600–3000 IU/day
Level 20–30 ng/mL despite above increase: increase to max 4000 IU/day
Level ≤ 20 ng/mL (50 nmol/L): maximum 4000 IU/day
Referral to specialist
Level < 30 ng/mL (75 nmol/L) despite max treatment
Children and adolescents ≥ 10 years old
Initial vitamin D3 dose: 800–1000 IU
Level 20–30 ng/mL (50–75 nmol/L): increase to 1600–6000 IU/day
Level 20–30 ng/mL despite above increase: increase to max 10,000 IU/day
Level ≤ 20 ng/mL (50 nmol/L): maximum 10,000 IU/day
Referral to specialist
Level < 30 ng/mL (75 nmol/L) despite max treatment

Adapted from Tangprichaa et al. [264]

PTH parathyroid hormone

cerebri [224]. Patients with CF who have serum retinal levels of up to 110 micrograms/dL have better lung function [225]. Vitamin A deficiency should be assessed via fasting serum retinol. Reduced serum retinol levels may occur in PS [226]. Vitamin A concentration should not be measured during pulmonary exacerbations, which decreases values [227]. There are currently no recommendations on the monitoring of vitamin A, but it would be prudent to survey this annually. The CFF recommends the following daily doses in CF patients: 0–12 months, 1500 IU; 1–3 years, 5000 IU; 4–8 years, 5000–10,000 IU; 9 years and older, 10,000 units. No randomized control trials on regular administration of vitamin A in CF patients exist; thus, recommendations and guidelines on its supplementations are not readily available [228, 229].

Table 13.11 Metabolic bone disease in CF: screening and management

Screening for reduced bone mineral density (BMD)		
Dual energy X-ray absorptiometry (DEXA)		
Age ≥ 18 years: screen all		
Age < 18 years: screen if 1 or more present: ideal body weight < 90%, FEV1 < 50% predicted, glucocorticoid intake ≥5 mg/day for ≥90 days/year, delayed puberty, history of fractures		
BMD reporting:	Age < 18 years:	Z score
	Age 18–30 years:	Z or T score
	Age ≥ 30 years:	T score
Treatment for DEXA T/Z score ≥ −1.0		
Supplement vitamin D, calcium, and vitamin K Achieve a target body mass index >25th percentile Encourage weight-bearing exercise Repeat DEXA every 5 years		
Treatment for DEXA − 1.0 > T/Z score > −2.0		
Supplement micronutrients, as above		
Treat pulmonary pathology:	Treat pulmonary infection	
	Minimize steroid dosing	
Treat endocrine pathology:	Treat CF-related diabetes	
	Refer for delayed puberty, hypogonadism	
Bisphosphonates for fragility fractures, transplant list, or BMD >3–5%/year		
Repeat DEXA every 2–4 years		
Treatment for DEXA T/Z score ≤ −2.0		

Supplement micronutrients, as above
Treat pulmonary and endocrine pathology, as above
Consider bisphosphonates
  Alendronate 70 mg weekly or 10 mg daily
  Risedronate 35 mg weekly or 5 mg daily
  Pamidronate 30 mg in 500-mL saline infused over 3 h, every 3 mos
  Zoledronic acid 4–5 mg infused over 15–20 min, yearly
  Zoledronic acid 2 mg every 3 mos for 2 years
Repeat DEXA annually		

Adapted from Aris et al. [279]
CF cystic fibrosis, *DEXA* dual-energy X-ray absorptiometry

Vitamin E

Vitamin E is an antioxidant and is important for development, cell membrane stability, and the prevention of hemolysis. The prevalence of vitamin E deficiency in CF is uncertain, but neurologic symptoms related to vitamin E deficiency are rarely observed in CF since the introduction of PERT and vitamin supplementation [230–232]. The CFF recommends the following daily vitamin E doses: 0–12 months, 40–50 IU; 1–3 years, 80–150 IU; 4–8 years, 100–200 IU; and 9 years and older, 200–400 IU. Newborn screening can identify vitamin E deficiency, which can be quickly corrected with supplementation and PERT [226, 233–235]. Vitamin E levels are dependent on serum lipid levels, and clinicians can assess for deficiency by ratios of serum vitamin E to either total lipid or cholesterol. Vitamin E deficiency is defined by ratios of vitamin E/total lipids <0.8 mg/dL, vitamin E/cholesterol <2.5 mg/g, or vitamin E/cholesterol <5.4 mg/g [236–238]. The CFF recommends 100–400 IU/day, but results of recent studies suggest that these doses may be too high with no proven benefit in children and adolescents [232, 239].

Vitamin K

The prevalence of vitamin K deficiency is quite high in the CF population [240–243] due to malabsorption, inadequate intake, the long-term effects of antibiotics on gut microbiota, and its ability to produce vitamin K [244]. There is no biomarker of vitamin K deficiency. Prothrombin time and international normalized ratio (INR) are surrogate markers that reflect vitamin K-dependent blood clotting times, useful for detecting severe deficiency [244]. The CFF recommends 300–500 ug/day of vitamin K for all age groups. Minimal evidence is available to guide the management of vitamin K deficiency in CF [245–248]. Recommended doses of vitamin K from international societies vary, ranging from 0.5 mg daily to 10 mg weekly [169, 239, 249, 250].

Vitamin D and Bone Health

The prevalence of vitamin D deficiency in CF varies but occurs in up to 90% of patients [251–254]. Vitamin D is important in calcium homeostasis [255], innate and adaptive immunity, bone health [256, 257], and insulin secretion and sensitivity [258, 259]. Numerous factors may cause vitamin D deficiency in CF: PI, decreased exposure to sunlight due to illness and use of photosensitive antibiotics, decreased appetite, increased vitamin D catabolism, altered biosynthesis of cholecalciferol, and frequent corticosteroid use [243, 260–263]. The North American CFF issued guidelines for the screening, diagnosis, and management of vitamin D deficiency in CF in 2012 [264] (Table 13.10).

Bone disease, manifested as osteoporosis, osteopenia, fractures, and/or arthritis/arthropathy, is the fourth most common extrapulmonary comorbidity of CF [265]. The 2017 CFF Patient Registry reports a 17.8% prevalence of bone disease among CF patients [265], which increases with age [265]. The pathophysiology of CF-related bone disease is multifactorial involving nutrition, endocrine, genetic, and environmental factors. Bone disease in CF results in poor bone mass accrual during puberty and accelerated bone loss during adulthood [254, 266–268]. Table 13.11 outlines the screening and management of bone disease in CF. Nutritional management of CF includes maintaining an optimal weight for height and assessing body mass index at every clinic visit. Dietary intake of energy, protein, and key micronutrients important for bone health should be assessed annually. Low vitamin K is associated with increased risk for bone disease in the general population, and supplementation, as described above, may lead to improved bone health [269–271].

Summary of Screening and Treatment of PI in CF

- *Severe PI* (>7 g fecal fat/24 h) in the majority of CF population
- *PS in ~15%, screen for progression to PI*

  – FE-1 testing: simple screen for severe PI

    Early in life to diagnose severe PI
    FE-1 ≤ 50 ug/g stool = PI, initiate PERT
    FE-1 > 50 ≤ 100 ug/g stool = possible PI

    - Ideal approach: confirm PI with 72-h quantitative fecal fat
    - Alternate option: initiate PERT, do annual FE-1

    FE-1 > 100 ug/g stool = PS, do annual FE-1

  – 72-h quantitative fecal fat test

    Consider:

    - PI possible, not definite (FE-1 > 50 ≤ 100 ug/g stool)
    - Liquid or semi-formed stool (FE-1 inaccurate)
    - Assess response to PERT therapy

    Diagnosis of severe PI

    - Children and adults: >7 g fecal fat/24 h
    - Infants: >15 g fecal fat/24 h

- *Pancrelipase*

  – Initiation:

    At diagnosis of severe PI (FE-1 ≤ 50 ug/g stool)
    If severe PI likely based on genotype (Table 13.1 or www.cftr2.org), particularly in children, FE-1 not necessary to initiate PERT

  – Dosing

    Dietary fat-based dosing (varies by age)
    Weight-based dosing (varies by age)
    Max dosage:

    - 2500 USP lipase units/kg/meal
    - 10,000 USP lipase units/kg/day
    - <4000 USP lipase units/g dietary fat/day

- Timing

  < 10 years old: "just before" meals
  >10 years old: during meals (*1/4 of dose with first few bites of meal, 1/2 during the meal, and 1/4 with last bites of meal*)

- Response to treatment

  Clinical assessment: weight, BMI, micronutrients, measurement of CFA
  Symptoms unreliable markers of response

- Approach to ineffective therapy

  Dose, timing
  Assess adherence (fecal chymotrypsin)
  Acid suppression
  Other causes: bacterial overgrowth, etc. (Table 13.6)
  Overlooked causes of luminal pancreatic enzyme deficiency (Table 13.5)

- *Fat-soluble vitamins* (A, D, E, K)

  - Screening: early in life and at least annually
  - Test more frequently (~3 months) to assess response to replacement therapy

- *Bone Health*

  - DEXA screening: all ≥18 years old or < 18 years old with risk factors (Table 13.11)
  - Treatment based on T/Z score (Table 13.11)

- *Weight loss/failure to thrive*

  - PERT:

    If appropriate genotype (see Table 13.1 or www.cftr2.org)
    FE-1 ≤ 50 ug/g stool (see above)

  - Consult with registered dietician, gastroenterologist, others

Future Considerations

More research is necessary to answer common clinical questions, including the frequency and risk factors of fibrosing colonopathy in CF patients taking PERT (study ongoing; trial, clinicaltrials.gov #NCT01652157), the appropriate dosing and timing of ingesting PERT, and diet. Performing clinical trials could be better accomplished if there was a simple method to assess exocrine pancreatic function. A potentially novel and less cumbersome test compared to quantitative fecal fat testing is a malabsorption blood test of oral coadministration of the free fatty acid pentadecanoic acid (PA) and the triglyceride triheptadecanoic acid (which requires lipase for absorption) and quantitating differences in relative absorption as a marker of PI [272, 273]. The full impact of CFTR modulation on exocrine pancreatic function will not be understood until children with PI due to CF who receive this therapy grow to adulthood.

Acknowledgments We thank Dr. Eugene P. DiMagno for his review of the chapter and his outstanding suggestions.

References

1. Quinton PM. Physiological basis of cystic fibrosis: a historical perspective. Physiol Rev. 1999;79(1 Suppl):S3–s22.
2. Busch R. On the history of cystic fibrosis. Acta Univ Carol Med (Praha). 1990;36(1–4):13–5.
3. Andersen DH, Hodges RG. Celiac syndrome; genetics of cystic fibrosis of the pancreas, with a consideration of etiology. Am J Dis Child. 1946;72:62–80.
4. Di Sant'Agnese PA, Darling RC, Perera GA, Shea E. Abnormal electrolyte composition of sweat in cystic fibrosis of the pancreas; clinical significance and relationship to the disease. Pediatrics. 1953;12(5):549–63.
5. Kerem B, Rommens JM, Buchanan JA, Markiewicz D, Cox TK, Chakravarti A, et al. Identification of the cystic fibrosis gene: genetic analysis. Science. 1989;245(4922):1073–80.
6. Riordan JR, Rommens JM, Kerem B, Alon N, Rozmahel R, Grzelczak Z, et al. Identification of the cystic fibrosis gene: cloning and characterization of complementary DNA. Science. 1989;245(4922):1066–73.
7. Rommens JM, Iannuzzi MC, Kerem B, Drumm ML, Melmer G, Dean M, et al. Identification of the cystic fibrosis gene: chromosome walking and jumping. Science. 1989;245(4922):1059–65.
8. Choi JY, Muallem D, Kiselyov K, Lee MG, Thomas PJ, Muallem S. Aberrant CFTR-dependent HCO3 – transport in mutations associated with cystic fibrosis. Nature. 2001;410(6824):94–7.
9. Barreto SG, Carati CJ, Toouli J, Saccone GT. The islet-acinar axis of the pancreas: more than just insulin. Am J Physiol Gastrointest Liver Physiol. 2010;299(1):G10–22.
10. Scheele G, Bartelt D, Bieger W. Characterization of human exocrine pancreatic proteins by two-dimensional isoelectric focusing/sodium dodecyl sulfate gel electrophoresis. Gastroenterology. 1981;80(3):461–73.
11. Owyang C, Logsdon CD. New insights into neurohormonal regulation of pancreatic secretion. Gastroenterology. 2004;127(3):957–69.
12. Owyang C, Williams JA. Pancreatic secretion. In Podolsky PK, Fitz JG, Kalloo AN, Shanahan F, Wang TC, Camilleri M, editors. Textbook of Gastroenterology. 6th ed. New York: John Wiley & Sons, Ltd, 2015. p. 450–473.
13. Rinderknecht H. Activation of pancreatic zymogens. Normal activation, premature intrapancreatic activation, protective mechanisms against inappropriate activation. Dig Dis Sci. 1986;31(3):314–21.
14. DiMagno EP, Malagelada JR, Go VL, Moertel CG. Fate of orally ingested enzymes in pancreatic insufficiency. Comparison of two dosage schedules. N Engl J Med. 1977;296(23):1318–22.
15. Heizer WD, Cleaveland CR, Iber FL. Gastric inactivation of pancreatic supplements. Bull Johns Hopkins Hosp. 1965;116:261–70.
16. Thiese N. Pancreas. In: Kumar V, Abbas AK, Aster JC, Robbins SL, editors. Robbins basic pathology. 9th ed. Philadelphia: Elsevier/Saunders; 2018. p. 679–89.
17. Marino CR, Matovcik LM, Gorelick FS, Cohn JA. Localization of the cystic fibrosis transmembrane conductance regulator in pancreas. J Clin Invest. 1991;88(2):712–6.
18. Cystic Fibrosis Mutation Database [Webpage]. [updated April 25th, 2011. Available from: http://www.genet.sickkids.on.ca/StatisticsPage.html.

19. The Clinical and Functional Translation of CFTR (CFTR2) [updated August 31st, 2018]. Available from: https://www.cftr2.org/.
20. De Boeck K, Amaral MD. Progress in therapies for cystic fibrosis. Lancet Respir Med. 2016;4(8):662–74.
21. Ahmed N, Corey M, Forstner G, Zielenski J, Tsui LC, Ellis L, et al. Molecular consequences of cystic fibrosis transmembrane regulator (CFTR) gene mutations in the exocrine pancreas. Gut. 2003;52(8):1159–64.
22. Kerem E, Corey M, Kerem BS, Rommens J, Markiewicz D, Levison H, et al. The relation between genotype and phenotype in cystic fibrosis--analysis of the most common mutation (delta F508). N Engl J Med. 1990;323(22):1517–22.
23. Kristidis P, Bozon D, Corey M, Markiewicz D, Rommens J, Tsui LC, et al. Genetic determination of exocrine pancreatic function in cystic fibrosis. Am J Hum Genet. 1992;50(6):1178–84.
24. Oppenheimer EH, Esterly JR. Cystic fibrosis of the pancreas. Morphologic findings in infants with and without diagnostic pancreatic lesions. Arch Pathol. 1973;96(3):149–54.
25. Allen RA, Baggenstoss AH. The pathogenesis of fibrocystic disease of the pancreas: study of the ducts by serial sections. Am J Pathol. 1955;31(2):337.
26. Lebenthal E, Lerner A, Rolston D. The pancreas in cystic fibrosis. In: Go VL, DiMagno EP, Gardner J, Lebenthal E, Reber H, Scheele G, editors. The pancreas: biology, pathophysiology, and disease. New York: Raven Press, Ltd; 1993. p. 1041–81.
27. Couper RT, Corey M, Durie PR, Forstner GG, Moore DJ. Longitudinal evaluation of serum trypsinogen measurement in pancreatic-insufficient and pancreatic-sufficient patients with cystic fibrosis. J Pediatr. 1995;127(3):408–13.
28. Imrie JR, Fagan DG, Sturgess JM. Quantitative evaluation of the development of the exocrine pancreas in cystic fibrosis and control infants. Am J Pathol. 1979;95(3):697–708.
29. Kopito LE, Shwachman H. The pancreas in cystic fibrosis: chemical composition and comparative morphology. Pediatr Res. 1976;10(8):742–9.
30. Marshall B. Cystic Fibrosis Foundation Annual Patient Registry Report, 2016 Cystic Fibrosis Foundation 2016 [updated 2016]. Available from: https://www.cff.org/.
31. Borowitz D, Baker SS, Duffy L, Baker RD, Fitzpatrick L, Gyamfi J, et al. Use of fecal elastase-1 to classify pancreatic status in patients with cystic fibrosis. J Pediatr. 2004;145(3):322–6.
32. Waters DL, Dorney SF, Gaskin KJ, Gruca MA, O'Halloran M, Wilcken B. Pancreatic function in infants identified as having cystic fibrosis in a neonatal screening program. N Engl J Med. 1990;322(5):303–8.
33. Barraclough M, Taylor C. Twenty-four hour ambulatory gastric and duodenal pH profiles in cystic fibrosis: effect of duodenal hyperacidity on pancreatic enzyme function and fat absorption. J Pediatr Gastroenterol Nutr. 1996;23(1):45–50.
34. Davidson G, Kirubakaran C, Ratcliffe G, Cooper D, Robb T. Abnormal pancreatic electrolyte secretion in cystic fibrosis: reliability as a diagnostic marker. Acta Paediatr. 1986;75(1):145–50.
35. Gaskin K, Durie P, Lee L, Hill R, Forstner G. Colipase and lipase secretion in childhood-onset pancreatic insufficiency: delineation of patients with steatorrhea secondary to relative colipase deficiency. Gastroenterology. 1984;86(1):1–7.
36. Hadorn B, Johansen P, Anderson C. Pancreozymin-secretin test of exocrine pancreatic function in cystic fibrosis and the significance of the result for the pathogenesis of the disease. J Paediatr Child Health. 1968;4(1):8–22.
37. Hadorn B, Zoppi G, Shmerling D, Prader A, McIntyre I, Anderson CM. Quantitative assessment of exocrine pancreatic function in infants and children. J Pediatr. 1968;73(1):39–50.
38. Kopelman H, Corey M, Gaskin K, Durie P, Weizman Z, Forstner G. Impaired chloride secretion, as well as bicarbonate secretion, underlies the fluid secretory defect in the cystic fibrosis pancreas. Gastroenterology. 1988;95(2):349–55.
39. Kopelman H, Durie P, Gaskin K, Weizman Z, Forstner G. Pancreatic fluid secretion and protein hyperconcentration in cystic fibrosis. N Engl J Med. 1985;312(6):329–34.
40. Kopelman H, Forstner G, Durie P, Corey M. Origins of chloride and bicarbonate secretory defects in the cystic fibrosis pancreas, as suggested by pancreatic function studies on control and CF subjects with preserved pancreatic function. Clin Invest Med. 1989;12(3):207–11.

41. Shwachman H, Lebenthal E, Khaw K-T. Recurrent acute pancreatitis in patients with cystic fibrosis with normal pancreatic enzymes. Pediatrics. 1975;55(1):86–95.
42. Wong L, Turtle S, Davidson A. Secretin pancreozymin stimulation test and confirmation of the diagnosis of cystic fibrosis. Gut. 1982;23(9):744–50.
43. Di Sant'Agnese PA. Fibrocystic disease of the pancreas with normal or partial pancreatic function; current views on pathogenesis and diagnosis. Pediatrics. 1955;15(6):683–97.
44. Dooley RR, Guilmette F, Leubner H, Patterson PR, Shwachman H, Weil C. Cystic fibrosis of the pancreas with varying degrees of pancreatic insufficiency. AMA J Dis Child. 1956;92(4):347–68.
45. Freedman SD, Kern HF, Scheele GA. Pancreatic acinar cell dysfunction in CFTR(−/−) mice is associated with impairments in luminal pH and endocytosis. Gastroenterology. 2001;121(4):950–7.
46. Fukuoka S, Freedman SD, Yu H, Sukhatme VP, Scheele GA. GP-2/THP gene family encodes self-binding glycosylphosphatidylinositol-anchored proteins in apical secretory compartments of pancreas and kidney. Proc Natl Acad Sci. 1992;89(4):1189–93.
47. Scheele GA, Fukuoka S-I, Kern HF, Freedman SD. Pancreatic dysfunction in cystic fibrosis occurs as a result of impairments in luminal pH, apical trafficking of zymogen granule membranes, and solubilization of secretory enzymes. Pancreas. 1996;12(1):1–9.
48. DiMagno MJ, Lee S-H, Hao Y, Zhou S-Y, McKenna BJ, Owyang C. A proinflammatory, anti-apoptotic phenotype underlies the susceptibility to acute pancreatitis in cystic fibrosis transmembrane regulator (−/−) mice. Gastroenterology. 2005;129(2):665–81.
49. Fukuoka S, Freedman SD, Scheele GA. A single gene encodes membrane-bound and free forms of GP-2, the major glycoprotein in pancreatic secretory (zymogen) granule membranes. Proc Natl Acad Sci. 1991;88(7):2898–902.
50. Freeman AJ, Ooi CY. Pancreatitis and pancreatic cystosis in cystic fibrosis. J Cyst Fibros. 2017;16:S79–86.
51. De Boeck K, Weren M, Proesmans M, Kerem E. Pancreatitis among patients with cystic fibrosis: correlation with pancreatic status and genotype. Pediatrics. 2005;115(4):e463–e9.
52. Maisonneuve P, Campbell P III, Durie P, Lowenfels AB. Pancreatitis in hispanic patients with cystic fibrosis carrying the R334W mutation. Clin Gastroenterol Hepatol. 2004;2(6):504–9.
53. Bishop MD, Freedman SD, Zielenski J, Ahmed N, Dupuis A, Martin S, et al. The cystic fibrosis transmembrane conductance regulator gene and ion channel function in patients with idiopathic pancreatitis. Hum Genet. 2005;118(3–4):372–81.
54. Cohn JA, Friedman KJ, Noone PG, Knowles MR, Silverman LM, Jowell PS. Relation between mutations of the cystic fibrosis gene and idiopathic pancreatitis. N Engl J Med. 1998;339(10):653–8.
55. DiMagno EP. Gene mutations and idiopathic chronic pancreatitis: clinical implications and testing. Gastroenterology. 2001;121(6):1508–12.
56. Noone PG, Zhou Z, Silverman LM, Jowell PS, Knowles MR, Cohn JA. Cystic fibrosis gene mutations and pancreatitis risk: relation to epithelial ion transport and trypsin inhibitor gene mutations. Gastroenterology. 2001;121(6):1310–9.
57. Farrell PM, White TB, Ren CL, Hempstead SE, Accurso F, Derichs N, et al. Diagnosis of cystic fibrosis: consensus guidelines from the Cystic Fibrosis Foundation. J Pediatr. 2017;181S:S4–S15. e1
58. Ooi CY, Dorfman R, Cipolli M, Gonska T, Castellani C, Keenan K, et al. Type of CFTR mutation determines risk of pancreatitis in patients with cystic fibrosis. Gastroenterology. 2011;140(1):153–61.
59. Ooi CY, Gonska T, Durie PR, Freedman SD. Genetic testing in pancreatitis. Gastroenterology. 2010;138(7):2202–6.e1.
60. Freedman SD, Blanco PG, Zaman MM, Shea JC, Ollero M, Hopper IK, et al. Association of cystic fibrosis with abnormalities in fatty acid metabolism. N Engl J Med. 2004;350(6):560–9.
61. Strandvik B, Gronowitz E, Enlund F, Martinsson T, Wahlstrom J. Essential fatty acid deficiency in relation to genotype in patients with cystic fibrosis. J Pediatr. 2001;139(5):650–5.
62. Freedman SD, Blanco P, Shea JC, Alvarez JG. Mechanisms to explain pancreatic dysfunction in cystic fibrosis. Med Clin North Am. 2000;84(3):657–64, x.

63. Roulet M, Frascarolo P, Rappaz I, Pilet M. Essential fatty acid deficiency in well nourished young cystic fibrosis patients. Eur J Pediatr. 1997;156(12):952–6.
64. Freedman SD, Katz MH, Parker EM, Laposata M, Urman MY, Alvarez JG. A membrane lipid imbalance plays a role in the phenotypic expression of cystic fibrosis in cftr(−/−) mice. Proc Natl Acad Sci U S A. 1999;96(24):13995–4000.
65. Leggieri E, De Biase RV, Savi D, Zullo S, Halili I, Quattrucci S. Clinical effects of diet supplementation with DHA in pediatric patients suffering from cystic fibrosis. Minerva Pediatr. 2013;65(4):389–98.
66. Morin C, Cantin AM, Vezina FA, Fortin S. The efficacy of MAG-DHA for correcting AA/DHA imbalance of cystic fibrosis patients. Mar Drugs. 2018;16(6):1–10.
67. DiMagno EP, Go VL, Summerskill WH. Relations between pancreatic enzyme outputs and malabsorption in severe pancreatic insufficiency. N Engl J Med. 1973;288(16):813–5.
68. Lankisch PG. Function tests in the diagnosis of chronic pancreatitis. Critical evaluation. Int J Pancreatol. 1993;14(1):9–20.
69. Lankisch PG, Schreiber A, Otto J. Pancreolauryl test. Evaluation of a tubeless pancreatic function test in comparison with other indirect and direct tests for exocrine pancreatic function. Dig Dis Sci. 1983;28(6):490–3.
70. Stallings VA, Stark LJ, Robinson KA, Feranchak AP, Quinton H. Evidence-based practice recommendations for nutrition-related management of children and adults with cystic fibrosis and pancreatic insufficiency: results of a systematic review. J Am Diet Assoc. 2008;108(5):832–9.
71. Sullivan JS, Mascarenhas MR. Nutrition: prevention and management of nutritional failure in cystic fibrosis. J Cyst Fibros. 2017;16(Suppl 2):S87–s93.
72. Pencharz PB, Durie PR. Pathogenesis of malnutrition in cystic fibrosis, and its treatment. Clin Nutr. 2000;19(6):387–94.
73. El-Chammas KI, Rumman N, Goh VL, Quintero D, Goday PS. Rectal prolapse and cystic fibrosis. J Pediatr Gastroenterol Nutr. 2015;60(1):110–2.
74. Pitts-Tucker TJ, Miller MG, Littlewood JM. Finger clubbing in cystic fibrosis. Arch Dis Child. 1986;61(6):576–9.
75. Borowitz DS, Grand RJ, Durie PR. Use of pancreatic enzyme supplements for patients with cystic fibrosis in the context of fibrosing colonopathy. Consensus Committee. J Pediatr. 1995;127(5):681–4.
76. Chey WD, DiMagno MJ, Chey WY. Tests of gastric and exocrine pancreatic function and absorption. In: Textbook of gastroenterology. Wiley-Blackwell: Chichester; 2008. p. 3414–30.
77. DiMagno MJ. Pancreatic function tests. In: Johnson LR, Barrett K, et al., editors. Encylopedia of gastroenterology. San Diego: Elsevier Science; 2003.
78. Keller J, Aghdassi AA, Lerch MM, Mayerle JV, Layer P. Tests of pancreatic exocrine function – clinical significance in pancreatic and non-pancreatic disorders. Best Pract Res Clin Gastroenterol. 2009;23(3):425–39.
79. Adler M, Waye JD, Dreiling D. The pancreas, a correlation of function, structure and histopathology. Acta Gastroenterol Belg. 1976;39(11–12):502–8.
80. Burton P, Evans DG, Harper AA, Howath T, Oleesky S, Scott JE, et al. A test of pancreatic function in man based on the analysis of duodenal contents after administration of secretin and pancreozymin. Gut. 1960;1:111–24.
81. DiMagno EP, Malagelada JR, Moertel CG, Go VL. Prospective evaluation of the pancreatic secretion of immunoreactive carcinoembryonic antigen, enzyme, and bicarbonate in patients suspected of having pancreatic cancer. Gastroenterology. 1977;73(3):457–61.
82. DiMagno EP, Malagelada JR, Taylor WF, Go VL. A prospective comparison of current diagnostic tests for pancreatic cancer. N Engl J Med. 1977;297(14):737–42.
83. Dornberger GR, Comfort MW, et al. Pancreatic function as measured by analysis of duodenal contents before and after stimulation with secretin. Gastroenterology. 1948;11(5):701–13.
84. Dreiling DA Sr. Studies in pancreatic function. V. The use of the secretin test in the diagnosis of pancreatitis and in the demonstration of pancreatic insufficiencies in gastrointestinal disorders. Gastroenterology. 1953;24(4):540–55.

85. Hayakawa T, Kondo T, Shibata T, Noda A, Suzuki T, Nakano S. Relationship between pancreatic exocrine function and histological changes in chronic pancreatitis. Am J Gastroenterol. 1992;87(9):1170–4.
86. Heij HA, Obertop H, van Blankenstein M, ten Kate FW, Westbroek DL. Relationship between functional and histological changes in chronic pancreatitis. Dig Dis Sci. 1986;31(10):1009–13.
87. Waye JD, Adler M, Dreiling DA. The pancreas: a correlation of function and structure. Am J Gastroenterol. 1978;69(2):176–81.
88. Lundh G. Pancreatic exocrine function in neoplastic and inflammatory disease; a simple and reliable new test. Gastroenterology. 1962;42:275–80.
89. Braganza JM, Rao JJ. Disproportionate reduction in tryptic response to endogenous compared with exogenous stimulation in chronic pancreatitis. Br Med J. 1978;2(6134):392–4.
90. Levin GE, Youngs GR, Bouchier IA. Evaluation of the Lundh test in the diagnosis of pancreatic disease. J Clin Pathol. 1972;25(2):129–32.
91. Mottaleb A, Kapp F, Noguera EC, Kellock TD, Wiggins HS, Waller SL. The Lundh test in the diagnosis of pancreatic disease: a review of five years' experience. Gut. 1973;14(11):835–41.
92. Barry RE, Barry R, Ene MD, Parker G. Fluorescein dilaurate – tubeless test for pancreatic exocrine failure. Lancet. 1982;2(8301):742–4.
93. Delchier JC, Soule JC. BT-PABA test with plasma PABA measurements: evaluation of sensitivity and specificity. Gut. 1983;24(4):318–25.
94. Gyr K, Stalder GA, Schiffmann I, Fehr C, Vonderschmitt D, Fahrlaender H. Oral administration of a chymotrypsin-labile peptide – a new test of exocrine pancreatic function in man (PFT). Gut. 1976;17(1):27–32.
95. Lankisch PG, Brauneis J, Otto J, Goke B. Pancreolauryl and NBT-PABA tests. Are serum tests more practicable alternatives to urine tests in the diagnosis of exocrine pancreatic insufficiency? Gastroenterology. 1986;90(2):350–4.
96. Larsen B, Ekelund S, Jorgensen L, Bremmelgaard A. Determination of the exocrine pancreatic function with the NBT-PABA test using a novel dual isotope technique and gas chromatography-mass spectrometry. Scand J Clin Lab Invest. 1997;57(2):159–65.
97. Malfertheiner P, Buchler M, Muller A, Ditschuneit H. Fluorescein dilaurate serum test: a rapid tubeless pancreatic function test. Pancreas. 1987;2(1):53–60.
98. Niederau C, Grendell JH. Diagnosis of chronic pancreatitis. Gastroenterology. 1985;88(6):1973–95.
99. Otsuki M. Chronic pancreatitis. The problems of diagnostic criteria. Pancreatology. 2004;4(1):28–41.
100. Sziegoleit A. A novel proteinase from human pancreas. Biochem J. 1984;219(3):735–42.
101. Kalivianakis M, Verkade HJ, Stellaard F, van der Were M, Elzinga H, Vonk RJ. The 13C-mixed triglyceride breath test in healthy adults: determinants of the 13CO2 response. Eur J Clin Investig. 1997;27(5):434–42.
102. Vantrappen GR, Rutgeerts PJ, Ghoos YF, Hiele MI. Mixed triglyceride breath test: a noninvasive test of pancreatic lipase activity in the duodenum. Gastroenterology. 1989;96(4):1126–34.
103. Ventrucci M, Cipolla A, Ubalducci GM, Roda A, Roda E. 13C labelled cholesteryl octanoate breath test for assessing pancreatic exocrine insufficiency. Gut. 1998;42(1):81–7.
104. Dominguez-Munoz JE, Nieto L, Vilarino M, Lourido MV, Iglesias-Garcia J. Development and diagnostic accuracy of a breath test for pancreatic exocrine insufficiency in chronic pancreatitis. Pancreas. 2016;45(2):241–7.
105. Lembcke B, Braden B, Caspary WF. Exocrine pancreatic insufficiency: accuracy and clinical value of the uniformly labelled 13C-Hiolein breath test. Gut. 1996;39(5):668–74.
106. Loser C, Mollgaard A, Folsch UR. Faecal elastase 1: a novel, highly sensitive, and specific tubeless pancreatic function test. Gut. 1996;39(4):580–6.
107. Stevens T, Conwell D, Zuccaro G, Van Lente F, Khandwala F, Hanaway P, et al. Analysis of pancreatic elastase-1 concentrations in duodenal aspirates from healthy subjects and patients with chronic pancreatitis. Dig Dis Sci. 2004;49(9):1405–11.
108. Walkowiak J, Cichy WK, Herzig KH. Comparison of fecal elastase-1 determination with the secretin-cholecystokinin test in patients with cystic fibrosis. Scand J Gastroenterol. 1999;34(2):202–7.

109. Miendje Y, Maisin D, Sipewa MJ, Deprez P, Buts JP, De Nayer P, et al. Polyclonal versus monoclonal ELISA for the determination of fecal elastase 1: diagnostic value in cystic fibrosis and chronic pancreatic insufficiency. Clin Lab. 2004;50(7–8):419–24.
110. Borowitz D, Lin R, Baker SS. Comparison of monoclonal and polyclonal ELISAs for fecal elastase in patients with cystic fibrosis and pancreatic insufficiency. J Pediatr Gastroenterol Nutr. 2007;44(2):219–23.
111. Borowitz D, Robinson KA, Rosenfeld M, Davis SD, Sabadosa KA, Spear SL, et al. Cystic Fibrosis Foundation evidence-based guidelines for management of infants with cystic fibrosis. J Pediatr. 2009;155(6 Suppl):S73–93.
112. Turck D, Braegger CP, Colombo C, Declercq D, Morton A, Pancheva R, et al. ESPEN-ESPGHAN-ECFS guidelines on nutrition care for infants, children, and adults with cystic fibrosis. Clin Nutr. 2016;35(3):557–77.
113. Carroccio A, Verghi F, Santini B, Lucidi V, Iacono G, Cavataio F, et al. Diagnostic accuracy of fecal elastase 1 assay in patients with pancreatic maldigestion or intestinal malabsorption: a collaborative study of the Italian Society of Pediatric Gastroenterology and Hepatology. Dig Dis Sci. 2001;46(6):1335–42.
114. Stein J, Jung M, Sziegoleit A, Zeuzem S, Caspary WF, Lembcke B. Immunoreactive elastase I: clinical evaluation of a new noninvasive test of pancreatic function. Clin Chem. 1996;42(2):222–6.
115. Cade A, Walters MP, McGinley N, Firth J, Brownlee KG, Conway SP, et al. Evaluation of fecal pancreatic elastase-1 as a measure of pancreatic exocrine function in children with cystic fibrosis. Pediatr Pulmonol. 2000;29(3):172–6.
116. Daftary A, Acton J, Heubi J, Amin R. Fecal elastase-1: utility in pancreatic function in cystic fibrosis. J Cyst Fibros. 2006;5(2):71–6.
117. Hahn JU, Bochnig S, Kerner W, Koenig H, Sporleder B, Lankisch PG, et al. A new fecal elastase 1 test using polyclonal antibodies for the detection of exocrine pancreatic insufficiency. Pancreas. 2005;30(2):189–91.
118. Gonzalez-Sanchez V, Amrani R, Gonzalez V, Trigo C, Pico A, de-Madaria E. Diagnosis of exocrine pancreatic insufficiency in chronic pancreatitis: (13)C-mixed triglyceride breath test versus fecal elastase. Pancreatology. 2017;17(4):580–5.
119. Nousia-Arvanitakis S. Fecal elastase-1 concentration: an indirect test of exocrine pancreatic function and a marker of an enteropathy regardless of cause. J Pediatr Gastroenterol Nutr. 2003;36(3):314–5.
120. Salvatore S, Finazzi S, Barassi A, Verzelletti M, Tosi A, Melzi d'Eril GV, et al. Low fecal elastase: potentially related to transient small bowel damage resulting from enteric pathogens. J Pediatr Gastroenterol Nutr. 2003;36(3):392–6.
121. Schappi MG, Smith VV, Cubitt D, Milla PJ, Lindley KJ. Faecal elastase 1 concentration is a marker of duodenal enteropathy. Arch Dis Child. 2002;86(1):50–3.
122. Hahn JU, Kerner W, Maisonneuve P, Lowenfels AB, Lankisch PG. Low fecal elastase 1 levels do not indicate exocrine pancreatic insufficiency in type-1 diabetes mellitus. Pancreas. 2008;36(3):274–8.
123. Girella E, Faggionato P, Benetazzo D, Mastella G. The assay of chymotrypsin in stool as a simple and effective test of exocrine pancreatic activity in cystic fibrosis. Pancreas. 1988;3(3):254–62.
124. Scotta MS, Marzani MD, Maggiore G, De Giacomo C, Melzi D'Eril GV, Moratti R. Fecal chymotrypsin: a new diagnostic test for exocrine pancreatic insufficiency in children with cystic fibrosis. Clin Biochem. 1985;18(4):233–4.
125. Cavallini G, Benini L, Brocco G, Riela A, Bovo P, Pederzoli P, et al. The fecal chymotrypsin photometric assay in the evaluation of exocrine pancreatic capacity. Comparison with other direct and indirect pancreatic function tests. Pancreas. 1989;4(3):300–4.
126. Goldberg DM, Durie PR. Biochemical tests in the diagnosis of chronic pancreatitis and in the evaluation of pancreatic insufficiency. Clin Biochem. 1993;26(4):253–75.
127. Remtulla MA, Durie PR, Goldberg DM. Stool chymotrypsin activity measured by a spectrophotometric procedure to identify pancreatic disease in infants. Clin Biochem. 1986;19(6):341–7.

128. Durr HK, Otte M, Forell MM, Bode JC. Fecal chymotroypsin: a study on its diagnostic value by comparison with the secretin-cholecystokinin test. Digestion. 1978;17(5):404–9.
129. Ehrhardt-Schmelzer S, Otto J, Schlaeger R, Lankisch PG. Faecal chymotrypsin for investigation of exocrine pancreatic function: a comparison of two newly developed tests with the titrimetric method. Z Gastroenterol. 1984;22(11):647–51.
130. Walkowiak J, Herzig KH, Strzykala K, Przyslawski J, Krawczynski M. Fecal elastase-1 is superior to fecal chymotrypsin in the assessment of pancreatic involvement in cystic fibrosis. Pediatrics. 2002;110(1 Pt 1):e7.
131. Van De Kamer JH, Ten Bokkel Huinink H, Weyers HA. Rapid method for the determination of fat in feces. J Biol Chem. 1949;177(1):347–55.
132. Wollaeger EE, Comfort MW, Osterberg AE. Total solids, fat and nitrogen in the feces; a study of normal persons taking a test diet containing a moderate amount of fat: comparison with results obtained with normal persons taking a test diet containing a large amount of fat. Gastroenterology. 1947;9(3):272–83.
133. Chibnall AC, Rees MW, Williams EF. The total nitrogen content of egg albumin and other proteins. Biochem J. 1943;37(3):354–9.
134. DiMagno EP, Malagelada JR, Go VL. Relationship between alcoholism and pancreatic insufficiency. Ann N Y Acad Sci. 1975;252(1):200–7.
135. Bozkurt T, Braun U, Leferink S, Gilly G, Lux G. Comparison of pancreatic morphology and exocrine functional impairment in patients with chronic pancreatitis. Gut. 1994;35(8):1132–6.
136. Wagner MH, Bowser EK, Sherman JM, Francisco MP, Theriaque D, Novak DA. Comparison of steatocrit and fat absorption in persons with cystic fibrosis. J Pediatr Gastroenterol Nutr. 2002;35(2):202–5.
137. Walkowiak J, Lisowska A, Blask-Osipa A, Drzymala-Czyz S, Sobkowiak P, Cichy W, et al. Acid steatocrit determination is not helpful in cystic fibrosis patients without or with mild steatorrhea. Pediatr Pulmonol. 2010;45(3):249–54.
138. King LJ, Scurr ED, Murugan N, Williams SG, Westaby D, Healy JC. Hepatobiliary and pancreatic manifestations of cystic fibrosis: MR imaging appearances. Radiographics. 2000;20(3):767–77.
139. Fiel SB, Friedman AC, Caroline DF, Radecki PD, Faerber E, Grumbach K. Magnetic resonance imaging in young adults with cystic fibrosis. Chest. 1987;91(2):181–4.
140. Murayama S, Robinson A, Mulvihill D, Goyco P, Beckerman R, Hines M, et al. MR imaging of pancreas in cystic fibrosis. Pediatr Radiol. 1990;20(7):536–9.
141. Engjom T, Erchinger F, Tjora E, Laerum BN, Georg D, Gilja OH. Diagnostic accuracy of secretin-stimulated ultrasonography of the pancreas assessing exocrine pancreatic failure in cystic fibrosis and chronic pancreatitis. Scand J Gastroenterol. 2015;50(5):601–10.
142. Engjom T, Tjora E, Wathle G, Erchinger F, Laerum BN, Gilja OH, et al. Secretin-stimulated ultrasound estimation of pancreatic secretion in cystic fibrosis validated by magnetic resonance imaging. Eur Radiol. 2018;28(4):1495–503.
143. Rosenfeld M, Wainwright CE, Higgins M, Wang LT, McKee C, Campbell D, et al. Ivacaftor treatment of cystic fibrosis in children aged 12 to <24 months and with a CFTR gating mutation (ARRIVAL): a phase 3 single-arm study. Lancet Respir Med. 2018;6(7):545–53.
144. Davies JC, Cunningham S, Harris WT, Lapey A, Regelmann WE, Sawicki GS, et al. Safety, pharmacokinetics, and pharmacodynamics of ivacaftor in patients aged 2-5 years with cystic fibrosis and a CFTR gating mutation (KIWI): an open-label, single-arm study. Lancet Respir Med. 2016;4(2):107–15.
145. Kounis I, Levy P, Rebours V. Ivacaftor CFTR potentiator therapy is efficient for pancreatic manifestations in cystic fibrosis. Am J Gastroenterol. 2018;113(7):1058–9.
146. Borowitz D, Lubarsky B, Wilschanski M, Munck A, Gelfond D, Bodewes F, et al. Nutritional status improved in cystic fibrosis patients with the G551D mutation after treatment with ivacaftor. Dig Dis Sci. 2016;61(1):198–207.
147. Edgeworth D, Keating D, Ellis M, Button B, Williams E, Clark D, et al. Improvement in exercise duration, lung function and well-being in G551D-cystic fibrosis patients: a double-blind, placebo-controlled, randomized, cross-over study with ivacaftor treatment. Clin Sci (Lond). 2017;131(15):2037–45.

148. Guimbellot J, Solomon GM, Baines A, Heltshe SL, VanDalfsen J, Joseloff E, et al. Effectiveness of ivacaftor in cystic fibrosis patients with non-G551D gating mutations. J Cyst Fibros. 2019;18(1):102–9.

149. Ramsey BW, Davies J, McElvaney NG, Tullis E, Bell SC, Drevinek P, et al. A CFTR potentiator in patients with cystic fibrosis and the G551D mutation. N Engl J Med. 2011;365(18):1663–72.

150. Sawicki GS, McKone EF, Pasta DJ, Millar SJ, Wagener JS, Johnson CA, et al. Sustained Benefit from ivacaftor demonstrated by combining clinical trial and cystic fibrosis patient registry data. Am J Respir Crit Care Med. 2015;192(7):836–42.

151. Milla CE, Ratjen F, Marigowda G, Liu F, Waltz D, Rosenfeld M. Lumacaftor/ivacaftor in patients aged 6-11 years with cystic fibrosis and homozygous for F508del-CFTR. Am J Respir Crit Care Med. 2017;195(7):912–20.

152. Sermet-Gaudelus I, Delion M, Durieu I, Jacquot J, Hubert D. Bone demineralization is improved by ivacaftor in patients with cystic fibrosis carrying the p.Gly551Asp mutation. J Cyst Fibros. 2016;15(6):e67–e9.

153. Guo JH, Chen H, Ruan YC, Zhang XL, Zhang XH, Fok KL, et al. Glucose-induced electrical activities and insulin secretion in pancreatic islet beta-cells are modulated by CFTR. Nat Commun. 2014;5:4420.

154. Berg T, Johansen L, Brekke IB. Insulin potentiates cholecystokinin (CCK)-induced secretion of pancreatic kallikrein. Acta Physiol Scand. 1985;123(1):89–95.

155. Kanno T, Saito A. The potentiating influences of insulin on pancreozymin-induced hyperpolarization and amylase release in the pancreatic acinar cell. J Physiol. 1976;261(3):505–21.

156. Lee KY, Zhou L, Ren XS, Chang TM, Chey WY. An important role of endogenous insulin on exocrine pancreatic secretion in rats. Am J Phys. 1990;258(2 Pt 1):G268–74.

157. Pollard H, Miller L, Brewer W. The external secretion of the pancreas and diabetes mellitus. Am J Dig Dis. 1943;10(1):20–3.

158. Chey WY, Shay H, Shuman CR. External pancreatic secretion in diabetes mellitus. Ann Intern Med. 1963;59(6):812–21.

159. Frier B, Saunders J, Wormsley K, Bouchier I. Exocrine pancreatic function in juvenile-onset diabetes mellitus. Gut. 1976;17(9):685–91.

160. Hsu J-T, Yeh C-N, Mannes GA, Yamato M, Nagahama K, Kotani T, et al. Follow-up of exocrine pancreatic function in type-1 diabetes mellitus. Digestion. 2005;72(2–3):71–5.

161. Lankisch P, Manthey G, Otto J, Koop H, Talaulicar M, Willms B, et al. Exocrine pancreatic function in insulin-dependent diabetes mellitus. Digestion. 1982;25(3):211–6.

162. Bellin MD, Laguna T, Leschyshyn J, Regelmann W, Dunitz J, Billings J, et al. Insulin secretion improves in cystic fibrosis following ivacaftor correction of CFTR: a small pilot study. Pediatr Diabetes. 2013;14(6):417–21.

163. Hayes D Jr, McCoy KS, Sheikh SI. Resolution of cystic fibrosis-related diabetes with ivacaftor therapy. Am J Respir Crit Care Med. 2014;190(5):590–1.

164. Pancreatic enzyme replacement products. JAMA. 2017;318(19):1929.

165. Goebell H, Klotz U, Nehlsen B, Layer P. Oroileal transit of slow release 5-aminosalicylic acid. Gut. 1993;34(5):669–75.

166. Hardy JG, Healey JN, Lee SW, Reynolds JR. Gastrointestinal transit of an enteric-coated delayed-release 5-aminosalicylic acid tablet. Aliment Pharmacol Ther. 1987;1(3):209–16.

167. Meyer JH, Elashoff J, Porter-Fink V, Dressman J, Amidon GL. Human postprandial gastric emptying of 1-3-millimeter spheres. Gastroenterology. 1988;94(6):1315–25.

168. Stevens J, Wyatt C, Brown P, Patel D, Grujic D, Freedman SD. Absorption and safety with sustained use of RELiZORB evaluation (ASSURE) study in patients with cystic fibrosis receiving enteral feeding. J Pediatr Gastroenterol Nutr. 2018;67(4):527–32.

169. Borowitz D, Baker RD, Stallings V. Consensus report on nutrition for pediatric patients with cystic fibrosis. J Pediatr Gastroenterol Nutr. 2002;35(3):246–59.

170. Ramsey BW, Farrell PM, Pencharz P. Nutritional assessment and management in cystic fibrosis: a consensus report. The Consensus Committee. Am J Clin Nutr. 1992;55(1):108–16.

171. DiMagno EP, DiMagno MJ. Chronic pancreatitis: landmark papers, management decisions, and future. Pancreas. 2016;45(5):641–50.

172. Brady M, Rickard K, Yu P, Eigen H. Effectiveness of enteric coated pancreatic enzymes given before meals in reducing steatorrhea in children with cystic fibrosis. J Am Diet Assoc. 1992;92(7):813–7.
173. Maguiness K, Casey S, Fulton J, Luder E, McKenna A, Hazle L. Nutrition: pancreatic enzyme replacement in people with cystic fibrosis. 2006.
174. Naehrlich L. Pancreatic enzyme replacement therapy (PERT) for children and adolescents with cystic fibrosis. Q Health Editor NEMO Group.
175. Castellani C, Duff AJ, Bell SC, Heijerman HG, Munck A, Ratjen F, et al. ECFS best practice guidelines: the 2018 revision. J Cyst Fibros. 2018;17(2):153–78.
176. Somaraju UR, Solis-Moya A. Pancreatic enzyme replacement therapy for people with cystic fibrosis. Cochrane Database Syst Rev. 2014;10
177. Lankisch P, Lembcke B, Wemken G, Creutzfeldt W. Functional reserve capacity of the exocrine pancreas. Digestion. 1986;35(3):175–81.
178. Regan PT, Malagelada J-R, DiMagno EP, Glanzman SL, Go VLW. Comparative effects of antacids, cimetidine and enteric coating on the therapeutic response to oral enzymes in severe pancreatic insufficiency. N Engl J Med. 1977;297(16):854–8.
179. DiMagno MJ, Wamsteker EJ, Lee A. Chronic pancreatitis, in BMJ Point-of-Care 2018. 2018 October 26. Available from: www.pointofcare.bmj.com.
180. Freedman SD. Treatment of chronic pancreatitis. In: Whitcomb DC, editor. UpToDate. Waltham, MA: UpToDate Inc. https://www.uptodate.com. Accessed 2 Feb 2018.
181. Owyang C, DiMagno MJ. Chronic pancreatitis. In: Yamada T, editor. Textbook of gastroenterology. Philadelphia: Lippincott Williams and Wilkins; 2009. p. 1811–52.
182. Bornman PC, Botha J, Ramos J, Smith M, Van der Merwe S, Watermeyer G, et al. Guideline for the diagnosis and treatment of chronic pancreatitis. S Afr Med J. 2010;100(12):845–60.
183. Frulloni L, Falconi M, Gabbrielli A, Gaia E, Graziani R, Pezzilli R, et al. Italian consensus guidelines for chronic pancreatitis. Dig Liver Dis. 2010;42:S381–406.
184. De-Madaria E, Abad-González A, Aparicio J, Aparisi L, Boadas J, Boix E, et al. The Spanish Pancreatic Club's recommendations for the diagnosis and treatment of chronic pancreatitis: part 2 (treatment). Pancreatology. 2013;13(1):18–28.
185. Domínguez–Muñoz JE. Chronic pancreatitis and persistent steatorrhea: what is the correct dose of enzymes? Clin Gastroenterol Hepatol. 2011;9(7):541–6.
186. Layer P, Keller J. Lipase supplementation therapy: standards, alternatives, and perspectives. Pancreas. 2003;26(1):1–7.
187. Forsmark CE. Management of chronic pancreatitis. Gastroenterology. 2013;144(6):1282–91.
188. Hart PA, Conwell DL. Challenges and updates in the management of exocrine pancreatic insufficiency. Pancreas. 2016;45(1):1–4.
189. Kalser M, Leite C, Warren W, Harper CL, Jacobson J. Fat assimilation after massive distal pancreatectomy. N Engl J Med. 1968;279(11):570–6.
190. Domínguez-Muñoz J, Iglesias-García J, Iglesias-Rey M, Figueiras A, Vilariño-Insua M. Effect of the administration schedule on the therapeutic efficacy of oral pancreatic enzyme supplements in patients with exocrine pancreatic insufficiency: a randomized, three-way crossover study. Aliment Pharmacol Ther. 2005;21(8):993–1000.
191. Baker SS, Borowitz D, Duffy L, Fitzpatrick L, Gyamfi J, Baker RD. Pancreatic enzyme therapy and clinical outcomes in patients with cystic fibrosis. J Pediatr. 2005;146(2):189–93.
192. de la Iglesia-Garcia D, Huang W, Szatmary P, Baston-Rey I, Gonzalez-Lopez J, Prada-Ramallal G, et al. Efficacy of pancreatic enzyme replacement therapy in chronic pancreatitis: systematic review and meta-analysis. Gut. 2017;66(8):1354–5.
193. Shafiq N, Rana S, Bhasin D, Pandhi P, Srivastava P, Sehmby SS, et al. Pancreatic enzymes for chronic pancreatitis. The Cochrane Library. 2009.
194. Taylor J, Gardner T, Waljee A, DiMagno M, Schoenfeld P. Systematic review: efficacy and safety of pancreatic enzyme supplements for exocrine pancreatic insufficiency. Aliment Pharmacol Ther. 2010;31(1):57–72.
195. Waljee AK, DiMagno MJ, Wu BU, Schoenfeld PS, Conwell DL. Systematic review: pancreatic enzyme treatment of malabsorption associated with chronic pancreatitis. Aliment Pharmacol Ther. 2009;29(3):235–46.

196. Weber AM, Roy CC. Intraduodenal events in cystic fibrosis. J Pediatr Gastroenterol Nutr. 1984;3(Suppl 1):S113–9.
197. Ferrone M, Raimondo M, Scolapio JS. Pancreatic enzyme pharmacotherapy. Pharmacotherapy. 2007;27(6):910–20.
198. Kraisinger M, Hochhaus G, Stecenko A, Bowser E, Hendeles L. Clinical pharmacology of pancreatic enzymes in patients with cystic fibrosis and in vitro performance of microencapsulated formulations. J Clin Pharmacol. 1994;34(2):158–66.
199. Delchier JC, Vidon N, Saint-Marc Girardin MF, Soule JC, Moulin C, Huchet B, et al. Fate of orally ingested enzymes in pancreatic insufficiency: comparison of two pancreatic enzyme preparations. Aliment Pharmacol Ther. 1991;5(4):365–78.
200. Guarner L, Rodriguez R, Guarner F, Malagelada JR. Fate of oral enzymes in pancreatic insufficiency. Gut. 1993;34(5):708–12.
201. Gelfond D, Ma C, Semler J, Borowitz D. Intestinal pH and gastrointestinal transit profiles in cystic fibrosis patients measured by wireless motility capsule. Dig Dis Sci. 2013;58(8):2275–81.
202. Robinson P, Smith A, Sly P. Duodenal pH in cystic fibrosis and its relationship to fat malabsorption. Dig Dis Sci. 1990;35(10):1299–304.
203. Regan PT, Malagelada JR, DiMagno EP, Go VL. Reduced intraluminal bile acid concentrations and fat maldigestion in pancreatic insufficiency: correction by treatment. Gastroenterology. 1979;77(2):285–9.
204. Zentler-Munro PL, Fine DR, Batten JC, Northfield TC. Effect of cimetidine on enzyme inactivation, bile acid precipitation, and lipid solubilisation in pancreatic steatorrhoea due to cystic fibrosis. Gut. 1985;26(9):892–901.
205. Holtmann G, Kelly DG, Sternby B, DiMagno EP. Survival of human pancreatic enzymes during small bowel transit: effect of nutrients, bile acids, and enzymes. Am J Phys. 1997;273(2 Pt 1):G553–8.
206. Ng SM, Moore HS. Drug therapies for reducing gastric acidity in people with cystic fibrosis. Cochrane Database Syst Rev. 2016;8:CD003424.
207. Saunders JH, Drummond S, Wormsley KG. Inhibition of gastric secretion in treatment of pancreatic insufficiency. Br Med J. 1977;1(6058):418–9.
208. Bruno MJ, Rauws EA, Hoek FJ, Tytgat GN. Comparative effects of adjuvant cimetidine and omeprazole during pancreatic enzyme replacement therapy. Dig Dis Sci. 1994;39(5):988–92.
209. Carroccio A, Pardo F, Montalto G, Iapichino L, Soresi M, Averna MR, et al. Use of famotidine in severe exocrine pancreatic insufficiency with persistent maldigestion on enzymatic replacement therapy. A long-term study in cystic fibrosis. Dig Dis Sci. 1992;37(9):1441–6.
210. Durie PR, Bell L, Linton W, Corey ML, Forstner GG. Effect of cimetidine and sodium bicarbonate on pancreatic replacement therapy in cystic fibrosis. Gut. 1980;21(9):778–86.
211. Heijerman HG, Lamers CB, Bakker W. Omeprazole enhances the efficacy of pancreatin (pancrease) in cystic fibrosis. Ann Intern Med. 1991;114(3):200–1.
212. Proesmans M, De Boeck K. Omeprazole, a proton pump inhibitor, improves residual steatorrhoea in cystic fibrosis patients treated with high dose pancreatic enzymes. Eur J Pediatr. 2003;162(11):760–3.
213. Moayyedi P, Leontiadis GI. The risks of PPI therapy. Nat Rev Gastroenterol Hepatol. 2012;9(3):132.
214. DiMagno MJ, Forsmark CE. Chronic pancreatitis and small intestinal bacterial overgrowth. Pancreatology. 2018;18(4):360–2.
215. Lee A, Baker JR, Wamsteker E, Saad R, DiMagno MJ. Small intestinal bacterial overgrowth is common in chronic pancreatitis (CP) and associates with diabetes, CP severity, low zinc levels and opiate us. Am J Gastroenterol. 2019;114(7):1163–71.
216. FitzSimmons SC, Burkhart GA, Borowitz D, Grand RJ, Hammerstrom T, Durie PR, et al. High-dose pancreatic-enzyme supplements and fibrosing colonopathy in children with cystic fibrosis. N Engl J Med. 1997;336(18):1283–9.
217. Freiman JP, FitzSimmons SC. Colonic strictures in patients with cystic fibrosis: results of a survey of 114 cystic fibrosis care centers in the United States. J Pediatr Gastroenterol Nutr. 1996;22(2):153–6.

218. Smyth RL, van Velzen D, Smyth AR, Lloyd DA, Heaf DP. Strictures of ascending colon in cystic fibrosis and high-strength pancreatic enzymes. Lancet. 1994;343(8889):85–6.

219. Borowitz D, Parad RB, Sharp JK, Sabadosa KA, Robinson KA, Rock MJ, et al. Cystic Fibrosis Foundation practice guidelines for the management of infants with cystic fibrosis transmembrane conductance regulator-related metabolic syndrome during the first two years of life and beyond. J Pediatr. 2009;155(6 Suppl):S106–16.

220. Dodge JA. Pancreatic enzymes and Fibrosing Colonopathy. J Cyst Fibros. 2015;14(1):153.

221. O'Keefe SJ, Cariem AK, Levy M. The exacerbation of pancreatic endocrine dysfunction by potent pancreatic exocrine supplements in patients with chronic pancreatitis. J Clin Gastroenterol. 2001;32(4):319–23.

222. Stapleton FB, Kennedy J, Nousia-Arvanitakis S, Linshaw MA. Hyperuricosuria due to high-dose pancreatic extract therapy in cystic fibrosis. N Engl J Med. 1976;295(5):246–8.

223. Wallace CS, Hall M, Kuhn RJ. Pharmacologic management of cystic fibrosis. Clin Pharm. 1993;12(9):657–74; quiz 700–1.

224. Morrice G Jr, Havener WH, Kapetansky F. Vitamin A intoxication as a cause of pseudotumor cerebri. JAMA. 1960;173:1802–5.

225. Rivas-Crespo MF, Gonzalez Jimenez D, Acuna Quiros MD, Sojo Aguirre A, Heredia Gonzalez S, Diaz Martin JJ, et al. High serum retinol and lung function in young patients with cystic fibrosis. J Pediatr Gastroenterol Nutr. 2013;56(6):657–62.

226. Lancellotti L, D'Orazio C, Mastella G, Mazzi G, Lippi U. Deficiency of vitamins E and A in cystic fibrosis is independent of pancreatic function and current enzyme and vitamin supplementation. Eur J Pediatr. 1996;155(4):281–5.

227. Duggan C, Colin AA, Agil A, Higgins L, Rifai N. Vitamin A status in acute exacerbations of cystic fibrosis. Am J Clin Nutr. 1996;64(4):635–9.

228. de Vries JJ, Chang AB, Bonifant CM, Shevill E, Marchant JM. Vitamin A and beta (beta)-carotene supplementation for cystic fibrosis. Cochrane Database Syst Rev. 2018;8:CD006751.

229. Brei C, Simon A, Krawinkel MB, Naehrlich L. Individualized vitamin A supplementation for patients with cystic fibrosis. Clin Nutr. 2013;32(5):805–10.

230. Okebukola PO, Kansra S, Barrett J. Vitamin E supplementation in people with cystic fibrosis. Cochrane Database Syst Rev. 2017;3:CD009422.

231. Sapiejka E, Krzyzanowska-Jankowska P, Wenska-Chyzy E, Szczepanik M, Walkowiak D, Cofta S, et al. Vitamin E status and its determinants in patients with cystic fibrosis. Adv Med Sci. 2018;63(2):341–6.

232. Woestenenk JW, Broos N, Stellato RK, Arets HG, van der Ent CK, Houwen RH. Vitamin E intake, alpha-tocopherol levels and pulmonary function in children and adolescents with cystic fibrosis. Br J Nutr. 2015;113(7):1096–101.

233. Bines JE, Truby HD, Armstrong DS, Carzino R, Grimwood K. Vitamin A and E deficiency and lung disease in infants with cystic fibrosis. J Paediatr Child Health. 2005;41(12):663–8.

234. Feranchak AP, Sontag MK, Wagener JS, Hammond KB, Accurso FJ, Sokol RJ. Prospective, long-term study of fat-soluble vitamin status in children with cystic fibrosis identified by newborn screen. J Pediatr. 1999;135(5):601–10.

235. Sokol RJ, Reardon MC, Accurso FJ, Stall C, Narkewicz M, Abman SH, et al. Fat-soluble-vitamin status during the first year of life in infants with cystic fibrosis identified by screening of newborns. Am J Clin Nutr. 1989;50(5):1064–71.

236. Huang SH, Schall JI, Zemel BS, Stallings VA. Vitamin E status in children with cystic fibrosis and pancreatic insufficiency. J Pediatr. 2006;148(4):556–9.

237. James DR, Alfaham M, Goodchild MC. Increased susceptibility to peroxide-induced haemolysis with normal vitamin E concentrations in cystic fibrosis. Clin Chim Acta. 1991;204(1–3):279–90.

238. Sokol RJ, Heubi JE, Iannaccone ST, Bove KE, Balistreri WF. Vitamin E deficiency with normal serum vitamin E concentrations in children with chronic cholestasis. N Engl J Med. 1984;310(19):1209–12.

239. Sinaasappel M, Stern M, Littlewood J, Wolfe S, Steinkamp G, Heijerman HG, et al. Nutrition in patients with cystic fibrosis: a European Consensus. J Cyst Fibros. 2002;1(2):51–75.

240. Grey V, Atkinson S, Drury D, Casey L, Ferland G, Gundberg C, et al. Prevalence of low bone mass and deficiencies of vitamins D and K in pediatric patients with cystic fibrosis from 3 Canadian centers. Pediatrics. 2008;122(5):1014–20.
241. Krzyzanowska P, Drzymala-Czyz S, Rohovyk N, Bober L, Moczkco J, Rachel M, et al. Prevalence of vitamin K deficiency and associated factors in non-supplemented cystic fibrosis patients. Arch Argent Pediatr. 2018;116(1):e19–25.
242. Rashid M, Durie P, Andrew M, Kalnins D, Shin J, Corey M, et al. Prevalence of vitamin K deficiency in cystic fibrosis. Am J Clin Nutr. 1999;70(3):378–82.
243. Siwamogsatham O, Dong W, Binongo JN, Chowdhury R, Alvarez JA, Feinman SJ, et al. Relationship between fat-soluble vitamin supplementation and blood concentrations in adolescent and adult patients with cystic fibrosis. Nutr Clin Pract. 2014;29(4):491–7.
244. Conway SP. Vitamin K in cystic fibrosis. J R Soc Med. 2004;97(Suppl 44):48–51.
245. Beker LT, Ahrens RA, Fink RJ, O'Brien ME, Davidson KW, Sokoll LJ, et al. Effect of vitamin K1 supplementation on vitamin K status in cystic fibrosis patients. J Pediatr Gastroenterol Nutr. 1997;24(5):512–7.
246. Jagannath VA, Thaker V, Chang AB, Price AI. Vitamin K supplementation for cystic fibrosis. Cochrane Database Syst Rev. 2017;8:CD008482.
247. van Hoorn JH, Hendriks JJ, Vermeer C, Forget PP. Vitamin K supplementation in cystic fibrosis. Arch Dis Child. 2003;88(11):974–5.
248. Wilson DC, Rashid M, Durie PR, Tsang A, Kalnins D, Andrew M, et al. Treatment of vitamin K deficiency in cystic fibrosis: Effectiveness of a daily fat-soluble vitamin combination. J Pediatr. 2001;138(6):851–5.
249. Ruseckaite R, Pekin N, King S, Carr E, Ahern S, Oldroyd J, et al. Evaluating the impact of 2006 Australasian Clinical Practice Guidelines for nutrition in children with cystic fibrosis in Australia. Respir Med. 2018;142:7–14.
250. Yankaskas JR, Marshall BC, Sufian B, Simon RH, Rodman D. Cystic fibrosis adult care: consensus conference report. Chest. 2004;125(1 Suppl):1s–39s.
251. Chesdachai S, Tangpricha V. Treatment of vitamin D deficiency in cystic fibrosis. J Steroid Biochem Mol Biol. 2016;164:36–9.
252. Rovner AJ, Stallings VA, Schall JI, Leonard MB, Zemel BS. Vitamin D insufficiency in children, adolescents, and young adults with cystic fibrosis despite routine oral supplementation. Am J Clin Nutr. 2007;86(6):1694–9.
253. Siwamogsatham O, Alvarez JA, Tangpricha V. Diagnosis and treatment of endocrine comorbidities in patients with cystic fibrosis. Curr Opin Endocrinol Diabetes Obes. 2014;21(5):422–9.
254. Wolfenden LL, Judd SE, Shah R, Sanyal R, Ziegler TR, Tangpricha V. Vitamin D and bone health in adults with cystic fibrosis. Clin Endocrinol. 2008;69(3):374–81.
255. Fleet JC. The role of vitamin D in the endocrinology controlling calcium homeostasis. Mol Cell Endocrinol. 2017;453:36–45.
256. Aranow C. Vitamin D and the immune system. J Investig Med. 2011;59(6):881–6.
257. Pincikova T, Paquin-Proulx D, Sandberg JK, Flodstrom-Tullberg M, Hjelte L. Vitamin D treatment modulates immune activation in cystic fibrosis. Clin Exp Immunol. 2017;189(3):359–71.
258. Alvarez JA, Ashraf A. Role of vitamin d in insulin secretion and insulin sensitivity for glucose homeostasis. Int J Endocrinol. 2010;2010:351385.
259. Pincikova T, Nilsson K, Moen IE, Fluge G, Hollsing A, Knudsen PK, et al. Vitamin D deficiency as a risk factor for cystic fibrosis-related diabetes in the Scandinavian Cystic Fibrosis Nutritional Study. Diabetologia. 2011;54(12):3007–15.
260. Burdge DR, Nakielna EM, Rabin HR. Photosensitivity associated with ciprofloxacin use in adult patients with cystic fibrosis. Antimicrob Agents Chemother. 1995;39(3):793.
261. Hall WB, Sparks AA, Aris RM. Vitamin d deficiency in cystic fibrosis. Int J Endocrinol. 2010;2010:218691.
262. Lark RK, Lester GE, Ontjes DA, Blackwood AD, Hollis BW, Hensler MM, et al. Diminished and erratic absorption of ergocalciferol in adult cystic fibrosis patients. Am J Clin Nutr. 2001;73(3):602–6.

263. Rogiers V, Crokaert R, Vis HL. Altered phospholipid composition and changed fatty acid pattern of the various phospholipid fractions of red cell membranes of cystic fibrosis children with pancreatic insufficiency. Clin Chim Acta. 1980;105(1):105–15.

264. Tangpricha V, Kelly A, Stephenson A, Maguiness K, Enders J, Robinson KA, et al. An update on the screening, diagnosis, management, and treatment of vitamin D deficiency in individuals with cystic fibrosis: evidence-based recommendations from the Cystic Fibrosis Foundation. J Clin Endocrinol Metab. 2012;97(4):1082–93.

265. 2017 Annual Data Report [Internet]. 2017 [cited January 14th, 2019]. Available from: https://www.cff.org/Research/Researcher-Resources/Patient-Registry/2017-Patient-Registry-Annual-Data-Report.pdf.

266. Lucidi V, Bizzarri C, Alghisi F, Bella S, Russo B, Ubertini G, et al. Bone and body composition analyzed by Dual-energy X-ray Absorptiometry (DXA) in clinical and nutritional evaluation of young patients with cystic fibrosis: a cross-sectional study. BMC Pediatr. 2009;9:61.

267. Buntain HM, Schluter PJ, Bell SC, Greer RM, Wong JCH, Batch J, et al. Controlled longitudinal study of bone mass accrual in children and adolescents with cystic fibrosis. Thorax. 2006;61(2):146–54.

268. Stalvey MS, Havasi V, Tuggle KL, Wang D, Birket S, Rowe SM, et al. Reduced bone length, growth plate thickness, bone content, and IGF-I as a model for poor growth in the CFTR-deficient rat. PLoS One. 2017;12(11):e0188497.

269. Conway SP, Wolfe SP, Brownlee KG, White H, Oldroyd B, Truscott JG, et al. Vitamin K status among children with cystic fibrosis and its relationship to bone mineral density and bone turnover. Pediatrics. 2005;115(5):1325–31.

270. Nicolaidou P, Stavrinadis I, Loukou I, Papadopoulou A, Georgouli H, Douros K, et al. The effect of vitamin K supplementation on biochemical markers of bone formation in children and adolescents with cystic fibrosis. Eur J Pediatr. 2006;165(8):540–5.

271. Pearson DA. Bone health and osteoporosis: the role of vitamin K and potential antagonism by anticoagulants. Nutr Clin Pract. 2007;22(5):517–44.

272. Mascarenhas MR, Mondick J, Barrett JS, Wilson M, Stallings VA, Schall JI. Malabsorption blood test: assessing fat absorption in patients with cystic fibrosis and pancreatic insufficiency. J Clin Pharmacol. 2015;55(8):854–65.

273. Stallings VA, Mondick JT, Schall JI, Barrett JS, Wilson M, Mascarenhas MR. Diagnosing malabsorption with systemic lipid profiling: pharmacokinetics of pentadecanoic acid and triheptadecanoic acid following oral administration in healthy subjects and subjects with cystic fibrosis. Int J Clin Pharmacol Ther. 2013;51(4):263.

274. Wilschanski M, Zielenski J, Markiewicz D, Tsui LC, Corey M, Levison H, et al. Correlation of sweat chloride concentration with classes of the cystic fibrosis transmembrane conductance regulator gene mutations. J Pediatr. 1995;127(5):705–10.

275. Zielenski J, Tsui LC. Cystic fibrosis: genotypic and phenotypic variations. Annu Rev Genet. 1995;29:777–807.

276. Gibbs GE. Secretin tests with bilumen gastroduodenal drainage in infants and children. Pediatrics. 1950;5(6):941–6.

277. Engjom T, Erchinger F, Laerum BN, Tjora E, Aksnes L, Gilja OH, et al. Diagnostic accuracy of a short endoscopic secretin test in patients with cystic fibrosis. Pancreas. 2015;44(8):1266–72.

278. Rick W. Untersuchung zur exokrinen Funktion des Pankreas bei zystischer Pankreasfibrose. Med Welt. 1963;42:2158.

279. Aris RM, Merkel PA, Bachrach LK, Borowitz DS, Boyle MP, Elkin SL, et al. Guide to bone health and disease in cystic fibrosis. J Clin Endocrinol Metab. 2005;90(3):1888–96.

Chapter 14
Hepatobiliary Involvement in Cystic Fibrosis

Anna Bertolini, Frank A. J. A. Bodewes, Mordechai Slae, and Michael Wilschanski

The improved management of respiratory complications and malnutrition in CF over the past decades has led to an increase in median life expectancy, which is now 44 years of age in the USA [1]. With increased life expectancy, the clinical relevance of extrapulmonary complications of CF, such as liver disease, has increased, leading to a new need for preventative, diagnostic, and therapeutic tools.

Definition and Classification

Most patients with CF have evidence of hepatobiliary involvement, although with no clinical consequences for the vast majority. CF patients may present with a variety of hepatobiliary signs, symptoms, and clinical disease patterns, ranging from isolated elevated liver enzymes, biliary disease, steatosis, to fibrosis and cirrhosis (Table 14.1). Although clinically relevant hepatobiliary involvement in CF is frequently gathered under the umbrella term cystic fibrosis liver disease (CFLD), the definition of CFLD is not clearly demarcated. Likewise, there is no definite classification of hepatobiliary involvement in CF. Precise and functional definitions and classifications are important for use in establishing the natural course of the disease, for selecting patients in clinical trials and for use in patient registries.

A. Bertolini
Department of Pediatrics, University Medical Center Groningen, Groningen, The Netherlands

F. A. J. A. Bodewes
Pediatric Gastroenterology, Department of Pediatrics, University Medical Center Groningen, Groningen, The Netherlands

M. Slae · M. Wilschanski (✉)
Pediatric Gastroenterology Unit, Department of Pediatrics, Hadassah Hebrew University Medical Center, Jerusalem, Israel
e-mail: michaelwil@hadassah.org.il

© Springer Nature Switzerland AG 2020
S. D. Davis et al. (eds.), *Cystic Fibrosis*, Respiratory Medicine,
https://doi.org/10.1007/978-3-030-42382-7_14

Table 14.1 Hepatobiliary involvement in CF: classification based on phenotypical presentations

A	Persistent increase in liver enzymes GGT, ALT, and AST

B	Liver parenchyma ultrasound abnormalities
	  Increased echogenicity (associated with steatosis)
	  Inhomogeneous (associated with fibrosis)
	  Nodular deformation (associated with cirrhosis)

C	Portal hypertension (splenomegaly, variceal bleeding)
	  Cirrhotic
	  Non-cirrhotic

D	Cholangiopathies and biliary disease
	  Bile duct stones, gallstones
	  Microgallbladder
	  Bile duct stenosis

E	Malignancies
	  Hepatocellular carcinoma
	  Biliary tract cancer

Table 14.2 2011 "Debray–Colombo" criteria for CFLD diagnosis [2]

CF patients are considered to have developed CFLD if at least two of the following conditions are present:

1. Hepatomegaly (increase in liver span relative to age or liver edge palpable more than 2 cm below the costal margin on the midclavicular line), confirmed by ultrasonography

2. Elevated serum liver enzyme levels, consisting of elevation above the upper normal limits of two of the following: aspartate aminotransferase (AST), alanine aminotransferase (ALT), and y-glutamyltransferase (GGT), on at least three consecutive occasions over 12 months, after excluding other causes of liver disease

3. Ultrasound abnormalities other than hepatomegaly (i.e., increased, heterogeneous echogenicity, nodularity, irregular margins, biliary abnormalities, splenomegaly)
A liver biopsy is indicated in case of diagnostic doubt

The most commonly used definition of CFLD was described by Debray and Colombo [2], in which CFLD diagnosis is based on a combination of the presence of at least two conditions among (1) hepatomegaly; (2) persistent elevation of plasma AST, ALT, and GGT; and (3) abnormalities on liver ultrasound (Table 14.2). This classification has been frequently used to select patient that may be eligible for treatment with ursodeoxycholic acid. Although well-established in clinical practice, the Debray–Colombo criteria for CFLD diagnosis present some shortcomings. Whereas it is unknown whether hepatomegaly reflects clinically relevant liver involvement in CF, elevations in liver enzymes during routine follow-up, in particular the transaminases AST and ALT, are a very frequent observation in CF patients [3]. However, abnormal liver enzyme levels are not demonstrated to universally precede more severe forms of liver involvement in CF, in particular cirrhosis, and may often be due to other causes, such as antibiotics usage [4]. Persistent increases in serum GGT, on the other hand, were found to be a predictor for the development of cirrhosis and portal hypertension [5]. It is not clear whether the heterogeneous phenotypes diagnosed as CFLD by these criteria relate to clinically relevant cirrhosis or portal hypertension.

Another approach to classify hepatobiliary involvement in CF is based on the various phenotypical presentations, as shown in Table 14.1. This classification does not imply any causal relation between the various phenotypes. However, it includes a complete spectrum of currently described clinical presentations, separated based on clinical consequences and severity.

Epidemiology

Within the CF population, CFLD prevalence ranges between 10% and 41% [6–12], and between 4% and 28% of patients are reported to have *severe* CFLD [6, 7, 11–14]. This great variation depends on the population studied and the diagnostic criteria utilized.

The mean age at diagnosis ranges between 10 and 35 years across studies [9–12, 15–18], with most studies reporting disease onset at the end of the first decade of life but the recent recognition that a second wave of CFLD onset may occur later in life, possibly due to distinct pathophysiological mechanisms.

Risk Factors

The most frequently reported risk factors for the development of clinically severe CFLD are male gender [6, 11, 12, 18–20], meconium ileus [6, 8, 11, 12, 17–19], and severe genotype [6, 12, 16, 17, 19, 21–23]. Why only a minority of patients with the same severe (class I, II, and III) CFTR mutations progresses to clinically significant liver disease is unclear. It has been hypothesized that inheritance of non-CF modifier genes, such as polymorphisms in genes that upregulate inflammation, fibrosis, or oxidative stress, confers an increased susceptibility. In a multinational gene modifier study of different candidate genes, the SERPINA 1 Z allele of alpha-1 antitrypsin was found to be strongly associated with severe CFLD [20]. This supports the hypothesis that severe CFLD is a result of a double-hit pathogenesis; however, only a minority of CF patients are carriers. Hitherto undefined environmental factors are also likely to be involved.

Etiology and Pathogenesis

The pathogenesis of liver disease in CF is not yet completely understood. Besides the basic CFTR secretory defect, the multi-organ complexity of CF disease offers numerous factors that could contribute to damage and dysfunction of the hepatobiliary tract. A multifactorial pathophysiology, combined with the role of modifier genes and environmental factors, could explain the heterogeneous epidemiology and spectrum of disease that are observed in this patient population.

In the normal hepatobiliary tract, CFTR is expressed on the apical membrane of cholangiocytes lining both intrahepatic and extrahepatic bile ducts [24], as well as in the gallbladder [25], and is not found in hepatocytes or other types of liver cells. In the bile ducts, CFTR fulfils a role in bile flow. Along with other chloride channels such as anoctamin-1 (ANO-1 or TMEM16A), CFTR exports chloride ions to the lumen to drive the secretion of water and bicarbonate into bile [26]. In addition to regulating epithelial efflux of chloride, bicarbonate, and water, CFTR is also known to regulate sodium absorption, glutathione transport, as well as mucin secretion and maturation, via incompletely understood pathways.

Fibrosis and Cirrhosis

The mechanisms leading to fibrosis and cirrhosis are of major interest, as these lesions represent the most clinically relevant manifestations of CF liver involvement.

The oldest and most widely accepted theory directly blames defective CFTR secretory function in cholangiocytes to result in inspissated bile. As deducible from the functional role of CFTR in biliary epithelia, loss of CFTR is expected to result in less hydrated and less alkalinized bile. These characteristics could also impede proper mucin maturation [27]. The resulting inspissated bile would then reduce bile flow, causing more or less severe ductal cholestasis and exposing cholangiocytes to the cytotoxic effects of bile acids. Inflammation resulting from cytotoxicity would then progress to focal biliary fibrosis mediated by activated stellate cells [28]. Bridging of multiple fibrotic foci could then eventually lead to multilobular cirrhosis and its related complications [29]. Supporting this theory, excessive mucus was found in intrahepatic ducts of some infants with CF, although it was only occasionally associated with periportal changes or cholestasis [30]. Other studies reported that bile inspissation is found infrequently in patients [31, 32] and in mice with CFLD [33]. Furthermore, the highly variable presentation of fibrosis and cirrhosis across patients is not fully elucidated by this theory.

Hepatic stellate cell activation could also arise as a consequence of increased cytotoxicity of bile in CF due to a more hydrophobic composition of biliary bile acids [34, 35], linked or not with inspissation of bile and thus prolonged exposure to hydrophobic bile acids. Studies in CF patients and mice have found that their bile contains a higher proportion of primary, more hydrophobic bile acids [36]. This shift in biliary bile acid composition could stem from the yet unexplained disruption of the enterohepatic circulation of bile acids in CF [37], which could deplete bile of secondary bile acids and stimulate hepatic production of primary bile acids. Deficiency of glutathione and fat-soluble antioxidants in CF could worsen oxidative stress in response to cytotoxicity [38]. However, a study in CF mice found that the development of liver disease was unrelated to the hydrophobicity of bile, which was in fact decreased in this study [39]. A higher biliary bile acid-to-phospholipid ratio was found in CF mice and was proposed to promote cell damage in combination with a more hydrophobic bile [40]; however, these findings were not confirmed in subsequent studies [39, 41].

A series of studies reported that CFTR deficiency in cholangiocytes promotes inflammation in response to gut-derived bacterial endotoxins, suggesting a role of CFTR in the regulation of inflammatory responses resulting in prolonged and more vigorous TLR4 responses [42–44]. Patients with primary sclerosing cholangitis (PSC), a rare liver disease with histological findings similar to CFLD, have an increased probability to carry CFTR polymorphisms [45]. PSC is often accompanied by inflammatory bowel disease (IBD) [46]. Both CF and IBD patients have an intestinal phenotype that features inflammation, dysbiosis, and increased permeability [46, 47], characteristics that increase the likelihood of intermittent translocation of bacterial products from the gut to the liver (portal bacteremia). This gut–liver axis hypothesis in which the CF gut promotes translocation of bacterial by-products to the liver [48] was supported by the increased finding of macroscopic intestinal lesions in CF patients with cirrhosis compared to those without liver disease [49], as well as a different gut microbiota composition among the two groups. Unfortunately, this study was unable to determine causality, as intestinal lesions and altered microbiota could also arise after the development of cirrhosis and portal hypertension. Furthermore, differences in intestinal permeability or calprotectin were not found between patients with cirrhosis and without liver disease [49]. It is however likely that increased portal bacteremia could play a role in the development or progression of CFLD.

Finally, because the development of portal hypertension in CF patients has been frequently observed before the onset of overt cirrhosis [50–52], vascular changes, namely, obliteration of portal vein branches with fibrosis, have been observed and suggested to lead to portal hypertension in this patient population [50, 52–54]. However, such vascular changes were not observed in another study in patients with non-cirrhotic portal hypertension [55].

Steatosis

The pathophysiological mechanisms leading to the increased prevalence of steatosis in CF are still unclear and are likely distinct from those leading to fibrosis and cirrhosis. Whether steatosis in CF progresses to cirrhosis is not clear, and although steatosis in CF, especially when mild, has long been considered a benign condition, the discovery that nonalcoholic steatohepatitis can progress to cirrhosis has led to reconsideration of the risk.

Several pathophysiological mechanisms have been proposed. Deficiencies of essential fatty acids, which are common in CF [56, 57], are associated with hepatic steatosis [58, 59] and were reported to correlate with steatosis in CF patients [60]. However, in one study, essential fatty acids supplementation did not prevent steatosis progression in patients [61], whereas in another, administration of docosahexaenoic acid was observed to reduce periportal inflammation in CF mice; however, no effect on steatosis was reported [62]. It must be noted that CF mice are pancreatic-sufficient and only develop steatosis upon feeding of lipid-rich (liquid) diets. Interestingly, they may be more prone to developing steatosis than wild-type mice upon this diet [63].

This finding may suggest that dietary factors are important in the development of steatosis in CF, as they are for the general population, especially in the light of the high-fat, often unbalanced diet followed by CF patients [64]. An association between overweight in CF and hepato-steatosis has been reported [65]. The prevalence of overweight and obesity in CF are, respectively, 6–15% and 1–8% [66–68].

Other dietary deficiencies suggested to contribute to steatosis in CF are those of carnitine [69], choline [70], and trace elements [19]. Administration of choline did not decrease liver lipid levels in CF [71].

Low-grade chronic systemic inflammation, which is present in CF [72], was suggested to contribute to steatosis in non-CF patients [73]. However, chronic pseudomonas colonization was not associated with hepatic steatosis in a study [65]. Although hepato-steatosis is associated with insulin resistance and type 2 diabetes in the general population [74], no association between steatosis and CF-related diabetes was found [65], likely because the pancreatic component predominates over insulin resistance in CFRD. Dysregulations in bile acid metabolism have been recently implicated in the development of NAFLD [75]; NAFLD patients exhibit a deficiency in fibroblast growth factor 19 (FGF19) [76], which is implicated in lipids homeostasis. Interestingly, reduced serum levels of FGF19 were also found in CF patients [77] and are thought to be linked to intestinal bile acid malabsorption. FGF19 was shown to ameliorate hepato-steatosis and fibrosis in animal models of NAFLD [78]. The role of extrahepatic factors in the development of liver steatosis in CF is supported by the finding that steatosis is common in allograft liver biopsies of liver transplants of CF patients, solely in patients with preexisting steatosis in their explant. Of note, steatohepatitis was also common following liver transplant [79].

Further studies will be needed to elucidate the pathophysiology, as well as the clinical relevance of hepato-steatosis in CF.

Clinical Presentation

CF Liver Involvement with Fibrosis and Cirrhosis

Liver involvement with fibrosis and cirrhosis is the most severe form of CF-related liver involvement. The pathological hepatic feature is focal biliary cirrhosis (Fig. 14.1). There are often no clinical features before the development of portal hypertension. Complications are discussed below.

Non-cirrhotic Portal Hypertension in CF

Recent publications reported that portal hypertension in CF may also develop independently of extensive fibrosis or cirrhosis [50, 54]. These patients had all the classical features of portal hypertension, such as splenomegaly, thrombocytopenia, and

Fig. 14.1 Histology (Masson trichrome staining) of explanted liver of a 12-year-old CF patient transplanted for cirrhosis-related hepatopulmonary syndrome, clearly demonstrating biliary nodular cirrhotic pattern

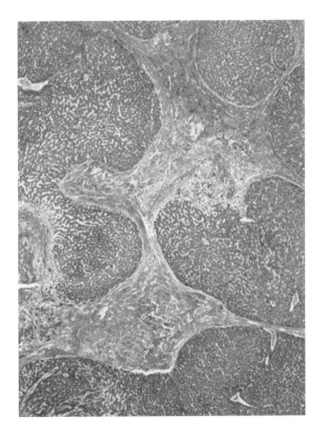

esophageal varices. This form of non-cirrhotic portal hypertension [80] has been defined as a disease of uncertain etiology characterized by periportal fibrosis and involvement of small and medium branches of the portal vein, resulting in the development of portal hypertension.

Biliary Tract Disease

There have been numerous reports of a variety of intrahepatic and extrahepatic abnormalities of the biliary tree in CF, although the incidence of these findings is controversial. These findings include irregularities and tapering of the small intrahepatic ducts, as well as stricturing, beading, and segmental dilation of the larger extrahepatic ducts, similar to primary sclerosing cholangitis [81]. There is also an increased risk of biliary tract cancer in CF, also before transplantation. The risk increased even more after solid-organ transplantation and the consequent need for immunosuppressive therapy. Based on these findings, it was recommended to screen CF patients over 40 years old for biliary tract cancer using abdominal ultrasound, magnetic resonance cholangiopancreatography, or endoscopic ultrasonography [82].

Cholestasis develops rarely in CF infants and may be the presenting feature, often together with meconium ileus [83]. Gallbladder abnormalities have been frequently reported and include either microgallbladders or distended gallbladders featuring defective function and requiring no treatment. Of clinical relevance, an increased incidence of gallbladder and intrahepatic stones was reported [21].

Diagnosis and Follow-Up

Diagnosis

The evidence of liver disease in CF is often subclinical until complications develop.

When clinical signs are present, physical examination is directed at the detection of hepato- and splenomegaly and other signs of chronic liver disease. Serum biomarkers are useful in detecting complications; for instance, persistent thrombocytopenia in combination with splenomegaly suggests portal hypertension. However, as elevated serum liver enzymes in CF patients are common, nonspecific, and may reflect different underlying etiologies, as discussed above, routine biochemistry is generally not helpful in reliably identifying patients with multilobular cirrhosis or in predicting the development of end-stage liver disease [2, 51]. Persistently elevated GGT predicted cirrhosis [5], and portal hypertension was predicted accurately by various indexes that combine demographic values with plasma biomarkers such as Hepascore, AST to Platelet Ratio Index (APRI), and Forns index (Forns index combines age, GGT, cholesterol, and platelet count), although cutoff scores are variable and more studies are needed for validation (reviewed in [84]).

The major challenge in the diagnosis of liver involvement in CF is distinguishing patients who will progress to clinically relevant complications such as cirrhosis and portal hypertension. Since this is not clear, although practice varies among institutions, international guidelines recommend screening every CF patient every year with a hepatobiliary ultrasound [1], including Doppler measurements of flow in the portal vein. However, the positive predictive value of a normal scan and sensitivity is low [85]. The gold standard for diagnosing fibrosis and cirrhosis in CF is liver biopsy, including two biopsies rather than one large biopsy [51] to circumvent the focal nature of disease. Because liver biopsy is an invasive procedure with inherent risks, numerous studies are being performed to identify noninvasive methods to detect early CF liver involvement which may clinically progress. MRI is valuable [86], but costs are a concern, and it is reserved, as CT, in cases of diagnostic doubt. Since the degree of histological liver fibrosis can predict the development of portal hypertension [51], noninvasive tests such as transient elastography (TE, Fibroscan[R]) and acoustic radiation force impulse (ARFI), both of which measure liver stiffness as a surrogate measure for fibrosis, are being studied in CF patients. Although these tests had low sensitivities in detecting earlier liver changes, they seem fairly accurate in detecting portal hypertension and cirrhosis [84] and may become implemented in the screening and follow-up of CF liver involvement, once cutoff values are defined and likely in combination with other tests. MRI, scintigraphy of the hepatobiliary tract, and magnetic resonance cholangiography are useful for visualizing bile duct and gallbladder disease. Because the clinical relevance of biliary tract abnormalities in CF is unclear, these tests do not find a place in the annual screening, which instead usually include clinical examination, abdominal ultrasound, and serum biochemistry.

Differential Diagnosis of Liver Involvement in CF

In CF patients that present with signs of liver involvement, e.g., persistent elevation of liver enzymes, it is imperative to consider a general differential diagnosis including, e.g., hepatitis (viral or autoimmune), alpha-1 antitrypsin deficiency, celiac disease, and Wilson disease. In the case of steatosis, other causes of steatosis like malnutrition and diabetes mellitus need to be considered. Interestingly, a subgroup of patients with primary sclerosing cholangitis may have electrophysiological and genetic similarities with CF patients [45]. In the work of liver involvement, liver biopsy may have to be considered to diagnose or exclude other cause of liver disease besides CF.

Follow-Up

It is useful to follow-up patients with early, subclinical liver involvement annually to screen for development of cirrhosis and/or portal hypertension. Patients with cirrhosis and/or portal hypertension are followed up to assess treatment efficacy and to prevent complications such as variceal bleeding (Table 14.3). In these patients, screening for hepatocellular carcinoma is recommended with ultrasound and plasma alpha-fetoprotein levels [2].

Management: Prevention and Treatment

UDCA

Debray et al. [2] recommended that treatment with the bile acid ursodeoxycholic acid (UDCA) should be initiated at the time of CFLD diagnosis (according to the Debray–Colombo criteria, Table 14.1) at a daily dose of 20 mg/kg/day to delay

Table 14.3 Complications of CF liver involvement with cirrhosis

Complications of portal hypertension
GI tract variceal bleeding
Ascites
Spontaneous bacterial peritonitis (SPB)
Hepatopulmonary syndrome (HPS)
Porto-pulmonary hypertension (PPH)
Signs and symptoms of functional liver decompensation
Hepatic protein synthesis defects (e.g., hypoalbuminemia)
Vitamin K-independent coagulopathy
Liver detoxification defects
Jaundice
Hypoglycemia
Hepatocellular carcinoma

progression. UDCA aims to induce a bicarbonate-rich bile that flows more easily, as well as to reduce the hydrophobicity of the bile acid pool [87]. However, a Cochrane review revealed that there is insufficient evidence to support the use of UDCA in CF [88]. UDCA treatment was associated with slight improvements in serum liver enzymes in the short term [89–93]. Moreover, long-term studies suggested benefits of UDCA on CFLD progression as assessed by ultrasonography; unfortunately, a control group was missing [94, 95]. Long-term controlled trials showing effectiveness of UDCA in delaying CFLD progression, preventing cirrhosis, liver transplantation, or death, are lacking. Furthermore, UDCA treatment and in particular the recommended dose have been questioned after a trial of high-dose UDCA in primary sclerosing cholangitis was terminated due to increased risk of severe side effects [96]. These limitations of UDCA therapy in CFLD have highlighted the need of novel preventative and therapeutic options.

CFTR Modulators

The emergence of novel targeted agents that directly modulate CFTR folding or function has led to new treatment opportunities for patients with class II (misfolded protein) and class III (reduced protein function) mutations. Bicarbonate secretion, intestinal inflammation, as well as other factors that may be contributing to CFLD may be, at least partially, improved by CFTR modulators. It should be possible to reliably follow their effect on liver fibrosis by transient elastography. These studies are still lacking but are expected to be included in further clinical trials. Ivacaftor treatment was reported to reverse hepatic steatosis, a liver complication frequently seen in CF patients, in one patient [97]. On the other hand, there have been reports of raised liver enzymes in some trials, but no detrimental clinical effect [98]. Monitoring of liver function upon CFTR modulators is warranted, especially in patients with raised liver enzymes.

Other Targets

A number of investigational avenues targeting different pathophysiological aspects of liver disease are being explored:

1. Bile acid analogues: norUDCA (a side chain-shortened homologue of UDCA with one less methylene group) undergoes cholehepatic shunting leading to a bicarbonate-rich hyperchloresis. This drug has direct anti-inflammatory, antifibrotic, and antiproliferative properties and stimulates alternative bile acid detoxification and elimination routes. It has shown encouraging effects improving serum liver tests in primary sclerosing cholangitis, an immune-mediated liver disease with biliary morphological similarities to CFLD [99], although it did not decrease biliary injury in a CF mouse model with liver pathology prompted by inducing colitis [43].
2. Farnesoid X receptor (FXR) agonists: activation of FXR, a nuclear receptor, suppresses bile acid synthesis via fibroblast growth factor 19 (FGF19), stimulates bile acid and bicarbonate secretion, modulates fibrosis, and regulates lipid and glucose metabolism [100].
3. Fibroblast growth factor 1 (FGF1) is a peroxisome proliferator-activated receptor gamma (PPARγ) target in visceral adipose tissue and is critical to adipose remodeling [101]. FGF1 improved hepatic inflammation, steatosis, and damage in leptin-deficient ob/ob and choline-deficient mice, two etiologically different NAFLD models [102].
4. Vitamin D receptors also offer potential for treatment intervention with their activation implicated in preventing hepatic fibrosis involving transforming growth factor beta 1 (TGFβ1) signaling via pro-fibrotic genes [103].

Moreover, supplementation of docosahexaenoic acid and stimulation of peroxisome proliferator-activated receptor, as well as Src inhibition, have been used with success in a mouse model of CF, where they reduced bile duct injury [44, 104, 105]. However, these treatments are in an early experimental stage, and, besides effectiveness in patients, their safety is to be explored.

Treatment of Complications of Cirrhosis

The management of GI varices in CF is according to general guidelines [106]. However, prophylactic treatment of variceal bleeding with nonselective beta blockers may be contraindicated in CF due to pulmonary side effects. The treatment of choice for bleeding varices is injection sclerotherapy or band ligation. Both transjugular intrahepatic portosystemic shunt (TIPS) and surgical portosystemic shunts are used in CF patients to relieve, endoscopic uncontrollable, GI bleeding due to portal hypertension. However, these procedures may present with a high rate of complication due to shunt obstruction and hepatic encephalopathy. Therefore it is advisable that, in this specific complicated clinical scenario, liver transplantation is also considered as a treatment option [107].

Liver Transplantation

End-stage liver disease in CF or otherwise not treatable life-threatening complications of liver disease (e.g., hepatopulmonary syndrome) in CF is an accepted indication for liver transplantation. However, CF is an exceptional indication for liver transplantation, as it is a multi-organ disease including, lung, pancreas, and gut complications. Disease presentation in these organs will not be cured by a single organ liver transplantation. The latter may be the reason why liver transplantation in cystic fibrosis is associated with poorer long-term patient survival compared to non-cystic fibrosis patients [108]. The need for immunosuppression following liver transplantation, which increases the risk for pulmonary infections, should also be taken into consideration while considering and planning liver transplantation.

Outcomes

Liver involvement in CF is regarded as relatively benign, with low prevalence of complications and progression [10, 14, 109], although it accounts for 2.1% of the mortality of CF patients in Europe, representing the third CF-related leading cause of death, and 3.4% in North America [1, 7]. Furthermore, CFLD is an independent risk factor for mortality [8, 110].

The most clinically prominent features and complications of CF liver disease with portal hypertension are related to severe portal hypertension (Table 14.3). The splenomegaly can be striking and may cause mechanical and abdominal complaints. The secondary thrombocytopenia may be associated with bleeding and epistaxis. CF patients with portal hypertension are at risk for variceal bleeding in the gastrointestinal tract. A recent report based on the US CF Foundation Patient Registry found that variceal bleeding episodes occur in ~6% of CF patients with cirrhosis, although without increasing mortality [111]. Moreover, there have been reports of hepatopulmonary syndrome [112].

Comparable to cirrhotic disease in other patient populations, CF patient with cirrhosis may develop hepatocellular carcinoma [113–115]. Accordingly, CF patient with cirrhosis should be screened for hepatocellular carcinoma by periodical liver ultrasound and alpha-fetoprotein testing.

Although CF patients with cirrhosis seldom develop end-stage liver disease [109], adverse liver outcomes are frequent after cirrhosis has been diagnosed in CF patients [111]. Additionally, CF patients with cirrhosis reportedly have a poorer survival [116].

Whether lung function is influenced by CFLD is a matter of debate, with studies reporting worsened [6, 109, 117, 118], unchanged [19, 22, 119], and even improved [120, 121] lung function. Severe CF-related diabetes (CFRD) was reported to occur more frequently in CFLD patients than in the general CF population [109]. CFLD did not seem associated with bone mineralization abnormalities in a study [117].

Research Tools and Directions

Clinical Studies

There are currently no therapeutic clinical trials directly targeting liver disease in CF. When considering clinical trials for CFLD, there are two potential directions.

First, the effects of the relatively new CFTR protein modulators on CFLD progression could be studied. In the currently performed trials for, e.g., ivacaftor, ivacaftor/lumacaftor, or tezacaftor–ivacaftor combination therapies, CFLD patients, in particular those with cirrhosis/or portal hypertension, were excluded. Furthermore, liver function was not reported as an outcome parameter. On the other hand, liver enzymes are monitored in clinical trials to evaluate liver toxicity and adverse events. It would be of great clinical and scientific interest to include CFLD-related outcome measures in future clinical trials with CFTR protein modulators, such as elastography and liver function tests including AST, ALT, alkaline phosphatase, bilirubin, and GTT, to gather information on whether these drugs are able to prevent the evolution to liver fibrosis or to reverse disease if present. In case patients with liver cirrhosis are included, markers of liver protein synthesis (e.g., albumin, clotting factors) or liver detoxification (total bilirubin, ammonia) as biomarkers of liver function could be added. Additionally, new outcome measures for liver function are currently evaluated. For example, in a recent study, it was demonstrated that the change in 7α-hydroxy-4-cholesten-3-one (C4), which is used as a surrogate marker for BA synthesis, can be used to monitor the effect of CFTR modulation on hepatic bile acid synthesis in CF [77, 122].

A second direction for clinical trials in CFLD may include new antifibrotic agents or novel therapies that target bile acid receptors and metabolism to improve liver disease. Clinical trials for these new drugs are currently performed in non-CF-related liver disease, including primary sclerosing cholangitis, primary biliary cholangitis, viral hepatitis, and NASH. If proven successful or effective, these new treatment options could also be considered for CFLD patients.

An international agreement on the definition, classification, and diagnostic criteria of CF liver involvement and CFLD is urgently needed to consistently select patients for clinical trials and for use in patient registries.

Animal Models

Since 1992, a great number of animal models of CF have been created utilizing small animals such as the mouse, rat, ferret, and rabbit, as well as large animals such as the pig and the sheep. In each animal model, the most prominent manifestation of disease is a severe intestinal phenotype characterized by meconium ileus and/or postweaning intestinal obstruction. The extent and nature of liver disease vary across animal models, being milder in small and severer in large animal models.

Several mouse models of CF are available, on different genetic backgrounds, which cover CFTR defects class I (including various knockouts with none or residual CFTR function and a conditional knockout), class II (including models carrying the F508del or G480C mutation), class III (G551D mutation), and class IV (R117H mutation) (reviewed in [123, 124]). The intestinal phenotype is particularly severe in *Cftr*-null strains, which show high rates of intestinal obstruction at weaning. CF mice do not usually develop spontaneous pulmonary nor pancreatic disease, although reports of these conditions in *Cftr*-null mice exist [33]. Reports of absent liver pathology in the various CF mouse models predominate. However, 20% of *Cftr*^{G551D} mice show hyperplasia of the bile duct epithelium [125]. *Cftr*-null mice were reported to have focal biliary and even lobular cirrhosis [33, 39], and about half of aged *Cftr*^{F508del} mice exhibited mild patchy cholangiopathy in a study [40]. Induction of colitis in *Cftr*-null mice leads to more severe bile duct injury compared with wild-type mice [126]. The liver phenotype of CF mice may to some extent depend on environmental factors, such as the diet administered. CF mouse strains at high risk for intestinal obstruction have been maintained on either a liquid diet or chow with added polyethylene glycol in drinking water. The development of steatosis was observed in CF mice to a greater extent than wild types upon liquid diet [33, 63] and an 11% fat diet [40], as that of cholangiopathy [127]. The gallbladder was reported to be enlarged and sometimes filled with black bile in some strains [125, 128, 129].

In a CF rat model, about 70% of *Cftr*-null rats developed intestinal obstruction around weaning, but no histological liver abnormalities were noted [130].

Besides CF mice and rats, a *Cftr*-null ferret was created by Sun et al. [131] to take advantage of fast breeding and more similar lung physiology of the ferret to humans. The *Cftr*-null kits displayed a severe intestinal phenotype, as about 75% developed meconium ileus, as well as pancreatic disease and failure to thrive. Despite no evidence for other hepatic histological changes indicating cholestasis or focal biliary cirrhosis, *Cftr*-null kits with or without MI had increased plasma levels of alanine aminotransferase (ALT) and direct and indirect bilirubin, similar to human CF infants [60], which improved upon treatment with ursodeoxycholic acid (UDCA) in combination with an osmotic laxative and antibiotics. This treatment regimen did not improve the nutritional status, which was instead improved by proton pump inhibitor treatment in combination with a liquid elemental diet and pancreatic enzyme replacement. The authors additionally attempted to improve the intestinal phenotype by expressing the human CFTR in the intestine only. Only one such transgenic kit with the highest CFTR protein expression did not develop MI and survived. Liver function tests were not reported for the gut-corrected kits.

In addition to the *Cftr*-null ferret model, Sun et al. also created *Cftr*-null rabbits and are currently developing rabbits with the F508del mutation. The intestinal and liver phenotype of CF rabbits has not been characterized yet.

Both the *Cftr*-null [132] and F508del [133] pig models have meconium ileus with 100% penetrance and develop pancreatic insufficiency. The liver showed infrequent histological changes consistent with early focal biliary cirrhosis. As in some patient studies [21, 134], the piglets displayed a microgallbladder, which was often filled with congealed bile, as were the bile ducts. Uc et al. reported that the baseline bile volume was unchanged in newborn *Cftr*-null piglets; however, upon stimulation with secretin, CF pigs failed to increase bile secretion. Bile was thick and contained more proteins, and the pH was somewhat lower in CF piglets than in wild types [135]. Transgenic expression of porcine CFTR restricted to the intestine alleviated meconium ileus, but did not ameliorate the liver and gallbladder phenotype [136, 137]. By relieving meconium ileus with an ileostomy or cecostomy, the pigs aged to develop hepatic steatosis [133] and lung disease [138] by 2–3 months of age.

Like the CF pig, recently created *Cftr*-null sheep showed 100% penetrance of meconium ileus. The liver phenotype was severe, although distinct form other animal models. Most lambs had (neonatal) intrahepatic cholestasis, which is rare in humans [139], with biliary and periportal fibrosis, and excessive hepatic glycogen accumulation. The gallbladder was hypoplastic and often empty.

Animal models of CF have been valuable in understanding the role of CFTR in cholangiocytes. Moreover, they have permitted the study of changes in biliary physiology in CF and the dysregulated response to inflammation of CF cholangiocytes. However, an animal model that reliably mirrors human CFLD is still lacking.

Summary

Due to the improved management of nutritional and pulmonary issues and increased life expectancy, the relevance and prevalence of liver disease in CF have increased. About one-third of CF patients have evidence of liver involvement, although only a minority develops complications, which are mostly related to portal hypertension. Definite diagnostic criteria that are linked to clinical outcomes are lacking. Because pathophysiological understanding is incomplete, effective treatment is not yet available. Although treatment commencement with ursodeoxycholic acid at diagnosis is recommended, its efficacy is not proven. The management of complications of portal hypertension and liver function failure are generally similar to non-CF patients. Scientific efforts are needed to elucidate the etiology and pathogenesis and to establish safe and effective prevention and treatment.

References

1. Cystic Fibrosis Foundation. 2017 patient registry: annual data report. Bethesda. 2018.
2. Debray D, Kelly D, Houwen R, Strandvik B, Colombo C. Best practice guidance for the diagnosis and management of cystic fibrosis-associated liver disease. J Cyst Fibros. 2011;10:S29–36.
3. Woodruff SA, Sontag MK, Accurso FJ, Sokol RJ, Narkewicz MR. Prevalence of elevated liver enzymes in children with cystic fibrosis diagnosed by newborn screen. J Cyst Fibros. 2017;16:139–45.
4. Jong T, Geake J, Yerkovich S, Bell SC. Idiosyncratic reactions are the most common cause of abnormal liver function tests in patients with cystic fibrosis. Intern Med J. 2015;45:395–401.
5. Bodewes FAJA, van der Doef HPJ, Houwen RHJ, Verkade HJ. Increase of serum gamma glutamyltransferase (GGT) associated with the development of cirrhotic cystic fibrosis liver disease. J Pediatr Gastroenterol Nutr. 2015;61:113–8.
6. Boëlle P-Y, Debray D, Guillot L, Clement A, Corvol H. Cystic fibrosis liver disease: outcomes and risk factors in a large cohort of French patients. Hepatology. 2019;69(4):1648–56.
7. European Cystic Fibrosis Society. ECFS patient registry annual data report. Karup. 2016.
8. Chryssostalis A, Hubert D, Coste J, Kanaan R, Burgel PR, Desmazes-Dufeu N, Soubrane O, Dusser D, Sogni P. Liver disease in adult patients with cystic fibrosis: a frequent and independent prognostic factor associated with death or lung transplantation. J Hepatol. 2011;55:1377–82.
9. Bhardwaj S, Canlas K, Kahi C, Temkit M, Molleston J, Ober M, Howenstine M, Kwo PY. Hepatobiliary abnormalities and disease in cystic fibrosis. J Clin Gastroenterol. 2009;43:858–64.
10. Desmond CP, Wilson J, Bailey M, Clark D, Roberts SK. The benign course of liver disease in adults with cystic fibrosis and the effect of ursodeoxycholic acid. Liver Int. 2007;27:1402–8.
11. Lamireau T, Monnereau S, Martin S, Marcotte J-E, Winnock M, Alvarez F. Epidemiology of liver disease in cystic fibrosis: a longitudinal study. J Hepatol. 2004;41:920–5.
12. Efrati O, Barak A, Modan-Moses D, Augarten A, Vilozni D, Katznelson D, Szeinberg A, Yahav J, Bujanover Y. Liver cirrhosis and portal hypertension in cystic fibrosis. Eur J Gastroenterol Hepatol. 2003;15:1073–8.
13. Parkins MD, Parkins VM, Rendall JC, Elborn S. Changing epidemiology and clinical issues arising in an ageing cystic fibrosis population. Ther Adv Respir Dis. 2011;5:105–19.
14. Nash KL, Allison ME, McKeon D, Lomas DJ, Haworth CS, Bilton D, Alexander GJM. A single centre experience of liver disease in adults with cystic fibrosis 1995–2006. J Cyst Fibros. 2008;7:252–7.
15. Koh C, Sakiani S, Surana P, et al. Adult-onset cystic fibrosis liver disease: diagnosis and characterization of an underappreciated entity. Hepatology. 2017;66:591–601.
16. Stonebraker JR, Ooi CY, Pace RG, Corvol H, Knowles MR, Durie PR, Ling SC. Features of severe liver disease with portal hypertension in patients with cystic fibrosis. Clin Gastroenterol Hepatol. 2016;14:1207–1215.e3.
17. Ciucă IM, Pop L, Tămaş L, Tăban S. Cystic fibrosis liver disease - from diagnosis to risk factors. Romanian J Morphol Embryol. 2014;55:91–5.
18. Colombo C, Apostolo MG, Ferrari M, Seia M, Genoni S, Giunta A, Piceni Sereni L. Analysis of risk factors for the development of liver disease associated with cystic fibrosis. J Pediatr. 1994;124:393–9.
19. Colombo C, Battezzati PM, Crosignani A, Morabito A, Costantini D, Padoan R, Giunta A. Liver disease in cystic fibrosis: a prospective study on incidence, risk factors, and outcome. Hepatology. 2002;36:1374–82.
20. Bartlett JR. Genetic modifiers of liver disease in cystic fibrosis. JAMA. 2009;302:1076–83.
21. Flass T, Narkewicz MR. Cirrhosis and other liver disease in cystic fibrosis. J Cyst Fibros. 2013;12:116–24.

22. Wilschanski M, Rivlin J, Cohen S, et al. Clinical and genetic risk factors for cystic fibrosis-related liver disease. Pediatrics. 1999;103:52–7.
23. Slieker MG, Deckers-Kocken JM, Uiterwaal CSPM, van der Ent CK, Houwen RHJ. Risk factors for the development of cystic fibrosis related liver disease. Hepatology. 2003;38: 775–6.
24. Cohn JA, Strong TV, Picciotto MR, Nairn AC, Collins FS, Fitz JG. Localization of the cystic fibrosis transmembrane conductance regulator in human bile duct epithelial cells. Gastroenterology. 1993;105:1857–64.
25. Strong TV, Boehm K, Collins FS. Localization of cystic fibrosis transmembrane conductance regulator mRNA in the human gastrointestinal tract by in situ hybridization. J Clin Invest. 1994;93:347–54.
26. Concepcion AR, Lopez M, Ardura-Fabregat A, Medina JF. Role of AE2 for pHi regulation in biliary epithelial cells. Front Physiol. 2014;4:1–7.
27. Yang N, Garcia MAS, Quinton PM. Normal mucus formation requires cAMP-dependent HCO3- secretion and Ca2+-mediated mucin exocytosis. J Physiol. 2013;591:4581–93.
28. Lewindon PJ, Pereira TN, Hoskins AC, Bridle KR, Williamson RM, Shepherd RW, Ramm GA. The role of hepatic stellate cells and transforming growth factor-beta(1) in cystic fibrosis liver disease. Am J Pathol. 2002;160:1705–15.
29. Feranchak AP, Sokol RJ. Cholangiocyte biology and cystic fibrosis liver disease. Semin Liver Dis. 2001;21:471–88.
30. Oppenheimer EH, Esterly JR. Hepatic changes in young infants with cystic fibrosis: possible relation to focal biliary cirrhosis. J Pediatr. 1975;86:683–9.
31. Potter CJ, Fishbein M, Hammond S, McCoy K, Qualman S. Can the histologic changes of cystic fibrosis-associated hepatobiliary disease be predicted by clinical criteria ? J Pediatr Gastroenterol Nutr. 1997;25:32–6.
32. Lindblad A, Hultcrantz R, Strandvik B. Bile-duct destruction and collagen deposition: a prominent ultrastructural feature of the liver in cystic fibrosis. Hepatology. 1992;16:372–81.
33. Durie PR, Kent G, Phillips MJ, Ackerley CA. Characteristic multiorgan pathology of cystic fibrosis in a long-living cystic fibrosis transmembrane regulator knockout murine model. Am J Pathol. 2004;164:1481–93.
34. Ramm GA, Shepherd RW, Hoskins AC, et al. Fibrogenesis in pediatric cholestatic liver disease: role of taurocholate and hepatocyte-derived monocyte chemotaxis protein-1 in hepatic stellate cell recruitment. Hepatology. 2009;49:533–44.
35. Pozniak KN, Pearen MA, Pereira TN, et al. Taurocholate induces biliary differentiation of liver progenitor cells causing hepatic stellate cell chemotaxis in the ductular reaction: role in pediatric cystic fibrosis liver disease. Am J Pathol. 2017;187:2744–57.
36. Strandvik B, Einarsson K, Lindblad A, Angelin B. Bile acid kinetics and biliary lipid composition in cystic fibrosis. J Hepatol. 1996;25:43–8.
37. O'Brien S, Mulcahy H, Fenlon H, O'Broin A, Casey M, Burke A, FitzGerald MX, Hegarty JE. Intestinal bile acid malabsorption in cystic fibrosis. Gut. 1993;34:1137–41.
38. Galli F, Battistoni A, Gambari R, Pompella A, Bragonzi A, Pilolli F, Iuliano L, Piroddi M, Dechecchi MC, Cabrini G. Oxidative stress and antioxidant therapy in cystic fibrosis. Biochim Biophys Acta Mol basis Dis. 2012;1822:690–713.
39. Bodewes FAJA, van der Wulp MYM, Beharry S, Doktorova M, Havinga R, Boverhof R, James Phillips M, Durie PRR, Verkade HJJ. Altered intestinal bile salt biotransformation in a cystic fibrosis (Cftr-/-) mouse model with hepato-biliary pathology. J Cyst Fibros. 2015;14:440–6.
40. Freudenberg F, Broderick AL, Yu BB, Leonard MR, Glickman JN, Carey MC. Pathophysiological basis of liver disease in cystic fibrosis employing a DeltaF508 mouse model. Am J Physiol Gastrointest Liver Physiol. 2008;294:G1411–20.
41. Bodewes FAJAJA, Bijvelds MJ, De Vries W, Baller JFWW, Gouw ASHH, De Jonge HR, Verkade HJ. Cholic acid induces a Cftr dependent biliary secretion and liver growth response in mice. PLoS One. 2015;10:1–14.

42. Bruscia EM, Zhang P-X, Satoh A, Caputo C, Medzhitov R, Shenoy A, Egan ME, Krause DS. Abnormal trafficking and degradation of TLR4 underlie the elevated inflammatory response in cystic fibrosis. J Immunol. 2011;186:6990–8.

43. Fiorotto R, Scirpo R, Trauner M, Fabris L, Hoque R, Spirli C, Strazzabosco M. Loss of CFTR affects biliary epithelium innate immunity and causes TLR4NF-κB-mediated inflammatory response in mice. Gastroenterology. 2011;141:1498–1508.e5.

44. Fiorotto R, Villani A, Kourtidis A, Scirpo R, Amenduni M, Geibel PJ, Cadamuro M, Spirli C, Anastasiadis PZ, Strazzabosco M. The cystic fibrosis transmembrane conductance regulator controls biliary epithelial inflammation and permeability by regulating Src tyrosine kinase activity. Hepatology. 2016;64:2118–34.

45. Werlin S, Scotet V, Uguen K, et al. Primary sclerosing cholangitis is associated with abnormalities in CFTR. J Cyst Fibros. 2018;17:666–71.

46. Karlsen TH, Folseraas T, Thorburn D, Vesterhus M. Primary sclerosing cholangitis – a comprehensive review. J Hepatol. 2017;67:1298–323.

47. De Lisle RC, Borowitz D. The cystic fibrosis intestine. Cold Spring Harb Perspect Med. 2013;3:1–17.

48. Fiorotto R, Strazzabosco M. Cystic fibrosis-related liver diseases: new paradigm for treatment based on pathophysiology. Clin Liver Dis. 2016;8:113–6.

49. Flass T, Tong S, Frank DN, et al. Intestinal lesions are associated with altered intestinal microbiome and are more frequent in children and young adults with cystic fibrosis and cirrhosis. PLoS One. 2015;10:e0116967.

50. Witters P, Libbrecht L, Roskams T, et al. Liver disease in cystic fibrosis presents as noncirrhotic portal hypertension. J Cyst Fibros. 2017;16:e11–3.

51. Lewindon PJ, Shepherd RW, Walsh MJ, Greer RM, Williamson R, Pereira TN, Frawley K, Bell SC, Smith JL, Ramm GA. Importance of hepatic fibrosis in cystic fibrosis and the predictive value of liver biopsy. Hepatology. 2011;53:193–201.

52. Witters P, Libbrecht L, Roskams T, et al. Noncirrhotic presinusoidal portal hypertension is common in cystic fibrosis-associated liver disease. Hepatology. 2011;53:1064–5.

53. Wu H, Vu M, Dhingra S, Ackah R, Goss JA, Rana A, Quintanilla N, Patel K, Leung DH. Obliterative portal venopathy without cirrhosis is prevalent in pediatric cystic fibrosis liver disease with portal hypertension. Clin Gastroenterol Hepatol. 2019;17(10):2134–6.

54. Hillaire S, Cazals-Hatem D, Bruno O, et al. Liver transplantation in adult cystic fibrosis: clinical, imaging, and pathological evidence of obliterative portal venopathy. Liver Transpl. 2017;23:1342–7.

55. Lewindon PJ, Ramm GA. Cystic fibrosis-cirrhosis, portal hypertension, and liver biopsy: reply. Hepatology. 2011;53:1065–6.

56. Witters P, Dupont L, Vermeulen F, Proesmans M, Cassiman D, Wallemacq P, De Boeck K. Lung transplantation in cystic fibrosis normalizes essential fatty acid profiles. J Cyst Fibros. 2013;12:222–8.

57. Lloyd-Still JD. Essential fatty acid deficiency and nutritional supplementation in cystic fibrosis. J Pediatr. 2002;141:157–9.

58. Werner A. Essential fatty acid deficiency in mice is associated with hepatic steatosis and secretion of large VLDL particles. Am J Physiol Gastrointest Liver Physiol. 2005;288:G1150–8.

59. Ducheix S, Montagner A, Polizzi A, et al. Essential fatty acids deficiency promotes lipogenic gene expression and hepatic steatosis through the liver X receptor. J Hepatol. 2013;58:984–92.

60. Lindblad A, Glaumann H, Strandvik B. Natural history of liver disease in cystic fibrosis. Hepatology. 1999;30:1151–8.

61. Strandvik B, Hultcrantz R. Liver function and morphology during long-term fatty acid supplementation in cystic fibrosis. Liver. 2008;14:32–6.

62. Beharry S, Ackerley C, Corey M, et al. Long-term docosahexaenoic acid therapy in a congenic murine model of cystic fibrosis. Am J Physiol Gastrointest Liver Physiol. 2007;292:G839–48.

63. Cottart CH, Bonvin E, Rey C, et al. Impact of nutrition on phenotype in CFTR-deficient mice. Pediatr Res. 2007;62:528–32.

64. Smith C, Winn A, Seddon P, Ranganathan S. A fat lot of good: balance and trends in fat intake in children with cystic fibrosis. J Cyst Fibros. 2012;11:154–7.
65. Ayoub F, Trillo-Alvarez C, Morelli G, Lascano J. Risk factors for hepatic steatosis in adults with cystic fibrosis: similarities to non-alcoholic fatty liver disease. World J Hepatol. 2018;10:34–40.
66. Hanna RM, Weiner DJ. Overweight and obesity in patients with cystic fibrosis: a center-based analysis. Pediatr Pulmonol. 2015;50:35–41.
67. González Jiménez D, Muñoz-Codoceo R, Garriga-García M, et al. Excess weight in patients with cystic fibrosis: is it always beneficial? Nutr Hosp. 2017;34:578.
68. Kastner-Cole D, Palmer CNA, Ogston SA, Mehta A, Mukhopadhyay S. Overweight and obesity in ΔF508 homozygous cystic fibrosis. J Pediatr. 2005;147:402–4.
69. Treem WR, Stanley CA. Massive hepatomegaly, steatosis, and secondary plasma carnitine deficiency in an infant with cystic fibrosis. Pediatrics. 1989;83:993–7.
70. Innis SM, Hasman D. Evidence of choline depletion and reduced betaine and dimethylglycine with increased homocysteine in plasma of children with cystic fibrosis. J Nutr. 2006;136:2226–31.
71. Schall JI, Mascarenhas MR, Maqbool A, et al. Choline supplementation with a structured lipid in children with cystic fibrosis: a randomized placebo-controlled trial. J Pediatr Gastroenterol Nutr. 2016;62:618–26.
72. Terheggen-Lagro S, de Jager W, Prakken B, van der Ent CK. Multiplex cytokine profile detection in young children with cystic fibrosis. J Cyst Fibros. 2007;6:S30.
73. Tarantino G, Savastano S, Colao A. Hepatic steatosis, low-grade chronic inflammation and hormone/growth factor/adipokine imbalance. World J Gastroenterol. 2010;16:4773–83.
74. Capeau J. Insulin resistance and steatosis in humans. Diabetes Metab. 2008;34:649–57.
75. Arab JP, Karpen SJ, Dawson PA, Arrese M, Trauner M. Bile acids and nonalcoholic fatty liver disease: molecular insights and therapeutic perspectives. Hepatology. 2017;65:350–62.
76. Alisi A, Ceccarelli S, Panera N, et al. Association between serum atypical fibroblast growth factors 21 and 19 and pediatric nonalcoholic fatty liver disease. PLoS One. 2013;8:e67160.
77. Van De Peppel IP, Doktorova M, Berkers G, de Jonge HR, Houwen RHJJ, Verkade HJ, Jonker JW, Bodewes FAJA. IVACAFTOR restores FGF19 regulated bile acid homeostasis in cystic fibrosis patients with an S1251N or a G551D gating mutation. J Cyst Fibros. 2018;50:297.
78. Zhou M, Learned RM, Rossi SJ, DePaoli AM, Tian H, Ling L. Engineered FGF19 eliminates bile acid toxicity and lipotoxicity leading to resolution of steatohepatitis and fibrosis in mice. Hepatol Commun. 2017;1:1024–42.
79. Cortes-Santiago N, Leung DH, Castro E, Finegold M, Wu H, Patel K. Hepatic steatosis is prevalent following orthotopic liver transplantation in children with cystic fibrosis. J Pediatr Gastroenterol Nutr. 2018;68:96–103.
80. Hillaire S, Bonte E, Denninger MH, Casadevall N, Cadranel JF, Lebrec D, Valla D, Degott C. Idiopathic non-cirrhotic intrahepatic portal hypertension in the West: a re-evaluation in 28 patients. Gut. 2002;51:275–80.
81. King LJ, Scurr ED, Murugan N, Williams SGJ, Westaby D, Healy JC. Hepatobiliary and pancreatic manifestations of cystic fibrosis: MR imaging appearances. Radiographics. 2000;20:767–77.
82. Yamada A, Komaki Y, Komaki F, Micic D, Zullow S, Sakuraba A. Risk of gastrointestinal cancers in patients with cystic fibrosis: a systematic review and meta-analysis. Lancet Oncol. 2018;19:758–67.
83. Lykavieris P, Bernard O, Hadchouel M. Neonatal cholestasis as the presenting feature in cystic fibrosis. Arch Dis Child. 1996;75:67–70.
84. Van De Peppel IP, Bertolini A, Jonker JW, Bodewes FAJAJA, Verkade HJ. Diagnosis, follow-up and treatment of cystic fibrosis-related liver disease. Curr Opin Pulm Med. 2017;23:562–9.
85. Mueller-Abt PR, Frawley KJ, Greer RM, Lewindon PJ. Comparison of ultrasound and biopsy findings in children with cystic fibrosis related liver disease. J Cyst Fibros. 2008;7:215–21.

86. Lemaitre C, Dominique S, Billoud E, et al. Relevance of 3D cholangiography and transient elastography to assess cystic fibrosis-associated liver disease? Can Respir J. 2016; 2016:1–8.

87. Erlinger S, Dumont M. Influence of ursodeoxycholic acid on bile secretion. In: Paumgartner G, Stiehl A, Barbara L, Roda E, editors. Strategies for the treatment of hepatobiliary disease. Dordrecht: Kluwer Academic; 1990. p. 35–42.

88. Cheng K, Ashby D, Smyth RL. Ursodeoxycholic acid for cystic fibrosis-related liver disease. Cochrane Database Syst Rev. 2017. https://doi.org/10.1002/14651858.CD000222.pub4.

89. Colombo C, Crosignani A, Alicandro G, Zhang W, Biffi A, Motta V, Corti F, Setchell KDR. Long-term ursodeoxycholic acid therapy does not alter lithocholic acid levels in patients with cystic fibrosis with associated liver disease. J Pediatr. 2016;177:59–65.e1.

90. Merli M, Bertasi S, Servi R, Diamanti S, Martino F, De Santis A, Goffredo F, Quattrucci S, Antonelli M, Angelico M. Effect of a medium dose of ursodeoxycholic acid with or without taurine supplementation on the nutritional status of patients with cystic fibrosis: a randomized, placebo-controlled, crossover trial. J Pediatr Gastroenterol Nutr. 1994;19:198–203.

91. O'Brien S, Fitzgerald M, Hegarty JE. A controlled trial of ursodeoxycholic acid treatment in cystic fibrosis-related liver disease. Eur J Gastroenterol Hepatol. 1992;4:857–63.

92. van der Feen C, van der Doef HPJ, van der Ent CK, Houwen RHJ. Ursodeoxycholic acid treatment is associated with improvement of liver stiffness in cystic fibrosis patients. J Cyst Fibros. 2016;15:834–8.

93. Lindblad A, Glaumann H, Strandvik B. A two-year prospective study of the effect of ursodeoxycholic acid on urinary bile acid excretion and liver morphology in cystic fibrosis- associated liver disease. Hepatology. 1998;27:166–74.

94. Ciucă IM, Pop L, Ranetti E, Popescu IM, Almajan-Guta B, Malita IM, Anghel I. Ursodeoxycholic acid effects on cystic fibrosis liver disease. Farmacia. 2015;63:2–6.

95. Nousia-Arvanitakis S, Fotoulaki M, Economou H, Xefteri M, Galli-Tsinopoulou A. Long-term prospective study of the effect of ursodeoxycholic acid on cystic fibrosis-related liver disease. J Clin Gastroenterol. 2001;32:324–8.

96. Ooi CY, Nightingale S, Durie PR, Freedman SD. Ursodeoxycholic acid in cystic fibrosis-associated liver disease. J Cyst Fibros. 2012;11:72–3.

97. Hayes D, Warren PS, McCoy KS, Sheikh SI. Improvement of hepatic steatosis in cystic fibrosis with ivacaftor therapy. J Pediatr Gastroenterol Nutr. 2015;60:578–9.

98. Davies JC, Cunningham S, Harris WT, et al. Safety, pharmacokinetics, and pharmacodynamics of ivacaftor in patients aged 2-years with cystic fibrosis and a CFTR gating mutation (KIWI): an open-label, single-arm study. Lancet Respir Med. 2016;4:107–15.

99. Fickert P, Hirschfield GM, Denk G, et al. norUrsodeoxycholic acid improves cholestasis in primary sclerosing cholangitis. J Hepatol. 2017;67:549–58.

100. Beuers U, Trauner M, Jansen P, Poupon R. New paradigms in the treatment of hepatic cholestasis: from UDCA to FXR, PXR and beyond. J Hepatol. 2015;62:S25–37.

101. Jonker JW, Suh JM, Atkins AR, et al. A PPARγ-FGF1 axis is required for adaptive adipose remodelling and metabolic homeostasis. Nature. 2012;485:391–4.

102. Liu W, Struik D, Nies VJM, et al. Effective treatment of steatosis and steatohepatitis by fibroblast growth factor 1 in mouse models of nonalcoholic fatty liver disease. Proc Natl Acad Sci. 2016;113:2288–93.

103. Ding N, Yu RT, Subramaniam N, et al. A vitamin D receptor/SMAD genomic circuit gates hepatic fibrotic response. Cell. 2013;153:601–13.

104. Scirpo R, Fiorotto R, Villani A, Amenduni M, Spirli C, Strazzabosco M. Stimulation of nuclear receptor peroxisome proliferator-activated receptor-γ limits NF-κB-dependent inflammation in mouse cystic fibrosis biliary epithelium. Hepatology. 2015;62:1551–62.

105. Fiorotto R, Amenduni M, Mariotti V, Fabris L, Spirli C, Strazzabosco M. Src kinase inhibition reduces inflammatory and cytoskeletal changes in ΔF508 human cholangiocytes and improves cystic fibrosis transmembrane conductance regulator correctors efficacy. Hepatology. 2018;67:972–88.

106. Garcia-Tsao G, Abraldes JG, Berzigotti A, Bosch J. Portal hypertensive bleeding in cirrhosis: risk stratification, diagnosis, and management: 2016 practice guidance by the American Association for the Study of Liver Diseases. Hepatology. 2017;65:310–35.
107. Palaniappan SK, Than NN, Thein AW, Moe S, van Mourik I. Interventions for preventing and managing advanced liver disease in cystic fibrosis. Cochrane Database Syst Rev. 2017;8:CD012056.
108. Black SM, Woodley FW, Tumin D, Mumtaz K, Whitson BA, Tobias JD, Hayes D. Cystic fibrosis associated with worse survival after liver transplantation. Dig Dis Sci. 2016;61:1178–85.
109. Rowland M, Gallagher CG, Ó'Laoide R, et al. Outcome in cystic fibrosis liver disease. Am J Gastroenterol. 2011;106:104–9.
110. Rowland M, Gallagher C, Gallagher CG, et al. Outcome in patients with cystic fibrosis liver disease. J Cyst Fibros. 2015;14:120–6.
111. Ye W, Narkewicz MR, Leung DH, Karnsakul W, Murray KF, Alonso EM, Magee JC, Schwarzenberg SJ, Weymann A, Molleston JP. Variceal hemorrhage and adverse liver outcomes in patients with cystic fibrosis cirrhosis. J Pediatr Gastroenterol Nutr. 2018;66: 122–7.
112. Breuer O, Shteyer E, Wilschanski M, Perles Z, Cohen-Cymberknoh M, Kerem E, Shoseyov D. Hepatopulmonary syndrome in patients with cystic fibrosis and liver disease. Chest. 2016;149:e35–8.
113. O'Donnell DH, Ryan R, Hayes B, Fennelly D, Gibney RG. Hepatocellular carcinoma complicating cystic fibrosis related liver disease. J Cyst Fibros. 2009;8:288–90.
114. Kelleher T, Staunton M, O'Mahony S, McCormick PA. Advanced hepatocellular carcinoma associated with cystic fibrosis. Eur J Gastroenterol Hepatol. 2005;17:1123–4.
115. Mckeon D, Day A, Parmar J, Alexander G, Bilton D. Hepatocellular carcinoma in association with cirrhosis in a patient with cystic fibrosis. J Cyst Fibros. 2004;3:193–5.
116. Pals FH, Verkade HJ, Gulmans VAM, et al. Cirrhosis associated with decreased survival and a 10-year lower median age at death of cystic fibrosis patients in the Netherlands. J Cyst Fibros. 2019;18(3):385–9.
117. Alex G, Catto-Smith AG, Ditchfield M, Roseby R, Robinson PJ, Cameron FJ, Oliver MR. Is significant cystic fibrosis-related liver disease a risk factor in the development of bone mineralization abnormalities? Pediatr Pulmonol. 2006;41:338–44.
118. Corbett K, Kelleher S, Rowland M, Daly L, Drumm B, Canny G, Greally P, Hayes R, Bourke B. Cystic fibrosis-associated liver disease: a population-based study. J Pediatr. 2004;145:327–32.
119. Polineni D, Piccorelli AV, Hannah WB, Dalrymple SN, Pace RG, Durie PR, Ling SC, Knowles MR, Stonebraker JR. Analysis of a large cohort of cystic fibrosis patients with severe liver disease indicates lung function decline does not significantly differ from that of the general cystic fibrosis population. PLoS One. 2018;13:e0205257.
120. Slieker MG, van der Doef HPJ, Deckers-Kocken JM, van der Ent CK, Houwen RHJ. Pulmonary prognosis in cystic fibrosis patients with liver disease. J Pediatr. 2006;149:144.
121. Tabernero da Veiga S, González Lama Y, Lama More R, Martínez Carrasco MC, Antelo Landeria MC, Jara Vega P. Chronic liver disease associated with cystic fibrosis: energy expenditure at rest, risk factors, and impact on the course of the disease. Nutr Hosp. 2004;19:19–27.
122. Gälman C, Arvidsson I, Angelin B, Rudling M. Monitoring hepatic cholesterol 7α-hydroxylase activity by assay of the stable bile acid intermediate 7α-hydroxy-4-cholesten-3-one in peripheral blood. J Lipid Res. 2003;44:859–66.
123. Guilbault C, Saeed Z, Downey GP, Radzioch D. Cystic fibrosis mouse models. Am J Respir Cell Mol Biol. 2007;36:1–7.
124. Wilke M, Buijs-Offerman RM, Aarbiou J, Colledge WH, Sheppard DN, Touqui L, Bot A, Jorna H, De Jonge HR, Scholte BJ. Mouse models of cystic fibrosis: phenotypic analysis and research applications. J Cyst Fibros. 2011;10:S152–71.
125. Delaney SJ, Alton EW, Smith SN, et al. Cystic fibrosis mice carrying the missense mutation G551D replicate human genotype-phenotype correlations. EMBO J. 1996;15:955–63.

126. Blanco PG, Zaman MM, Junaidi O, Sheth S, Yantiss RK, Nasser IA, Freedman SD. Induction of colitis in cftr −/− mice results in bile duct injury. Am J Physiol Gastrointest Liver Physiol. 2004;287:G491–6.

127. Debray D, El Mourabit H, Merabtene F, et al. Diet-induced dysbiosis and genetic background synergize with cystic fibrosis transmembrane conductance regulator deficiency to promote cholangiopathy in mice. Hepatol Commun. 2018;2:1533–49.

128. Snouwaert J, Brigman K, Latour A. An animal fibrosis made for model by gene cystic targeting. Science (80-). 1992;257:1083–8.

129. Debray D, Rainteau D, Barbu V, et al. Defects in gallbladder emptying and bile acid homeostasis in mice with cystic fibrosis transmembrane conductance regulator deficiencies. Gastroenterology. 2012;142:1581–1591.e6.

130. Tuggle KL, Birket SE, Cui X, et al. Characterization of defects in ion transport and tissue development in cystic fibrosis transmembrane conductance regulator (CFTR)-knockout rats. PLoS One. 2014;9:e91253.

131. Sun X, Sui H, Fisher JT, et al. Disease phenotype of a ferret CFTR-knockout model of cystic fibrosis. J Clin Invest. 2010;120:3149–60.

132. Rogers CS, Stoltz DA, Meyerholz DK, et al. Disruption of the CFTR gene produces a model of cystic fibrosis in newborn pigs. Science (80-). 2008;321:1837–41.

133. Ostedgaard LS, Meyerholz DK, Chen JH, et al. The ΔF508 mutation causes CFTR misprocessing and cystic fibrosis-like disease in pigs. Sci Transl Med. 2011;3:74–98.

134. Wilschanski M, Durie PR. Patterns of GI disease in adulthood associated with mutations in the CFTR gene. Gut. 2007;56:1153–63.

135. Uc A, Giriyappa R, Meyerholz DK, et al. Pancreatic and biliary secretion are both altered in cystic fibrosis pigs. Am J Physiol Gastrointest Liver Physiol. 2012;303:G961–8.

136. Stoltz DA, Rokhlina T, Ernst SE, et al. Intestinal CFTR expression alleviates meconium ileus in cystic fibrosis pigs. J Clin Invest. 2013;123:2685–93.

137. Ballard ST, Evans JW, Drag HS, Schuler M. Pathophysiologic evaluation of the transgenic CFTR "gut-corrected" porcine model of cystic fibrosis. Am J Physiol Lung Cell Mol Physiol. 2016;311:L779–87.

138. Stoltz DA, Meyerholz DK, Pezzulo AA, et al. Cystic fibrosis pigs develop lung disease and exhibit defective bacterial eradication at birth. Sci Transl Med. 2010;2:29–31.

139. Leeuwen L, Fitzgerald DA, Gaskin KJ. Liver disease in cystic fibrosis. Paediatr Respir Rev. 2014;15:69–74.

Chapter 15
Gastrointestinal Complications

Adam C. Stein, Nicole Green, and Sarah Jane Schwarzenberg

Introduction

Cystic fibrosis (CF) is the result of mutations to the cystic fibrosis transmembrane conductance regulator (CFTR) that lead to dysfunction. CFTR is expressed throughout the gastrointestinal and pancreaticobiliary systems including the intrahepatic bile ducts. Corresponding gastrointestinal manifestations have a significant impact on the well-being of people with CF, increasing complaints of pain [1]. While there is no systematic characterization of the incidence and prevalence of gastrointestinal manifestations of CF on a population level, single-center studies show that the majority of people with CF will report some gastrointestinal symptoms or history of complications at some point during their lifetimes [2]. GI-related issues can lead to the diagnosis of CF, as seen with meconium ileus (MI) during infancy, and other digestive health problems can occur at any point during childhood or as an adult.

The pathophysiology of gastrointestinal disease in CF can be linked, in part, to abnormal mucus buildup with potential inflammatory responses, directly related to dysfunction in CFTR, which is expressed throughout the gastrointestinal system. Ion exchange (chloride and bicarbonate) is impacted, which leads to decrease in the

A. C. Stein
Division of Gastroenterology and Hepatology, Northwestern Medicine, Chicago, IL, USA
e-mail: Adam.stein@northwestern.edu

N. Green
Division of Gastroenterology and Hepatology, Department of Pediatrics,
Seattle Children's Hospital-University of Washington, Seattle, WA, USA
e-mail: Nicole.green@seattlechildrens.org

S. J. Schwarzenberg (✉)
University of Minnesota Masonic Children's Hospital, Department of Pediatrics,
Minneapolis, MN, USA
e-mail: schwa005@umn.edu

© Springer Nature Switzerland AG 2020
S. D. Davis et al. (eds.), *Cystic Fibrosis*, Respiratory Medicine,
https://doi.org/10.1007/978-3-030-42382-7_15

pH of the intestinal lumen, as well as the pancreaticobiliary system [3]. In regard to the small bowel and colon, this increase in acidity leads to dehydration of the intestinal mucous layer that is in direct contact with the surface epithelium, leading to increased mucous viscosity and even stasis. Pancreaticobiliary mucous changes leads to decreased bile and pancreatic exocrine enzyme release into the small bowel, further contributing to malabsorption and gastrointestinal symptoms. Also impacted is the intestinal microbiota, with dysbiosis leading to further symptoms [4]. To date, therapy has largely been symptomatic or targeted endpoint treatment (such as pancreatic exocrine enzyme replacement therapy). It is yet to be seen how the newer CFTR modulators impact overall digestive health [5].

With improvement in life expectancy and overall functionality of people with CF, recognition of gastrointestinal complications is increasingly important as a factor impacting physical and mental health. Nonetheless, gastrointestinal signs and symptoms may be underreported or minimized during a CF-related visit. As such, the CF provider must recognize gastrointestinal-related problems, be able to initiate an initial workup, and know when to refer to a gastroenterologist/hepatologist (ideally an individual with experience in CF, if available).

Meconium Ileus

Meconium ileus (MI) is intestinal obstruction that occurs in the neonatal period as a result of inspissated intraluminal meconium. Before newborn screening, it was often the presenting symptom of cystic fibrosis (CF), occurring in approximately 20% of neonates diagnosed with CF [3]. Estimates of the likelihood that a baby with MI has CF range from 54% to 90% depending on the studies. Prematurity and low birth weight may be responsible for MI in patients without CF [6]. Interestingly, MI can result in a false-negative newborn screen based on immunoreactive trypsinogen levels, so sweat testing and genetic evaluation should be performed [7]. Clinically, MI can present in two forms: (1) simple obstruction with failure to pass meconium as viscid meconium physically obstructs the terminal ileum resulting in proximal dilation of the small intestine and (2) complex MI in which secondary complications occur, such as perforation, meconium peritonitis, volvulus, ischemic necrosis, and/or intestinal atresia [3].

Meconium ileus and meconium peritonitis are often detected on prenatal ultrasound based on the presence of hyperechoic bowel or peritoneal calcifications [8]. If MI is not identified prenatally, symptoms of intestinal obstruction may be observed within hours of birth. Symptoms include bilious emesis with feeding, abdominal distension, and, in the case of meconium peritonitis, abdominal tenderness, fever, and shock [9]. Other infants may display milder symptoms with only delayed passage of meconium. The differential diagnosis in these cases includes meconium plug (inspissated meconium in the colon, which is difficult to pass), Hirschsprung's disease, intestinal atresia, volvulus, and bowel perforation.

Abdominal films often show dilated loops of bowel with or without air-fluid levels. In the case of complete obstruction, air may not be present in the rectum. In a contained intestinal perforation, abdominal calcifications may be present. The "soap-bubble" sign describes the radiographic appearance of meconium mixing with swallowed air that may be appreciated in the distal small intestine [10]. The presence of peritoneal signs or hemodynamic instability is a medical emergency. If the infant is stable, a contrast enema can identify microcolon distal to the terminal ileum obstruction and resultant colonic disuse.

Medical management of simple meconium ileus involves hyperosmolar enemas under fluoroscopic guidance to ensure solution reaches the terminal ileum [11]. IV hydration is imperative during hyperosmolar enema administration to avoid hypovolemia. If the hyperosmolar enema is unsuccessful, surgical intervention is required to irrigate the terminal ileum and disimpact the meconium [12, 13]. An enterostomy can be created to allow for ongoing irrigation of the terminal ileum if needed. Bowel resection may be required in complex cases depending on the extent of bowel injury. Many infants, especially those with complex MI who undergo surgical resection, may require parenteral nutrition and lipids initially to support growth. However, enteral nutrition should be started as soon as possible after resolution of MI.

The most common risk associated with a history MI in CF is the later development of distal intestinal obstruction syndrome (DIOS), a condition characterized by the accumulation of inspissated fecal material in the distal ileum and proximal colon resulting in partial or complete obstruction. This risk of DIOS in CF patients with a history of MI is approximately 50% versus 15% in the general CF population [3, 9]. Patients who require surgical intervention for their MI are at risk for subsequent postsurgical complications (e.g., adhesions, small bowel obstruction, anastomotic ulcers, strictures). Patients with a history of MI may also be at higher risk for delayed small bowel transit time due to history of compromised bowel.

Early diagnosis and management of MI by a multidisciplinary team with experience in CF (pediatric surgeons, neonatologists, pulmonologists, gastroenterologists, dietitians) is imperative and has been demonstrated to improve both short- and long-term outcomes for these patients [14–16].

Constipation and Distal Intestinal Obstruction Syndrome (DIOS)

Constipation is one of the most common gastrointestinal manifestations of CF. Constipation is associated with pancreatic insufficiency, history of MI, and fat malabsorption. The European Society for Pediatric Gastroenterology, Hepatology, and Nutrition (ESPGHAN) CF Working Group published definitions for constipation, which emphasize a slow period of development of symptoms (weeks or months), with increased consistency of stools and decreased frequency of bowel movements [17].

History is sufficient for diagnosis of constipation, and abdominal imaging should be used only to exclude other diagnoses, including DIOS. Therapy for constipation is individualized and often provider dependent, often requiring a combination of medications. Initial therapy is usually an osmotic laxative (polyethylene glycol), with or without a mild stimulant, such as senna. Other medications, such as the intestinal secretagogue lubiprostone, have been studied in small numbers of people with CF [18]. If constipation remains refractory to conservative treatment, referral to a gastroenterologist, preferably one with experience in CF, may be warranted.

In terms of specific medical management for constipation, first-line therapy is typically osmotic laxatives with polyethylene glycol (PEG)-based solutions. Intestinal secretagogues may have a role as preventative agents in certain CF patients [19]. These include lubiprostone and linaclotide. Lubiprostone is a type 2 chloride channel (CIC-2) activator that induces intestinal chloride secretion and decreases transit time [20]. Furthermore, there is some debate about the efficacy of lubiprostone in patients with CF as there is suggestion that induced chloride secretion requires the presence of functional CFTR despite the medication working on an unrelated chloride-activating pathway [21]. Linaclotide is a guanylate cyclase-C (GC-C) ligand agonist which binds to the GC-C receptor located on the luminal surface of intestinal enterocytes. Binding increases intracellular levels of cyclic guanosine monophosphate (cGMP), stimulating intestinal fluid secretion through activation of CFTR, resulting in secretion of chloride and bicarbonate into the intestinal lumen as well as decreased transit time. Linaclotide has not been formally studied in CF, and anecdotal experience reports variable efficacy. Lubiprostone and linaclotide are not approved for use in children in the United States.

Differentiating DIOS from constipation can be difficult. Symptoms of DIOS are typically more acute than those of constipation, with more acute worsening of abdominal pain and/or abdominal distension [22, 23]. Diagnosis is usually a combination of presenting history and imaging. The ESPGHAN CF Working Group definition for DIOS emphasizes pain and/or distention associated with an ileocecal fecal mass and evidence of intestinal obstruction [17]. In select circumstances, CT may be indicated to help distinguish DIOS from other mimickers, such as intestinal intussusception or appendicitis [19, 22]. DIOS treatment protocols vary among centers with use of oral lavage, rectal-/enema-based lavage, or a combination of both [17]. According to the Cystic Fibrosis Foundation DIOS Task Force Clinical Pathway, in the setting of symptoms reflective of complete DIOS (i.e., bilious vomiting, inability to pass stool or flatus, severe abdominal pain, and distension), hospitalization with bowel rest and nasogastric decompression is recommended [21]. Consultation with gastroenterology (and, if peritoneal signs are present, surgery) is appropriate.

Patients with prior episodes of DIOS may be ten times more likely to experience a subsequent episode [22]. Following a DIOS episode, the importance of a consistent osmotic laxative regimen should be emphasized to minimize reoccurrence [22]. However, there is no single validated strategy for prevention of DIOS recurrence [19]. General recommendations include ensuring adequate hydration and activity.

Fiber in CF patients is generally not thought to be beneficial given their baseline delayed intestinal transit and propensity for more viscous stool. Ensuring adherence to pancreatic enzyme replacement therapy (PERT) is critical for these patients.

Gastroesophageal Reflux

Gastroesophageal reflux is the effortless movement of gastric contents into the esophagus. This is a normal physiologic event occurring several times a day in most people. When reflux produces bothersome symptoms, for example, esophagitis, reduced food intake, vomiting, or pneumonia, it is termed gastroesophageal reflux *disease* [24, 25]. Reflux symptoms or complications may be esophageal (e.g., heartburn, bleeding, esophageal stricture) or extra-esophageal (e.g., pneumonia, wheezing, coughing).

Gastroesophageal reflux and gastroesophageal reflux disease are common in people with cystic fibrosis. Studies of reflux in CF have been difficult to interpret, as most are small, single-center studies, some examining adults and others children, and using a variety of techniques to assess reflux. Multichannel intraluminal esophageal impedance and pH monitoring detects both acidic and nonacidic or weakly acidic reflux. Using this tool, gastroesophageal reflux is found in 67% of children with CF and 87% of adults with CF [26–28]. Most exhibit acid reflux; a smaller group has weakly acidic reflux. Not all are symptomatic.

There are many risks for people with gastroesophageal reflux, including pain from heartburn, loss of weight from pain with eating, and the cancer risk associated with Barrett's esophagus [24, 25]. Without diminishing the risk of these esophageal symptoms in people with CF, the greatest concern for people with CF is the risk of pulmonary injury and impairment associated with reflux. The most convincing evidence of the risk of reflux to the lung in CF comes from studies in lung transplant recipients. People with CF who have had lung transplantation have a high prevalence of gastroesophageal reflux, with a significant proportion having bile in the refluxate [29]. Bilious refluxate is associated with bronchiolitis obliterans after lung transplantation, raising concerns that untreated reflux may imperil successful lung transplantation. Acid suppression has not been effective in prevention of reflux after lung transplant. Some have suggested fundoplication as a means to protect the transplanted lung, but this remains controversial [30].

Diagnosis of gastroesophageal reflux is difficult because of the large differential for abdominal pain with or without vomiting (Table 15.1) and the many diagnostic modalities for reflux. No one study can unequivocally demonstrate that reflux is the cause of impaired lung disease. Reflux in individuals with heartburn, abdominal pain, water brash (increased salivation with regurgitation), or other esophageal symptoms is often diagnosed clinically, at least initially. If the patient does not have high-risk factors such as gastrointestinal bleeding, intractable pain, or intractable vomiting, a 6–8-week trial of proton pump inhibitor treatment is acceptable.

Table 15.1 Common conditions confused with gastroesophageal reflux

Eosinophilic esophagitis, food allergy
Intestinal partial obstruction
Delayed gastric emptying
Peptic ulcer disease
Celiac disease
Gallbladder disease or gallstones
Urinary tract infection
Increased intracranial pressure
Achalasia
Pancreatitis
Esophageal cancer
Gastric bezoar
Factitious disorder by patient or by proxy

This table is not exhaustive. For further differential diagnosis discussion, the reader is referred to Rosen (2015) and Katz (2013) [31, 32]

If the patient's symptoms are unresponsive to initial acid suppression, examination by 24 hour multichannel intraluminal esophageal impedance and pH monitoring, with or without endoscopy to examine histopathology, may be warranted. If it is suspected that reflux is impairing pulmonary function, referral to a gastroenterologist is necessary. Guidelines for diagnosis and management of reflux in adults and children are published [31, 32].

For individuals with infrequent symptoms, acid neutralization medications (antacids) or occasional H2 antagonist use can be suggested. For patients with extra-esophageal symptoms, a short trial of PPI is often suggested, but these patients should have an early referral to gastroenterology to evaluate the need for fundoplication.

Much has been written lately about the potential harm of long-term PPI therapy [33]. It has been difficult to confirm many of the complications attributed to PPIs; however, it is important to be cautious in the use of any medication long term. A good guideline is to carefully assess the need for long-term PPI by periodic withdrawal of the drug and to weigh the risk of untreated reflux against those of long-term PPI. It should be noted that PPI and H2 antagonists, when used for more than a few weeks, must be weaned over 1–4 weeks, rather than abruptly stopped, to avoid rebound hyperacidity in the stomach [34].

Colorectal Cancer

Colorectal cancer (CRC) is one of the leading causes of cancer-related death in adults in the general population, with the incidence increasing with advancing age. The Cystic Fibrosis Foundation (CFF) patient registry analysis shows there is an increased risk of CRC as well as other digestive tract cancers among adults with CF as compared to the general population [35]. In this population-level study, the overall risk as compared to a general population (as measured using standardized incidence ratio (SIR)) is 3.5 (95% confidence interval (CI) 2.6–4.7) for all digestive cancers, with the SIR for colon cancer at 4.2 (95% CI 4.2–9.0) [35]. This risk is further amplified after lung and liver transplant, with an SIR of 18.4 (95% CI 5.9–44.5) for all digestive cancers and colon cancer specifically at 26.7 (95% CI 4.5–88.1) [35].

There is some suggestion in animal models that CFTR may play a role as a tumor-suppressing gene and could be implicated in digestive tract cancer development [36]. Increased risk of CRC may also be related to changes in the microbiome, altered mucus, low-level inflammation (with increased intestinal cell turnover), and nutritional deficiencies [19]. However, the exact pathophysiology remains elusive.

To address this increased risk of CRC, a task force convened by the CFF published consensus recommendations in 2018 [37]. The cornerstone recommendation is to start screening colonoscopy for CRC screening early (at age 40), with repeat colonoscopy intervals no longer than 5 years or sooner based on findings [37]. In the posttransplant population, if a transplant recipient is 30 years of age or older and adequately recovered from surgery, screening colonoscopy is recommended within 2 years of transplant if a colonoscopy was not done within the past 5 years [37].

Special consideration must be paid to bowel preparation for screening/surveillance colonoscopy in CF, as more intense preparations are typically required [37]. While there is no consensus CF-related bowel prep, the 2018 consensus recommendations suggest split-dose prep, several smaller volume washes, limited delay from time finishing prep to colonoscopy, and patient education stressing the importance of the prep to have a complete examination [37].

Diarrhea

Chronic or acute diarrhea is commonly seen in CF and may alternate with constipation [2]. The differential can be classified based on the etiology of symptoms, which are divided into malabsorptive, infectious, inflammatory, and functional. Differentiation can be accomplished with a careful history, medication review, and, if needed, stool studies (Table 15.2).

Malabsorptive diarrhea is a risk for anyone with undiagnosed exocrine pancreatic insufficiency [38]. With reduction in bicarbonate secretion into the pancreatic duct from lack of CFTR, the ductal fluid becomes more acidic and thick, leading to reduced solubility and flow of digestive enzymes into the small intestine as well as intraluminal obstruction and damage to the pancreatic tissue [39]. Clinically, this is manifested by steatorrhea or fatty stools. Stools may be more frequent and are typically loose with visible fat/grease in the stool or toilet. This type of stool can take on a frothy/foamy appearance and can often be difficult to flush and leave a residue on the toilet bowl itself. Diagnosis is suspected based on symptoms and can be confirmed with a coefficient of fecal fat test, measuring fat in the stool over 72 hours while on a high-fat diet (greater than 70 g/fat per day). Commonly 7 g of fat in a

Table 15.2 Differential diagnosis of diarrhea and evaluation

Type	Examples	Chronicity	History	Evaluation
Malabsorptive	Fat Sugar (lactose, etc.)	Chronic Acute exacerbations	Known pancreatic insufficiency Worse with food Visible fat/grease Floating stool Frothy appearance Difficult to flush Noncompliance with enzymes	24–72 hour stool collection for fat, electrolytes Empiric increase in pancreatic enzymes
Infectious	Bacterial Viral	Acute > chronic	Infectious exposure Antibiotic use (e.g., clindamycin) Associated vomiting Blood in stool Nocturnal bowel movements Fever	Stool studies for infection Biopsies (small bowel, colon)
Inflammatory	Celiac Crohn's disease Ulcerative colitis Autoimmune enteritis	Chronic Acute exacerbations	Urgency Blood in stool Abdominal pain Skin or joint problems Nocturnal bowel movements	Stool studies for infection Colonoscopy Endoscopy Labs for inflammatory markers (CRP), celiac serologies, fecal calprotectin
Functional	Chronic constipation with overflow Irritable bowel syndrome Pelvic floor dysfunction	Chronic Acute exacerbations Intermittent symptoms	Bloating Abdominal pain improved with laxation Urgency Incontinence Rectal prolapse	Breath test Anorectal manometry

24 hour period is considered elevated [40]. Because of the difficulty of collecting stool in very young children, and the resistance to stool collection on the part of most patients, pancreatic insufficiency is screened for by measuring fecal elastase, with a low value representative of insufficiency. Stool collected for fecal elastase measurement cannot be loose or liquid, as this may give a false-positive result.

Treatment of pancreatic exocrine insufficiency consists of taking exogenous pancreatic enzymes before and during meals, with dosing typically measured by units of lipase per kilogram and/or based on grams of fat consumed. Recommended initial dose as well as dose limits are debated and outside the scope of this chapter (see Chapter "Nutrition"). Correct dosing can be monitored by symptoms and evidence of growth, although a stool collection for fat on a regular diet with enzyme coverage can be done if needed. People with pancreatic insufficiency who report diarrhea should be evaluated for adherence to enzyme replacement therapy. Consideration should also be given to other causes of diarrhea, including small intestinal bacterial overgrowth (SIBO) [41]. One concern with pancreatic enzyme replacement therapy is a potential relationship of very high doses of pancreatic enzymes with fibrosing colonopathy, a condition leading to fibrosis of the colon that can necessitate surgical therapy [42]. While there has been some evidence put forth of the association, the relationship remains speculative.

Diarrhea with more rapid onset, or a more rapid change in bowel habits to looser stools, can be an indicator of enteric infection or antibiotic-associated diarrhea. People with CF have increased risk factors for both community and healthcare-associated infectious diarrhea, including antibiotic therapy, exposure to the healthcare system (hospitals, clinics, caregivers, etc.), and potentially exposure to others with infectious illness. If suspected, stool studies for infectious organisms should be sent and focused based on exposure. Of note, there is a high carriage rate of *Clostridium difficile* in CF, so testing in clinically asymptomatic patients should be avoided [43]. Other pathogens specific to the individual presentation can be sent, such as sending giardia antigen if a person develops diarrhea after a hiking trip in the mountains. Occasionally duodenal biopsies are helpful if atypical infections are considerations [44]. Treatment will depend on the pathogen, with targeted therapy when applicable.

Noninfectious intestinal inflammation in cystic fibrosis is increasingly recognized as a common occurrence with improvement in the ability to visualize the bowel (such as with video capsule endoscopy) as well as more accurate stool tests for inflammation (fecal calprotectin) [45]. This inflammatory change seems to be seen in both pancreatic-insufficient and pancreatic-sufficient patients; however, there is some suggestion that there could be an increased rate of inflammation in pancreatic-insufficient patients [45, 46]. There are no robust population-level studies to suggest that there is an increased risk or link between CF and inflammatory bowel disease (Crohn's disease, ulcerative colitis) specifically, so it is unclear if this represents some sort of pathophysiologic overlap.

Celiac disease may coexist with CF and should be evaluated in a person with CF and undiagnosed chronic diarrhea and/or poor weight gain. As the celiac serologic tests measure immunoglobulins, and in certain scenarios in CF the total number of immunoglobulins (including immunoglobulin A) can be significantly elevated, there is the potential for falsely positive serologic markers [47].

Diarrhea and fecal incontinence from functional disorders, including pelvic floor disorders, overflow incontinence, and irritable bowel syndrome, are seen in CF [48, 49]. Unfortunately very little population-level data is available regarding the prevalence of these disorders, and there are no widely accepted CF-specific screening tools in use.

Pancreatitis and Pancreatic Cystosis

Pancreatitis in CF is uncommon and occurs almost exclusively in pancreatic-sufficient (PS) patients. Approximately 20% of PS CF patients will develop pancreatitis during their lifetime, typically in teens or adulthood, and of these patients the majority will develop acute recurrent pancreatitis or chronic pancreatitis [50, 51].

The risk of developing pancreatitis is significantly higher in those patients with a milder CF genotype [50]. However, mutations in CFTR alone are not thought to be sufficient for the development of pancreatitis and likely require the addition of other modifying factors. Pancreatitis is more frequently seen in patients with recurrent pulmonary exacerbations, viral infections, or after surgery. The additional risk factors are the same as those seen in non-CF-associated pancreatitis and include ethanol, smoking, drugs/toxins, hypertriglyceridemia, anatomic abnormalities (e.g., pancreatic divisum), and genetic modifiers (SPINK, PRSS1, CTRC) [52].

In order to diagnose pancreatitis, the patient must meet two of the following three criteria: (1) upper abdominal pain consistent with pancreatitis, (2) amylase and/or lipase $\geq 3 \times$ the upper limit of normal, and/or (3) abdominal imaging consistent with pancreatitis. Pancreatitis may be the sole or initial manifestation of CF prior to its diagnosis [52].

General pancreatitis management guidelines should be employed when a CF patient presents with pancreatitis, and it is recommended that a gastroenterologist is consulted during any episode of pancreatitis [52]. Initial management of acute pancreatitis focuses on supportive care, aggressive fluid resuscitation, correction of electrolyte derangements, and adequate pain control [53, 54]. Early reintroduction of enteral nutrition is encouraged within the first 48 hours once a patient is hemodynamically stable unless there are other contraindications (e.g., ileus or bowel obstruction). Patients with acute recurrent pancreatitis or chronic pancreatitis should be considered for a more in-depth evaluation including genetic testing and assessment of anatomy [55, 56].

Pancreatic cysts can be seen in CF patients. Pancreatic cystosis refers to a condition where the pancreatic parenchyma is replaced by multiple cysts of abnormal pancreatic tissue [57]. Patients tend to be asymptomatic and present during the second decade of life with incidental findings on imaging. Some patients may express vague symptoms of abdominal pain, nausea, and/or early satiety [58]. Symptoms are thought to be secondary to mass effect, vascular compromise, or hemorrhage of the cyst [59]. Management is based purely on symptoms. Surgical interventions and endoscopic cyst gastrostomy are available options for those with symptoms which warrant intervention.

Summary

There are a variety of gastrointestinal manifestations in CF, presenting throughout life. It is important for all providers, not just gastroenterologists, to be familiar with these conditions as this will hopefully lead to early recognition and evaluation with appropriate treatment. We hope that with continued improvements in the medical care of gastrointestinal manifestations, there is a significant positive impact in the life of people with CF.

References

1. Masson A, Kirszenbaum M, Sermet-Gaudelus I. Pain is an underestimated symptom in cystic fibrosis. Curr Opin Pulm Med. 2017;23(6):570–3. https://doi.org/10.1097/MCP.0000000000000427.

2. Tabori H, Arnold C, Jaudszus A, Mentzel HJ, Renz DM, Reinsch S, Lorenz M, Michl R, Gerber A, Lehmann T, Mainz JG. Abdominal symptoms in cystic fibrosis and their relation to genotype, history, clinical and laboratory findings. PLoS One. 2017;12(5):e0174463. https://doi.org/10.1371/journal.pone.0174463.

3. Sathe M, Houwen R. Meconium ileus in Cystic Fibrosis. J Cyst Fibros. 2017;16 Suppl 2:S32–9. https://doi.org/10.1016/j.jcf.2017.06.007.

4. Dorsey J, Gonska T. Bacterial overgrowth, dysbiosis, inflammation, and dysmotility in the Cystic Fibrosis intestine. J Cyst Fibros. 2017;16 Suppl 2:S14–23. https://doi.org/10.1016/j.jcf.2017.07.014.

5. Gelfond D, Heltshe S, Ma C, Rowe SM, Frederick C, Uluer A, Sicilian L, Konstan M, Tullis E, Roach RN, Griffin K, Joseloff E, Borowitz D. Impact of CFTR modulation on intestinal pH, motility, and clinical outcomes in patients with cystic fibrosis and the G551D mutation. Clin Transl Gastroenterol. 2017;8(3):e81. https://doi.org/10.1038/ctg.2017.10.

6. Gorter RR, Karimi A, Sleeboom C, Kneepkens CM, Heij HA. Clinical and genetic characteristics of meconium ileus in newborns with and without cystic fibrosis. J Pediatr Gastroenterol Nutr. 2010;50(5):569–72. https://doi.org/10.1097/MPG.0b013e3181bb3427.

7. Rusakow LS, Abman SH, Sokol RJ, Seltzer W, Hammond K, Accurso FJ. Immunoreactive trypsinogen levels in infants with cystic fibrosis complicated by meconium ileus. Screening. 1993;2(1):13–7.

8. Scotet V, Dugueperoux I, Audrezet MP, Audebert-Bellanger S, Muller M, Blayau M, Ferec C. Focus on cystic fibrosis and other disorders evidenced in fetuses with sonographic finding of echogenic bowel: 16-year report from Brittany, France. Am J Obstet Gynecol. 2010;203(6):592. e591-596. https://doi.org/10.1016/j.ajog.2010.08.033.

9. Escobar MA, Grosfeld JL, Burdick JJ, Powell RL, Jay CL, Wait AD, West KW, Billmire DF, Scherer LR 3rd, Engum SA, Rouse TM, Ladd AP, Rescorla FJ. Surgical considerations in cystic fibrosis: a 32-year evaluation of outcomes. Surgery. 2005;138(4):560–71; discussion 571-562. https://doi.org/10.1016/j.surg.2005.06.049.

10. Neuhauser EB. Roentgen changes associated with pancreatic insufficiency in early life. Radiology. 1946;46:319–28. https://doi.org/10.1148/46.4.319.

11. Noblett HR. Treatment of uncomplicated meconium ileus by Gastrografin enema: a preliminary report. J Pediatr Surg. 1969;4(2):190–7.

12. Hiatt RB, Wilson PE. Celiac syndrome; therapy of meconium ileus, report of eight cases with a review of the literature. Surg Gynecol Obstet. 1948;87(3):317–27.

13. Burke MS, Ragi JM, Karamanoukian HL, Kotter M, Brisseau GF, Borowitz DS, Ryan ME, Irish MS, Glick PL. New strategies in nonoperative management of meconium ileus. J Pediatr Surg. 2002;37(5):760–4.

14. Munck A, Gerardin M, Alberti C, Ajzenman C, Lebourgeois M, Aigrain Y, Navarro J. Clinical outcome of cystic fibrosis presenting with or without meconium ileus: a matched cohort study. J Pediatr Surg. 2006;41(9):1556–60. https://doi.org/10.1016/j.jpedsurg.2006.05.014.

15. Efrati O, Nir J, Fraser D, Cohen-Cymberknoh M, Shoseyov D, Vilozni D, Modan-Moses D, Levy R, Szeinberg A, Kerem E, Rivlin J. Meconium ileus in patients with cystic fibrosis is not a risk factor for clinical deterioration and survival: the Israeli Multicenter Study. J Pediatr Gastroenterol Nutr. 2010;50(2):173–8. https://doi.org/10.1097/MPG.0b013e3181a3bfdd.

16. Johnson JA, Bush A, Buchdahl R. Does presenting with meconium ileus affect the prognosis of children with cystic fibrosis? Pediatr Pulmonol. 2010;45(10):951–8. https://doi.org/10.1002/ppul.21271.

17. Houwen RH, van der Doef HP, Sermet I, Munck A, Hauser B, Walkowiak J, Robberecht E, Colombo C, Sinaasappel M, Wilschanski M, Group ECFW. Defining DIOS and constipation in cystic fibrosis with a multicentre study on the incidence, characteristics, and treatment of DIOS. J Pediatr Gastroenterol Nutr. 2010;50(1):38–42. https://doi.org/10.1097/MPG.0b013e3181a6e01d.

18. Assis DN, Freedman SD. Gastrointestinal disorders in cystic fibrosis. Clin Chest Med. 2016;37(1):109–18. https://doi.org/10.1016/j.ccm.2015.11.004.

19. Abraham JM, Taylor CJ. Cystic Fibrosis & disorders of the large intestine: DIOS, constipation, and colorectal cancer. J Cyst Fibros. 2017;16 Suppl 2:S40–9. https://doi.org/10.1016/j.jcf.2017.06.013.

20. O'Brien CE, Anderson PJ, Stowe CD. Lubiprostone for constipation in adults with cystic fibrosis: a pilot study. Ann Pharmacother. 2011;45(9):1061–6. https://doi.org/10.1345/aph.1Q219.

21. Bijvelds MJ, Bot AG, Escher JC, De Jonge HR. Activation of intestinal Cl- secretion by lubiprostone requires the cystic fibrosis transmembrane conductance regulator. Gastroenterology. 2009;137(3):976–85. https://doi.org/10.1053/j.gastro.2009.05.037.

22. Colombo C, Ellemunter H, Houwen R, Munck A, Taylor C, Wilschanski M, ECFS. Guidelines for the diagnosis and management of distal intestinal obstruction syndrome in cystic fibrosis patients. J Cyst Fibros. 2011;10 Suppl 2:S24–8. https://doi.org/10.1016/S1569-1993(11)60005-2.

23. van der Doef HP, Kokke FT, van der Ent CK, Houwen RH. Intestinal obstruction syndromes in cystic fibrosis: meconium ileus, distal intestinal obstruction syndrome, and constipation. Curr Gastroenterol Rep. 2011;13(3):265–70. https://doi.org/10.1007/s11894-011-0185-9.

24. Sherman PM, Hassall E, Fagundes-Neto U, Gold BD, Kato S, Koletzko S, Orenstein S, Rudolph C, Vakil N, Vandenplas Y. A global, evidence-based consensus on the definition of gastroesophageal reflux disease in the pediatric population. Am J Gastroenterol. 2009;104(5):1278–95;. quiz 1296. https://doi.org/10.1038/ajg.2009.129.

25. Vakil N, van Zanten SV, Kahrilas P, Dent J, Jones R, Global Consensus G. The Montreal definition and classification of gastroesophageal reflux disease: a global evidence-based consensus. Am J Gastroenterol. 2006;101(8):1900–20; quiz 1943. https://doi.org/10.1111/j.1572-0241.2006.00630.x.

26. Blondeau K, Pauwels A, Dupont L, Mertens V, Proesmans M, Orel R, Brecelj J, Lopez-Alonso M, Moya M, Malfroot A, De Wachter E, Vandenplas Y, Hauser B, Sifrim D. Characteristics of gastroesophageal reflux and potential risk of gastric content aspiration in children with cystic fibrosis. J Pediatr Gastroenterol Nutr. 2010;50(2):161–6. https://doi.org/10.1097/MPG.0b013e3181acae98.

27. Blondeau K, Dupont LJ, Mertens V, Verleden G, Malfroot A, Vandenplas Y, Hauser B, Sifrim D. Gastro-oesophageal reflux and aspiration of gastric contents in adult patients with cystic fibrosis. Gut. 2008;57(8):1049–55. https://doi.org/10.1136/gut.2007.146134.

28. Pauwels A, Blondeau K, Mertens V, Farre R, Verbeke K, Dupont LJ, Sifrim D. Gastric emptying and different types of reflux in adult patients with cystic fibrosis. Aliment Pharmacol Ther. 2011;34(7):799–807. https://doi.org/10.1111/j.1365-2036.2011.04786.x.

29. Blondeau K, Mertens V, Vanaudenaerde BA, Verleden GM, Van Raemdonck DE, Sifrim D, Dupont LJ. Gastro-oesophageal reflux and gastric aspiration in lung transplant patients with or without chronic rejection. Eur Respir J. 2008;31(4):707–13. https://doi.org/10.1183/09031936.00064807.

30. Biswas Roy S, Elnahas S, Serrone R, Haworth C, Olson MT, Kang P, Smith MA, Bremner RM, Huang JL. Early fundoplication is associated with slower decline in lung function after lung transplantation in patients with gastroesophageal reflux disease. J Thorac Cardiovasc Surg. 2018;155(6):2762–71. e2761. https://doi.org/10.1016/j.jtcvs.2018.02.009.

31. Katz PO, Gerson LB, Vela MF. Guidelines for the diagnosis and management of gastroesophageal reflux disease. Am J Gastroenterol. 2013;108(3):308–28;. quiz 329. https://doi.org/10.1038/ajg.2012.444.

32. Rosen R, Vandenplas Y, Singendonk M, Cabana M, DiLorenzo C, Gottrand F, Gupta S, Langendam M, Staiano A, Thapar N, Tipnis N, Tabbers M. Pediatric Gastroesophageal Reflux

Clinical Practice Guidelines: Joint Recommendations of the North American Society for Pediatric Gastroenterology, Hepatology, and Nutrition and the European Society for Pediatric Gastroenterology, Hepatology, and Nutrition. J Pediatr Gastroenterol Nutr. 2018;66(3):516–54. https://doi.org/10.1097/MPG.0000000000001889.
33. Vaezi MF, Yang YX, Howden CW. Complications of proton pump inhibitor therapy. Gastroenterology. 2017;153(1):35–48. https://doi.org/10.1053/j.gastro.2017.04.047.
34. Kim J, Blackett JW, Jodorkovsky D. Strategies for effective discontinuation of proton pump inhibitors. Curr Gastroenterol Rep. 2018;20(6):27. https://doi.org/10.1007/s11894-018-0632-y.
35. Maisonneuve P, Marshall BC, Knapp EA, Lowenfels AB. Cancer risk in cystic fibrosis: a 20-year nationwide study from the United States. J Natl Cancer Inst. 2013;105(2):122–9. https://doi.org/10.1093/jnci/djs481.
36. Than BLN, Linnekamp JF, Starr TK, Largaespada DA, Rod A, Zhang Y, Bruner V, Abrahante J, Schumann A, Luczak T, Walter J, Niemczyk A, O'Sullivan MG, Medema JP, Fijneman RJA, Meijer GA, Van den Broek E, Hodges CA, Scott PM, Vermeulen L, Cormier RT. CFTR is a tumor suppressor gene in murine and human intestinal cancer. Oncogene. 2017;36(24):3504. https://doi.org/10.1038/onc.2017.3.
37. Hadjiliadis D, Khoruts A, Zauber AG, Hempstead SE, Maisonneuve P, Lowenfels AB, Cystic Fibrosis Colorectal Cancer Screening Task F. Cystic fibrosis colorectal cancer screening consensus recommendations. Gastroenterology. 2018;154(3):736–45. e714. https://doi.org/10.1053/j.gastro.2017.12.012.
38. Wilschanski M, Durie PR. Pathology of pancreatic and intestinal disorders in cystic fibrosis. J R Soc Med. 1998;91 Suppl 34:40–9.
39. Wilschanski M, Durie PR. Patterns of GI disease in adulthood associated with mutations in the CFTR gene. Gut. 2007;56(8):1153–63. https://doi.org/10.1136/gut.2004.062786.
40. Singh VK, Schwarzenberg SJ. Pancreatic insufficiency in Cystic Fibrosis. J Cyst Fibros. 2017;16 Suppl 2:S70–8. https://doi.org/10.1016/j.jcf.2017.06.011.
41. Fridge JL, Conrad C, Gerson L, Castillo RO, Cox K. Risk factors for small bowel bacterial overgrowth in cystic fibrosis. J Pediatr Gastroenterol Nutr. 2007;44(2):212–8. https://doi.org/10.1097/MPG.0b013e31802c0ceb.
42. FitzSimmons SC, Burkhart GA, Borowitz D, Grand RJ, Hammerstrom T, Durie PR, Lloyd-Still JD, Lowenfels AB. High-dose pancreatic-enzyme supplements and fibrosing colonopathy in children with cystic fibrosis. N Engl J Med. 1997;336(18):1283–9. https://doi.org/10.1056/NEJM199705013361803.
43. Burke DG, Harrison MJ, Fleming C, McCarthy M, Shortt C, Sulaiman I, Murphy DM, Eustace JA, Shanahan F, Hill C, Stanton C, Rea MC, Ross RP, Plant BJ. Clostridium difficile carriage in adult cystic fibrosis (CF); implications for patients with CF and the potential for transmission of nosocomial infection. J Cyst Fibros. 2017;16(2):291–8. https://doi.org/10.1016/j.jcf.2016.09.008.
44. Serra S, Jani PA. An approach to duodenal biopsies. J Clin Pathol. 2006;59(11):1133–50. https://doi.org/10.1136/jcp.2005.031260.
45. Werlin SL, Benuri-Silbiger I, Kerem E, Adler SN, Goldin E, Zimmerman J, Malka N, Cohen L, Armoni S, Yatzkan-Israelit Y, Bergwerk A, Aviram M, Bentur L, Mussaffi H, Bjarnasson I, Wilschanski M. Evidence of intestinal inflammation in patients with cystic fibrosis. J Pediatr Gastroenterol Nutr. 2010;51(3):304–8. https://doi.org/10.1097/MPG.0b013e3181d1b013.
46. Rumman N, Sultan M, El-Chammas K, Goh V, Salzman N, Quintero D, Werlin S. Calprotectin in cystic fibrosis. BMC Pediatr. 2014;14:133. https://doi.org/10.1186/1471-2431-14-133.
47. Hodson ME, Morris L, Batten JC. Serum immunoglobulins and immunoglobulin G subclasses in cystic fibrosis related to the clinical state of the patient. Eur Respir J. 1988;1(8):701–5.
48. Benezech A, Desmazes-Dufeu N, Baumstarck K, Bouvier M, Coltey B, Reynaud-Gaubert M, Vitton V. Prevalence of fecal incontinence in adults with cystic fibrosis. Dig Dis Sci. 2018;63(4):982–8. https://doi.org/10.1007/s10620-017-4825-2.
49. Neemuchwala F, Ahmed F, Nasr SZ. Prevalence of pelvic incontinence in patients with cystic fibrosis. Glob Pediatr Health. 2017;4:2333794X17743424. https://doi.org/10.1177/2333794X17743424.

50. Ooi CY, Dorfman R, Cipolli M, Gonska T, Castellani C, Keenan K, Freedman SD, Zielenski J, Berthiaume Y, Corey M, Schibli S, Tullis E, Durie PR. Type of CFTR mutation determines risk of pancreatitis in patients with cystic fibrosis. Gastroenterology. 2011;140(1):153–61. https://doi.org/10.1053/j.gastro.2010.09.046.
51. Hegyi P, Wilschanski M, Muallem S, Lukacs GL, Sahin-Toth M, Uc A, Gray MA, Rakonczay Z Jr, Maleth J. CFTR: a new horizon in the pathomechanism and treatment of pancreatitis. Rev Physiol Biochem Pharmacol. 2016;170:37–66. https://doi.org/10.1007/112_2015_5002.
52. Freeman AJ, Ooi CY. Pancreatitis and pancreatic cystosis in Cystic Fibrosis. J Cyst Fibros. 2017;16 Suppl 2:S79–86. https://doi.org/10.1016/j.jcf.2017.07.004.
53. Abu-El-Haija M, Lin TK, Palermo J. Update to the management of pediatric acute pancreatitis: highlighting areas in need of research. J Pediatr Gastroenterol Nutr. 2014;58(6):689–93. https://doi.org/10.1097/MPG.0000000000000360.
54. American Gastroenterological Association Institute on "Management of Acute Pancreatits" Clinical P, Economics C, Board AGAIG. AGA Institute medical position statement on acute pancreatitis. Gastroenterology. 2007;132(5):2019–21. https://doi.org/10.1053/j.gastro.2007.03.066.
55. Majumder S, Chari ST. Chronic pancreatitis. Lancet. 2016;387(10031):1957–66. https://doi.org/10.1016/S0140-6736(16)00097-0.
56. Gariepy CE, Heyman MB, Lowe ME, Pohl JF, Werlin SL, Wilschanski M, Barth B, Fishman DS, Freedman SD, Giefer MJ, Gonska T, Himes R, Husain SZ, Morinville VD, Ooi CY, Schwarzenberg SJ, Troendle DM, Yen E, Uc A. Causal evaluation of acute recurrent and chronic pancreatitis in children: consensus from the INSPPIRE group. J Pediatr Gastroenterol Nutr. 2017;64(1):95–103. https://doi.org/10.1097/MPG.0000000000001446.
57. Monti L, Salerno T, Lucidi V, Fariello G, Orazi C, Manfredi R, Bella S, Castro M. Pancreatic cystosis in cystic fibrosis: case report. Abdom Imaging. 2001;26(6):648–50. https://doi.org/10.1007/s00261-001-0027-6.
58. Freeman AJ, Giles HW, Nowicki MJ. Image of the month. Pancreatic cystosis complicating cystic fibrosis. Clin Gastroenterol Hepatol. 2010;8(2):e18–9. https://doi.org/10.1016/j.cgh.2009.09.027.
59. van Rijn RR, Schilte PP, Wiarda BM, Taminiau JA, Stoker J. Case 113: pancreatic cystosis. Radiology. 2007;243(2):598–602. https://doi.org/10.1148/radiol.2432040915.

Part IV
Other Organ System Manifestations

Chapter 16
Cystic Fibrosis-Related Diabetes

Andrea Granados and Kara S. Hughan

Abbreviations

ADA	American Diabetes Association
BMI	Body mass index
CF	Cystic fibrosis
CFF	Cystic Fibrosis Foundation
CFRD	Cystic fibrosis-related diabetes
CFTR	Cystic fibrosis transmembrane conductance regulator
CGM	Continuous glucose monitoring
FA	Fructosamine
GA	Glycated albumin
HbA1c	Glycated hemoglobin
IFG	Impaired fasting glucose
IGT	Impaired glucose tolerance

A. Granados (✉)
Washington University School of Medicine in St. Louis, St. Louis Children's Hospital, Department of Pediatrics, Division of Pediatric Endocrinology and Diabetes, One Children's Place, St. Louis, MO, USA
e-mail: agranados@wustl.edu

K. S. Hughan
Department of Pediatrics, Pittsburgh Heart, Lung, Blood and Vascular Medicine Institute, University of Pittsburgh, UPMC Children's Hospital of Pittsburgh, Division of Pediatric Endocrinology and Diabetes, Pittsburgh, PA, USA
e-mail: kara.hughan@chp.edu

© Springer Nature Switzerland AG 2020
S. D. Davis et al. (eds.), *Cystic Fibrosis*, Respiratory Medicine,
https://doi.org/10.1007/978-3-030-42382-7_16

INDET	Indeterminate glycemia
NGT	Normal glucose tolerance
OGTT	Oral glucose tolerance test

Patient Perspective

Living with cystic fibrosis (CF) can be challenging, and the additional diagnosis of cystic fibrosis related diabetes (CFRD) can be overwhelming. In addition to engaging in the complex care demanded in routine CF management, patients diagnosed with CFRD must complete blood sugar monitoring, watch carefully what they eat, count carbohydrates and manage insulin administration. Usually the diagnosis of CFRD is received with surprise and frustration, although some patients can tell that something is wrong with their overall health prior to learning that they have CFRD. They may receive messages from their primary pulmonologist about worsening of lung function, poor weight gain and abnormal glucose levels during routine oral glucose tolerance test screening years prior to the overt diagnosis of CFRD. New responsibilities are added to individuals living with CFRD including checking blood sugars to monitor the fluctuating blood glucose levels several times per day and injecting insulin. Injecting insulin is often the factor that causes more distress to the patient compared to the other diabetes related tasks.

The CFRD diagnosis may be received with fear. Many times patients with CF are already acclimated to a routine of medications, treatments, clinic visits, and hospitalizations; therefore, incorporating CFRD into the existing structure of CF does not seem as difficult. As they learn more, as time goes by, as they adjust, and as they make new decisions, the way they feel changes a lot too. Patients need to make lifestyle changes and a slow step-by-step approach helps, starting with small things such as being more aware of what they eat everyday.

Given the complexity of these two diagnoses, patients rely on the care of health professionals from multiple specialties. They seek doctors and health professionals that truly listen and are willing to learn from the patient's experiences and interactions. Patients want health care providers that allow the patients to educate them on their limitations and providers who are supportive despite the patient's struggles. Patients appreciate how much the medical emphasis has changed—more teamwork with a multidisciplinary approach including pulmonologists, endocrinologists, gastroenterologists, dieticians, social workers, physical therapists, respiratory therapists, psychologists and research staff. Patients expect that this integrative approach and the collective energy be applied to the ultimate goal of CFRD prevention and the improvement of the quality of life of those living with CFRD.

—Anonymous

Introduction

Cystic fibrosis (CF) is the most common autosomal recessive disorder among Caucasians. CF occurs as a result of mutations in the cystic fibrosis transmembrane conductance regulator (CFTR) gene that causes thick and viscous mucous secretions that lead to obstruction of epithelium-lined ducts in multiple mucin-producing organs [1]. Consequently, patients with CF develop characteristic lung disease as well as problems in the gastrointestinal tract, the exocrine and endocrine pancreas, and the reproductive system.

Cystic fibrosis-related diabetes (CFRD) has emerged as a common comorbidity in CF as life expectancy continues to improve. Patients with CFRD are typically asymptomatic for many years, and annual glycemic screening by 10 years of age is recommended. The importance of an early diagnosis primarily resides in the association of CFRD with worse health outcomes.

Over the past two decades, much research has focused on the basic pathogenesis of CFRD and implications of treatment at all stages of glucose intolerance. The purpose of this chapter is to provide an updated overview of the pathogenesis and methods of diagnosis and treatment of CFRD.

Natural History of CFRD

The prevalence of CFRD increases with age and affects approximately 10% of children by 10 years of age, 20% of adolescents, and 40–50% of adults (Fig. 16.1) [2]. Since the predicted survival of individuals with CF is increasing each year [3], the proportion of patients with abnormal glucose tolerance may continue to increase. However, with introduction of new CFTR modulator and potentiator therapies, we may continue to observe a change in the prevalence of CFRD.

Fig. 16.1 CFRD prevalence by age. (Adapted from Cystic Fibrosis–Related Diabetes: Current Trends in Prevalence, Incidence, and Mortality [2])

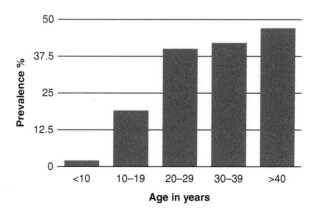

Table 16.1 Risk factors
associated with CFRD

Advancing age
Female sex
CFTR gene mutations in classes I and II
Pancreatic exocrine insufficiency
Hepatobiliary disease
Solid organ transplantation
Corticosteroid use

Close to 80% of middle-age individuals with CF who were diagnosed with pancreatic insufficiency during the first year of life develop CFRD [4, 5]. Risk factors associated with the development of CFRD are presented in Table 16.1 [4, 6–8].

The presentation of diabetes in CF is generally silent. Thus, routine annual screening using the gold standard oral glucose tolerance test (OGTT) by 10 years of age is indicated in all patients with CF [9]. In those with CFRD, insulin secretion is delayed and blunted during an OGTT, primarily due to the loss of the first phase of insulin secretion [10].

The diagnosis of CFRD has significant implications on the overall health of patients with CF. CFRD is associated with increased frequency of pulmonary exacerbations, greater reduction in lung function, poorer nutritional status, and increased mortality [11]. Several retrospective studies have clearly demonstrated that the rate of decline of percent predicted forced expiratory volume at 1 second is greater in individuals with CF over a 2- to 4-year period prior to the diagnosis of CFRD [12–14]. In one study, the rate of decline in pulmonary function was directly proportional to the severity of glucose intolerance and the degree of insulin deficiency [15].

Nutritional status is also compromised in CFRD. An insidious decline in body mass index (BMI) and weight has been recognized as glucose intolerance develops, particularly in the 4 years prior to the diagnosis of CFRD [2]. In addition, numerous studies in individuals with CF have described a depletion of fat-free mass, independent of BMI or body weight, which is associated with reduced lung function, increased pulmonary exacerbations, and increased inflammation [16–19]. Poor glycemic control and gradual loss of the anabolic effects of insulin are likely contributors to this decline, and treatment with insulin partially reverses the deterioration of the BMI [20].

While median age of survival has overall improved in CF, CFRD is associated with increased mortality [2]. More recent data from 2008 to 2012 has demonstrated a 3.5-fold increased mortality in those with CFRD compared to patients with CF without diabetes and higher age-adjusted mortality among those 30 years and older [4].

Pathophysiology and Potential Mechanisms Underlying the Development of CFRD

Reduced β-cell mass The mechanisms underlying CFRD development remain incompletely defined. Impaired insulin secretion has historically been attributed to "collateral damage," i.e., β-cell destruction due to pancreatic exocrine tissue fibrosis and scarring [5]. Abnormal expression of CFTR in intralobular duct cells and pancreatic centroacinar cells manifests as reduced chloride and bicarbonate ion transport leading to reduced fluid secretion into the pancreaticobiliary ducts [21]. Pancreatic proteins, which include enzymes, become concentrated within the pancreatic ducts, causing protein precipitation and ductal obstruction. Obstruction of the pancreatic ducts causes interstitial edema, which impairs blood flow within the pancreatic tissue and leads to ischemia. Accordingly, patients with exocrine pancreatic insufficiency have a higher risk of developing glucose intolerance and CFRD and present with more severe insulin deficiency compared to CF pancreatic sufficient subjects and healthy controls [22].

Insulin resistance Patients with CF appear to have some degree of insulin resistance, although the molecular and cellular basis that explains this process is not fully understood. Insulin resistance is variable and is likely dependent on clinical status. During times of illness, cytokines (e.g., tumor necrosis factor-α, interleukin-6) or corticosteroid administration can precipitate hyperglycemia by inciting an insulin-resistant state [23]. In addition, patients with CF do not appropriately suppress protein breakdown in the postprandial (hyperinsulinemic) state, which results in protein catabolism instead of preservation of protein mass [24].

Abnormalities in the enteroinsular axis Other data suggests that mechanisms in addition to islet destruction, fibrosis, and insulin resistance may play a role in the development of CFRD. Studies in animal models of CF have shown evidence of abnormalities in insular and enteroinsular hormone axis regulation. Incretins, including glucagon-like peptide-1 and gastric inhibitory polypeptide, are gastrointestinal hormones that augment insulin secretion in response to an oral glucose load and with nutrient digestion. In human studies, active glucagon-like peptide-1 levels in the postprandial state are lower in CF and CFRD patients compared with non-CF controls. Given this, impaired incretin secretion likely contributes to the postprandial hyperglycemia noted in CF [25]. Pancreatic enzyme supplementation markedly improves postprandial hyperglycemia by slowing gastric emptying and augmenting incretin hormone secretion, but fat digestion remains incomplete even with enzyme replacement [26].

Intrinsic pancreatic β-cell defects due to CFTR gene mutations could involve mechanisms such as alterations in cellular membranes that potentially affect insulin secretion [27]. Several groups have reported the presence of CFTR protein in human and mouse pancreatic β-cells and α-cells [28, 29]. A recent treatment study with ivacaftor, a novel drug therapy that potentiates CFTR function, directly addressed the question about the role of CFTR function on glucose homeostasis. The effects of ivacaftor therapy on insulin secretion were evaluated in CF subjects with normal and mildly impaired glucose tolerance. Improved insulin secretion and glucagon secretion regulation were demonstrated after 4 months of ivacaftor, while incretin secretion was unchanged, suggesting improved β-cell and α-cell function and not alterations in incretin secretion [30]. Another small open-label pilot study was conducted in CF patients with impaired glucose tolerance following ivacaftor therapy, and the majority of patients improved insulin secretion by 51–346% [31]. These findings suggest that reported improvements in glucose tolerance following iva-caftor therapy may be conferred through improved β-cell and α-cell function. Whether this effect arises directly from regulation of pancreatic CFTR or indirectly, through reduced islet inflammation, is not known. Improved insulin secretion is a promising finding, considering that CFTR modulators are now approved in young subjects with CF.

Oxidative stress Mutations in CFTR can render β-cells more susceptible to oxidative stress. β-cell lines in which CFTR is silenced display higher levels of lipid peroxides, NF-κB signaling, and reduced antioxidant enzyme activity (superoxide dismutase, catalase, and glutathione peroxidase), especially following incubation with oxygen radical-generating iron/ascorbate. Furthermore, basal and glucose-stimulated insulin secretion were decreased, and apoptosis rate was raised in response to iron/ascorbate in CFTR-silenced β-cells [32].

Chronic inflammation Islet cell inflammation has been identified in subjects with CF with and without diabetes, measured by IL-1β immunoreactivity [33]. IL-1β is known to contribute to impaired islet function and viability [34]. Interestingly, IL-1β immunoreactivity was observed in subjects <10 years of age [33], suggesting that islet inflammation could begin very early in CF patients, consistent with clinical studies showing derangements in glucose tolerance and β-cell function in young subjects with CF [35, 36].

Genetics of CFRD

CFTR expression on human pancreatic β-cells and the role that CFTR plays in β-cell function and development of CFRD are highly controversial. CFTR genotypes in which no functional CFTR protein is created or where CFTR is misfolded, including the Class I and II CFTR mutations, confer increased risk for CFRD more than other genotypes [4]. However, the increased CFRD risk may also be secondary to pancreatic exocrine damage [7].

Given the primary defect in CFRD is decreased insulin secretion, there is pathophysiologic overlap with type 1 diabetes. A large portion of familial clustering of type 1 diabetes is attributed to variation of alleles in the human leukocyte antigen (HLA) DR region, with different DR types conferring susceptibility vs. resistance to type 1 diabetes. Evaluation of human leukocyte antigen haplotype and diabetes in CF patients demonstrated the HLA-DR types were similarly distributed among nondiabetic CF patients, diabetic CF patients, and healthy controls [37]. This suggests the HLA haplotype distribution in CF does not confer an increased susceptibility nor resistance to diabetes as the HLA-DR haplotypes do that characterize type 1 diabetes.

Heritability of diabetes in general does not appear to strongly influence development of CFRD, as a positive family history of any diabetes in CF patients is highly variable, ranging from 1% to 44% [37, 38]. However, family history of type 2 diabetes in non-CF family members significantly increases CFRD risk [39]. Therefore, susceptibility genes associated with type 2 diabetes have been explored. Polymorphisms in transcription factor 7-like 2 (TCF7L2) and calpain 10 (CAPN10), genes involved in β-cell proliferation and insulin secretion [40, 41], increase the risk of CFRD and decrease the age at diagnosis [39, 42]. More recently, several known susceptibility alleles for type 2 diabetes were identified as novel genetic modifiers of CFRD onset, including SLC26A9, CDKAL1, CDKN2A/B, and IGFBP2 [42], while no associations of known type 2 diabetes polymorphisms in KCNJ11, PPARY, Kir6.2, HHEX, or SLC30A8 were found with diabetes in CF [41, 42].

The role of cytokines in β-cell destruction and insulin resistance in CF has been examined. Heat shock protein 70, an intracellular polypeptide involved in protection against cytotoxic damage, maps near the HLA region that associates with type 1 diabetes and has also been examined in CF. The patterns of polymorphisms in the cytokine gene tumor necrosis factor (TNF)-β and heat shock protein 70 were similar in CF patients with diabetes to those with insulin-dependent diabetes mellitus, suggesting these polymorphisms may be involved in the pathogenesis of diabetes in CF [37]. In contrast, the allele frequencies of the inflammatory cytokines interleukin-1β, TNF-α, IL-6, and IL-18 did not differ in CF patients with and without diabetes, patients with insulin-dependent diabetes mellitus, and healthy controls [37, 41].

In conclusion, CFRD shares pathologic features of both type 1 and type 2 diabetes. However, current work suggests that CF patients with more severe classes of CFTR mutations, a family history of type 2 diabetes, and polymorphisms in several key genes associated with type 2 diabetes may be more susceptible to developing diabetes.

Screening and Diagnosis of CFRD

Routine screening of CFRD is critical due to the association of this diagnosis with poor clinical outcomes coupled with the insidious onset of symptoms. The current recommendation is to obtain a standard 2-hour 75 g OGTT (1.75 g/kg body weight of oral glucose up to 75 g maximum) in all patients with CF at the age of 10 years. According to the current clinical practice guideline from the Cystic Fibrosis Foundation (CFF) and the position statement by the American Diabetes Association (ADA) [9], CFRD can be diagnosed during stable baseline health based on the criteria presented in Table 16.2. However, a glycated hemoglobin (HbA1c) of <6.5% does not rule out CFRD, because this value is often spuriously low in CF.

CF patients with acute pulmonary exacerbation requiring intravenous antibiotics and/or systemic glucocorticoids should be screened for CFRD by monitoring fasting and 2-hour postprandial plasma glucose levels for the first 48 hours while on these therapies. If elevated blood glucose levels are found by self-monitoring of blood glucose over 48 hours, the results must be confirmed by a plasma glucose in a certified laboratory [9].

Table 16.2 Diagnostic criteria of CFRD

Diagnostic test	Diagnostic criteria
2-Hour OGTT glucose	$\geq$200 mg/dL ($\geq$11.1 mmol/L)
Fasting plasma glucose	$\geq$126 mg/dL ($\geq$7.0 mmol/L)
Hemoglobin A1c (HbA1c)	$\geq$6.5% ($\geq$48 mmol/mol)
Random plasma glucose	$\geq$200 mg/dL ($\geq$11.1 mmol/L) + classical symptoms of diabetes (polyuria and polydipsia)

Other available methods for the diagnosis of diabetes have been studied in CF. Both fasting blood glucose and HbA1c levels, which are used in the screening of diabetes mellitus, are unsuitable for diagnosing CFRD. CFRD patients typically experience transient postprandial hyperglycemia, while fasting hyperglycemia rarely develops at the early stages of the disease and generally presents years following initial diagnosis [15]. HbA1c measures average glycemic status over 90 days, the life span of a red blood cell. CFRD patients typically experience postprandial hyperglycemia that does not significantly affect the glycation status of red blood cells, and HbA1c can be spuriously low in patients with CF. There has been speculation about the possibility of an increased red blood cell turnover [43]. However, the evidence for these explanations is limited, and the exact reasons why HbA1c might perform differently in individuals with CF are not well understood. In fact, HbA1c has a sensitivity of 50% in detecting CFRD when compared to the gold standard, the OGTT [44, 45]. HbA1c is still the method of choice once the diagnosis of CFRD has been established for monitoring of diabetes control [9].

There is growing interest in the use of alternate markers of glycemia such as fructosamine (FA), glycated albumin (GA), and 1,5-anhydroglucitol for diabetes screening and glucose management, but these methods have had limited investigation in CF [46]. A recent study evaluated the relationships among glycemic markers including HbA1c, FA, %GA, and 1,5-anhydroglucitol and minute-to-minute glucoses measured by continuous glucose monitoring (CGM) in CF and hypothesized that alternate markers would better predict average CGM than HbA1c [47]. The authors reported that HbA1C and %GA strongly correlated with the average CGM ($r = 0.86$ and $r = 0.83$, respectively; $P \leq 0.01$ for both). However, the authors did not explore whether these alternate glycemic measurements correlated with the diagnosis of CFRD.

CGM systems, an emerging diabetes management technology, allow frequent subcutaneous interstitial fluid glucose measurements to monitor glycemic trends in real time. CGMs have been studied in CFRD, and this technology is a safe and effective replacement to conventional self-monitoring of blood glucose. Recent studies have shown that in pediatric and adult patients with CF, CGM systems identified a greater degree of impaired glucose tolerance than the gold standard 2-hour OGTT [48–50]. The increased frequency of monitoring glucose changes during real-life settings for up to 10–14 days improves the chance to detect more glycemic abnormalities during basal and postprandial conditions compared to other short-timed methods [49, 50]. The use of CGM systems as diagnostic tools is still in development. More work is needed to establish and validate screening parameters and thresholds and more importantly to correlate these measurements with clinical outcomes in CF.

Significance of Early Glucose Abnormalities

While the significance of CFRD is relatively clear, investigators are also evaluating the impact of several prediabetes glucose tolerance categories on clinical outcomes (Table 16.3). Recent evidence suggests that these early glucose abnormalities are associated with clinical deterioration of pulmonary function and nutritional status [12, 14] and are predictors of future CFRD [51]. The CFF has recognized that impaired glucose tolerance (IGT) and indeterminate glycemia (INDET) may be important for the clinical status of patients with CF, but the impact of these conditions is unknown. Therefore, no specific guidelines for management have been recommended, except for close follow-up to detect the onset of CFRD [52].

The possibility that early insulin therapy may contribute to a sustained clinical state of mild glucose abnormalities in CF patients is inferred. Controlled clinical trials are in progress to determine the possible benefits of early insulin therapy (clinicaltrials.gov NCT01100892) or dipeptidyl peptidase-4 inhibitors (DPP-IV inhibitors, clinicaltrials.gov NCT01879228) in the CF population with IGT, INDET [53], or early CFRD. Similar studies using oral insulin secretagogues are needed.

Individuals with CF can also experience hypoglycemia following the OGTT and postprandially. It has been hypothesized that this may represent a stage preceding the onset of CFRD. However, several studies have failed to prove this hypothesis [54, 55]. The prevalence of hypoglycemia in CF patients during the OGTT varies in the literature and has been reported as high as 29% [55]. The etiology of hypoglycemia in CF is unknown, but may be caused by delayed first-phase insulin secretion together with a diminished glucagon response [5].

Table 16.3 Glucose tolerance categories in CF

Glucose tolerance category	Fasting glucose	1-Hour glucose	2-Hour glucose
Normal glucose tolerance (NGT)	<100 mg/dL (<5.5 mmol/L)	<140 mg/dL (<7.8 mmol/L)	<140 mg/dL (<7.8 mmol/L)
Impaired fasting glucose (IFG)	100–125 mg/dL (5.5–6.9 mmol/L)	N/A	<140 mg/dL (<7.8 mmol/L)
Impaired glucose tolerance (IGT)	< 100 mg/dL (<5.5 mmol/L)	N/A	140–199 mg/dL (7.8–11.1 mmol/L)
Indeterminate glycemia (INDET)	<126 mg/dL (<7.0 mmol/L)	≥200 mg/dL (11.1 mmol/L)	<140 mg/dL (<7.8 mmol/L)

Therapeutic Strategies in CFRD

Insulin Therapy

Insulin remains the only recommended treatment for CFRD [9, 56]. Insulin therapy improves glycemic control, nutritional parameters, and pulmonary function of patients with CFRD [20]. Patients with CFRD without fasting hyperglycemia may be treated with fast acting "bolus" insulin given preprandially. Bolus insulin is personalized and is calculated using an insulin-to-carbohydrate ratio or the ratio of the grams of carbohydrate that will be covered by one unit of fast-acting insulin. In patients with fasting hyperglycemia, long-acting "basal" insulin in combination with preprandial bolus insulin, delivered via injections or a pump device, should be considered. Frequently, a nocturnal feeding schedule is part of the routine of patients with CF. Therefore, the use of intermediate-acting NPH insulin together with regular insulin is a good choice in an effort to minimize sleep interruptions and optimize glucose control [5].

Insulin pumps are a particularly attractive option for patients with CFRD. The use of insulin pumps to provide multiple daily boluses may be advantageous to patients with CFRD who are often encouraged to consume frequent meals and snacks throughout the day to maintain a high caloric intake.

During acute pulmonary exacerbations or when using steroids, CFRD may initially manifest, and patients with existing CFRD typically require significantly higher doses of insulin due to increased insulin resistance. The insulin requirements may decrease rapidly once the acute exacerbation resolves; therefore, close monitoring of glycemic control is indicated to reduce the risk of hypoglycemia.

Use of Oral Antidiabetic Drugs and Incretin Mimetics in CF

The use of oral antidiabetic drugs in patients with CFRD is not currently recommended [9, 57]. As insulin resistance is not the major etiological factor in the development of CFRD, insulin sensitizers such as metformin are unlikely to control blood glucose in CFRD, and minimal studies have been conducted in individuals with CFRD [58–61]. Insulin resistance is more prevalent in the acute setting (i.e., CF exacerbations). However, metformin is not currently recommended in this setting due to a potential increased risk of lactic acidosis, concern for weight loss, and gastrointestinal side effects, as has been reported in individuals with type 2 diabetes mellitus.

Repaglinide is an oral hypoglycemic agent that has a short half-life and is used for postprandial glycemic control in type 2 diabetes. The largest clinical trial in subjects with CFRD or abnormal glucose tolerance compared therapy with either repaglinide, premeal insulin, or oral placebo [20]. All participants had weight loss in the year preceding treatment; however, the repaglinide-treated group had initial weight gain, but this was not sustained throughout the 6 months of therapy.

In the insulin-treated group, this pattern was reversed, and patients gained 0.39 BMI units after 1 year of therapy ($P < 0.02$). The placebo group continued to lose weight.

Incretin-based therapy, including glucagon-like peptide-1 receptor agonists and dipeptidyl peptidase-4 inhibitors, is routinely used in the management of type 2 diabetes [62]. The incretin hormones, glucagon-like peptide-1, and gastric inhibitory polypeptide, released from the gut in response to nutrients, regulate postprandial glycemia through an increase in insulin secretion [63]. Glucagon-like peptide-1 agonists have a lower risk of hypoglycemia compared to insulin, but have a potential risk of weight loss due to appetite reduction and the increased risk for pancreatitis with some of these medications. The weight loss and pancreatitis risks are significant drawbacks of glucagon-like peptide-1 receptor agonists that dipeptidyl peptidase-4 inhibitors are not associated with. However, there is no published data on glucagon-like peptide-1 agonists or dipeptidyl peptidase-4 inhibitors in the treatment of CFRD, and therefore, they are not currently recommended for CFRD treatment outside the context of clinical trials [56].

Nutritional Management

Nutritional management in CFRD includes maintenance of the recommended caloric intake [64]. The diagnosis of CFRD does not alter the usual CF dietary recommendations. CF patients require a very high-calorie, high-protein, high-fat, and high-salt diet that is 120–150% of the daily recommended caloric intake for age to compensate for both increased resting energy expenditure and increased loss of calories through malabsorption. Caloric restriction, unlike in patients with type 2 diabetes, is not recommended.

It is crucial to optimize pancreatic enzyme replacement because the fat maldigestion observed in patients with CF accelerates the absorption of carbohydrates resulting in postprandial hyperglycemia. Treatment of exocrine pancreatic insufficiency with pancreatic enzyme supplements has the benefit of reducing postprandial hyperglycemia, slowing gastric emptying, and augmenting incretin hormone secretion [26, 65].

Patients with CF may also present with hypoglycemia in the absence of glucose-lowering therapies, and nutritional strategies that address this issue have been published [66, 67]. The recommendations include a reduction in refined sugars if these are consumed in isolation between meals [66] and consuming carbohydrate-containing meals every 2 to 3 hours [67].

Management Goals

The ADA recommends that all patients on insulin therapy perform self-monitoring of blood glucose at least three times daily [9]. Continuous glucose monitoring has been validated in CF and may be useful for diabetes control in this population [68].

Current recommended blood glucose targets include a fasting or premeal glucose between 70 and 130 mg/dL in adults and a 2–3 hour postprandial glucose <180 in adolescents and adults and <200 mg/dL in children [9]. HbA1c is the standard method for assessing long-term glycemic control in CFRD. A HbA1c treatment goal of ≤7% (53 mmol/mol) is currently recommended to reduce the risk of microvascular complications, although the goal is not based upon CF-specific outcome studies [9].

Complications Associated with CFRD

Macrovascular complications are rarely seen in CF. Hypertriglyceridemia has been commonly described in CF patients, whereas cholesterol concentrations are generally low [69]. Hypertriglyceridemia may be related to chronic low-grade inflammation and has also been associated with increased insulin secretion but similar glucose excursion following ingestion of oral glucose solution in an OGTT, a pattern suggestive of insulin resistance [70]. Whether hypertriglyceridemia increases the risk of cardiovascular disease in individuals with CF is unknown, but as CF patients live longer, cardiovascular disease may emerge.

Microvascular complications have been observed in patients with the diagnosis of CFRD for longer than 10 years [71]. A study of 79 subjects with CFRD found that the prevalence of microalbuminuria was 21% and retinopathy was 10% [72]. Another recent study reported a prevalence of retinopathy of 42% in adult patients with CFRD [73]. Autonomic neuropathy was reported in 52% of patients with or without fasting hyperglycemia, and it was not clear if this was diabetes specific or related to CF [71]. Current ADA and CFF clinical care guidelines recommend starting annual screening for microvascular complications 5 years after diagnosis. If the exact time of diagnosis is unknown, screening should begin when fasting hyperglycemia is first diagnosed [9]. Measurement of blood pressure at quarterly diabetes visits is recommended per ADA guidelines. An annual lipid profile is only recommended in individuals with CFRD with pancreatic sufficiency or obesity, in those treated with immunosuppressive drugs following transplantation, or in those with a family history of coronary artery disease [9].

Future Perspectives

In recent decades, there has been a significant and remarkable improvement in the medical care of CF. These incredible efforts have resulted in a notable decrease in morbidity and progressive increase of survival time. The longer life expectancy and improved compliance with screening methods have made the early recognition and treatment of CFRD possible.

A clear priority is to identify ways to preserve β-cell function and to better understand the transition from early glucose abnormalities to the development of CFRD. It is important to ascertain new CFRD screening methods that lessen the burden currently encountered with the standard OGTT (cost, inconvenience, access to care). Screening enables detection of mild abnormalities in glucose and provides the opportunity for early intervention. Although mild glucose abnormalities are associated with poor clinical outcomes in CF, it is not known if early intervention in patients with CF with dysglycemia is beneficial to outcomes or preserving beta-cell function.

As new therapies continue to improve patient care in CF, particularly the use of CFTR modulators and potentiators from an early age, further studies are needed to explore the effects of these therapies on glucose tolerance and insulin secretion. Additionally, the contribution of incretin hormones in CFRD remains unclear, and the role of incretin-based medications needs to be further examined in CFRD. It is also important to establish whether alternative therapies are useful in CFRD and prospectively study the development of microvascular and macrovascular complications in this population.

References

1. Rowe S, Miller S, Sorscher E. Cystic fibrosis. N Engl J Med. 2005;352(19):1992–2001. https://doi.org/10.1136/bmj.39188.741944.47.
2. Moran A, Dunitz J, Nathan B, Saeed A, Holme B, Thomas W. Cystic fibrosis-related diabetes: current trends in prevalence, incidence, and mortality. Diabetes Care. 2009;32(9):1626–31. https://doi.org/10.2337/dc09-0586.
3. Stephenson AL, Sykes J, Stanojevic S, et al. Survival comparison of patients with cystic fibrosis in Canada and the United States: a population-based cohort study. Ann Intern Med. 2017; https://doi.org/10.7326/M16-0858.
4. Lewis C, Blackman SM, Nelson A, et al. Diabetes-related mortality in adults with cystic fibrosis. Role of genotype and sex. Am J Respir Crit Care Med. 2015;191(2):194–200. https://doi.org/10.1164/rccm.201403-0576OC.
5. Kelly A, Moran A. Update on cystic fibrosis-related diabetes. J Cyst Fibros. 2013;12(4):318–31. https://doi.org/10.1016/j.jcf.2013.02.008.
6. Marshall BC, Butler SM, Stoddard M, Moran AM, Liou TG, Morgan WJ. Epidemiology of cystic fibrosis-related diabetes. J Pediatr. 2005;146(5):681–7. https://doi.org/10.1016/j.jpeds.2004.12.039.
7. Adler AI, Shine BSF, Chamnan P, Haworth CS, Bilton D. Genetic determinants and epidemiology of cystic fibrosis-related diabetes: results from a British cohort of children and adults. Diabetes Care. 2008;31(9):1789–94. https://doi.org/10.2337/dc08-0466.
8. Bradbury RA, Shirkhedkar D, Glanville AR, Campbell LV. Prior diabetes mellitus is associated with increased morbidity in cystic fibrosis patients undergoing bilateral lung transplantation: an "orphan" area? A retrospective case-control study. Intern Med J. 2009; https://doi.org/10.1111/j.1445-5994.2008.01786.x.
9. Moran A, Brunzell C, Cohen RC, et al. Clinical care guidelines for cystic fibrosis-related diabetes: a position statement of the American Diabetes Association and a clinical practice guideline of the Cystic Fibrosis Foundation, endorsed by the Pediatric Endocrine Society. Diabetes Care. 2010;33(12):2697–708. https://doi.org/10.2337/dc10-1768.

10. Cucinotta D, De Luca F, Arrigo T, et al. First-phase insulin response to intravenous glucose in cystic fibrosis patients with different degrees of glucose tolerance. J Pediatr Endocrinol Metab. 1994;7(1):13–7. https://doi.org/10.1515/JPEM.1994.7.1.13.

11. Moran A, Becker D, Casella SJ, et al. Epidemiology, pathophysiology, and prognostic implications of cystic fibrosis-related diabetes: a technical review. Diabetes Care. 2010;33(12):2677–83. https://doi.org/10.2337/dc10-1279.

12. Finkelstein SM, Wielinski CL, Elliott GR, et al. Diabetes mellitus associated with cystic fibrosis. J Pediatr. 1988;112(3):373–7. https://doi.org/10.1016/S0022-3476(88)80315-9.

13. Lanng S, Thorsteinsson B, Røder ME, Nerup J, Koch C. Insulin sensitivity and insulin clearance in cystic fibrosis patients with normal and diabetic glucose tolerance. Clin Endocrinol. 1994;41(2):217–23. http://www.ncbi.nlm.nih.gov/pubmed/7923827. Accessed 13 April 2017.

14. Lanng S, Thorsteinsson B, Nerup J, Koch C. Influence of the development of diabetes mellitus on clinical status in patients with cystic fibrosis. Eur J Pediatr. 1992;151(9):684–7. http://www.ncbi.nlm.nih.gov/pubmed/1396931. Accessed 31 Jan 2016.

15. Milla CE, Warwick WJ, Moran A. Trends in pulmonary function in patients with cystic fibrosis correlate with the degree of glucose intolerance at baseline. Am J Respir Crit Care Med. 2000;162(3 Pt 1):891–5. https://doi.org/10.1164/ajrccm.162.3.9904075.

16. Ionescu AA, Evans WD, Pettit RJ, Nixon LS, Stone MD, Shale DJ. Hidden depletion of fat-free mass and bone mineral density in adults with cystic fibrosis. Chest. 2003;124(6):2220–8. https://doi.org/10.1378/chest.124.6.2220.

17. King SJ, Nyulasi IB, Strauss BJG, Kotsimbos T, Bailey M, Wilson JW. Fat-free mass depletion in cystic fibrosis: associated with lung disease severity but poorly detected by body mass index. Nutrition. 2010;26(7–8):753–9. https://doi.org/10.1016/j.nut.2009.06.026.

18. Engelen MPKJ, Schroder R, Van der Hoorn K, Deutz NEP, Com G. Use of body mass index percentile to identify fat-free mass depletion in children with cystic fibrosis. Clin Nutr. 2012;31(6):927–33. https://doi.org/10.1016/j.clnu.2012.04.012.

19. King SJ, Nyulasi IB, Bailey M, Kotsimbos T, Wilson JW. Loss of fat-free mass over four years in adult cystic fibrosis is associated with high serum interleukin-6 levels but not tumour necrosis factor-alpha. Clin Nutr. 2014;33(1):150. https://doi.org/10.1016/j.clnu.2013.04.012.

20. Moran A, Pekow P, Grover P, et al. Insulin therapy to improve BMI in cystic fibrosis-related diabetes without fasting hyperglycemia: results of the cystic fibrosis related diabetes therapy trial. Diabetes Care. 2009;32(10):1783–8. https://doi.org/10.2337/dc09-0585.

21. Kopelman H, Corey M, Gaskin K, Durie P, Weizman Z, Forstner G. Impaired chloride secretion, as well as bicarbonate secretion, underlies the fluid secretory defect in the cystic fibrosis pancreas. Gastroenterology. 1988;95(2):349–55. http://www.ncbi.nlm.nih.gov/pubmed/3391365. Accessed 28 Dec 2015.

22. Sheikh S, Gudipaty L, De Leon DD, et al. Reduced β-cell secretory capacity in pancreatic-insufficient, but not pancreatic-sufficient, cystic fibrosis despite normal glucose tolerance. Diabetes. 2017;19(7):1173–82. https://doi.org/10.2337/db16-0394.

23. Moran A, Pyzdrowski KL, Weinreb J, et al. Insulin sensitivity in cystic fibrosis. Diabetes. 1994;43(8):1020–6. http://www.ncbi.nlm.nih.gov/pubmed/8039595. Accessed 16 Feb 2017.

24. Moran A, Milla C, Ducret R, Nair KS. Protein metabolism in clinically stable adult cystic fibrosis patients with abnormal glucose tolerance. Diabetes. 2001;50(6):1336–43. https://doi.org/10.2337/diabetes.50.6.1336.

25. Hillman M, Eriksson L, Mared L, Helgesson K, Landin-Olsson M. Reduced levels of active GLP-1 in patients with cystic fibrosis with and without diabetes mellitus. J Cyst Fibros. 2012;11(2):144–9. https://doi.org/10.1016/j.jcf.2011.11.001.

26. Kuo P, Stevens JE, Russo A, et al. Gastric emptying, incretin hormone secretion, and postprandial glycemia in cystic fibrosis - effects of pancreatic enzyme supplementation. J Clin Endocrinol Metab. 2011;96(5):E851–5. https://doi.org/10.1210/jc.2010-2460.

27. Koivula FNM, McClenaghan NH, Harper AGS, Kelly C. Islet-intrinsic effects of CFTR mutation. Diabetologia. 2016;59(7):1350–5. https://doi.org/10.1007/s00125-016-3936-1.

28. Edlund A, Esguerra JLS, Wendt A, Flodström-Tullberg M, Eliasson L. CFTR and Anoctamin 1 (ANO1) contribute to cAMP amplified exocytosis and insulin secretion in human and murine pancreatic beta-cells. BMC Med. 2014;12:87. https://doi.org/10.1186/1741-7015-12-87.

29. Edlund A, Pedersen MG, Lindqvist A, Wierup N, Flodström-Tullberg M, Eliasson L. CFTR is involved in the regulation of glucagon secretion in human and rodent alpha cells. Sci Rep. 2017;7(1):90. https://doi.org/10.1038/s41598-017-00098-8.

30. Kelly A, DeLeon D, Sheikh S, et al. Islet hormone and incretin secretion in cystic fibrosis following 4-months of Ivacaftor therapy. Am J Respir Crit Care Med. 2018;199(3):342–51. https://doi.org/10.1164/rccm.201806-1018OC.

31. Bellin MD, Laguna T, Leschyshyn J, et al. Insulin secretion improves in cystic fibrosis following ivacaftor correction of CFTR: a small pilot study. Pediatr Diabetes. 2013;14(6):417–21. https://doi.org/10.1111/pedi.12026.

32. Ntimbane T, Mailhot G, Spahis S, et al. CFTR silencing in pancreatic β-cells reveals a functional impact on glucose-stimulated insulin secretion and oxidative stress response. Am J Physiol Endocrinol Metab. 2016;310(3):E200–12. https://doi.org/10.1152/ajpendo.00333.2015.

33. Hull RL, Gibson RL, McNamara S, et al. Islet interleukin-1β immunoreactivity is an early feature of cystic fibrosis that may contribute to β-cell failure. Diabetes Care. 2018;41(4):823–30. https://doi.org/10.2337/dc17-1387.

34. Cnop M, Welsh N, Jonas J-C, Jorns A, Lenzen S, Eizirik DL. Mechanisms of pancreatic -cell death in type 1 and type 2 diabetes: many differences, few similarities. Diabetes. 2005;54(Suppl 2):S97–107. https://doi.org/10.2337/diabetes.54.suppl_2.S97.

35. Ode KL, Frohnert B, Laguna T, et al. Oral glucose tolerance testing in children with cystic fibrosis Ode et al. Pediatr Diabetes. 2010;11(7):487–92. https://doi.org/10.1111/j.1399-5448.2009.00632.x.

36. Yi Y, Norris AW, Wang K, et al. Abnormal glucose tolerance in infants and young children with cystic fibrosis. Am J Respir Crit Care Med. 2016;194(8):974–80. https://doi.org/10.1164/rccm.201512-2518OC.

37. Lanng S, Thorsteinsson B, Pociot F, et al. Diabetes mellitus in cystic fibrosis: genetic and immunological markers. Acta Paediatr. 1993;82(2):150–4. https://doi.org/10.1111/j.1651-2227.1993.tb12628.x.

38. Charles RN, Kelley ML. Occurrence of diabetes mellitus in families of patients with cystic fibrosis of the pancreas. J Chronic Dis. 1961;14(4):381.

39. Blackman SM, Hsu S, Ritter SE, et al. A susceptibility gene for type 2 diabetes confers substantial risk for diabetes complicating cystic fibrosis. Diabetologia. 2009;52(9):1858–65. https://doi.org/10.1007/s00125-009-1436-2.

40. Jin T. Current understanding on role of the Wnt signaling pathway effector TCF7L2 in glucose homeostasis. Endocr Rev. 2016;37(3):254.

41. Derbel S, Doumaguet C, Hubert D, et al. Calpain 10 and development of diabetes mellitus in cystic fibrosis. J Cyst Fibros. 2006;5(1):47–51. https://doi.org/10.1016/j.jcf.2005.09.011.

42. Blackman SM, Commander CW, Watson C, et al. Genetic modifiers of cystic fibrosis-related diabetes. Diabetes. 2013; https://doi.org/10.2337/db13-0510.

43. Hardin DS, Grilley K, Baron BHK. Accelerated red blood cell turnover can invalidate the use of hemoglobin A1c as a diagnostic test for cystic fibrosis related diabetes (abstract). Pediatr Res. 1999;45:90A.

44. Lee KMN, Miller RJH, Rosenberg FM, Kreisman SH. Evaluation of glucose tolerance in cystic fibrosis: comparison of 50-g and 75-g tests. J Cyst Fibros. 2007;6(4):274–6. https://doi.org/10.1016/j.jcf.2006.10.008.

45. Godbout A, Hammana I, Potvin S, et al. No relationship between mean plasma glucose and glycated haemoglobin in patients with cystic fibrosis-related diabetes. Diabetes Metab. 2008;34(6 Pt 1):568–73. https://doi.org/10.1016/j.diabet.2008.05.010.

46. Selvin E, Francis LMA, Ballantyne CM, et al. Nontraditional markers of glycemia: Associations with microvascular conditions. Diabetes Care. 2011;34(4):960–7. https://doi.org/10.2337/dc10-1945.

47. Chan CL, Hope E, Thurston J, et al. Hemoglobin A1c accurately predicts continuous glucose monitoring-derived average glucose in youth and young adults with cystic fibrosis. Diabetes Care. 2018;41(7):1406–13. https://doi.org/10.2337/dc17-2419.
48. Clemente León M, Bilbao Gassó L, Moreno-Galdó A, et al. Oral glucose tolerance test and continuous glucose monitoring to assess diabetes development in cystic fibrosis patients. Endocrinol Diabetes Nutr. 2017;65(1):45–51. https://doi.org/10.1016/j.endinu.2017.08.008.
49. Taylor-Cousar JL, Janssen JS, Wilson A, et al. Glucose >200 mg/dL during continuous glucose monitoring identifies adult patients at risk for development of cystic fibrosis related diabetes. J Diabetes Res. 2016;2016:1527932. https://doi.org/10.1155/2016/1527932.
50. Leclercq A, Gauthier B, Rosner V, et al. Early assessment of glucose abnormalities during continuous glucose monitoring associated with lung function impairment in cystic fibrosis patients. J Cyst Fibros. 2014;13(4):478–84. https://doi.org/10.1016/j.jcf.2013.11.005.
51. Schmid K, Fink K, Holl RW, Hebestreit H, Ballmann M. Predictors for future cystic fibrosis-related diabetes by oral glucose tolerance test. J Cyst Fibros. 2014;13(1):80–5. https://doi.org/10.1016/j.jcf.2013.06.001.
52. Lavie M, Fisher D, Vilozni D, et al. Glucose intolerance in cystic fibrosis as a determinant of pulmonary function and clinical status. Diabetes Res Clin Pract. 2015;110(3):276–84. https://doi.org/10.1016/j.diabres.2015.10.007.
53. Moran A. The impact of insulin therapy on protein turnover in pre-diabetic cystic fibrosis patients. https://clinicaltrials.gov/ct2/show/record/NCT02496780?term=moran+antoinete&rank=1.
54. Radike K, Molz K, Holl RW, Poeter B, Hebestreit H, Ballmann M. Prognostic relevance of hypoglycemia following an oral glucose challenge for cystic fibrosis-related diabetes. Diabetes Care. 2011;34(4):e43. https://doi.org/10.2337/dc10-2286.
55. Mannik LA, Chang KA, Annoh PQK, et al. Prevalence of hypoglycemia during oral glucose tolerance testing in adults with cystic fibrosis and risk of developing cystic fibrosis-related diabetes. J Cyst Fibros. 2018;17(4):536–41. https://doi.org/10.1016/j.jcf.2018.03.009.
56. Moran A, Pillay K, Becker D, Granados A, Hameed S, Acerini CL. ISPAD clinical practice consensus guidelines 2018: management of cystic fibrosis-related diabetes in children and adolescents. Pediatr Diabetes. 2018;19(Suppl 27):64–74.
57. Mayer-Davis EJ, Kahkoska AR, Jefferies C, et al. ISPAD clinical practice consensus guidelines 2018: definition, epidemiology, and classification of diabetes in children and adolescents. Pediatr Diabetes. 2018;19:7–19. https://doi.org/10.1111/pedi.12773.
58. van den Berg HGH JM. Proof of principle. Treatment of cystic fibrosis-related diabetes: a possible role for complementary metformin? J Cyst Fibros. 2009;8:S82.
59. de Lind van Wijngaarden-van den Berg JMW, van der Meer R, HGMH. WS6.4. A placebo-controlled trial of insulin therapy with or without adjuvant metformin in patients with cystic fibrosis-related diabetes (CFRD). J Cyst Fibros. 2014;13:S12.
60. Onady GM, Stolfi A. Insulin and oral agents for managing cystic fibrosis-related diabetes. Cochrane Database Syst Rev. 2016; https://doi.org/10.1002/14651858.CD004730.pub4.
61. Brennan A, Elisaus P, Bianco B, Cottam S, Pickles J, Toffec K et al. Metformin tolerability in patients with CF. J Cyst Fibros. 2019;18(supplem) S142.
62. Dorsey JL, Becker MH, Al E. Standards of medical care in diabetes—2019. Diabetes Care/Am Diabetes Assoc. 2019;42(Suppl 1):S61–70. https://doi.org/10.2337/dc19-S006.
63. Ma J, Rayner CK, Jones KL, Horowitz M. Insulin secretion in healthy subjects and patients with type 2 diabetes - role of the gastrointestinal tract. Best Pract Res Clin Endocrinol Metab. 2009;23(4):413–24. https://doi.org/10.1016/j.beem.2009.03.009.
64. Borowitz D, Baker RD, Stallings V, et al. Consensus report on nutrition for pediatric patients with cystic fibrosis. J Pediatr Gastroenterol Nutr. 2002;35(3):246–59. https://doi.org/10.1097/01.MPG.0000025580.85615.14.
65. Perano S, Rayner CK, Couper J, Martin J, Horowitz M. Cystic fibrosis related diabetes - a new perspective on the optimal management of postprandial glycemia. J Diabetes Complicat. 2014;28(6):904–11. https://doi.org/10.1016/j.jdiacomp.2014.06.012.

66. Armaghanian N, Brand-Miller JC, Markovic TP, Steinbeck KS. Hypoglycaemia in cystic fibrosis in the absence of diabetes: a systematic review. J Cyst Fibros. 2016;15(3):274–84. https://doi.org/10.1016/j.jcf.2016.02.012.
67. Brunzell C, Hardin DS, Kogler A, Moran A, Schindler T. Managing Cystic Fibrosis-Related Diabetets (CFRD) - an instruction guide for patients and families. Cyst Fibros Found. 2015.
68. O'Riordan SMP, Hindmarsh P, Hill NR, et al. Validation of continuous glucose monitoring in children and adolescents with cystic fibrosis. Diabetes Care. 2009;32(6). http://care.diabetes-journals.org/content/32/6/1020.long. Accessed 7 April 2017.
69. Figueroa V, Milla C, Parks EJ, Schwarzenberg SJ, Moran A. Abnormal lipid concentrations in cystic fibrosis. Am J Clin Nutr. 2002;75(6):1005–11. https://doi.org/10.1093/ajcn/75.6.1005.
70. Ishimo MC, Belson L, Ziai S, et al. Hypertriglyceridemia is associated with insulin levels in adult cystic fibrosis patients. J Cyst Fibros. 2013;12(3):271–6. https://doi.org/10.1016/j.jcf.2012.08.012.
71. Schwarzenberg SJ, Thomas W, Olsen TW, et al. Microvascular complications in cystic fibrosis-related diabetes. Diabetes Care. 2007;30(5):1056–61. https://doi.org/10.2337/dc06-1576.
72. van den Berg JMW, Morton AM, Kok SW, Pijl H, Conway SP, Heijerman HGM. Microvascular complications in patients with cystic fibrosis-related diabetes (CFRD). J Cyst Fibros. 2008;7(6):515–9. https://doi.org/10.1016/j.jcf.2008.05.008.
73. Roberts R, Speight L, Lee J, et al. Retinal screening of patients with cystic fibrosis-related diabetes in Wales - a real eye opener. J Cyst Fibros. 2015; https://doi.org/10.1016/j.jcf.2014.07.014.

Chapter 17
Cystic Fibrosis-Related Bone Disease: Current Knowledge and Future Directions

Sophie Guérin, Isabelle Durieu, and Isabelle Sermet-Gaudelus

Patient Perspective

I am a 26 year old patient with cystic fibrosis. I was diagnosed at the age of 15 months, a few weeks after my brother was diagnosed, as newborn screening was not available at that time in France. My doctors always focused on the pulmonary and digestive problems that can occur in CF patients. During my childhood, my disease was very mild. I barely had any difficulties with pulmonary infection, and I do not have pancreatic insufficiency. My first significant pulmonary infection occurred when I was 18, necessitating my first intravenous antibiotic course.

I decided to begin medical studies and a fellowship in pediatrics. It was a very difficult time. I did all my internships at the hospital without telling anyone about my CF. I burnt myself out, and my infections started to become increasingly more frequent. I am now a pediatric resident, and over the years, I have learnt to talk about myself and my CF during my internships.

I underwent my first bone densitometry in 2016 when I transferred to the adult clinic. The results showed that I had osteoporosis, but I never had any previous symptoms. In 2017, my doctors detected bronchopulmonary aspergillosis and decided to start corticosteroid treatment in October 2017 at 60 mg per day for 1 month. The dosage was then decreased progressively to 15 mg, which I continued from January 2018 to December 2018, and now I take 12 mg per day.

S. Guérin
Service de Pneumologie et Allergologie Pédiatrique, Hôpital Necker Enfants Malades, Paris, France

I. Durieu
Centre de Reference de la Mucoviscidose, Centre Hospitalier Lyon Sud, Lyon, France

I. Sermet-Gaudelus (✉)
Service de Pneumologie et Allergologie Pédiatrique, Hôpital Necker Enfants Malades, Paris, France

Institut Necker Enfants Malades, INSERM U1151, Paris, France
e-mail: Isabelle.sermet@aphp.fr

© Springer Nature Switzerland AG 2020
S. D. Davis et al. (eds.), *Cystic Fibrosis*, Respiratory Medicine,
https://doi.org/10.1007/978-3-030-42382-7_17

In October 2018, I experienced my first spontaneous rib fracture. I had an x-ray which showed that my 8th right rib was broken. It was a terrible shock to me to accept that I had broken a bone spontaneously without any traumatic cause. My pain was very intense, barely tolerable. I had to use drugs like Tramadol and Nefopam. The pain started to decrease after 2 weeks, a 2 week period during which I was lying in my bed; every single motion was terribly painful, and coughing was torture (not practical for a CF patient!).

The 22nd December 2018, during a party with friends, I suddenly felt the exact same pain, at the exact same place in my chest. I had a panic attack; the idea of a fracture terrified me. I had difficulty breathing, and the pain started to become more intense. My brother took me to the nearest emergency center where they made the diagnosis: I had another rib fracture, the 9th rib this time, but still on the right side.

I was mentally destroyed. The idea of feeling the same pain was unbearable. This fracture happened to be less painful than the first one. I stayed at home for a few weeks as it healed, but I was more capable of moving and coughing than the first time.

In January 2019, I felt a terrible pain in my back after a cough. I could not move. After a few hours, the pain started to decrease, and I had a very normal day. But, in the evening when I laid in my bed, the pain started again. It was impossible for me to move in a lying position. It was excruciating. The days were ok; I could do pretty much everything. But, it was impossible for me to sleep. I had tough nights, crying because I was exhausted and unable to sleep because of the pain.

I had an MRI which confirmed the vertebral fracture (T11) and showed another old fracture (T8). I began a treatment using TERIPARATIDE (Forsteo) in February 2019. Later that month, during a cold, I broke a rib again, the 8th rib on the right side. This time, it was as painful as the first one in October, and I had to stay in bed, not moving, breathing gently and waiting for the pain to subside.

This is my experience as a CF patient. I probably always had osteoporosis, but started to have fractures only after corticosteroid treatment. I wanted to share it with you because I think that, maybe, I could have avoided these multiple fractures. Indeed, had I known that I already had osteoporosis prior to starting corticosteroid treatment, perhaps I could have started an anti-osteoporosis treatment at the same time, and I would not have had to experience all of this pain.

I think it is important to understand what patients with CF endure during periods of fractures. From the outside, we think that it is just a bone fracture, and everything will be ok; it will pass eventually. But from the inside, the pain, the shock, the inability to move and cough as we would like, is a terrible experience.

–Anonymous

Introduction

Cystic fibrosis (CF) affects over 70,000 patients worldwide. It is caused by the defect in cystic fibrosis transmembrane conductance regulator (CFTR) protein, a cAMP-dependent ion channel that is one of the main regulators of the transepithelial solute flow. An absent or a malfunctioning CFTR protein causes consequent imbalance in ion and fluid transport and, as a main clinical consequence, chronic infected obstructive bronchopathy [1]. The increased life span of patients with CF has led to the detection of new complications such as bone disease [2]. First reported in 1979, abnormal bone mineral density (BMD) is now evidenced in ~ 20% adults with CF, and its complications can cause difficulties in treatment management [3]. Recent investigations, however, suggest that these problems actually begin during childhood, especially at puberty [4].

Although nutritional deficits, chronic infection, vitamin D deficiency, hypogonadism, delayed puberty, and reduced physical activity may all jeopardize bone health in this population, the pathogenesis of low BMD in individuals with CF still remains uncertain. This chapter will review current pharmacologic interventions.

Epidemiology of CF-Related Bone Disease

Adult Studies

More than 70 reports have observed low bone mass and fractures in individuals with CF. In a systematic review involving 1055 patients with a median age of 28 years, the pooled prevalence of osteoporosis was 23.5% in 2010 (95% CI, 16.6–31.0) [5]. More recent cross-sectional studies reported that 20% of adults with CF have standard Z-scores (age-adjusted standard deviation scores) < −2 [6, 7], while 10–20% have T-scores (standard deviations compared with young healthy adults) < −2.5 [6, 8–10]. The prevalence of osteopenia defined by a T-score between −1 and −2.5 SDs has been reported to range from 34% [6] to 45% [9] and up to 58% [10]. Longitudinal cohort studies have demonstrated overall improvement in bone density, as highlighted by Conway et al., who compared BMD status in a cohort of adults followed in the same center between 2000 and 2012 [11]. In this center, prevalence of osteoporosis decreased from 18% to 6% and osteopenia from 48% to 33%. This was mainly due to improvements in respiratory and nutritional status. Several studies demonstrated a positive correlation between BMD and both forced expiratory volume in 1 second percent predicted (FEV$_1$%pred) and body mass index (BMI) [2, 11–13]. In patients with moderate CF disease, annual losses in BMD approach those experienced by women (from non-CF cohorts) following menopause, averaging losses of 0.1–0.5% per year at lumbar spine and 1 to 1.8% at total hip BMD [2, 14, 15].

Pediatric Studies

In children, several studies demonstrated that BMD may be defective in childhood [4, 16–18]. However most of the prepubertal children with mild disease do not display low BMD [19–24]. Deficits in BMD become apparent in adolescence [23].

Longitudinal studies make it possible to analyze the course of bone mass over time [25–27]. They suggest that inadequate bone mass accrual begins in childhood, where it is half that of healthy children [18] and may be aggravated during adolescence because of inadequate peak bone mass [28], with a loss of approximately one standard deviation (SD) every 6–8 years from the age of 5 years onward [29]. Another study reports no catch up for either lumbar spine (LS) or femoral neck (FN) BMD Z-scores over a 2-year period in mildly ill children or adolescents with low BMD Z-scores at the beginning of the study [16]. Although young people with CF may be maintaining normal growth in height, bone accrual is impaired in those with the poorest nutritional status and lung function [25]. Altogether, these data suggest that children and adolescents with CF fail to achieve adequate bone mass compared to their healthy counterparts.

Clinical Manifestations and Monitoring of Bone Disease in CF

Fractures

Several cross-sectional studies have observed a higher incidence of fractures in individuals with CF [2, 26]. More recent studies have confirmed excess fractures particularly in the vertebral spine (21% prevalence in a Canadian study and 27% in an Italian study) [27, 30]. In a German study, the fracture rate was 9.2-fold higher compared to an age-matched healthy control population. The probability of remaining free of any fracture for patients with CF at 25 years was significantly reduced to 40% compared to 84.6% in healthy controls ($p < 0.001$) [31]. Children with CF do not appear to be at increased risk for fractures [32].

Screening and Monitoring for Bone Mineral Content in CF-Related Bone Disease

Measurements of Bone Mineral Content

Dual-energy x-ray absorptiometry (DEXA) is the gold standard method for measuring bone mineral content (BMC) and bone mineral density (BMD) [33]. It provides measurement of areal (two-dimensional) bone mineral density (BMD, g/cm^2), that is, BMC within the bone envelope of the region of the skeleton scanned divided by its projected bone area. BMD is measured at the lumbar spine, the femoral neck but can be assessed for the total body. It is expressed as a T-score in comparison with bone density in young healthy adults. Osteoporosis is defined as a BMD more than 2.5 T-scores below the mean for age- and sex-matched normal values and osteopenia as BMD between 1 and 2.5 T-scores below the same mean.

However, while DEXA measurements have been shown to predict a fracture risk in postmenopausal women, this is not the case for children and younger adults. Measurements of BMD in children and young adults must be scored by Z-scores related to an age- and gender-matched population. In children, demineralization is classed as moderate for a Z-score between −1 and −2 and severe for a Z-score below −2. The current recommendations are to use Z-scores up to age 30 and T-scores for those older than 30 years [34].

A major caveat for areal BMD measurement in pediatric populations is that it fails to distinguish between changes in mineral density and bone size in growing children, because the depth, and therefore the volume, of the scanned bone is not measured. Most frequently in CF, the decrease in skeletal size and therefore bone area is more severe than the decrease in BMC, so that BMD deficits may be artifactually overestimated in the pediatric population [35]. Correction for height or bone size using bone mineral apparent density (BMAD) may improve the accuracy of the measurement [34].

Quantitative computed tomography (QCT) which provides a three-dimensional image allows assessment of bone microstructure using high-resolution peripheral QCT (HR-pQCT). These measurements show that tibial total trabecular and cortical volumetric BMD are significantly lower with fewer, more widely spaced trabecular plates, lower trabecular connectivity, and lower axial and torsional stiffness independent to limb length [36]. Studies in children also display controversial inconsistencies in findings [37, 38].

Monitoring BMD in CF Patients

Although screening and monitoring of BMD will vary between centers, children with more severe disease must be screened earlier. American guidelines recommend determining a baseline BMD in all adults with cystic fibrosis at age 18 and in children over the age of 8 with risk factors for poor bone health (ideal body weight below 90%, FEV_1%pred <50%, glucocorticoids >5 mg/d for more than 90 days/year, delayed puberty, or history of fractures) [39]. European and French guidelines recommend a first baseline assessment at 8 years of age [34]. Individuals with T- or Z-scores of −1 or better should not need repeat DEXA monitoring for 5 years unless there is a change in risk factors. Individuals between −1 and −2 should have a repeat DEXA scan every 2–4 years and every year for those below −2 [34, 39].

Risk Factors for CF-Related Bone Disease and Prevention Strategies

Preventive care is based on a multifaceted approach including maintenance of good respiratory function and nutrition and treatment of bronchial exacerbations while aggressively promoting maintenance of lean body mass [34, 39]. Oral and even inhaled steroids should be avoided as much as possible based on a wealth of information mostly outside the arena of CF research.

Physical Activity

Physical activity is positively correlated to bone mineralization in CF [40]. Weight-bearing activity maintains bone mass at the proximal femur by a heightened anabolic skeletal response to mechanical force [41]. Weight-bearing activity is recommended and may be associated with gains in BMD [42–44].

Nutrition

Low BMD is significantly associated with malnutrition [4, 34]; however, significant demineralization is also reported in normal-weight patients with normal nutritional status highlighting the relationship between BMD and lean body mass (LBM) [4, 45, 46]. This may reflect the role of the muscle in bone health by exerting mechanical forces on the bone [47] but also indirectly the deficit of insulin-like growth factor-1 (IGF-1), a growth factor implicated simultaneously in protein anabolism and in endocrine and paracrine regulation of osteoblast proliferation and differentiation [48].

Calcium Metabolism

A calcium-rich diet is imperative, especially in adolescence, where increased requirements lay vital foundations for bone development. High urine calcium can be observed linked to high natriuresis because of CF patients' high-salt diet [49]. Calcium accretion may be diminished, possibly related to a deficit of IGF-1 but also because of inadequate osteocalcin and leptin, especially in prepubertal and late-pubertal girls [50].

Vitamin D

The prevalence of vitamin D insufficiency (serum 25-hydroxyvitamin D 25(OH)D <30 ng/ml) and deficiency (serum 25(OH)D <20 ng/ml) in CF is high [32, 51]. Concentrations of 25(OH)D <30 ng/ml cause parathyroid stimulation, impair intestinal Ca absorption, and induce bone resorption [52]. There is no relation between serum vitamin D concentration and BMD [23, 53–55]. But vitamin D may also modulate non-skeletal functions, including muscle strength, innate antimicrobial defense by upregulating antimicrobial peptides such as human cathelicidin [56], immune response [57], and control of chronic inflammatory response [58]. This may be especially important, with regard to pulmonary disease severity, as suggested by Vanstone [59].

High-dose vitamin D may improve outcomes of pulmonary exacerbation, including increased survival and number of hospital-free days over 1 year, with more patients returning to their pre-exacerbation FEV_1 values in comparison with placebo controls. This was associated with a decrease in inflammatory markers including tumor necrosis factor-α (TNFα) and interleukin-6 (IL-6) [60]. The recommended doses are 800 IU in infants, 800–1200 IU daily in children older than 1 year, 50,000 IU once a month, or 100,000 IU every quarter [34, 39]. This is inadequate for patients with vitamin D deficiency (usually defined as a 25(OH)D concentration below the normative range) or vitamin D insufficiency (<30 ng/ml).

Ergocalciferol (vitamin D2) is less efficient than cholecalciferol (vitamin D3) in increasing serum 25(OH)D [61]. In reported cases of low concentration, loading doses of 50,000 IU weekly for 8 weeks [62] or 100,000 UI weekly [63] resulted in marked improvements in 25(OH)D concentrations. Alternatively, more polar compounds, such as calcifediol or calcitriol, may be more effective in improving calcium homeostasis [64]. In terms of appropriate dosing, the response to vitamin D may also depend on several other factors such as variations in genes involved in vitamin D metabolism or function, and thus a given dose will not necessarily translate into the same serum 25(OH)D concentrations. Moreover, higher doses than those currently recommended for bone health may be needed to observe modulation of immune and inflammatory responses. Finally, it must be kept in mind that high serum concentrations above 30 ng/ml can be associated with hypercalciuria and increased risk of nephrolithiasis. Moreover, the 30 ng/ml cutoff proposed by Holick is designed to keep parathyroid hormone (PTH) concentrations as low as possible [52]. This is beneficial in cases where the bone defect is due to increased bone resorption. This may however be detrimental in children and young adults where PTH concentration in the high normal range is needed to stimulate bone formation, highlighting the need to monitor 25(OH)D and PTH [65]. Studies are needed to evaluate the potential role of vitamin D as adjunctive therapy in CF beyond its impact upon bone density and to consider the long-term consequences of maintaining 25(OH)D concentrations above 30 ng/ml in the context of the increased survival of adults with CF.

Vitamin K

Vitamin K is a carboxylase cofactor transforming glutamate into gamma-carboxylated residues. The non-carboxylated prothrombin and osteocalcin are functionally inactive. A deficiency in carboxylated-functional osteocalcin is frequently found in patients with CF together with low BMD and reduced bone formation markers [66].

Vitamin K supplementation increases carboxylated osteocalcin after 1 month of daily supplementation with 1 mg of vitamin K [67]. However, the only study published thus far shows an increase in carboxylated serum osteocalcin, without any effect on bone mineralization [68]. A supplementation of 1 mg/d or 10 mg/week increased to 1–5 mg/d in cases of low vitamin K level is recommended [34]. These doses have been shown to improve bone biochemical markers leading to reduced bone resorption and improved bone formation in CF. In the absence of studies, European guidelines recommend a higher dose with a starting dose in infants with CF of at least 0.5 mg to 2 mg/day and in children above 1 year of age to adults with CF of at least 1–10 mg/day.

Gaps in Knowledge and Future Directions

Bone is permanently remodeled in a process where old bone is replaced by new bone. After resorption of mineralized bone, recruited osteoblasts form new bone which is further mineralized in these resorption cavities. In the growing child, the bone shape and structure is sculpted by bone modeling. In the young adult, bone resorption equals bone formation resulting in remodeling balance (Fig. 17.1). Endocrine disorders and inflammation result in a negative remodeling balance. The decision and choice of medication in those patients with severe bone defect should be made on a case-by-case basis considering the patient's history in collaboration with an endocrinologist.

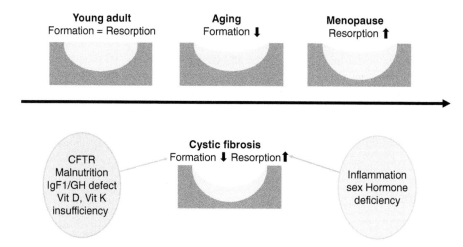

Fig. 17.1 Complex pathogenesis of cystic fibrosis-related bone disease

Endocrine Disorders

Low Bone Turnover, Delayed Puberty, and Sex Hormone Deficiency

The amount of bone mineral content is linked to body size, and peak bone accrual is influenced by both sex steroids and growth hormone [68]. Thus, endocrine disorders impact bone health. Puberty is a crucial period for the development of bone density because peak bone accrual occurs during the time of peak growth velocity [69]. The reduction in bone formation at this age may be due to delayed puberty. In a recent study, the age of peak height velocity (HV) as a marker of the onset of puberty was delayed by 9–10 months in boys and 10–14 months in girls. Girls with CF reach menarche 2 years later than their healthy peers [70]. However, a recent retrospective study including 729 contemporary children with CF showed that delayed onset of puberty was not a common occurrence [71].

Indeed, pubertal delay in CF has been usually attributed to chronic disease and/or poor nutrition [72]; however, it could also occur in the setting of good nutritional and clinical status. This finding along with recent evidence that CFTR can directly modulate the reproductive endocrine axis raises the possibility that some of pubertal delay in CF could stem directly from alterations in CFTR function and increased level of proinflammatory cytokines that affect the hypothalamic-pituitary-gonadal axis and induce growth hormone (GH) resistance [73].

All these data strongly suggest that pubertal delay of CF children may play an important role in suboptimal peak bone mass acquisition leading to particular risk for osteoporosis in these patients. Delayed puberty in patients with CF is associated with reduced concentrations of sex hormones in adolescents with CF compared to age-matched controls [74]. However, no studies with hormone replacement therapy have been conducted thus far to determine the benefits on bone mass content.

Growth Impairment and Growth Hormone Defects

Studies of growth in CF suggests that nutritional issues and pulmonary disease are not sufficient to explain growth abnormalities. Poor growth in CF is already seen in the neonatal period, as well as a reduction in systemic IGF-1 on blood spot screening [75, 76]. Whether this is due to underlying chronic inflammation or other unknown factors is unclear. In adolescence, further worsening of pubertal disorders and CF-related diabetes may herald or worsen the onset of CF-related bone disease. The complex interplay between CFTR genotype, inflammation, and nutritional and endocrine perturbations on the bone requires further investigation. Low IGF-1 and IGF binding protein-2 or IGF binding protein-3 (IGFBP-2 or IGFBP-3) are reported in studies in children with CF in association with lean body mass and poor growth. Alternatively, "normal" IGF-1 in the context of growth failure in CF could also point to IGF-1 resistance [77, 78].

Intervention targeted to improve growth may be beneficial for bone health in CF, and therefore recombinant human growth hormone (rhGH) treatment, first limited to GH deficient children, is now expanded to other clinical conditions not necessarily related to short stature. To date, there are six RCTs of rhGH therapy on linear growth in children with CF. Change in height standard deviation score (SDS) with rhGH treatment over 12 months in CF demonstrated that height velocity peaks up to 180% higher than the control group. rhGH treatment can be associated with pubertal progression, reduction in the number of IV courses, significant improvement in exercise tolerance, and maximal oxygen uptake increase in FVC%pred [79–82]. The latter might be related to an increase in absolute lung volume as a result of increased growth, improvement in lean body mass via the potential anabolic effect of rhGH, as well as possible role of macrophage killing capacity and even a potential role of IGF-1 on CFTR expression [83, 84].

For all these reasons, GH treatment could be an important therapy for patients with CF with insufficient bone mineral content. However, all studies conducted thus far have not yet clarified issues about patient selection and appropriate long-term use.

Accelerated Bone Resorption, Inflammation, and Antiresorptive Drugs

Inflammation

Studies of biochemical markers of bone turnover suggest an imbalance with bone resorption exceeding formation. Accelerated bone resorption occurs while serum undercarboxylated osteocalcin concentrations are low [85, 86].

Increased inflammatory cytokines such as TNFα, PTH, vascular endothelial growth factor (VEGF), and interleukins IL-1, IL-6, and IL-11 cause bone breakdown during bronchial exacerbations by stimulating osteoclast precursors [85–87]. This is illustrated by the association between serum concentrations of IL-6, IL-1, TNFα, and the bone resorption markers N-telopeptide (NTx) and deoxypyridinoline (Dpd) [88] and annual declines in BMD [87]. All of these abnormalities improve dramatically after antibiotic treatment of bronchial exacerbations. Serum RANK-L (molecule receptor activator of NFκB ligand) also follows the same pattern [6, 86, 89]. This proinflammatory cytokine is expressed by osteogenic cells including osteoblasts and by binding its RANK receptor onto osteoclast progenitor cells promotes osteoclast differentiation and consequent bone resorption. Osteoprotegerin (OPG), a soluble decoy receptor that binds to RANK ligand (RANKL) and inhibits its resorptive effect, seems to be decreased in patients with CF as compared to controls [85, 89]. This imbalance between RANK/RANKL and OPG is a major determinant of bone resorption in CF, as already also demonstrated in other inflammatory diseases [68].

Specificity of the Transplanted Patient

Pre-transplant patients with CF frequently have low reported BMD [90]. Immunosuppression may exacerbate pre-existing low BMD, and lung transplant recipients have declines of 1–5% in spinal and femoral BMD during the first 6–12 months after transplant [91]. However, these studies have included only a few individuals with CF, and it appears that BMD tends to remain more stable for adults with CF after lung transplantation than for other patient groups despite immunosuppression and may even improve. This suggests that the benefits of removing suppurative lungs counterbalance the adverse impact of immunosuppressants on the bone [92, 93].

Antiresorptive Agents

Antiresorptive agents inhibit the recruitment and the activity of osteoclasts. This in turn reduces the number of resorption cavities, thus decreasing the rate of remodeling which is in turn associated with secondary mineralization of the bone.

Bisphosphonates

Nine clinical trials assessing treatment with bisphosphonates for osteoporosis in people with CF were identified in a Cochrane review. Seven studies (with a total of 237 adult participants) were included, including 1 in lung transplant patients [94]. Pamidronate (30 mg IV every 3 months) was the first bisphosphonate used in adults with CF because it circumvented the potential problems related to malabsorption of an oral bisphosphonate [95]. The other bisphosphonates tested were oral alendronate, 10 mg once daily [94] or 70 mg once weekly [14]. Zoledronic acid, a new-generation IV bisphosphonate, showed benefit in a 2-year, multicenter Australian trial, but bone pain led to 20% patient dropout [15].

There was no significant reduction in fractures between treatment and control groups at 12 and 24 months. Studies reported significant improvement at 6, 12, and 24 months in bone mineral density of the lumbar spine, the hip, or the femur, with the more potent zoledronate. In participants with a lung transplant, although intravenous pamidronate did not change the number of new fractures, bone mineral density increased in the lumbar spine [92].

Although clinical trials show positive data, there are also many reports of failure of bisphosphonates to improve BMD, highlighting the need to clarify the indications of these drugs in the context of CF. Severe bone pain and flu-like symptoms may occur with intravenous agents which may possibly be prevented by steroids. Bisphosphonates can lead to potential severe complications such as jaw osteonecrosis, and most importantly in children, it can lead to brittle bones with long-term use, as has been shown in osteogenesis imperfecta and cerebral palsy-related osteoporosis. Moreover in this population, long-term adverse effects are not known, such as potential effects on developing fetal skeleton if subsequent pregnancy in life. Currently it is unclear when to stop giving these medications. The drugs are still excreted in the urine 8 years after stopping [96]. Thus, additional trials are needed to determine a long-term strategy (e.g., to determine the optimal (shortest) duration and indication for "drug holidays"). The European Guidelines recommend indication of bisphosphonates in children and adolescents with reductions in bone mass/density associated with low-trauma extremity fractures and symptomatic vertebral compression and for patients with BMD < −2 Z-score on the transplant list in anticipation of high-dose steroid therapy [34].

Denosumab

Denosumab is a human monoclonal antibody which acts as a RANKL inhibitor. The great advantage is subcutaneous administration every 6 months. Its potent effect on BMD increases over 10 years of treatment [97]. Studies on populations other than postmenopausal women are lacking.

Reduced Bone Formation, CFTR Defect, and Anabolic Drugs

Anabolic skeletal effects can be achieved through increase in bone formation or bone remodeling.

Bone Remodeling and Anabolic Agents

Teriparatide is a recombinant protein form of PTH, consisting of the first 34 amino acids, which is the bioactive portion of the hormone. When administered daily by subcutaneous injection for 18–24 months, it reduces the risk of fracture [98]. A small number of patients have been treated with success [99]. Abaloparatide, a synthetic analogue of parathyroid hormone-related protein (PTHrP), has skeletal effects similar to teriparatide.

Bone Modeling and CFTR Defect

Murine animal models of CF bone disease where lung infections did not develop have allowed the study of bone biology without the confounding effect of systemic inflammation. These would suggest a primary bone defect due to the absence of CFTR [100–103]. Recent findings in the young *Cftr−/−* rats demonstrated a reduced size of the growth plate and decreased IGF-1 concentrations for this phenotype

[104]. Mechanistically, keratin 8 (Krt8) deletion in F508del-Cftr mice corrected overactive NFκB signaling and decreased Wnt-β-catenin signaling induced by the F508del-Cftr mutation in osteoblasts. Disruption of the Krt8-F508del-Cftr interaction corrected the abnormal NFκB and Wnt-β-catenin signaling and the altered phenotypic gene expression in F508del-Cftr osteoblasts and normalized bone formation in F508del-Cftr mice [105, 106].

CFTR seems to be expressed in osteoblasts but not osteoclasts [107]. Resting CF osteoblasts demonstrate a strong expression of RANKL, whereas OPG production is defective under TNFα stimulation, leading to an elevated RANKL-to-OPG protein ratio in CF osteoblasts in inflammatory conditions. The link to CFTR defect is provided by the fact that (i) these observations are replicated by pharmacological inhibition of CFTR chloride channel conductance in non-CF osteoblasts and (ii) CFTR correctors such as C18 significantly reduce the production of RANKL by CF osteoblasts [108]. Recent studies suggest an improvement of bone disease upon treatment with ivacaftor [109]. Altogether these data suggest an intrinsic role of CFTR in bone formation and an indirect role in promoting bone resorption.

Conclusion

Altogether, decreased bone mineralization is clearly one of the characteristic features of adults with CF. Efforts to obtain and maintain normal bone status is one element for maintaining a good quality of life for these patients. The opportunity to influence bone mineralization appears to be greatest during childhood and adolescence. We recommend that all patients with CF undergo assessment of BMD to make it possible to target those who need active care. Complete elucidation of the mechanisms causing this bone defect should help to redefine therapeutic strategies. There is urgent need for studies to assess the impact of CFTR modulation on bone health and medications other than bisphosphonates, in patients with severe bone defects.

References

1. Rowe SM, Miller S, Sorscher EJ. Cystic fibrosis. N Engl J Med. 2005;352:1992–2001.
2. Haworth CS, Selby PL, Webb AK, et al. Low bone mineral density in adults with cystic fibrosis. Thorax. 1999;54:961–7.
3. Mischler EH, Chesney PJ, Chesney RW, et al. Demineralization in cystic fibrosis detected by direct photon absorptiometry. Am J Dis Child. 1979;133:632–5.
4. Sermet-Gaudelus I, Souberbielle JC, Ruiz JC, et al. Low bone mineral density in young children with cystic fibrosis. Am J Respir Crit Care Med. 2007;175:951–7.
5. Paccou J, Zeboulon N, Combescure C, et al. The prevalence of osteoporosis, osteopenia, and fractures among adults with cystic fibrosis: a systematic literature review with meta-analysis. Calcif Tissue Int. 2010;86:1–7.

6. Gensburger D, Boutroy S, Chapurlat R, et al. Reduced bone volumetric density and weak correlation between infection and bone markers in cystic fibrosis adult patients. Osteoporos Int. 2016;27:2803–13.

7. Vanacor R, Raimundo FV, Marcondes NA, et al. Prevalence of low bone mineral density in adolescents and adults with cystic fibrosis. Rev Assoc Med Bras (1992). 2014;60:53–8.

8. Putman MS, Baker JF, Uluer A, et al. Trends in bone mineral density in young adults with cystic fibrosis over a 15 year period. J Cyst Fibros. 2015;14:526–32.

9. Sheikh S, Gemma S, Patel A. Factors associated with low bone mineral density in patients with cystic fibrosis. J Bone Miner Metab. 2015;33:180–5.

10. Legroux-Gérot I, Leroy S, Prudhomme C, et al. Bone loss in adults with cystic fibrosis: prevalence, associated factors, and usefulness of biological markers. Joint Bone Spine. 2012;79:73–7.

11. Conway SP, Morton AM, Oldroyd B, et al. Osteoporosis and osteopenia in adults and adolescents with cystic fibrosis: prevalence and associated factors. Thorax. 2000;55:798–804.

12. Mathiesen IH, Pressler T, Oturai P, et al. Osteoporosis is associated with deteriorating clinical status in adults with cystic fibrosis. Int J Endocrinol. 2018;2018:4803974.

13. Smith N, Lim A, Yap M, et al. Bone mineral density is related to lung function outcomes in young people with cystic fibrosis-a retrospective study. Pediatr Pulmonol. 2017;52:1558–64.

14. Papaioannou A, Kennedy CC, Freitag A, et al. Alendronate once weekly for the prevention and treatment of bone loss in Canadian adult cystic fibrosis patients (CFOS trial). Chest. 2008;134:794–800.

15. Chapman I, Greville H, Ebeling PR, et al. Intravenous zoledronate improves bone density in adults with cystic fibrosis (CF). Clin Endocrinol. 2009;70:838–46.

16. Gronowitz E, Garemo M, Lindblad A, et al. Decreased bone mineral density in normal-growing patients with cystic fibrosis. Acta Paediatr. 2003;92:688–93.

17. Ujhelyi R, Treszl A, Vásárhelyi B, et al. Bone mineral density and bone acquisition in children and young adults with cystic fibrosis: a follow-up study. J Pediatr Gastroenterol Nutr. 2004;38:401–6.

18. Bianchi ML, Romano G, Saraifoger S, et al. BMD and body composition in children and young patients affected by cystic fibrosis. J Bone Miner Res. 2006;21:388–96.

19. Grey V, Atkinson S, Drury D, et al. Prevalence of low bone mass and deficiencies of vitamins D and K in pediatric patients with cystic fibrosis from 3 Canadian centers. Pediatrics. 2008;122:1014–20.

20. Caldeira RJ do A, Fonseca V de M, Gomes SCDS, et al. Prevalence of bone mineral disease among adolescents with cystic fibrosis. J Pediatr. 2008;84:18–25.

21. Donadio MVF, de Souza GC, Tiecher G, et al. Bone mineral density, pulmonary function, chronological age, and age at diagnosis in children and adolescents with cystic fibrosis. J Pediatr. 2013;89:151–7.

22. Lucidi V, Bizzarri C, Alghisi F, et al. Bone and body composition analyzed by Dual-energy X-ray Absorptiometry (DXA) in clinical and nutritional evaluation of young patients with Cystic Fibrosis: a cross-sectional study. BMC Pediatr. 2009;9:61.

23. Buntain HM, Greer RM, Schluter PJ, et al. Bone mineral density in Australian children, adolescents and adults with cystic fibrosis: a controlled cross sectional study. Thorax. 2004;59:149–55.

24. Bravo MP, Balboa P, Torrejón C, et al. Bone mineral density, lung function, vitamin D and body composition in children and adolescents with cystic fibrosis: a multicenter study. Nutr Hosp. 2018;35:789–95.

25. Sharma S, Jaksic M, Fenwick S, et al. Accrual of bone mass in children and adolescents with cystic fibrosis. J Clin Endocrinol Metab. 2017;102:1734–9.

26. Elkin SL, Fairney A, Burnett S, et al. Vertebral deformities and low bone mineral density in adults with cystic fibrosis: a cross-sectional study. Osteoporos Int. 2001;12:366–72.

27. Papaioannou A, Kennedy CC, Freitag A, et al. Longitudinal analysis of vertebral fracture and BMD in a Canadian cohort of adult cystic fibrosis patients. BMC Musculoskelet Disord. 2008;9:125.
28. Bhudhikanok GS, Wang MC, Marcus R, et al. Bone acquisition and loss in children and adults with cystic fibrosis: a longitudinal study. J Pediatr. 1998;133:18–27.
29. Henderson RC, Madsen CD. Bone density in children and adolescents with cystic fibrosis. J Pediatr. 1996;128:28–34.
30. Rossini M, Viapiana O, Del Marco A, et al. Quantitative ultrasound in adults with cystic fibrosis: correlation with bone mineral density and risk of vertebral fractures. Calcif Tissue Int. 2007;80:44–9.
31. Stahl M, Holfelder C, Kneppo C, et al. Multiple prevalent fractures in relation to macroscopic bone architecture in patients with cystic fibrosis. J Cyst Fibros. 2018;17:114–20.
32. Rovner AJ, Zemel BS, Leonard MB, et al. Mild to moderate cystic fibrosis is not associated with increased fracture risk in children and adolescents. J Pediatr. 2005;147:327–31.
33. Raisz LG. Clinical practice. Screening for osteoporosis. N Engl J Med. 2005;353:164–71.
34. Sermet-Gaudelus I, Bianchi ML, Garabédian M, et al. European cystic fibrosis bone mineralisation guidelines. J Cyst Fibros. 2011;10(Suppl 2):S16–23.
35. Schoenau E, Land C, Stabrey A, et al. The bone mass concept: problems in short stature. Eur J Endocrinol. 2004;151 Suppl 1:S87–91.
36. Nishiyama KK, Agarwal S, Kepley A, et al. Adults with cystic fibrosis have deficits in bone structure and strength at the distal tibia despite similar size and measuring standard and relative sites. Bone. 2018;107:181–7.
37. O'Brien CE, Com G, Fowlkes J, et al. Peripheral quantitative computed tomography detects differences at the radius in prepubertal children with cystic fibrosis compared to healthy controls. PLoS One. 2018;13:e0191013.
38. Braun C, Bacchetta J, Braillon P, et al. Children and adolescents with cystic fibrosis display moderate bone microarchitecture abnormalities: data from high-resolution peripheral quantitative computed tomography. Osteoporos Int. 2017;28:3179–88.
39. Aris RM, Merkel PA, Bachrach LK, et al. Guide to bone health and disease in cystic fibrosis. J Clin Endocrinol Metab. 2005;90:1888–96.
40. Tejero S, Cejudo P, Quintana-Gallego E, et al. The role of daily physical activity and nutritional status on bone turnover in cystic fibrosis: a cross-sectional study. Braz J Phys Ther. 2016;20:206–12.
41. Dodd JD, Barry SC, Barry RBM, et al. Bone mineral density in cystic fibrosis: benefit of exercise capacity. J Clin Densitom. 2008;11:537–42.
42. MacKelvie KJ, Petit MA, Khan KM, et al. Bone mass and structure are enhanced following a 2-year randomized controlled trial of exercise in prepubertal boys. Bone. 2004;34:755–64.
43. Frangolias DD, Paré PD, Kendler DL, et al. Role of exercise and nutrition status on bone mineral density in cystic fibrosis. J Cyst Fibros. 2003;2:163–70.
44. Britto MT, Garrett JM, Konrad TR, et al. Comparison of physical activity in adolescents with cystic fibrosis versus age-matched controls. Pediatr Pulmonol. 2000;30:86–91.
45. Ionescu AA, Evans WD, Pettit RJ, et al. Hidden depletion of fat-free mass and bone mineral density in adults with cystic fibrosis. Chest. 2003;124:2220–8.
46. Baker JF, Putman MS, Herlyn K, et al. Body composition, lung function, and prevalent and progressive bone deficits among adults with cystic fibrosis. Joint Bone Spine. 2016;83:207–11.
47. Kelly A, Schall J, Stallings VA, et al. Trabecular and cortical bone deficits are present in children and adolescents with cystic fibrosis. Bone. 2016;90:7–14.
48. Yakar S, Werner H, Rosen CJ. Insulin-like growth factors: actions on the skeleton. J Mol Endocrinol. 2018;61:T115–37.
49. Turner MA, Goldwater D, David TJ. Oxalate and calcium excretion in cystic fibrosis. Arch Dis Child. 2000;83:244–7.

50. Schulze KJ, Cutchins C, Rosenstein BJ, et al. Calcium acquisition rates do not support age-appropriate gains in total body bone mineral content in prepuberty and late puberty in girls with cystic fibrosis. Osteoporos Int. 2006;17:731–40.

51. Wolfenden LL, Judd SE, Shah R, et al. Vitamin D and bone health in adults with cystic fibrosis. Clin Endocrinol. 2008;69:374–81.

52. Holick MF. Vitamin D deficiency. N Engl J Med. 2007;357:266–81.

53. Buntain HM, Schluter PJ, Bell SC, et al. Controlled longitudinal study of bone mass accrual in children and adolescents with cystic fibrosis. Thorax. 2006;61:146–54.

54. Stephenson A, Brotherwood M, Robert R, et al. Cholecalciferol significantly increases 25-hydroxyvitamin D concentrations in adults with cystic fibrosis. Am J Clin Nutr. 2007;85:1307–11.

55. Greer RM, Buntain HM, Potter JM, et al. Abnormalities of the PTH-vitamin D axis and bone turnover markers in children, adolescents and adults with cystic fibrosis: comparison with healthy controls. Osteoporos Int. 2003;14:404–11.

56. Yim S, Dhawan P, Ragunath C, et al. Induction of cathelicidin in normal and CF bronchial epithelial cells by 1,25-dihydroxyvitamin D(3). J Cyst Fibros. 2007;6:403–10.

57. Hewison M. Vitamin D and the intracrinology of innate immunity. Mol Cell Endocrinol. 2010;321:103–11.

58. Herscovitch K, Dauletbaev N, Lands LC. Vitamin D as an anti-microbial and anti-inflammatory therapy for Cystic Fibrosis. Paediatr Respir Rev. 2014;15:154–62.

59. Vanstone MB, Egan ME, Zhang JH, et al. Association between serum 25-hydroxyvitamin D level and pulmonary exacerbations in cystic fibrosis. Pediatr Pulmonol. 2015;50:441–6.

60. Grossmann RE, Zughaier SM, Kumari M, et al. Pilot study of vitamin D supplementation in adults with cystic fibrosis pulmonary exacerbation: a randomized, controlled trial. Dermatoendocrinol. 2012;4:191–7.

61. Khazai NB, Judd SE, Jeng L, et al. Treatment and prevention of vitamin D insufficiency in cystic fibrosis patients: comparative efficacy of ergocalciferol, cholecalciferol, and UV light. J Clin Endocrinol Metab. 2009;94:2037–43.

62. Simoneau T, Sawicki GS, Milliren CE, et al. A randomized controlled trial of vitamin D replacement strategies in pediatric CF patients. J Cyst Fibros. 2016;15:234–41.

63. Sermet-Gaudelus I, Castanet M, Souberbielle J-C, et al. [Bone health in cystic fibrosis]. Arch Pediatr. 2009;16:616–18.

64. Brown SA, Ontjes DA, Lester GE, et al. Short-term calcitriol administration improves calcium homeostasis in adults with cystic fibrosis. Osteoporos Int. 2003;14:442–9.

65. Chapelon E, Garabedian M, Brousse V, et al. Osteopenia and vitamin D deficiency in children with sickle cell disease. Eur J Haematol. 2009;83:572–8.

66. Fewtrell MS, Benden C, Williams JE, et al. Undercarboxylated osteocalcin and bone mass in 8-12 year old children with cystic fibrosis. J Cyst Fibros. 2008;7:307–12.

67. Drury D, Grey VL, Ferland G, et al. Efficacy of high dose phylloquinone in correcting vitamin K deficiency in cystic fibrosis. J Cyst Fibros. 2008;7:457–9.

68. Compston JE, McClung MR, Leslie WD. Osteoporosis. Lancet. 2019;393:364–76.

69. Saggese G, Baroncelli GI, Bertelloni S. Puberty and bone development. Best Pract Res Clin Endocrinol Metab. 2002;16:53–64.

70. Umławska W, Sands D, Zielińska A. Age of menarche in girls with cystic fibrosis. Folia Histochem Cytobiol. 2010;48:185–90.

71. Bournez M, Bellis G, Huet F. Growth during puberty in cystic fibrosis: a retrospective evaluation of a French cohort. Arch Dis Child. 2012;97:714–20.

72. Johannesson M, Gottlieb C, Hjelte L. Delayed puberty in girls with cystic fibrosis despite good clinical status. Pediatrics. 1997;99:29–34.

73. Street ME, Spaggiari C, Volta C, et al. The IGF system and cytokine interactions and relationships with longitudinal growth in prepubertal patients with cystic fibrosis. Clin Endocrinol. 2009;70:593–8.

74. Moshang T, Holsclaw DS. Menarchal determinants in cystic fibrosis. Am J Dis Child. 1980;134:1139–42.
75. Festini F, Taccetti G, Repetto T, et al. Gestational and neonatal characteristics of children with cystic fibrosis: a cohort study. J Pediatr. 2005;147:316–20.
76. Rogan MP, Reznikov LR, Pezzulo AA, et al. Pigs and humans with cystic fibrosis have reduced insulin-like growth factor 1 (IGF1) levels at birth. Proc Natl Acad Sci U S A. 2010;107:20571–5.
77. Switzer M, Rice J, Rice M, et al. Insulin-like growth factor-I levels predict weight, height and protein catabolism in children and adolescents with cystic fibrosis. J Pediatr Endocrinol Metab. 2009;22:417–24.
78. Sermet-Gaudelus I, Souberbielle JC, Azhar I, et al. Insulin-like growth factor I correlates with lean body mass in cystic fibrosis patients. Arch Dis Child. 2003;88:956–61.
79. Stalvey MS, Anbar RD, Konstan MW, et al. A multi-center controlled trial of growth hormone treatment in children with cystic fibrosis. Pediatr Pulmonol. 2012;47:252–63.
80. Hardin DS, Adams-Huet B, Brown D, et al. Growth hormone treatment improves growth and clinical status in prepubertal children with cystic fibrosis: results of a multicenter randomized controlled trial. J Clin Endocrinol Metab. 2006;91:4925–9.
81. Wong SC, Dobie R, Altowati MA, et al. Growth and the growth hormone-insulin like growth factor 1 Axis in children with chronic inflammation: current evidence, gaps in knowledge, and future directions. Endocr Rev. 2016;37:62–110.
82. Schnabel D, Grasemann C, Staab D, et al. A multicenter, randomized, double-blind, placebo-controlled trial to evaluate the metabolic and respiratory effects of growth hormone in children with cystic fibrosis. Pediatrics. 2007;119:e1230–8.
83. Bessich JL, Nymon AB, Moulton LA, et al. Low levels of insulin-like growth factor-1 contribute to alveolar macrophage dysfunction in cystic fibrosis. J Immunol. 2013;191:378–85.
84. Lee HW, Cheng J, Kovbasnjuk O, et al. Insulin-like growth factor 1 (IGF-1) enhances the protein expression of CFTR. PLoS One. 2013;8:e59992.
85. Shead EF, Haworth CS, Barker H, et al. Osteoclast function, bone turnover and inflammatory cytokines during infective exacerbations of cystic fibrosis. J Cyst Fibros. 2010;9:93–8.
86. Haworth CS, Selby PL, Webb AK, et al. Inflammatory related changes in bone mineral content in adults with cystic fibrosis. Thorax. 2004;59:613–7.
87. Shead EF, Haworth CS, Gunn E, et al. Osteoclastogenesis during infective exacerbations in patients with cystic fibrosis. Am J Respir Crit Care Med. 2006;174:306–11.
88. Aris RM, Stephens AR, Ontjes DA, et al. Adverse alterations in bone metabolism are associated with lung infection in adults with cystic fibrosis. Am J Respir Crit Care Med. 2000;162:1674–8.
89. Ambroszkiewicz J, Sands D, Gajewska J, et al. Bone turnover markers, osteoprotegerin and RANKL cytokines in children with cystic fibrosis. Adv Med Sci. 2013;58:338–43.
90. Cairoli E, Eller-Vainicher C, Morlacchi LC, et al. Bone involvement in young adults with cystic fibrosis awaiting lung transplantation for end-stage respiratory failure. Osteoporos Int. Epub ahead of print 23 February 2019. https://doi.org/10.1007/s00198-019-04893-z.
91. Aris RM, Neuringer IP, Weiner MA, et al. Severe osteoporosis before and after lung transplantation. Chest. 1996;109:1176–83.
92. Aris RM, Lester GE, Renner JB, et al. Efficacy of pamidronate for osteoporosis in patients with cystic fibrosis following lung transplantation. Am J Respir Crit Care Med. 2000;162:941–6.
93. Hubert G, Chung TT, Prosser C, et al. Bone mineral density and fat-soluble vitamin status in adults with cystic fibrosis undergoing lung transplantation: a pilot study. Can J Diet Pract Res. 2016;77:199–202.
94. Conwell LS, Chang AB. Bisphosphonates for osteoporosis in people with cystic fibrosis. Cochrane Database Syst Rev. 2014; CD002010.
95. Haworth CS, Selby PL, Adams JE, et al. Effect of intravenous pamidronate on bone mineral density in adults with cystic fibrosis. Thorax. 2001;56:314–6.

96. Land C, Rauch F, Glorieux FH. Cyclical intravenous pamidronate treatment affects metaphyseal modeling in growing patients with osteogenesis imperfecta. J Bone Miner Res. 2006;21(3):374–9. Proposed additional reference.
97. Cummings SR, San Martin J, McClung MR, et al. Denosumab for prevention of fractures in postmenopausal women with osteoporosis. N Engl J Med. 2009;361:756–65.
98. Neer RM, Arnaud CD, Zanchetta JR, et al. Effect of parathyroid hormone (1-34) on fractures and bone mineral density in postmenopausal women with osteoporosis. N Engl J Med. 2001;344:1434–41.
99. Siwamogsatham O, Stephens K, Tangpricha V. Evaluation of teriparatide for treatment of osteoporosis in four patients with cystic fibrosis: a case series. Case Rep Endocrinol. 2014;2014:893589.
100. Dif F, Marty C, Baudoin C, et al. Severe osteopenia in CFTR-null mice. Bone. 2004;35:595–603.
101. Haston CK, Li W, Li A, et al. Persistent osteopenia in adult cystic fibrosis transmembrane conductance regulator-deficient mice. Am J Respir Crit Care Med. 2008;177:309–15.
102. Pashuck TD, Franz SE, Altman MK, et al. Murine model for cystic fibrosis bone disease demonstrates osteopenia and sex-related differences in bone formation. Pediatr Res. 2009;65:311–6.
103. Le Henaff C, Haÿ E, Velard F, et al. Enhanced F508del-CFTR channel activity ameliorates bone pathology in murine cystic fibrosis. Am J Pathol. 2014;184:1132–41.
104. Stalvey MS, Havasi V, Tuggle KL, et al. Reduced bone length, growth plate thickness, bone content, and IGF-I as a model for poor growth in the CFTR-deficient rat. PLoS One. 2017;12:e0188497.
105. Le Henaff C, Faria Da Cunha M, Hatton A, et al. Genetic deletion of keratin 8 corrects the altered bone formation and osteopenia in a mouse model of cystic fibrosis. Hum Mol Genet. 2016;25:1281–93.
106. Le Henaff C, Mansouri R, Modrowski D, et al. Increased NF-κB activity and decreased Wnt/β-catenin signaling mediate reduced osteoblast differentiation and function in ΔF508 cystic fibrosis transmembrane conductance regulator (CFTR) mice. J Biol Chem. 2015;290:18009–17.
107. Shead EF, Haworth CS, Condliffe AM, et al. Cystic fibrosis transmembrane conductance regulator (CFTR) is expressed in human bone. Thorax. 2007;62:650–1.
108. Delion M, Braux J, Jourdain M-L, et al. Overexpression of RANKL in osteoblasts: a possible mechanism of susceptibility to bone disease in cystic fibrosis. J Pathol. 2016;240:50–60.
109. Sermet-Gaudelus I, Delion M, Durieu I, et al. Bone demineralization is improved by ivacaftor in patients with cystic fibrosis carrying the p.Gly551Asp mutation. J Cyst Fibros. 2016;15:e67–9.

Chapter 18
Rheumatologic Manifestations of CF

Amanda Reis and Andrew J. White

Patient Perspective

No one knows the hospital better than me; I have been in and out of it my whole life. I know almost everyone by name, especially the nurses. I remember my nurses singing to me for my sixth birthday party, and comforting me through the tears of missing the first day of fourth grade. Throughout my childhood, it was always my lungs that gave me problems. It wasn't until I was 14 that I started having joint pain.

The first time it happened, I thought I had just injured my knee while playing with my brother. I had been feeling otherwise well and hadn't been in the hospital in more than a month. It started with an ache one evening, but by the next morning, my knee was swollen and very painful. My mom called one of my doctors, and he recommended we go to the emergency room. There, they stuck a huge needle into my knee to look for an infection. I was scared. I always knew my lungs got infections, but this was different. I had to stay in the hospital overnight and get antibiotics, but it was on a different floor than usual, without any of my usual nurses. The next morning, there were red bumps on my legs, too. The doctors still couldn't tell us what was going on. I could barely move my leg, and my knee looked huge. Lots of different doctors came and saw me. Two days later, they told us no bacteria were growing and stopped the antibiotics. I still had to keep asking for more pain medicine, and I was confused and worried that I wouldn't get better. Fortunately, the next morning my knee started looking better. The day after that, I was able to walk again. Eventually, the doctors told us that it was a type of arthritis. I thought only old people got that, but they told me it was just another part of my cystic fibrosis.

Since then, it's happened four more times. Sometimes one knee, sometimes both knees, and one time my ankle. At least I don't have to go to the hospital every time

A. Reis · A. J. White (✉)
Saint Louis Children's Hospital, Department of Pediatrics, Washington University School of Medicine, Saint Louis, MO, USA
e-mail: white_a@wustl.edu

© Springer Nature Switzerland AG 2020
S. D. Davis et al. (eds.), *Cystic Fibrosis*, Respiratory Medicine,
https://doi.org/10.1007/978-3-030-42382-7_18

anymore – we just call my doctor and he says to take Motrin and rest until it goes away. I sometimes have to miss a few days of school. In between, though, my knees don't bother me at all. I can still walk and kick around a soccer ball with my brother. I think it's important for doctors to know about cystic fibrosis arthritis so that they can help the children who have it, and so they don't have to scare them and do so many extra tests. Us CF patients get poked enough!

–Anonymous

Cystic Fibrosis Arthropathy (CFA)

Description

CFA (also referred to as cystic fibrosis-related arthropathy or episodic arthropathy of cystic fibrosis) refers to a pattern of severely painful, episodic arthropathy that occurs in patients with CF [1–12]. It may be mono-, pauci-, or polyarticular. Both large and small joints may be involved, although knees seem to be the most commonly affected, followed by ankles, wrists, shoulders, elbows, and hips [1, 3, 4, 6, 8, 10].

Occurrences of this arthropathy usually last 5–7 days, although a range of several hours to 2 weeks has been reported. Symptoms may recur as often as multiple times per week [9] but more commonly recur every few months [1, 2, 10, 11]. In the majority of case studies, joint pain has been described to remit completely between episodes, though one small case series reported that some patients progress to chronic arthritis [9]. Joint inflammation and effusions are frequently seen during episodes of pain. Most case series report no associated erosions [1, 3, 6, 8, 12], with occasional exceptions [9]. This seems to hold true even when more modern imaging techniques, such as MRI, are employed [3].

For most patients with CFA, joint exacerbations do not correlate with pulmonary exacerbations and the severity of arthropathy does not correlate with the severity of pulmonary disease [1, 2, 4–6, 9, 10]. However, in some case series, a minority of patients did seem to have increased joint symptoms during or after times of increased pulmonary disease activity [7, 11].

In a subset of patients, joint erythema and swelling are associated with one of two types of rashes: either a painful, nodular rash over the forearms or shins resembling erythema nodosum or a nonspecific erythematous maculopapular rash, often near involved joints [2, 6, 8–10, 12]. The rash tends to remit with improvement in joint symptoms. A fever may occur along with joint pain in some patients [2, 8, 12].

Epidemiology Prevalence of CFA in patients with CF has been estimated to be between 3% and 12.9% in various cohorts of children and adults [1, 3, 4, 7, 13, 14]. Predictably, prevalence increases with age. Mean age of onset has been most frequently reported to be in the mid-teens [1, 2, 9, 11] with a range of 2–41 years [3, 6, 8]. Males and females are affected in approximately equal numbers, though some authors have noted a younger age of onset for females as opposed to males [9].

Laboratory findings Laboratory findings in CFA tend to be nonspecific. Multiple case series have reported normal to mildly elevated ESR [1, 2, 4, 6, 8] with normal [3] or mildly elevated [4] CRP. WBC count is often normal, though may be slightly elevated [1, 2, 8]. Uric acid levels are normal [1, 6, 8, 9], which can be helpful in distinguishing initial presentations of CFA from gout, which can also complicate CF [15]. Complement levels tend to be normal [2, 6, 9–11]. Rheumatoid factor (RF) is also generally negative [4, 6–10]. Interestingly, some of the few RF+ patients who presented with what initially seemed to be CFA had a more progressive disease course with eventual joint damage, though these patients may or may not have ultimately met the criteria for classic juvenile rheumatoid arthritis (JRA) or rheumatoid arthritis [7, 9, 11]. In most cases, patients with symptoms characteristic for CFA have negative ANA [3, 6, 10], and the presence of ANA in patients with CF is not correlated with development of arthropathy symptoms [4]. In contrast to many auto-immune pathologies, the HLA distribution in CFA has not suggested an association with any particular haplotype [1, 2, 8, 10]. Joint fluid, when obtained, has demonstrated sterile fluid without crystals, with either no cells [1] or WBC counts in the 4000–56,000 range [7, 9].

Diagnosis There are no clear clinical or laboratory criteria for the diagnosis of CFA. The diagnosis should be considered in any patient with CF presenting with sudden onset, severe joint pain, with or without swelling. Other causes of joint pain and swelling, such as septic arthritis, mechanical injury, gout, and JRA, should be ruled out before making a diagnosis of CFA. If an erythematous rash is seen, cellulitis should be considered in the differential. For an erythema nodosum-type rash, other common diseases associated with erythema nodosum, such as group A streptococcus, tuberculosis, mycoplasma, chlamydia trachomatis, histoplasmosis, blastomycosis, mononucleosis, pregnancy, sarcoidosis, and malignancy, should be considered [16, 17].

Treatment While the pain and swelling of CFA resolves without intervention within days to weeks, nonsteroidal anti-inflammatory drugs (NSAIDs) have frequently been used to decrease pain and improve mobility during acute exacerbations [2, 5, 8, 10, 14]. In various case reports, prednisone has been helpful with symptoms not sufficiently alleviated by NSAIDs [2, 8]. Disease-modifying anti-rheumatic drugs such as sulfasalazine, hydroxychloroquine, and methotrexate have also been reportedly used in some refractory patients [14]. Unfortunately, no conclusions about the safety or efficacy of these second- and third-line treatments can be drawn, or dosing guidelines recommended, given the small numbers of patients involved and the lack of randomized trials [18, 19]. Careful consideration of side effects is especially important in populations prone to infections, renal toxicity, and medication interactions, such as patients with underlying CF.

Prognosis Most patients with CFA report intermittent symptoms for years, although some patients may experience only rare recurrences or none at all [1, 2, 8]. As discussed above, severity of the arthropathy does not correlate with severity of pulmonary disease. It has not been shown to have any impact on survival [20];

but, interestingly, arthropathy was found to be associated with worse post-lung transplant survival [21]. However, the overall number of patients with arthropathy in this study was small, and replication of these results with other cohorts will be necessary before making robust conclusions.

Future Directions Further investigation of causative factors in CFA and more thorough comparisons of various treatment regimens would be of use in diagnosis and management of this disorder. Randomized trials would be helpful in determining optimal medical management, especially in patients who do not report sufficient pain relief with NSAIDs [19].

Hypertrophic Pulmonary Osteoarthropathy (HPOA)

Description

HPOA describes a condition characterized by joint pain along with digital clubbing and periosteal elevations at the end of long bones [22]. Secondary HPOA can be seen in CF as well as in a variety of other diseases, such as pulmonary malignancies, chronic infections, and congenital cyanotic heart defects [23, 24].

Compared to patients with CFA or age- and sex-matched controls with CF, patients with HPOA tend to have poorer lung function [2, 5, 8, 9, 25]. Similarly, exacerbations of joint symptoms tend to correlate with exacerbations of pulmonary disease in most [2, 8, 9, 26, 27], but not all [25], cases. Pain tends to progressively worsen over time as pulmonary status worsens. While symptoms often wane between exacerbations, they often do not entirely disappear.

Joint involvement is generally symmetric, with large joints such as knees, ankles, and wrists most commonly affected and elbows or proximal interphalangeal joints occasionally involved [2, 8, 25, 28, 29]. Swelling is often seen, and long bone pain may also be present [2, 8, 27, 28]. Some case series have reported an association with gynecomastia in men and mastalgia in women [8, 27], although in other cohorts this has not been reported [9].

X-ray findings of periosteal elevations at the distal ends of long bones, or findings of periosteal new bone formation on bone scans, are classic for HPOA [2, 8, 9, 25–28, 30, 31]. FDG-PET imaging in patients with characteristic clinical symptoms has also demonstrated increased distal periosteal uptake, indicating increased metabolic activity in these areas [32]. While there have been reports that these imaging changes can be found in asymptomatic patients [28], larger cohorts have reported that these imaging findings are rare in patients without clinical features [25]. Also rarely, patients may lack these characteristic imaging findings, yet demonstrate a clinical course that fits with HPOA [25].

While the mechanism underlying HPOA is not yet proven, the leading theories on its pathogenesis suggest that megakaryocytes, platelets, and some related growth factors (e.g., platelet-derived growth factor [PDGF] and vascular endothelial growth factor [VEGF]), which are usually broken down in the lung, escape degradation in severe lung disease, thereby enabling entrance into the systemic circulation. The involvement of prostaglandin E in this process has also been postulated [33].

Platelets and megakaryocytes have been thought to be involved in the etiology of digital clubbing for some time [34]. More recently, VEGF has been implicated as playing a key role in activating fibroblasts and osteoblasts [35, 36], leading to bone remodeling [37, 38]. This may relate to the periosteal elevations seen in HPOA.

Epidemiology Given that HPOA depends on lung disease severity in the population, prevalence estimates are difficult to generalize. One group estimated a prevalence of 1.9% in their patients with CF under the age of 16 years and 2.9% in those who are older [9]. Another group reported that 8% of their CF patients had characteristic clinical symptoms and X-ray findings consistent with HPOA [25]. Unlike CFA, HPOA has a male predominance with a male/female ratio of approximately 2:1 [8, 25, 29]. Mean age of onset has been reported to be generally in the range of 15–23 years [2, 8, 9], although these numbers are based on data from the 1980s. Prevalence as well as mean age of onset is likely to change over time as our ability to treat the underlying pathology in CF becomes more advanced.

Laboratory findings Laboratory findings in HPOA are nonspecific. Mildly elevated WBC count and ESR may be present [2, 26]. As in CFA, ANA and RF are generally negative [2, 9]. HLA distribution tends to be consistent with the general population [2], uric acid levels are normal [9], C3 is normal, and C4 may be normal to decreased [2, 9]. Joint fluid, when obtained, is sterile, without crystals, and has generally fewer than 1000 WBC with a lymphocytic predominance [2, 26, 30]. As alluded to above, FEV_1 tends to be lower in CF patients with HPOA compared to similarly aged CF patients without HPOA-type joint pain [8, 9, 25]. This relationship is likely not causative but rather a reflection of the finding that HPOA tends to occur in patients with poor lung function.

Diagnosis The diagnostic criteria for HPOA include finger clubbing, chronic symmetric joint pain and/or long bone pain, and characteristic imaging findings (periosteal elevations at the distal ends of long bones on X-ray or distal periosteal new bone formation on bone scan) [2, 8, 9]. Correlation of musculoskeletal symptoms with respiratory exacerbations is also suggestive of the diagnosis.

As finger clubbing is present in the majority of CF patients, this criterion is of limited utility in this population [2, 29, 31]. There has been some heterogeneity about whether imaging findings are essential to the diagnosis or whether history and exam findings are sufficient. Interestingly, one study found that patients with symptoms of HPOA and classic X-ray findings had significantly worse FEV_1 compared not only to CF controls without joint pain but also compared to a cohort of CF patients with HPOA-type joint pain but normal X-rays [25]. This suggests that patients with HPOA symptoms but no findings on imaging may either be earlier in their disease process or have a different prognosis compared to patients with HPOA symptoms and imaging findings. When considering the diagnosis of HPOA, the following diagnoses should also be included in the differential: episodic CFA, osteomyelitis, fracture, and other mechanical injuries [24].

Treatment As HPOA generally correlates in severity to underlying lung pathology, optimizing treatment of pulmonary symptoms, such as with antibiotics and increased respiratory clearance, is the optimal method of decreasing musculoskeletal symptoms [8, 9, 18, 26, 38, 39]. For symptomatic relief, NSAIDs are commonly used [2, 25, 26, 30, 40–42]. Their antiprostaglandin effects may contribute to pain relief [41, 42].

Isolated case reports describe treating with subcutaneous octreotide [43, 44] and anticholinergic medicines such as atropine or propranolol/phenoxybenzamine [45, 46] to decrease symptoms of HPOA, though not specifically in patients with CF. Corticosteroids have also been attempted, with limited success [44]. Historically, partial or complete severing of the vagus nerve was noted to lead to symptomatic relief and radiographic improvement in patients with HPOA [39, 47, 48]. However, this type of surgical intervention would only be considered a last resort in refractory cases.

Recently, there have been reports of the successful use of oral or intravenous bisphosphonates to control HPOA symptoms in patients with various underlying pathologies, including CF [49–54]. A proposed mechanism for the efficacy of bisphosphonates is control of the excessive osteoclast and osteoblast activation induced by VEGF [36]. Further controlled trials will be useful in determining efficacy and safety of this potentially promising new treatment option.

Prognosis HPOA is a chronic and progressive disease, which generally reflects the severity of the patient's underlying lung disease [2, 18]. Although HPOA itself is unlikely to directly impact mortality, those who develop this complication have higher mortality rate in the years following diagnosis compared to CF patients of similar age. One group found a 36% mortality rate over 3 years in patients with both symptoms and X-ray findings of HPOA, compared with 9% in patients with symptoms but no imaging findings, and 5% in age- and sex-matched asymptomatic CF controls [25]. Another case study reported 29% mortality within 3 years of HPOA diagnosis, although no control group was available for comparison [8]. These case series were both conducted in the 1980s, however, and therefore may not accurately reflect mortality in the present era, when more advanced therapies are available to control lung disease in patients with CF.

Future directions While the use of bisphosphonates to control the symptoms of HPOA seems promising, it is currently an off-label use with no randomized, controlled trials exploring efficacy, potential side effects, or optimal dosing. Further research is necessary to evaluate the efficacy of bisphosphonates and other treatments for this potentially debilitating arthropathy associated with CF.

Idiopathic Vasculitic Rash Associated with CF

Description

There are many case reports and case series of people with CF developing idiopathic vasculitic rashes. The rash sometimes presents at the time of a pulmonary exacerbation but most often independently [55–57]. In a subset of cases, the rash can present along with joint pain that may be due to episodic arthropathy [10, 29, 55].

These rashes are often petechial and purpuric in nature and often regress spontaneously with recurrences at several week to month intervals [8, 10, 55–61]. The dorsums of the feet, ankles, and the anterior tibial surface of the leg tend to be most heavily involved [8, 10, 56, 57, 59, 61, 62], although the rash can extend up the legs and occasionally involve the upper extremities as well [8, 56, 59, 62]. Some patients report pruritis, edema, and painful burning sensation with the onset of the rash [10, 56, 58, 61]. The speed of onset has not been widely discussed, but in one case report, the rash was described as developing over 2–3 days [58]. It tends to remit spontaneously in 3–10 days [10, 57, 59], but longer durations of 2–5 weeks have been reported [55, 56, 62]. In all but two [59, 62] reported cases, no findings of systemic vasculitis were present.

The exact etiology of the idiopathic vasculitic rash seen in CF remains unclear. Some studies have suggested an association with high levels of circulating immune complexes [63], while others have highlighted the association with atypical ANCA, specifically antibodies against bactericidal/permeability-increasing protein (BPI) [18, 55, 64]. This protein is part of the azurophilic granule of neutrophils and is particularly active in opsonization of gram-negative bacilli such as *Pseudomonas aeruginosa* [64–68], a common cause of infection in patients with CF. As other types of ANCA are associated with other forms of vasculitis, and CF patients with vasculitis are more likely to be ANCA-positive than age- and sex-matched controls [62], some theorize that anti-BPI antibodies may relate to the pathogenesis of cutaneous vasculitis in CF. While many of the older case reports do not comment on the presence of anti-BPI ANCA specifically, it is probable that many of these would have had anti-BPI antibodies if tested, as more recent studies have found that in patients with vasculitis and ANCA positivity that is not MPO or PR3, almost half are anti-BPI [69]. Anti-BPI antibodies may be involved in the cycle of chronic inflammation often seen in patients with CF [65] and have been shown to act on vasculature [70, 71], suggesting a possible role in the pathogenesis of the vasculitic rash of CF.

Nevertheless, it is also worth noting that anti-BPI antibodies are common in the CF population. Estimates range from 70% of patients with CF (age range 3–50 years, 6% with vasculitic rash) [72] to 77% of children with CF (not reported if any had vasculitic rash) [65] to 91% of adult CF patients with FEV_1 values <50% predicted (only 10% of whom had a vasculitic rash) [73]. While the prevalence depends on the method of detection and debility of the population, the presence of anti-BPI antibodies is clearly not a specific marker for diagnosis of the vasculitic rash associated with CF.

Epidemiology Compared to the number of patients with CFA and HPOA, the appearance of a vasculitic rash is rare. Prevalence has been roughly estimated at 2–3% of patients with CF, based on two case series [1, 10]. The age of onset in case reports and case series seems to usually be in the late teens to early twenties [10, 29, 56, 57, 59–62], although it has been seen in children as young as 9 [10]. No clear male or female predominance has been identified [29].

Laboratory findings Serologic findings tend to be nonspecific. WBC count may be normal to slightly elevated [10], and ESR is often normal unless the patient has coexisting exacerbation of pulmonary symptoms [59, 62].

ANA and RF are most often negative but may be positive [8, 55, 57, 61, 62]. As discussed above, ANCA is often positive, though the pattern is more often anti-BPI antibodies or atypical versus MPO or PR3 type [55, 59]. C3 and C4 are generally normal to slightly elevated [56, 58, 60], with normal [61] to elevated [56, 58, 59, 62] C1q. In interpreting this data, it must be noted that patients with CF are more likely than healthy controls to have elevated immune complexes even in the absence of vasculitis [74]. Most patients with CF and vasculitis in whom immunoglobulin levels have been checked have had elevated IgG, slightly elevated IgA and IgM, and most often normal IgE [8, 10, 27, 56, 58, 60–62]; although again, it is unclear the extent to which this differs from CF patients without vasculitis [75]. In contrast to patients with Henoch-Schonlein purpura (HSP), which can produce a similar vasculitic rash, urinalysis and creatinine in patients with the idiopathic rash of CF are normal, consistent with normal kidney function [10, 58, 62].

Most biopsy specimens have a perivenular, neutrophil-predominant leukocytoclastic vasculitis [10, 55, 56, 59–61]. Sometimes, IgA and/or IgG deposits are found in the dermis [56, 60], dermal–epidermal junction [56], or, in one case report, the vessel wall [61].

Diagnosis The diagnosis of idiopathic vasculitic rash in patients with CF depends on excluding other known causes of cutaneous vasculitis. Importantly, the vasculitic rash of CF is generally exclusively cutaneous. Two case reports exist which each describe a CF patient being diagnosed with what appears to be only a cutaneous rash but who later develops serious systemic manifestations [59, 62]. It is unclear if these cases represent a true idiopathic CF vasculitis or whether another pathology contributed to the findings.

Important differential diagnoses include (i) other primary vasculidites – especially HSP, which also causes a purpuric rash of the lower extremities, as well as granulomatosis with polyangiitis (associated with PR3 ANCA, generally associated with systemic involvement); (ii) microscopic polyangiitis (associated with MPO-ANCA, generally associated with systemic involvement); (iii) eosinophilic granulomatosis with polyangiitis (associated with MPO ANCA and elevated IgE levels as well as systemic symptoms); (iv) hypersensitivity vasculitis (often presents with fever, urticaria, lymphadenopathy, and arthralgias, but no IgA deposits); (v) hypergammaglobulinemic purpura (similar presentation but would present with positive rheumatoid factor [76]); and (vi) vascular inflammation due to hepatitis B or C.

As the first step in diagnosis, a thorough physical exam should be undertaken assessing for joint, mucous membrane, abdominal, and skin involvement. In order to exclude systemic vasculitis, a CBC, CMP, urinalysis, and PT/PTT should be obtained to assess for an inadequate platelet count, eosinophilia, liver inflammation or dysfunction, and kidney involvement. Hepatitis B sAb, sAg, Hepatitis C ab, and HIV testing are important to rule out infectious causes of vasculitis. ANCA testing revealing a nonspecific or BPI pattern, while not diagnostic, would be characteristic of the idiopathic vasculitic rash of CF. In contrast, MPO or PR3 ANCA positivity would likely indicate a different vasculitis.

Treatment No clear treatment guidelines exist. The most common treatment has been prednisone, which has reportedly resulted in partial improvement in many cases, but has not been shown to prevent recurrences [55, 56, 58, 59, 62]. NSAIDs and antihistamines have been trialed to relieve the burning and itching that can sometimes accompany rash onset but have proven unsuccessful in doing so [10]. Immunomodulatory therapies show some preliminary promise. Immune suppression with azathioprine resulted in improvement in two case reports [57, 59], and, more recently, chloroquine was used successfully to improve vasculitic rash in one patient with CF [55]. However, controlled and larger studies are necessary before these therapies can be recommended.

Prognosis While the idiopathic vasculitic rash of CF is not generally associated with systemic vasculitis, it is nevertheless associated with a poor overall prognosis. In case reports, a majority of patients do not live longer than 2 years after the initial presentation of the vasculitic rash [8, 10, 56, 57, 60–62]. Nevertheless, without a control group, these data are difficult to interpret. Additionally, the majority of these case reports are from the 1980s to the 1990s, and our ability to treat CF and its complications has increased substantially since then [77, 78]. Interestingly, the presence and amount of anti-BPI antibodies themselves have also been shown to be associated with poor prognosis in patients with CF [78]. Further studies delineating the relationship between these variables (general CF treatment, anti-BPI antibodies, and the vasculitic rash) will be helpful in better understanding the prognosis of patients with the vasculitic rash of CF.

Future directions Currently, only case reports and case series exist to describe the vasculitic rash associated with CF. Much opportunity exists for further research into the pathogenesis, treatment options, and prognosis of this condition in the modern era.

Fluoroquinolone-Associated Arthropathy

Description

Fluoroquinolones are a commonly used class of antibiotics in the CF population. They are bactericidal and have broad-spectrum activity, including against *Pseudomonas aeruginosa* [79], a common cause of morbidity and mortality in patients with CF. They are well-absorbed via an oral route [80, 81] and have good tissue penetrance [82], including into the lungs [83–85]. There has been some concern, however, that they have the potential to induce cartilaginous damage and cause joint pain in children.

The initial concern was based on animal data, which showed that when fluoroquinolones were administered to juvenile rats, dogs, and nonhuman primates, irreversible cartilage damage was seen [86–90]. Even adult human cartilage has shown chondrocyte toxicity and necrosis when incubated in vitro with fluoroquinolones at concentrations that would be biologically realistic [91]. Clinical data, however, has been reassuring. In children, there have been reports of only transient arthralgias when taking fluoroquinolones. These arthralgias were mild to moderate in severity and resolved after cessation of therapy [4, 5, 92–98].

Arthralgias are a recognized side effect of fluoroquinolone treatment but occur rarely. In a systematic review which included over 16,000 pediatric patients receiving ciprofloxacin, arthralgias were reported in about 1.6% [99]. Children with CF may be at particular risk, given that they are often treated with prolonged courses of antibiotics. However, even in 1 review of over 1100 children with CF treated with oral ciprofloxacin for a mean of 23 days, the incidence of arthralgias was estimated at only 3.2%, and in all of these cases, symptoms resolved with cessation of drug therapy [100]. Other studies since that time have reported similar arthralgia incidences of 4–4.5% in patients with CF who were treated with oral ciprofloxacin [96, 98]. Higher incidence has been reported for IV ciprofloxacin in children with CF (22%), although this was no higher than the incidence of arthralgias in the control group treated with ceftazidime and tobramycin [94]. Incidence of arthralgias may be higher for children treated with pefloxacin compared to ciprofloxacin [93]. The arthralgias seem to be more common in female patients [93, 101].

Due to the concern for long-term harm, joint damage has been extensively investigated in children treated with fluoroquinolones. Knee circumference measurements in children before and after multiple courses of ciprofloxacin did not demonstrate swelling [92]. After 14–28-day courses of ciprofloxacin treatment in children, there was no visible pathology on X-ray [97, 102, 103] or on MRI during therapy [104], immediately after therapy [104], or 3 months to 7 years [104, 105] post-therapy. Long-term growth rates in children with CF are also not affected by fluoroquinolones [103]. Analysis of a database of over 6000 children who had received fluoroquinolones found no increased reports of tendon or joint disorders compared to children prescribed azithromycin [106]. Analysis of knee cartilage after autopsy of two children with CF who had received 2–12 weeks of oral ciprofloxacin revealed no macroscopic or microscopic changes to cartilage [107]. Overall, despite the concerns raised by animal studies, the potential for fluoroquinolones to cause long-term musculoskeletal damage in children has not been demonstrated. Due to the overall reassuring nature of clinical reports and studies in children, the benefits of the use of fluoroquinolones, especially to treat *Pseudomonas aeruginosa* in children with CF, outweigh the risks [100, 101, 108–112].

Osteoporosis

Description

For many decades, it has been recognized that patients with CF have lower bone mineral density (BMD) and bone mineral apparent density (BMAD), a measure of bone density that corrects for bone size, compared to healthy controls [113–134]. A recent meta-analysis estimated the prevalence of osteoporosis in CF to be 23.5% in adults [135]. While BMD z-scores compared to healthy controls tend to worsen with age [114, 115, 120, 129, 130, 136], even a significant percentage of children with CF have a decrease in BMD or bone mineralization compared to their peers [115, 117, 122, 126].

Low bone mineral density is of importance as it can increase risk for fractures [116, 121, 129, 137]. Of particular concern, rib fractures and atraumatic vertebral fractures are more common in patients with CF compared to controls [116, 124, 130]. One group estimates that the CF population is at a 10-fold increased risk of rib fractures and 100-fold increased risk of vertebral fractures compared to the general population [134]. This increase in fracture rate, while more pronounced in adults, can be seen as early as adolescence [138]. Rib fractures can lead to atelectasis [139] and pain with airway clearance regimens. Vertebral fractures, present in an estimated 14% of adults with CF [135], contribute toward kyphosis [121, 124, 134], which is common in patients with CF (estimated 5–19% of adults [5, 138]) and can lead to reduced lung volumes [140] and increased risk for atelectasis [141] as well as back pain [142].

There are likely multiple factors which contribute to poor bone health in children with CF. One of the main causes likely has to do with the high frequency of poor growth and low body mass index (BMI), which are known risk factors for osteoporosis [143, 144]. Low BMI and poor nutritional status have consistently been one of the most strongly associated factors with low BMD, BMAD, and total body bone mineral content in people with CF [113–115, 117–119, 124, 125, 127, 130]. In fact, two studies found that the effect of CF on BMD disappeared when children and adolescents with CF were compared to age-, sex-, and BMI-matched controls [145, 146].

Another strongly associated variable is severity of lung disease, often measured using percent predicted FEV_1 or Shwachman score [5, 113–115, 119, 121, 125, 126, 129, 132, 136]. For patients with disease severe enough to warrant workup for lung transplant, two studies found that fewer than 30% had normal bone mineral density at the lumbar spine and femoral neck [116, 147]. As with many of the variables associated with low BMD, the independent causality of this factor is unclear, as patients with poorer lung function are likely to have poorer BMI and nutrition as well as other risk factors for BMD, such as extensive glucocorticoid use. Glucocorticoid use has been associated with decreased bone mineral density in CF as well as other diseases [113, 114, 121, 148, 149].

There are multiple other possible contributing factors. Children with CF often undergo puberty later [150]; while this may to some extent reflect malnutrition [150], this effect has been seen even in well-nourished adolescents with CF [151]. This delayed puberty can result in delayed bone age [126], and two small studies found a correlation between delayed puberty in young adults with CF and lower bone mineral density later in life [114, 128]. Another study reported that patients with CF and gonadal dysfunction had lower BMD than other CF patients (although with the possible confounders that patients with gonadal dysfunction tended to have lower BMI and worse pulmonary function) [113].

Decreased physical activity may also play a role. Due to their illness, children with CF may also not be as physically active compared to other children their age which can lead to poorer bone formation from reduced weight bearing [152].

Pancreatic enzyme deficiency can lead to poor fat soluble vitamin uptake, and many patients with CF demonstrate low or borderline-low levels of 25-hydroxy vitamin D [113, 116, 118, 120, 121, 126, 127], even with pancreatic enzyme supplementation and/or vitamin supplements [123, 126, 130]. In some cases, low 25-hydroxy vitamin D levels or low 1–25 hydroxy vitamin D levels in patients with CF have been found to correlate with lower bone mineral density [113, 115, 116, 130], though in other cases, no correlation has been found [119, 127].

There is also some evidence that the delta F508 mutation may serve as an independent risk factor for lower BMD [131], though results have been equivocal with some studies finding no significant contribution of genotype [113, 125, 126].

Likely related to low activity levels, corticosteroid use, poor nutrition, and perhaps other factors such as genetics, patients with CF have been noted to have not only poorer bone formation but also higher bone resorption compared to age-matched controls, as measured by urinary levels of pyridinium, deoxypyridinoline crosslinks, or their precursor molecules [118, 124, 126, 129].

Epidemiology As described above, the rate of osteoporosis in patients with CF is estimated at approximately 23.5% [135] and increases with age. Interestingly, multiple studies have observed a higher rate of low BMD in men with CF compared to women with CF [121, 126, 129, 147], in contrast to the higher rate of osteoporosis in females in the general population [153, 154]. The etiology of this is not clear. Multiple studies have assessed for a relationship between low BMD and hypogonadism in men. Results have been mixed. Some studies have found normal mean testosterone levels in men with CF [126, 146] and that low testosterone levels were not correlated with BMD [127, 131]. Other studies have noted a large proportion of men with low free or total testosterone levels and that low levels correlated with lower BMD [113, 124]. Men with gonadal dysfunction, however, also had lower BMIs and worse pulmonary function, leading to concern for confounding factors. Further research is needed to delineate the contribution of gonadal dysfunction to BMD in men with CF.

Lab findings As discussed above, serum vitamin D and hormone levels may be abnormal in patients with CF and low BMD.

Diagnosis According to the consensus statement from the International Society for Clinical Densitometry, the diagnosis of osteoporosis in children should be made in the presence of both a "clinically significant fracture history" and low bone mineral content or BMD [155]. Multiple modalities exist for measuring bone health and strength. The most commonly used and preferred method [155] is Dual X-ray Absortiometry (DEXA, or DXA), with z-scores −1 to −2.0 concerning for osteopenia and z-scores less than −2.0 consistent with osteoporosis [155, 156].

Treatment Prevention of low BMD in children and adolescents with CF should focus on optimizing nutritional status, as children with a normal BMI have improved bone mineralization [115, 136, 145]. Weight-bearing exercise, especially during adolescence, is also important [152]. Due to the finding of low vitamin D levels in many patients with CF, increased calcitriol (1–25 hydroxy vitamin D) supplementation has been attempted in an effort to reduce BMD losses, with some encouraging preliminary results [157, 158] but no definitive evidence of benefit. Due to concern for hypogonadism, women may be treated with combined hormonal therapy with estrogen and progesterone, which in some case reports has resulted in increases in BMD [114]. However, estrogen therapy has the potential for negative side effects, especially in women with CF [159].

Many recent studies have focused on bisphosphonates for osteoporosis treatment in patients with CF. Intravenous pamidronate and oral alendronate or etidronate have been shown to increase BMD or decrease loss of BMD in patients with CF compared to control patients treated with only calcium and vitamin D [160–163]. Unfortunately, a significant proportion of patients receiving IV pamidronate experienced moderate-to-severe bone pain [163, 164], necessitating early termination of one trial. Interestingly, patients simultaneously treated with corticosteroids did not experience bone pain [161, 163]. Studies thus far have not been powered to detect a change in fracture rate in patients treated with bisphosphonates versus controls [165]. Bisphosphonates have been used in pediatric patients with osteoporosis, with some success at increasing bone mineral density [166], though no trials in children with CF have thus far been undertaken. More research will be necessary to further elucidate the risks, benefits, and side effect profiles of bisphosphonates in pediatric patients with CF.

References

1. Bourke S, Rooney M, Fitzgerald M, Bresnihan B. Episodic arthropathy in adult cystic fibrosis. Q J Med. 1987;64:651–9.
2. Dixey J, et al. The arthropathy of cystic fibrosis. Ann Rheum Dis. 1988;47:218–23.
3. Fitch G, et al. Ultrasound and magnetic resonance imaging assessment of joint disease in symptomatic patients with cystic fibrosis arthropathy. J Cyst Fibros. 2016;15:e35–40.
4. Koch A-K, Brömme S, Wollschläger B, Horneff G, Keyszer G. Musculoskeletal manifestations and rheumatic symptoms in patients with cystic fibrosis (CF) —no observations of CF-specific arthropathy. J Rheumatol. 2008;35:1882–91.
5. Massie RJ, et al. The musculoskeletal complications of cystic fibrosis. J Paediatr Child Health. 1998;34:467–70.
6. Newman AJ, Ansell BM. Episodic arthritis in children with cystic fibrosis. J Pediatr. 1979;94:594–6.
7. Pertuiset E, et al. Cystic fibrosis arthritis. A report of five cases. Br J Rheumatol. 1992;31:535–8.
8. Phillips BM, David TJ. Pathogenesis and management of arthropathy in cystic fibrosis. J R Soc Med. 1986;79:44–50.
9. Rush PJ, et al. The musculoskeletal manifestations of cystic fibrosis. Semin Arthritis Rheum. 1986;15:213–25.
10. Schidlow DV, Goldsmith DP, Palmer J, Huang NN. Arthritis in cystic fibrosis. Arch Dis Child. 1984;59:377–9.
11. Wulffraat NM, de Graeff-Meeder ER, Rijkers GT, van der Laag H, Kuis W. Prevalence of circulating immune complexes in patients with cystic fibrosis and arthritis. J Pediatr. 1994;125:374–8.
12. Summers GD, Webley M. Episodic arthritis in cystic fibrosis: a case report. Br J Rheumatol. 1986;25:393–5.

13. Simmonds NJ, Cullinan P, Hodson ME. Growing old with cystic fibrosis – the characteristics of long-term survivors of cystic fibrosis. Respir Med. 2009;103:629–35.
14. Jawad A, Pákozdi A, Watson D, Kuitert L. OP0112 cystic fibrosis related arthritis in adults in south East England. Ann Rheum Dis. 2013;71:91.
15. Horsley A, et al. Gout and hyperuricaemia in adults with cystic fibrosis. J R Soc Med. 2011;104:S36–9.
16. Gilchrist H, Patterson JW. Erythema nodosum and erythema induratum (nodular vasculitis): diagnosis and management. Dermatol Ther. 2010;23:320–7.
17. González-Gay MA, García-Porrúa C, Pujol RM, Salvarani C. Erythema nodosum: a clinical approach. Clin Exp Rheumatol. 2001;19:365–8.
18. Merkel PA. Rheumatic disease and cystic fibrosis. Arthritis Rheum. 1999;42:1563–71.
19. Thornton J, Rangaraj S. Anti-inflammatory drugs and analgesics for managing symptoms in people with cystic fibrosis-related arthritis. Cochrane Libr. 2016;1:1465–1858.
20. Liou TG, et al. Predictive 5-year survivorship model of cystic fibrosis. Am J Epidemiol. 2001;153:345–52.
21. Liou TG, Adler FR, Huang D. Use of lung transplantation survival models to refine patient selection in cystic fibrosis. Am J Respir Crit Care Med. 2005;171:1053–9.
22. Martínez-Lavín M, Matucci-Cerinic M, Jajic I, Pineda C. Hypertrophic osteoarthropathy: consensus on its definition, classification, assessment and diagnostic criteria. J Rheumatol. 1993;20:1386–7.
23. Bresnihan B. Cystic fibrosis, chronic bacterial infection, and rheumatic disease. Rheumatology. 1988;27:339–41.
24. Yao Q, Altman RD, Brahn E. Periostitis and hypertrophic pulmonary osteoarthropathy: report of 2 cases and review of the literature. Semin Arthritis Rheum. 2009;38:458–66.
25. Cohen AM, et al. Evaluation of pulmonary hypertrophic osteoarthropathy in cystic fibrosis: a comprehensive study. Am J Dis Child. 1986;140:74–7.
26. Athreya BH, Borns P, Rosenlund ML. Cystic fibrosis and hypertrophic osteoarthropathy in children: report of three cases. Am J Dis Child. 1975;129:634–7.
27. Braude S, Kennedy H, Hodson M, Batten J. Hypertrophic osteoarthropathy in cystic fibrosis. Br Med J Clin Res Ed. 1984;288:822–3.
28. Grossman H, Denning CR, Baker DH. Hyperthrophic osteoarthropathy in cystic fibrosis. Am J Dis Child. 1964;1960(107):1–6.
29. Turner MA, Baildam E, Patel L, David TJ. Joint disorders in cystic fibrosis. J R Soc Med. 1997;90(Suppl 31):13–20.
30. Matthay MA, Matthay RA, Mills DM, Lakshminarayan S, Cotton E. Hypertrophic osteoarthropathy in adults with cystic fibrosis. Thorax. 1976;31:572–5.
31. Nathanson I, Riddlesberger MM. Pulmonary hypertrophic osteoarthropathy in cystic fibrosis. Radiology. 1980;135:649–51.
32. Cengiz A, Eren MŞ, Polatli M, Yürekli Y. Hypertrophic pulmonary osteoarthropathy on bone scintigraphy and 18F-fluorodeoxyglucose positron emission tomography/computed tomography in a patient with lung adenocarcinoma. Indian J Nucl Med. 2015;30:251–3.
33. Letts M, Pang E, Simons J. Prostaglandin-induced neonatal periostitis. J Pediatr Orthop. 1994;14:809–13.
34. Dickinson CJ, Martin JF. Megakaryocytes and platelet clumps as the cause of finger clubbing. Lancet. 1987;330:1434–5.
35. Martinez-Lavin M. Exploring the cause of the most ancient clinical sign of medicine: finger clubbing. Semin Arthritis Rheum. 2007;36:380–5.
36. Silveira LH, et al. Vascular endothelial growth factor and hypertrophic osteoarthropathy. Clin Exp Rheumatol. 2000;18:57–62.
37. Atkinson S, Fox SB. Vascular endothelial growth factor (VEGF)-A and platelet-derived growth factor (PDGF) play a central role in the pathogenesis of digital clubbing. J Pathol. 2004;203:721–8.

38. Nguyen S, Hojjati M. Review of current therapies for secondary hypertrophic pulmonary osteoarthropathy. Clin Rheumatol. 2011;30:7–13.
39. Flavell G. Reversal of pulmonary hypertrophic osteoarthropathy by vagotomy. Lancet. 1956;270:260–2.
40. Blackwell N, Bangham L, Hughes M, Melzack D, Trotman I. Treatment of resistant pain in hypertrophic pulmonary arthropathy with ketorolac. Thorax. 1993;48:401.
41. Kozak KR, Milne GL, Morrow JD, Cuiffo BP. Hypertrophic osteoarthropathy pathogenesis: a case highlighting the potential role for cyclo-oxygenase-2-derived prostaglandin E2. Nat Clin Pract Rheumatol. 2006;2:452–6; quiz following 456.
42. Leung FW, Williams AJ, Fan P. Indomethacin therapy for hypertrophic pulmonary osteoarthropathy in patients with bronchogenic carcinoma. West J Med. 1985;142:345–7.
43. Angel-Moreno Maroto A, Martínez-Quintana E, Suárez-Castellano L, Pérez-Arellano J-L. Painful hypertrophic osteoarthropathy successfully treated with octreotide. The pathogenetic role of vascular endothelial growth factor (VEGF). Rheumatology. 2005;44:1326–7.
44. Johnson SA, Spiller PA, Faull CM. Treatment of resistant pain in hypertrophic pulmonary osteoarthropathy with subcutaneous octreotide. Thorax. 1997;52:298–9.
45. López-Enriquez E, Morales AR, Robert F. Effect of atropine sulfate in pulmonary hypertrophic osteoarthropathy. Arthritis Rheum. 1980;23:822–4.
46. Reardon G, Collins AJ, Bacon PA. The effect of adrenergic blockade in hypertrophic pulmonary osteoarthropathy (HPOA). Postgrad Med J. 1976;52:170–3.
47. Diner WC, Rock L. Hypertrophie osteoarthropathy: relief of symptoms by vagotomy in a patient with pulmonary metastases from a lympho-epithelioma of the nasopharynx. JAMA. 1962;181:555–7.
48. Ooi A, Saad RA, Moorjani N, Amer KM. Effective symptomatic relief of hypertrophic pulmonary osteoarthropathy by video-assisted thoracic surgery truncal vagotomy. Ann Thorac Surg. 2007;83:684–5.
49. Amital H, Applbaum YH, Vasiliev L, Rubinow A. Hypertrophic pulmonary osteoarthropathy: control of pain and symptoms with pamidronate. Clin Rheumatol. 2004;23:330–2.
50. Garske LA, Bell SC. Pamidronate results in symptom control of hypertrophic pulmonary osteoarthropathy in cystic fibrosis. Chest. 2002;121:1363–4.
51. Jayakar BA, Abelson AG, Yao Q. Treatment of hypertrophic osteoarthropathy with zoledronic acid: case report and review of the literature. Semin Arthritis Rheum. 2011;41:291–6.
52. King MM, Nelson DA. Hypertrophic osteoarthropathy effectively treated with zoledronic acid. Clin Lung Cancer. 2008;9:179–82.
53. Mauricio O, et al. Hypertrophic osteoarthropathy masquerading as lower extremity cellulitis and response to bisphosphonates. J Thorac Oncol. 2009;4:260–2.
54. Suzuma T, et al. Pamidronate-induced remission of pain associated with hypertrophic pulmonary osteoarthropathy in chemoendocrine therapy-refractory inoperable metastatic breast carcinoma. Anti-Cancer Drugs. 2001;12:731–4.
55. Molyneux ID, Moon T, Webb AK, Morice AH. Treatment of cystic fibrosis associated cutaneous vasculitis with chloroquine. J Cyst Fibros. 2010;9:439–41.
56. Soter NA, Mihm MC, Colten HR. Cutaneous necrotizing venulitis in patients with cystic fibrosis. J Pediatr. 1979;95:190–1.
57. Wujanto L, Ross C. Recurrent vasculitis in cystic fibrosis. BMJ Case Rep. 2010;2010
58. Garty BZ, Scanlin T, Goldsmith DP, Grunstein M. Cutaneous manifestations of cystic fibrosis: possible role of cryoglobulins. Br J Dermatol. 1989;121:655–8.
59. Hodson ME. Vasculitis and arthropathy in cystic fibrosis. J R Soc Med. 1992;85:38–40.
60. John EG, Medenis R, Rao S. Cutaneous necrotizing venulitis in patients with cystic fibrosis [letter]. J Pediatr. 1980;97:505.
61. Nielsen HE, Lundh S, Jacobsen SV, Høiby N. Hypergammagolbulinemic purpura in cystic fibrosis. Acta Paediatr. 1978;67:443–7.
62. Finnegan MJ, et al. Vasculitis complicating cystic fibrosis. Q J Med. 1989;72:609–21.

63. Hilton AM, et al. Cutaneous vasculitis and immune complexes in severe bronchiectasis. Thorax. 1984;39:185–91.
64. Schultz H, Weiss JP. The bactericidal/permeability-increasing protein (BPI) in infection and inflammatory disease. Clin Chim Acta. 2007;384:12–23.
65. Sedivá A, et al. Antineutrophil cytoplasmic autoantibodies (ANCA) in children with cystic fibrosis. J Autoimmun. 1998;11:185–90.
66. Iovine NM, Elsbach P, Weiss J. An opsonic function of the neutrophil bactericidal/permeability-increasing protein depends on both its N- and C-terminal domains. Proc Natl Acad Sci U S A. 1997;94:10973–8.
67. Elsbach P. The bactericidal/permeability-increasing protein (BPI) in antibacterial host defense. J Leukoc Biol. 1998;64:14–8.
68. Elsbach P, Weiss J. Role of the bactericidal/permeability-increasing protein in host defence. Curr Opin Immunol. 1998;10:45–9.
69. Zhao MH, Jones SJ, Lockwood CM. Bactericidal/permeability-increasing protein (BPI) is an important antigen for anti-neutrophil cytoplasmic autoantibodies (ANCA) in vasculitis. Clin Exp Immunol. 1995;99:49–56.
70. Van der Schaft DW, Toebes EA, Haseman JR, Mayo KH, Griffioen AW. Bactericidal/permeability-increasing protein (BPI) inhibits angiogenesis via induction of apoptosis in vascular endothelial cells. Blood. 2000;96:176–81.
71. Arditi M, et al. Bactericidal/permeability-increasing protein protects vascular endothelial cells from lipopolysaccharide-induced activation and injury. Infect Immun. 1994;62:3930–6.
72. Mahadeva R, et al. Anti-neutrophil cytoplasmic antibodies (ANCA) against bactericidal/permeability-increasing protein (BPI) and cystic fibrosis lung disease. Clin Exp Immunol. 1999;117:561–7.
73. Zhao MH, et al. Autoantibodies against bactericidal/permeability-increasing protein in patients with cystic fibrosis. QJM. 1996;89:259–65.
74. Döring G, Albus A, Høiby N. Immunologic aspects of cystic fibrosis. Chest. 1988;94:109S–14S.
75. Mathieu JP, Stack BH, Dick WC, Buchanan WW. Pulmonary infection and rheumatoid arthritis. Br J Dis Chest. 1978;72:57–61.
76. Finder KA, McCollough ML, Dixon SL, Majka AJ, Jaremko W. Hypergammaglobulinemic purpura of Waldenström. J Am Acad Dermatol. 1990;23:669–76.
77. Dodge JA, Lewis PA, Stanton M, Wilsher J. Cystic fibrosis mortality and survival in the UK: 1947-2003. Eur Respir J. 2007;29:522–6.
78. Lindberg U, Carlsson M, Löfdahl C-G, Segelmark M. BPI-ANCA and long-term prognosis among 46 adult CF patients: a prospective 10-year follow-up study. Clin Dev Immunol. 2012;2012:370107.
79. Wolfson JS, Hooper DC. The fluoroquinolones: structures, mechanisms of action and resistance, and spectra of activity in vitro. Antimicrob Agents Chemother. 1985;28:581–6.
80. Lode H, et al. Quinolone pharmacokinetics and metabolism. J Antimicrob Chemother. 1990;26(Suppl B):41–9.
81. Vance-Bryan K, Guay DRP, Rotschafer JC. Clinical pharmacokinetics of ciprofloxacin. Clin Pharmacokinet. 1990;19:434–61.
82. Hooper DC, Wolfson JS. The fluoroquinolones: pharmacology, clinical uses, and toxicities in humans. Antimicrob Agents Chemother. 1985;28:716–21.
83. Cook PJ, Andrews JM, Wise R, Honeybourne D, Moudgil H. Concentrations of OPC-17116, a new fluoroquinolone antibacterial, in serum and lung compartments. J Antimicrob Chemother. 1995;35:317–26.
84. Lee LJ, et al. Penetration of levofloxacin into lung tissue after oral administration to subjects undergoing lung biopsy or lobectomy. Pharmacotherapy. 1998;18:35–41.
85. Wise R, Baldwin DR, Andrews JM, Honeybourne D. Comparative pharmacokinetic disposition of fluoroquinolones in the lung. J Antimicrob Chemother. 1991;28(Suppl C):65–71.
86. Burkhardt JE, Hill MA, Carlton WW, Kesterson JW. Histologic and histochemical changes in articular cartilages of immature beagle dogs dosed with difloxacin, a fluoroquinolone. Vet Pathol. 1990;27:162–70.

87. Gough A, Barsoum NJ, Mitchell L, McGuire EJ, de la Iglesia FA. Juvenile canine drug-induced arthropathy: clinicopathological studies on articular lesions caused by oxolinic and pipemidic acids. Toxicol Appl Pharmacol. 1979;51:177–87.

88. Kato M, Onodera T. Morphological investigation of cavity formation in articular cartilage induced by ofloxacin in rats. Fundam Appl Toxicol. 1988;11:110–9.

89. Shakibaei M, et al. Comparative evaluation of ultrastructural changes in articular cartilage of ofloxacin-treated and magnesium-deficient immature rats. Toxicol Pathol. 1996;24:580–7.

90. Stahlmann R, et al. Ofloxacin in juvenile non-human primates and rats. Arthropathia and drug plasma concentrations. Arch Toxicol. 1990;64:193–204.

91. Menschik M, et al. Effects of ciprofloxacin and ofloxacin on adult human cartilage in vitro. Antimicrob Agents Chemother. 1997;41:2562–5.

92. Black A, Redmond AOB, Steen HJ, Oborska IT. Tolerance and safety of ciprofloxacin in paediatric patients. J Antimicrob Chemother. 1990;26:25–9.

93. Chalumeau M, et al. Fluoroquinolone safety in pediatric patients: a prospective, multicenter, comparative cohort study in France. Pediatrics. 2003;111:e714–9.

94. Church DA, et al. Sequential ciprofloxacin therapy in pediatric cystic fibrosis: comparative study vs. ceftazidime/tobramycin in the treatment of acute pulmonary exacerbations. Pediatr Infect Dis J. 1997;16:97.

95. Raeburn JA, et al. Ciprofloxacin therapy in cystic fibrosis. J Antimicrob Chemother. 1987;20:295–6.

96. Richard DA, et al. Oral ciprofloxacin vs intravenous ceftazidime plus tobramycin in pediatric cystic fibrosis patients: comparison of antipseudomonas efficacy and assessment of safety with ultrasonography and magnetic resonance imaging Cystic Fibrosis Study Group. Pediatr Infect Dis J. 1997;16:572–8.

97. Rubio TT. Ciprofloxacin in the treatment of Pseudomonas infection in children with cystic fibrosis. Diagn Microbiol Infect Dis. 1990;13:153–5.

98. Schaad UB, Wedgwood J, Ruedeberg A, Kraemer R, Hampel B. Ciprofloxacin as antipseudomonal treatment in patients with cystic fibrosis. Pediatr Infect Dis J. 1997;16:106–11; discussion 123–126.

99. Adefurin A, Sammons H, Jacqz-Aigrain E, Choonara I. Ciprofloxacin safety in paediatrics: a systematic review. Arch Dis Child. 2011;96:874–80.

100. Kubin R. Safety and efficacy of ciprofloxacin in paediatric patients--review. Infection. 1993;21:413–21.

101. Chyský V, et al. Safety of ciprofloxacin in children: worldwide clinical experience based on compassionate use. Emphasis on joint evaluation. Infection. 1991;19:289–96.

102. Cruciani M, et al. Prophylactic co-trimoxazole versus norfloxacin in neutropenic children--perspective randomized study. Infection. 1989;17:65–9.

103. Schaad UB, Wedgwood-Krucko J. Nalidixic acid in children: retrospective matched controlled study for cartilage toxicity. Infection. 1987;15:165–8.

104. Redmond A, et al. Oral ciprofloxacin in the treatment of pseudomonas exacerbations of paediatric cystic fibrosis: clinical efficacy and safety evaluation using magnetic resonance image scanning. J Int Med Res. 1998;26:304–12.

105. Aricò M, et al. Long-term magnetic resonance survey of cartilage damage in leukemic children treated with fluoroquinolones. Pediatr Infect Dis J. 1995;14:713–4.

106. Yee CL, Duffy C, Gerbino PG, Stryker S, Noel GJ. Tendon or joint disorders in children after treatment with fluoroquinolones or azithromycin. Pediatr Infect Dis J. 2002;21:525–9.

107. Schaad UB, Sander E, Wedgwood J, Schaffner T. Morphologic studies for skeletal toxicity after prolonged ciprofloxacin therapy in two juvenile cystic fibrosis patients. ET J. 1992;11:1047–9.

108. Adam D. Use of quinolones in pediatric patients. Rev Infect Dis. 1989;11(Suppl 5):S1113–6.

109. Jackson MA, Schutze GE, Committee on Infectious Diseases. The use of systemic and topical fluoroquinolones. Pediatrics. 2016;138:e20162706.

110. Schaad UB, et al. Use of fluoroquinolones in pediatrics: consensus report of an International Society of Chemotherapy commission. Pediatr Infect Dis J. 1995;14:1–9.

111. Velissariou IM. The use of fluoroquinolones in children: recent advances. Expert Rev Anti-Infect Ther. 2006;4:853–60.
112. Grady R. Safety profile of quinolone antibiotics in the pediatric population. Pediatr Infect Dis J. 2003;22:1128.
113. Bhudhikanok GS, et al. Correlates of osteopenia in patients with cystic fibrosis. Pediatrics. 1996;97:103–11.
114. Bhudhikanok GS, et al. Bone acquisition and loss in children and adults with cystic fibrosis: a longitudinal study. J Pediatr. 1998;133:18–27.
115. Henderson RC, Madsen CD. Bone density in children and adolescents with cystic fibrosis. J Pediatr. 1996;128:28–34.
116. Shane E, et al. Osteoporosis in lung transplantation candidates with end-stage pulmonary disease. Am J Med. 1996;101:262–9.
117. Gibbens DT, et al. Osteoporosis in cystic fibrosis. J Pediatr. 1988;113:295–300.
118. Grey AB, Ames RW, Matthews RD, Reid IR. Bone mineral density and body composition in adult patients with cystic fibrosis. Thorax. 1993;48:589–93.
119. Rochat T, Slosman DO, Pichard C, Belli DC. Body composition analysis by dual-energy X-ray absorptiometry in adults with cystic fibrosis. Chest. 1994;106:800–5.
120. Bachrach LK, Loutit CW, Moss RB. Osteopenia in adults with cystic fibrosis. Am J Med. 1994;96:27–34.
121. Conway S, et al. Osteoporosis and osteopenia in adults and adolescents with cystic fibrosis: prevalence and associated factors. Thorax. 2000;55:798–804.
122. Mischler EH, Chesney PJ, Chesney RW, Mazess RB. Demineralization in cystic fibrosis: detected by direct photon absorptiometry. Am J Dis Child. 1979;133:632–5.
123. Hahn TJ, Squires AE, Halstead LR, Strominger DB. Reduced serum 25-hydroxyvitamin D concentration and disordered mineral metabolism in patients with cystic fibrosis. J Pediatr. 1979;94:38–42.
124. Elkin SL, et al. Vertebral deformities and low bone mineral density in adults with cystic fibrosis: a cross-sectional study. Osteoporos Int. 2001;12:366–72.
125. Henderson RC, Madsen CD. Bone mineral content and body composition in children and young adults with cystic fibrosis. Pediatr Pulmonol. 1999;27:80–4.
126. Haworth CS, et al. Low bone mineral density in adults with cystic fibrosis. Thorax. 1999;54:961–7.
127. Tschopp O, et al. Osteoporosis before lung transplantation: association with low body mass index, but not with underlying disease. Am J Transplant. 2002;2:167–72.
128. Shaw N, Bedford C, Heaf D, Carty H, Dutton J. Osteopenia in adults with cystic fibrosis. Am J Med. 1995;99:690–2.
129. Baroncelli GI, et al. Bone demineralization in cystic fibrosis: evidence of imbalance between bone formation and degradation. Pediatr Res. 1997;41:397–403.
130. Donovan DS, et al. Bone mass and vitamin D deficiency in adults with advanced cystic fibrosis lung disease. Am J Respir Crit Care Med. 1998;157:1892–9.
131. King SJ, et al. Reduced bone density in cystic fibrosis: ΔF508 mutation is an independent risk factor. Eur Respir J. 2005;25:54–61.
132. Donadio MVF, et al. Bone mineral density, pulmonary function, chronological age, and age at diagnosis in children and adolescents with cystic fibrosis. J Pediatr. 2013;89:151–7.
133. Parasa RB, Maffulli N. Musculoskeletal involvement in cystic fibrosis. Bull Hosp Jt Dis N Y N. 1999;58:37–44.
134. Aris RM, et al. Increased rate of fractures and severe kyphosis: sequelae of living into adulthood with cystic fibrosis. Ann Intern Med. 1998;128:186–93.
135. Paccou J, Zeboulon N, Combescure C, Gossec L, Cortet B. The prevalence of osteoporosis, osteopenia, and fractures among adults with cystic fibrosis: a systematic literature review with meta-analysis. Calcif Tissue Int. 2010;86:1–7.
136. Laursen EM, Mølgaard C, Michaelsen KF, Koch C, Müller J. Bone mineral status in 134 patients with cystic fibrosis. Arch Dis Child. 1999;81:235–40.

137. Kanis JA. Diagnosis of osteoporosis and assessment of fracture risk. Lancet. 2002;359:1929–36.
138. Henderson RC, Specter BB. Kyphosis and fractures in children and young adults with cystic fibrosis. J Pediatr. 1994;125:208–12.
139. Sirmali M, et al. A comprehensive analysis of traumatic rib fractures: morbidity, mortality and management. Eur J Cardiothorac Surg. 2003;24:133–8.
140. Lorbergs AL, et al. Severity of kyphosis and decline in lung function: the Framingham study. J Gerontol A Biol Sci Med Sci. 2017;72:689–94.
141. Culham EG, Jimenez HA, King CE. Thoracic kyphosis, rib mobility, and lung volumes in normal women and women with osteoporosis. Spine. 1994;19:1250–5.
142. Ravilly S, Robinson W, Suresh S, Wohl ME, Berde CB. Chronic pain in cystic fibrosis. Pediatrics. 1996;98:741–7.
143. Felson DT, Zhang Y, Hannan MT, Anderson JJ. Effects of weight and body mass index on bone mineral density in men and women: the Framingham study. J Bone Miner Res. 1993;8:567–73.
144. Reid IR. Relationships between fat and bone. Osteoporos Int. 2008;19:595–606.
145. Salamoni F, et al. Bone mineral content in cystic fibrosis patients: correlation with fat-free mass. Arch Dis Child. 1996;74:314–8.
146. Hardin DS, Arumugam R, Seilheimer DK, LeBlanc A, Ellis KJ. Normal bone mineral density in cystic fibrosis. Arch Dis Child. 2001;84:363–8.
147. Aris RM, Neuringer IP, Weiner MA, Egan TM, Ontjes D. Severe osteoporosis before and after lung transplantation. Chest. 1996;109:1176–83.
148. Reid IR, Grey AB. Corticosteroid osteoporosis. Baillieres Clin Rheumatol. 1993;7:573–87.
149. Sambrook P, Lane NE. Corticosteroid osteoporosis. Best Pract Res Clin Rheumatol. 2001;15:401–13.
150. Borowitz D, Baker RD, Stallings V. Consensus report on nutrition for pediatric patients with cystic fibrosis. J Pediatr Gastroenterol Nutr. 2002;35:246.
151. Johannesson M, Gottlieb C, Hjelte L. Delayed puberty in girls with cystic fibrosis despite good clinical status. Pediatrics. 1997;99:29–34.
152. Bailey DA, Mckay HA, Mirwald RL, Crocker PRE, Faulkner RA. A six-year longitudinal study of the relationship of physical activity to bone mineral accrual in growing children: the University of Saskatchewan Bone Mineral Accrual Study. J Bone Miner Res. 1999;14:1672–9.
153. Alswat K, Gender A. Disparities in osteoporosis. J Clin Med Res. 2017;9:382–7.
154. Cawthon P, Gender M. Differences in osteoporosis and fractures. Clin Orthop. 2011;469:1900–5.
155. Baim S, et al. Official positions of the International Society for Clinical Densitometry and executive summary of the 2007 ISCD Pediatric Position Development Conference. J Clin Densitom. 2008;11:6–21.
156. Smith J, Shoukri K. Diagnosis of osteoporosis. Clin Cornerstone. 2000;2:22–30.
157. Brown SA, et al. Short-term calcitriol administration improves calcium homeostasis in adults with cystic fibrosis. Osteoporos Int. 2003;14:442–9.
158. Haworth CS, Jones AM, Adams JE, Selby PL, Webb AK. Randomised double blind placebo controlled trial investigating the effect of calcium and vitamin D supplementation on bone mineral density and bone metabolism in adult patients with cystic fibrosis. J Cyst Fibros. 2004;3:233–6.
159. Zeitlin PL. Cystic fibrosis and estrogens: a perfect storm. J Clin Invest. 2008;118:3841–4.
160. Aris RM, et al. Efficacy of alendronate in adults with cystic fibrosis with low bone density. Am J Respir Crit Care Med. 2004;169:77–82.
161. Aris RM, et al. Efficacy of pamidronate for osteoporosis in patients with cystic fibrosis following lung transplantation. Am J Respir Crit Care Med. 2000;162:941–6.
162. Conway SP, Oldroyd B, Morton A, Truscott JG, Peckham DG. Effect of oral bisphosphonates on bone mineral density and body composition in adult patients with cystic fibrosis: a pilot study. Thorax. 2004;59:699–703.

163. Haworth CS, et al. Effect of intravenous pamidronate on bone mineral density in adults with cystic fibrosis. Thorax. 2001;56:314–6.
164. Haworth CS, et al. Severe bone pain after intravenous pamidronate in adult patients with cystic fibrosis. Lancet. 1998;352:1753–4.
165. Conwell LS, Chang AB. Bisphosphonates for osteoporosis in people with cystic fibrosis. Cochrane Libr. 2014;3:1465–1858.
166. Bachrach LK, Ward LM. Bisphosphonate use in childhood osteoporosis. J Clin Endocrinol Metab. 2009;94:400–9.

Chapter 19
Impact of CF on the Kidneys

Andrew Prayle and Bradley S. Quon

Patient Perspective

1. *What were your feelings when you heard that you had been diagnosed with kidney disease?*

    I was first made aware of kidney disease shortly after my double lung transplant in 2008. My kidney function gradually declined and I was initially monitored by my transplant team. I was eventually referred to a nephrologist around 2 years post-transplant. At that stage I was not really worried, just aware that it was something we had to keep an eye on. As a CF patient who had already overcome a double lung transplant, the idea of dealing with kidney disease at first was not really worrisome. Shortly after being diagnosed, I was at a CF fundraiser and was fortunate to speak to another CF patient who had also undergone a heart-double lung transplant in addition to a kidney transplant. She reassured me by saying not to worry, that a kidney transplant was a "walk in the park" compared to a double lung transplant, and that she believed I would be just fine. As kidney disease can be slowly progressive, it wasn't a sudden diagnosis, and you can be diagnosed with CKD many years before it progresses to end stage – in my case it was about 7 years.

2. *Did you know anything about kidney disease before you were diagnosed?*

    I knew very little about my kidneys prior to being told they were showing a decline in function. I was only aware that the tobramycin I was on for many years could eventually cause some damage, but I was unaware of any damage until after my double lung transplant. Shortly after the diagnosis of end-stage

A. Prayle
The University of Nottingham, Child Health, Obstetrics and Gynaecology, Queens Medical Centre, Nottingham, UK

B. S. Quon (✉)
St. Paul's Hospital, University of British Columbia, Department of Medicine, Vancouver, BC, Canada
e-mail: BRADLEY.QUON@HLI.UBC.CA

© Springer Nature Switzerland AG 2020
S. D. Davis et al. (eds.), *Cystic Fibrosis*, Respiratory Medicine,
https://doi.org/10.1007/978-3-030-42382-7_19

disease, I was worked up for a kidney transplant. I had three people willing to be tested to see if they could be my donor. Unfortunately, none was a blood match, but we were told that the paired kidney exchange program could be an option. This is also known as a kidney swap and allows me to receive more compatible kidneys from an unrelated donor and another recipient also in need of a kidney to receive more compatible kidneys from one of my donors. Fortunately, my kidney function rebounded and stabilized for a couple more years and I was temporarily removed from the transplant program.

3. **How has this kidney disease impacted your life? How burdensome is the additional treatment for your kidney disease?**

   At this stage, now 8 years after the initial diagnosis of kidney disease, it has become quite burdensome. I am now required to do dialysis at home, overnight, for approx. 32 hours each week. The side effects of dialysis (i.e., headaches, nausea, restless leg syndrome, joint pain) have made things quite uncomfortable. The potential donors I had lined up 8 years ago have now moved on with their lives and are no longer able to be my donor. Instead, now my father has been worked up, and although he is not a blood match either, he has been approved for the paired exchange program. Now we just need to wait for a paired match to be made.

4. **Has your overall health changed since you developed kidney disease?**

   As far as I am aware, the rest of my organs are not suffering from the ESRD. In the first 7 years or so, there wasn't much change to my health at all. It was just a wait-and-see situation However, in the last year or so, my quality of life has declined significantly, first from the symptoms related to the kidney function declining and then, in the last 3–6 months, from the dialysis treatments.

5. **If you could speak directly to patients who were newly diagnosed with this, what would you want them to know?**

   From initial diagnosis through chronic kidney disease stages 3a, 3b, and 4, there is not much change; life was seemingly the same. By stage 5, things become much more complicated. Diet restrictions, symptoms of fatigue, and headaches and nausea all are signs that you need kidney replacement. My suggestion would be that if you can avoid dialysis by receiving a kidney transplant first, that would probably be your best choice.

6. **If you could speak directly to physicians who care for people with CF who develop kidney disease, what would you want them to know?**

   Push for a transplant before dialysis is required. If CF doctors could help encourage the nephrologist to start the transplant work up sooner and encourage patients to find friends or family willing to donate sooner, dialysis could be avoided.

7. **What is the most important thing that researchers could address about kidney disease that would improve your life?**

   I suppose other options for kidney replacement therapy. Improvements in the dialysis machines. Further research into the non-ABO compatible donation. Mechanical kidneys. And any other ideas that could replace failing kidneys.

   –Anonymous

Introduction

Renal issues are often an overlooked aspect of CF care, but based on a 40-year experience at the Royal Brompton Hospital, approximately 5% of adults with CF are impacted by some form of renal involvement [1]. With aging of the CF population and increased rates of lung transplantation, the prevalence is expected to rise in the future as many of the renal issues encountered by individuals with CF relate to comorbidities and/or medications as opposed to being primary to CF transmembrane conductance regulator (CFTR) dysfunction.

Role of CFTR in the Kidney

CFTR is abundantly expressed in all nephron segments, but its precise physiologic role in the kidney remains unclear. CFTR does not appear to play a primary role in kidney function, but it might be involved in the regulation of other ion channels (e.g., epithelial sodium channel [ENaC] and renal outer medullary potassium [ROMK]). Furthermore, it potentially interacts with other proteins located in proximal tubular (PT) cells to acidify endosomal vesicles, which is important for the endocytosis of low-molecular-weight (LMW) proteins [2–6]. It has been postulated that the lack of a clear-cut renal phenotype in CF is due to other renal transporters or proteins compensating for a lack of CFTR function. Interestingly, a functional isoform of CFTR referred to as TNR-CFTR capable of functioning like wild-type CFTR in vitro has been identified in the renal medulla of humans and CFTR knockout mice and may potentially replace some of its function when wild-type CFTR is absent or not functioning correctly [5].

Even though renal function is not believed to be directly affected by CFTR dysfunction, the renal clearance of several antibiotics (e.g., amikacin, ceftazidime, cloxacillin, ticarcillin, piperacillin, trimethoprim) has been shown to be increased in individuals with CF compared to the general population [7, 8]. As such, antibiotic doses to treat airway infection in CF are typically higher than that required for the general population [8]. While the precise mechanism for increased renal clearance in CF remains unclear for most antibiotics, increased glomerular filtration and enhanced tubular secretion are presumed contributors [8–10].

Additional insights into the potential physiologic role of CFTR in the kidney have been demonstrated in the study of non-CF pathologic conditions [11, 12]. CFTR is an important modifier gene in the pathogenesis of autosomal dominant polycystic kidney disease (ADPKD) by increasing fluid accumulation leading to cyst enlargement [11]. Based on clinical studies, individuals affected by both ADPKD and CF appear to have a milder PKD phenotype with smaller cysts, and thus CF might have a protective effect on kidney function in this condition [13, 14]. Emerging data has also implicated CFTR in the pathogenesis of unilateral ureteral obstruction-induced kidney fibrosis. Downregulation of CFTR in renal tubular epithelial cells results in higher Wnt/ß-catenin signaling, which induces epithelial-to-mesenchymal transition, critical to the progression of kidney fibrosis [15]. The implications of this finding for individuals with CF remains unclear but raises the possibility of dysregulated repair signaling in response to renal injury potentially leading to higher rates of fibrosis post-injury.

Diagnosing and Monitoring Renal Dysfunction in CF

As described by our patient, there are very few overt symptoms or signs during the early stages of chronic kidney disease. As such, renal disease may go unnoticed for a considerable period of time. Accurate but minimally burdensome screening for renal disease and measurement of renal function in CF are therefore of particular importance.

Measurement and Monitoring of Renal Function in CF

Serum creatinine and blood urea nitrate (BUN) are helpful in identifying acute kidney injury (AKI) in cystic fibrosis (such as AKI secondary to nephrotoxic drugs) and are routinely measured in the CF clinic. However, simple measurement of Cr and BUN and comparison to normal ranges cannot reliably identify chronic kidney disease, especially in chronic diseases such as CF when muscle mass is low (and when CKD is more important), as they do not identify patients with reduced glomerular filtration rate (GFR) [16]. Therefore, several more invasive (and complex) tests have been developed to monitor renal function.

From the perspective of the CF physician, the kidneys are central to pharmacokinetics (largely determined by glomerular function and the glomerular filtration rate [GFR]), electrolyte balance (largely determined by tubular function), and regulation of blood pressure. In late-stage chronic kidney disease, renal-related bone disease becomes important. However, assessments of GFR are perhaps most useful as a "global" measure of kidney function and, unfortunately, more difficult to assess. GFR is usually normalized to body surface area (usually expressed as mL per 1.73 m^2) to allow comparison of GFR between individuals. We next discuss the various approaches to measuring or estimating GFR, and then give some practical recommendations.

Ideal measurement of GFR uses a pharmacologically inert tracer substance which is freely filtered by the glomerulus, not reabsorbed by the tubule, and accurately assayed in the laboratory. In the classical clearance-based methods for evaluating GFR, the tracer is infused until a steady state is achieved and then the GFR calculated from the rate of infusion and the steady-state concentration. The original "gold standard" of inulin clearance is rarely undertaken in clinical practice, as it is cumbersome. Alternate methods, in order of accuracy include (i) the plasma disappearance method, usually employing radioisotopes, (ii) timed collections of urine to measure urinary creatinine clearance, and (iii) equations incorporating serum creatinine and body measurements to estimate glomerular filtration rate.

Plasma Disappearance Methods of Radioisotopes

Plasma disappearance methods have been used since the 1950s. There are multiple published protocols, and experienced centers have validated their own protocols. A tracer agent (such as ^{Cr51}EDTA or $^{Tc\text{-}99m}$DTPA) is administered as a bolus and then measured at timed intervals after the administration, and from this the pharmacokinetics of the elimination (or "disappearance") from the plasma is calculated. If the tracer is freely filtered, and not reabsorbed by the tubules, then its elimination from the plasma is a function of the glomerular filtration rate. More frequent plasma samples give a greater accuracy of measurement of the plasma elimination rate but at the cost of increased burden.

Radioisotopes are frequently used as tracers, as their concentration can be assayed in a rigorous and standardized manner. Choice of radioisotope is largely driven by local experience, and the regulatory environment. Additionally, there are intermittent international shortages of radioisotopes, which can significantly affect access to tests. The radiation exposure from a single GFR measurement is minimal, and less than a chest radiograph, although some precautions are required when disposing of urine. Radioisotope methods should only be undertaken in experienced accredited laboratories – there are numerous reports indicating that experience is key to accurate, reproducible results.

Creatinine Clearance

Timed 24-hour collections of urinary creatinine (the creatinine clearance, CrCl) allows calculation of the urinary CrCl, a proxy for GFR. The underlying physiology is that serum creatinine, produced by muscle, is produced at a relatively stable rate and is freely filtered by the glomerulus, and therefore the urinary clearance provides a good measure of GFR. There is a small amount of tubular secretion of creatinine, and therefore the method is not as accurate as plasma disappearance ones. However, inaccuracies in collecting a full 24 hours of urine are more likely to affect the results. Therefore, although this method is useful in highly motivated adults, it is seldom used in children, due to the difficulty in obtaining a full 24-hour urine collection.

Estimation of GFR from Plasma Creatinine

There have been multiple methods described to estimate GFR from a plasma sample of creatinine, using equations which take into account demographic and body habitus parameters. The most widely known are the Cockcroft and Gault (C&G) and MDRD formulae in adults and the Schwartz formula in children. Of particular concern is that individuals with reduced muscle mass have decreased creatinine, impacting upon the estimation. This is of particular importance in individuals with any chronic disease, especially in cystic fibrosis with severe lung disease, where

Table 19.1 Selected studies evaluating serum creatinine-based estimating equations comparing measured GFR with estimated GFR

N	Age group included	Reference standard	Creatinine-based estimating equation	Bias	95% Limits of agreement	Reference
20	Adults	**99mTcDTPA**	C&G	25.2	−26.5 to 76.5	[17]
20	Adults	**99mTcDTPA**	MDRD	−64.2	−211.3 to 82.9	[17]
27	Children	**99mTcDTPA**	Schwartz	−3.5	−51.1 to 44.1	[17]
80	Adults	**Creatinine clearance**	C&G	9.7	−24.9 to 43.9	[18]
80	Adults	**Creatinine clearance**	MDRD	4.0	−34.3 to 42.3	[18]
16	Adults	**51CrEDTA**	MDRD	0.73	−37.5 to 39.0	[19][a]
50	Children	**51CrEDTA**	Schwartz	−4.4	−74.2 to 65.4	[18][a]

The bias represents the systematic under or over estimation of the estimating equation. The 95% limits of agreement can be interpreted as a range of values above and below any individual estimate for which it is plausible that the actual GFR is. As can be seen, the creatinine-based estimating equations universally perform poorly. C&G, Cockcroft and Gault; MDRD, modified diet in renal disease
[a]Data presented, final manuscript currently under review

evaluating renal function has important implications for medication dosing. Several studies have evaluated formulas to estimate GFR in the setting of cystic fibrosis (Table 19.1) [17–19]. There is poor performance of estimating equations – the Bland Altman 95% limits of agreement provides an assessment of the plausible range within which a true GFR may lay, based on an estimated GFR. True GFR can be 50 ml/min/1.72 m^2 above or below the estimated GFR. Therefore, a single estimate of GFR from a creatinine-based formulae is unhelpful, but often in clinical practice, a low level is used as an indication to conduct a more formal test. However, a trend over time, especially in the relative short term while monitoring potentially nephrotoxic medications, may be more useful.

Cystatin C-Based Formulae

There has been intense effort in finding and evaluating minimally invasive and accurate methods of estimating GFR. In particular, cystatin C (CysC) has been proposed. CysC is produced by all nucleated cells at a relatively constant rate and is freely filtered from the plasma into the tubular fluid, where it is reabsorbed by the tubules but metabolized in this process, meaning that none returns to the circulation. As a result, plasma levels of CysC are related to the number of nucleated cells (not muscle mass), and therefore it is potentially more reliable than creatinine [20]. Originally, it was thought that CysC production was highly coupled to nuclear number alone, but in actual fact, CysC production can be influenced by other factors, such as administration of steroids. There are multiple assays for CysC, and only recently reference standards have been produced. Unfortunately, although CysC based formulae do outperform creatinine formulas (especially in children), the improvement is not sufficient to replace formal GFR measurement [17].

Novel Biomarkers

An accurate screening test for GFR would be immensely helpful, especially if it performed well in a cystic fibrosis cohort. We evaluated various urinary proteins which are traditionally thought of as biomarkers of acute kidney injury and found that elevated levels of Kidney Injury Molecule-1 (KIM-1), when taken during a period of stability off antibiotics, is associated with a 25% risk of a GFR less than 90 ml/min/1.73 m2 in our clinic population [21]. This could represent an approach to screening but requires further validation.

Imaging biomarkers may well be helpful in the future to detect early renal damage in CF. Several functional magnetic resonance imaging (MRI) techniques have been applied to the kidney, and many of these techniques do not require intravenous contrast or radiation making them particularly attractive for application in children [22–25]. MRI can measure a diverse range of parameters including renal blood flow, kidney oxygenation, and renal function. Quantitative diffusion tensor imaging (DTI) MRI techniques can measure the magnitude and directionality of water's movement through tissue, with reduced diffusion and lack of directionality indicating renal dysfunction [25]. A recent study has shown that medullary FA is decreased in CF patients compared to health controls despite "normal" renal function (based on eGFR) and therefore represents a promising early indicator of renal impairment (Fig. 19.1).

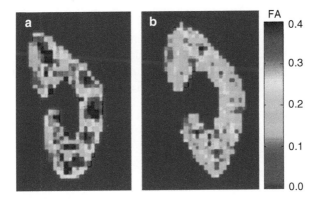

Fig. 19.1 Kidney diffusion MRI in cystic fibrosis. Diffusion MRI fractional anisotropy (FA) maps from (**a**) a healthy non-CF control subject and (**b**) an adult subject with CF-related diabetes. Note the altered medullary microstructure in the kidney of the subject with CF indicative of chronic kidney disease. Initial results suggest that these renal changes are associated with CF-related diabetes. (Images courtesy of Dr. Chris Flask and Dr. Kimberley McBennett from Case Western Reserve University)

A Practical Approach to Monitoring for Chronic Kidney Disease in CF

The preceding discussion is somewhat abstract; a practical discussion follows. For patients without known kidney disease, we would recommend an annual measurement of electrolytes, including magnesium, calcium, phosphate, and bicarbonate, to screen for tubulopathy, and a measurement of blood pressure (which is often omitted in pediatric clinics). A urine dip for urine protein creatinine ratio is also minimally invasive. Serum creatinine is easily measured, and an appropriate formula (such as the Schwartz formula in children) should be used to estimate GFR and should be compared to previous years looking for a trend.

For patients who have who have had an episode of AKI, we would recommend referral for a formal evaluation of GFR, which will usually involve a radioisotope method. Choice of measurement is largely dictated by local nephrology practice and regional availability of radioisotopes; In our centers we use Cr51EDTA, but other isotopes such as DTPA are frequently used. Laboratory experience, rather than choice of isotope, is a major determinant of accuracy. If the GFR is low (less than 90 ml/min/1.73 m2), we recommend an annual formal assessment of GFR and consideration of more intensive monitoring if frequent potentially nephrotoxic drugs are being used.

Acute Kidney Injury

Acute kidney injury (AKI) is the syndrome of rapid deterioration in kidney function, which can be conceptualized by a sudden reduction in glomerular filtration rate, disordered plasma homeostasis and electrolyte disturbance, and often reduced urine production. AKI in CF can be categorized as pre-renal, renal, or post-renal (Fig. 19.2).

Pre-renal AKI

Pre-renal AKI is characterized by reduced renal plasma flow and reduced kidney function. It is the extreme end of the spectrum of appropriate dehydration-induced oliguria to pre-renal AKI with abnormal urinary electrolytes but which rapidly improves with rehydration if recognized early. If left untreated, or in the presence of additional insults to the kidney (such as nephrotoxic medications), pre-renal AKI develops and evolves into AKI with kidney tissue damage.

People with CF are at particularly high risk of dehydration. Sweat sodium losses can be considerable in CF, reducing total body sodium, leading to dehydration and effective circulating volume reduction, decreased renal plasma flow, and pre-renal

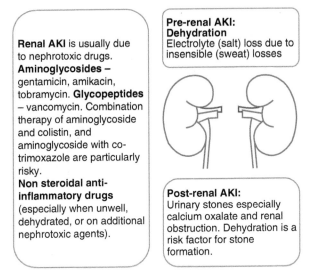

Fig. 19.2 Common causes of acute kidney injury in CF

acute renal failure. Normally an increase in serum osmolality accompanies hypotonic fluid loss, and this stimulates thirst, but the effect is dampened in CF due to sodium losses. Prevention is with adequate hydration and sodium supplementation in hot weather. Treatment is with fluid and electrolyte resuscitation.

Renal AKI

Intrinsic renal AKI in CF is predominantly caused by nephrotoxic antibiotics. Treatment regimens for important chronic infections, such as due to *Pseudomonas* and non-tuberculosis mycobacteria (NTM), frequently involve an aminoglycoside. Aminoglycosides have predictable dose-related nephrotoxicity, with a narrow therapeutic window necessitating careful prescribing. Other drugs can cause AKI via (for example) an interstitial nephritis. Often the diagnosis of drug-induced AKI is presumed, but there is a characteristic pattern on histology should a kidney biopsy be undertaken (Fig. 19.3).

In the UK, an observational study found that AKI is 100-fold more likely in the pediatric CF population compared to the general pediatric population [26]. Furthermore, the major risk factor for AKI in CF is exposure to aminoglycosides, with gentamicin more risky than tobramycin [27]. This study was performed prior to the routine treatment for NTM, and therefore it was not possible to compare the relative toxicity of amikacin and tobramycin.

AKI during exacerbations may be more common than is currently recognized, due to limitations in the current renal function monitoring. Many CF centers

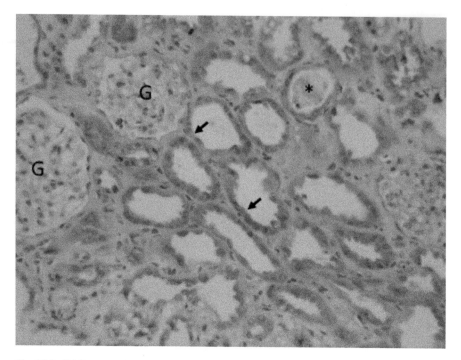

Fig. 19.3 H&E preparation of a renal biopsy in cystic fibrosis. AKI had developed over a 2-week period and required hemodialysis due to gentamicin exposure. Adjacent to the glomeruli (G), the tubules are clearly visible. Note that the usually cuboidal epithelia of the proximal tubules have lost their brush border and are showing significant flattening (arrows) leading to an apparent increase in luminal diameter. There is also debris (representing sloughed off epithelial material) in some of the tubular lumena (∗). (Image courtesy of Dr. Tom McCulloch, Consultant Histopathologist, Nottingham University Hospitals NHS Trust, UK)

measure serum creatinine at intervals during a 2-week (or longer) intravenous antibiotic course. However, daily measurement of serum creatinine has indicated that AKI may be more common, with an incidence of up to 22% of courses of IV antibiotics [28]. In addition to aminoglycosides, co-trimoxazole was also a risk factor for AKI in this study. Although other antibiotics traditionally considered to have high risk for nephrotoxicity, such as vancomycin, were not found to be risk factors for AKI in this study, we still advocate attention to the risk of nephrotoxicity and careful therapeutic drug monitoring (for aminoglycosides and glycopeptides) for all potentially nephrotoxic antibiotics.

Nonsteroidal anti-inflammatory drugs (NSAIDS) are well known to be associated with AKI. Ibuprofen is currently the only anti-inflammatory indicated to treat inflammation in CF lung disease, but there are several alternatives specifically in development. Ibuprofen is well recognized to be nephrotoxic. However, in the multicenter Canadian safety and effectiveness trial involving CF subjects, there was no increase in nephrotoxicity in the ibuprofen arm compared to the placebo arm over

2 years. However, it is worth noting that in that study, the trialists advised centers to cease ibuprofen use during periods of aminoglycoside treatment [29].

Small molecule disease-modifying drugs, also termed CFTR modulators, are now available for individuals with specific mutations, and the effectiveness in certain mutations (such as ivacaftor in G551D) is revolutionary. Currently all the approved modulators have excellent side effect profiles from the point of view of renal safety. However, future drugs do need careful evaluation. Although not FDA-approved due to lack of efficacy, Ataluren offers a cautionary example. This small molecule was developed to promote translational read-through of premature stop codon mutations. The efficacy of ataluren was unfortunately disappointing, but more concerning was the high incidence of AKI for individuals on active drug (15%) vs. placebo (<1%) [30]. The mechanism of AKI in ataluren is unclear, but it has structural similarity to aminoglycosides. The ataluren experience highlights the need for close monitoring on a population scale for side effects of new CF medications, ideally by following all patients on new medications through the various national registries.

Post-renal AKI: Nephrolithiasis

The mean prevalence of nephrolithiasis in CF reported across multiple studies is approximately 5%, and most cases tend to present during adolescence and early adulthood [31]. The risk of nephrolithiasis is estimated to be two- to fourfold higher than age-specific prevalence rates reported in individuals without CF [32]. Similar to the general population, the composition of renal stones in CF is typically calcium oxalate [33]. Patients can present clinically with renal colic, hematuria, or recurrent urinary tract infections.

Multiple factors contribute to the increased metabolic risk of calcium oxalate stones observed in CF, some of which are preventable. Conditions that tend to concentrate urinary calcium oxalate and favor stone formation include hyperoxaluria, hypocitraturia, hyperuricosuria, and low urine volume. While hypercalciuria has been described as a potential risk factor in CF, there is limited evidence of altered calcium homeostasis in CF [31].

Hyperoxaluria can occur in the setting of increased endogenous oxalate production or increased intestinal absorption of dietary oxalate. Net intestinal absorption depends on the balance between oxalate absorption and secretion; and there are CF-specific factors that lead to both increased oxalate absorption and decreased secretion. Systemic antibiotic use, frequently required to treat pulmonary exacerbations, reduces the quantity of oxalate-degrading bacteria in the gut (e.g., *Oxalobacter formigenes*), leading to increased intestinal oxalate and absorption [33]. Chronic malabsorption from inadequately treated pancreatic insufficiency can result in the binding of calcium to fatty acids rather than to oxalate, which increases the amount of free intestinal oxalate for absorption [34]. SLC26A6-mediated oxalate secretion is important for intestinal oxalate homeostasis, and, interestingly, SLC26A6 transport activity is stimulated by functioning CFTR. A recent study using a CF mouse model has demonstrated that loss of CFTR function reduces SLC26A6-mediated oxalate secretion, thus contributing to hyperoxaluria [35].

Citrate inhibits stone formation by binding calcium and thus hypocitraturia is an important lithogenic risk factor [31]. Hypocitraturia is a common finding in CF patients with nephrolithiasis and is attributed to metabolic acidosis stemming from increased gastrointestinal losses of bicarbonate leading to increased proximal renal tubular reabsorption of citrate and reduced urinary excretion [36]. Low total-body potassium stores (with or without hypokalemia) can also cause intracellular acidification and increased citrate reabsorption [31]. Other factors contributing to hypocitraturia in CF include hypomagnesemia from chronic diarrhea and increased dietary acid from the increased protein load ingested related to pancreatic enzyme replacement therapy [31, 37].

Hyperuricosuria can increase the risk of calcium oxalate stone formation by contributing to the nucleation of calcium oxalate. While hyperuricosuria was previously reported in CF in relation to the administration of high-dose purine-rich pancreatic extracts, advances in formulations in more recent years with microencapsulation and enteric coating have led to lower pancreatic enzyme dosing and purine ingestion, making the relative contribution of hyperuricosuria to stone formation uncertain but likely minimal [38]. Although understudied, excess sweat and stool fluid losses result in low urinary volume leading to supersaturation of calcium salts and uric acid; therefore, low urinary volume is undoubtedly an important factor leading to the increased risk of stone formation in CF [31].

Prevention and Treatment of AKI and Nephrolithiasis

A major risk factor for AKI in CF is intravenous aminoglycoside administration. These antibiotics are used in CF due to their excellent antimicrobial activity against *Pseudomonas*, NTM, and other airway pathogens. It is worth noting that there is very little evidence base on which to choose one antibiotic regimen over another in CF [39]. However, these antibiotics are firmly embedded into current practice, and therefore it is likely that they will be used to treat pulmonary exacerbations well into the future. We therefore need to develop evidence-based strategies for the safe use of these antibiotics.

We can make strong recommendations on the current evidence base to administer tobramycin in preference to gentamicin, and we can recommend a once-daily antibiotic regimen in preference to a multiple daily dosing one. Based on observational data, we suggest regular monitoring of serum creatinine, and recommend that clinics adopt a formal international definition of AKI, such as the KDIGO guidelines [40].

Within routine clinical practice, therapeutic drug monitoring is key. The gold standard for this is the calculation of individual patient's aminoglycoside pharmacokinetics in real time, with less complex methods including the use of cystic fibrosis specific nomograms, or alternatively monitoring for elevated trough tobramycin levels, or steady state levels of glycopeptides (such as vancomycin). There are no trials comparing these strategies. Adequate hydration when administering aminoglycosides is important – tachypnea and sputum loss during a pulmonary exacerbation, especially at presentation, can cause dehydration. Where possible, we recommend avoiding concomitant nephrotoxic drugs (e.g., ibuprofen). As the specific combination of intravenous tobramycin and colomycin may have synergistic toxicity, we also recommend avoiding this combination.

Several groups are actively undertaking work on reducing toxicity of antibiotic regimens. Early work suggests that the morning administration of aminoglycosides is preferable to evening administration; however, this is based on secondary endpoints of a pharmacokinetic clinical trial and therefore requires replication [41]. Elegant pre-clinical work suggests that statins may be able to reduce toxicity by reducing proximal tubular uptake, and the results of a phase II study is awaited [42].

A research priority setting program in the UK identified that complications of intravenous antibiotics are one of the top ten research priorities for people with CF [43]. Kidney injury remains a considerable source of iatrogenic disease in CF, and strategies to reduce toxicity while preserving efficacy of intravenous antibiotics are clearly required. For some agents such as aminoglycosides, it is the nephrotoxicity and ototoxicity that limit the dosage. Therefore, if effective strategies (such as c-administration of protective agents) are highly effective, it may become possible to administer higher doses safely, improving bacterial killing and enhancing effectiveness.

To reduce the risk of nephrolithiasis, malabsorption should be treated aggressively with pancreatic enzyme replacement therapy and calcium supplemented to bind intestinal oxalate and reduce the risk of free oxalate intestinal absorption and subsequent hyperoxaluria. Probiotic supplements containing *O. formigenes* to increase the intestinal oxalate-degrading capacity is an interesting approach, but processing and storage conditions must be further optimized so that formulations contain viable bacteria, a limitation of existing commercial products [44]. Adequate fluid intake should be encouraged to increase urinary fluid volume to decrease the supersaturation of calcium salts. Potassium replacement should be considered even in individuals without hypokalemia to increase urinary citrate which has stone-inhibiting properties. To reduce the risk of post-renal AKI, as persistent obstruction can lead to kidney damage, renal stones greater than 4 mm should be monitored closely with a low threshold to refer to urology for possible intervention as the likelihood of spontaneous passage decreases as the stone size increases [45, 46]. Proximal stones or those greater than 10 mm should be assessed by urology immediately as spontaneous passage is rare. Based on non-CF studies, the rate of spontaneous clearance for stones between 5 and 10 mm can be facilitated with the use of alpha blockers [47].

The wider effect of renal stones should not be underestimated – renal colic is particularly painful, and a significant episode of renal colic can prevent the patient's daily routine of physiotherapy. This hinders airway clearance, with a subsequent deterioration in pulmonary status. We advocate aggressive pain management.

Chronic Kidney Disease

The prevalence of chronic kidney disease (CKD) in the CF population varies based on age, lung transplant status, and method used to estimate renal function. From a study involving data from the CF Foundation (CFF) Patient Registry, the overall annualized disease prevalence of stage 3 or greater CKD (eGFR <60 ml/min/1.73 m^2 based on the Cockcroft–Gault formula standardized for body surface area) in CF adults without lung transplant was estimated at 2.3%, with a doubling in disease prevalence for every 10-year increase in age (Fig. 19.4) [48]. In comparison to the general population using National Health and Nutrition Examination Survey (NHANES) data, the age-adjusted prevalence of CKD was estimated to be twofold higher in CF. However, this likely represents a conservative estimate as renal function measurement based on eGFR tends to underestimate the true extent of renal damage in CF [49]. The risk of stage 3 or greater CKD increases dramatically post-transplant, with a prevalence of 23%, 35%, and 58% at 1, 2, and 5 years post-lung transplant, respectively [50]. As demonstrated by our patient, hemodialysis is not uncommon as up to 10% of CF patients with post-transplant CKD will progress to the point of requiring this intervention [50].

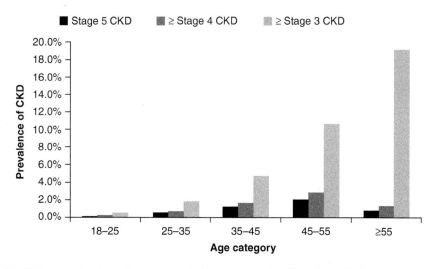

Fig. 19.4 Age-related prevalence of chronic kidney disease (CKD) in CF by CKD severity. Stage 3 CKD severity: estimated glomerular filtration rate (eGFR) less than 60 ml/min/1.73 m^2. Stage 4 CKD severity: eGFR less than 30 ml/min/1.73 m^2. Stage 5 CKD severity: eGFR less than 15 ml/min/1.73 m^2 (or need for hemodialysis). (Reprinted with permission of the American Thoracic Society. Copyright © 2018 American Thoracic Society. Quon et al. [48]. The *American Journal of Respiratory and Critical Care Medicine* is an official journal of the American Thoracic Society)

Causes of CKD

In the pre-lung transplant setting, we identified CF-related diabetes requiring insulin as one of the strongest risk factors for CKD [48]. While IV aminoglycosides and other nephrotoxic antibiotics (e.g., colistin, vancomycin) described above are well-established causes of acute kidney injury, evidence supporting their role in the development of CKD is conflicting [51]. Early reports describing renal pathology from autopsy cases suggested that renal tubulointerstitial disease (with lysosomal proliferation and tubular atrophy) might be attributed to chronic aminoglycoside exposure [52]. In support of this, in a study that focused on the renal function of 80 consecutive adults with CF and chronic *Pseudomonas* infection, there was a significant inverse correlation between measured creatinine clearance (24-h urine collection) and the number of lifetime nephrotoxic IV antibiotic courses [53]. However, a more recent study that focused on more contemporary once-daily aminoglycoside dosing demonstrated no significant relationship between frequency of IV tobramycin use and renal tubular function or estimated creatinine clearance [54]. Once-daily aminoglycoside dosing is now considered standard of care to reduce the risk of nephrotoxicity, particularly in children [55].

Other rarer causes of CKD reported in the CF literature include amyloid A (AA) amyloidosis, IgA nephropathy, and immune complex-related glomerulonephritis [1, 56, 57]. Inflammation-associated systemic amyloidosis (i.e., AA amyloidosis) is usually observed in the setting of chronic inflammation and infection resulting in the accumulation and deposition of serum amyloid A in various organs, including the kidneys [58]. Serum amyloid A is an acute phase reactant produced by the liver, and levels are increased prior to pulmonary exacerbation treatment and decrease with antibiotics and control of infection/inflammation. Several case reports have described AA amyloidosis involving CF patients, and this is considered a poor prognostic factor with most cases dying within 1 year of diagnosis, perhaps reflecting inadequate control of infection/inflammation [58]. While proteinuria with nephrotic syndrome and/or renal failure is the most common clinical presentation in CF, thyroid and hepatobiliary infiltration and hemorrhage due to blood vessel involvement have also been reported [57, 58]. Amyloidosis might be more common than clinically recognized, as a case series of 33 individuals with CF at autopsy identified amyloid deposits involving the spleen, liver, and kidneys in 33% of cases [59]. Also, driven by chronic infection and inflammation, IgA nephropathy and immune complex-mediated glomerular disease are also expected to be more common in CF than the general population, but there are relatively few reports in the literature in support of this [60–63].

In the post-lung transplant setting, risk factors for the development of stage 3 or greater CKD identified in the CFF Patient Registry include older age, female sex, pre-transplant renal dysfunction (eGFR 60–90 mL/min/1.73 m^2), insulin-requiring diabetes, and earlier year of lung transplantation (i.e., pre-2004) [50]. Interestingly, there was a stepwise decline observed in the risk of post-transplant CKD since 2002, perhaps related to the switch from cyclosporine to tacrolimus as the calcineurin inhibitor of choice, with the latter being related to less nephrotoxicity [64, 65].

Prevention and Treatment of CKD

Given the strong association between CFRD requiring insulin and the development of CKD both pre- and post-lung transplant, it is imperative to achieve tight glycemic control. Based on non-CF studies involving type 1 diabetics, intensive diabetes therapy reduces the risk of renal dysfunction and prevents nephropathy progression [66]. Individuals with CFRD should be closely monitored for hyperfiltration (often defined as GFR > 135 ml/min/1.72 m^2) with annual measurements of GFR (an early marker of diabetic nephropathy) and microalbuminuria as these findings may prompt the initiation of agents that block angiotensin (angiotensin converting enzyme [ACE] inhibitors or angiotensin II receptor blockers [ARBs]) to slow the rate of nephropathy progression. To reduce the risk of post-transplant CKD, CF physicians should use aminoglycosides sparingly, if possible, in the months leading up to lung transplant. To reduce the risk of other rarer causes of CKD (e.g., amyloidosis, IgA nephropathy), which are related to uncontrolled infection and inflammation, it is important to treat infection and pulmonary exacerbations aggressively.

A Rational Clinical Approach to Evaluating for Renal Disease in CF

The rates of kidney disease in CF likely vary from center to center, possibly due to local prescribing practices. However, an approach would be to identify patients at risk of CKD based on their clinical characteristics (such as age, presence of diabetes, and number of courses of antibiotics), blood pressure measurements, estimated GFR, urinalysis, and serum electrolytes (including magnesium and calcium) monitored on an annual basis. Those with low estimated GFR or other abnormal results should be referred for formal GFR measurement. When reduced GFR is identified, a review of medications should be undertaken. This will become increasingly important in the future, as there is currently limited experience of administering small molecular disease-modifying drugs such as potentiators and correctors in the setting of reduced renal clearance of these drugs. If the urinalysis shows blood, or if there is abdominal pain suggestive of urinary stones, then ultrasound should be performed. Given the increased risk of kidney disease after lung transplantation, GFR is ideally assessed in all transplant participants prior to and post-transplantation at regular intervals.

Summary and Future Directions

With aging of the CF population, the prevalence of renal disease is expected to grow. Risk factors for AKI including dehydration (pre-renal), nephrotoxic drugs (renal), and nephrolithiasis (post-renal) are all potentially preventable. CF-related diabetes is a major risk factor for chronic kidney disease both pre- and post-lung transplant. Therefore, until more CF-specific interventional data are available, we must adopt strategies proven to be beneficial in preventing or slowing the rate of nephropathy progression in type 1 diabetes, including intensive diabetes control and agents that block angiotensin.

Research priorities include the identification of more reliable ways to monitor renal function in CF as plasma creatinine-based estimating equations can be inaccurate. Emerging research has demonstrated that diffusion tensor imaging (DTI) MRI might be useful for the early detection of renal impairment in CF individuals with CFRD, and therefore, further validation studies are required [25]. Given the increased risk of renal disease for individuals with CFRD, strategies to reduce the risk of renal disease development and progression in this high-risk group should be prioritized.

Acknowledgments We would like to acknowledge and thank Lori Van Balkom for sharing her experience living with chronic kidney disease post-lung transplantation. We would also like to thank Dr. Chris Flask and Dr. Kimberley McBennett from Case Western Reserve University and Dr. Tom McCulloch from Nottingham University Hospitals NHS Trust for their contributions.

References

1. Wilcock MJ, Ruddick A, Gyi KM, Hodson ME. Renal diseases in adults with cystic fibrosis: a 40 year single Centre experience. J Nephrol. 2015;28(5):585–91.
2. Morales MM, Carroll TP, Morita T, Schwiebert EM, Devuyst O, Wilson PD, et al. Both the wild type and a functional isoform of CFTR are expressed in kidney. Am J Phys. 1996;270(6 Pt 2):F1038–48.
3. Crawford I, Maloney PC, Zeitlin PL, Guggino WB, Hyde SC, Turley H, et al. Immunocytochemical localization of the cystic fibrosis gene product CFTR. Proc Natl Acad Sci U S A. 1991;88(20):9262–6.
4. Devuyst O, Burrow CR, Schwiebert EM, Guggino WB, Wilson PD. Developmental regulation of CFTR expression during human nephrogenesis. Am J Phys. 1996;271(3 Pt 2):F723–35.
5. Souza-Menezes J, da Silva FG, Morales MM. CFTR and TNR-CFTR expression and function in the kidney. Biophys Rev. 2014;6(2):227–36.
6. Stanton BA. Cystic fibrosis transmembrane conductance regulator (CFTR) and renal function. Wien Klin Wochenschr. 1997;109(12–13):457–64.
7. Touw DJ. Clinical pharmacokinetics of antimicrobial drugs in cystic fibrosis. Pharm World Sci. 1998;20(4):149–60.
8. Rey E, Treluyer JM, Pons G. Drug disposition in cystic fibrosis. Clin Pharmacokinet. 1998;35(4):313–29.

9. Wang JP, Unadkat JD, al-Habet SM, O'Sullivan TA, Williams-Warren J, Smith AL, et al. Disposition of drugs in cystic fibrosis. IV. Mechanisms for enhanced renal clearance of ticarcillin. Clin Pharmacol Ther. 1993;54(3):293–302.

10. Vinks AA, Den Hollander JG, Overbeek SE, Jelliffe RW, Mouton JW. Population pharmacokinetic analysis of nonlinear behavior of piperacillin during intermittent or continuous infusion in patients with cystic fibrosis. Antimicrob Agents Chemother. 2003;47(2):541–7.

11. Li H, Yang W, Mendes F, Amaral MD, Sheppard DN. Impact of the cystic fibrosis mutation F508del-CFTR on renal cyst formation and growth. Am J Physiol Renal Physiol. 2012;303(8):F1176–86.

12. Hanaoka K, Devuyst O, Schwiebert EM, Wilson PD, Guggino WB. A role for CFTR in human autosomal dominant polycystic kidney disease. Am J Phys. 1996;270(1 Pt 1):C389–99.

13. O'Sullivan DA, Torres VE, Gabow PA, Thibodeau SN, King BF, Bergstralh EJ. Cystic fibrosis and the phenotypic expression of autosomal dominant polycystic kidney disease. Am J Kidney Dis. 1998;32(6):976–83.

14. Xu N, Glockner JF, Rossetti S, Babovich-Vuksanovic D, Harris PC, Torres VE. Autosomal dominant polycystic kidney disease coexisting with cystic fibrosis. J Nephrol. 2006;19(4):529–34.

15. Zhang JT, Wang Y, Chen JJ, Zhang XH, Dong JD, Tsang LL, et al. Defective CFTR leads to aberrant beta-catenin activation and kidney fibrosis. Sci Rep. 2017;7(1):5233.

16. Al-Aloul M, Miller H, Alapati S, Stockton P, Walshaw ML. Renal impairment in cystic fibrosis patients due to repeated intravenous aminoglycoside use. Pediatr Pulmonol. 2005;39(1):15–20.

17. Soulsby N, Greville H, Coulthard K, Doecke C. What is the best method for measuring renal function in adults and children with cystic fibrosis? J Cyst Fibros. 2010;9(2):124–9.

18. Al-Aloul M, Jackson M, Bell G, Ledson M, Walshaw M. Comparison of methods of assessment of renal function in cystic fibrosis (CF) patients. J Cyst Fibros. 2007;6(1):41–7.

19. Jain K, Prayle A, Lewis S, Watson A, Knox A, Dewar J, et al. Assessment of renal function in cystic fibrosis patients by estimated and measured glomerular filtration rate; a cross-sectional study. J Cyst Fibros. 2012;11:S52.

20. Tenstad O, Roald AB, Grubb A, Aukland K. Renal handling of radiolabelled human cystatin C in the rat. Scand J Clin Lab Invest. 1996;56(5):409–14.

21. Prayle AP, Jain K, Knox AJ, Watson AR, Smyth AR. Urinary kidney injury molecule-1 is superior to creatinine and cystatin-C based formulas at predicting chronic kidney disease in patients with cystic fibrosis. J Cyst Fibros. 2013;12:S13.

22. Mora-Gutierrez JM, Garcia-Fernandez N, Slon Roblero MF, Paramo JA, Escalada FJ, Wang DJ, et al. Arterial spin labeling MRI is able to detect early hemodynamic changes in diabetic nephropathy. J Magn Reson Imaging. 2017;46(6):1810–7.

23. Sugiyama K, Inoue T, Kozawa E, Ishikawa M, Shimada A, Kobayashi N, et al. Reduced oxygenation but not fibrosis defined by functional magnetic resonance imaging predicts the long-term progression of chronic kidney disease. Nephrol Dial Transplant. 2018. https://doi.org/10.1093/ndt/gfy324. [Epub ahead of print]. https://www.ncbi.nlm.nih.gov/pubmed/30418615.

24. Li LP, Tan H, Thacker JM, Li W, Zhou Y, Kohn O, et al. Evaluation of renal blood flow in chronic kidney disease using arterial spin labeling perfusion magnetic resonance imaging. Kidney Int Rep. 2017;2(1):36–43.

25. Lu L, Sedor JR, Gulani V, Schelling JR, O'Brien A, Flask CA, et al. Use of diffusion tensor MRI to identify early changes in diabetic nephropathy. Am J Nephrol. 2011;34(5):476–82.

26. Bertenshaw C, Watson AR, Lewis S, Smyth A. Survey of acute renal failure in patients with cystic fibrosis in the UK. Thorax. 2007;62(6):541–5.

27. Smyth A, Lewis S, Bertenshaw C, Choonara I, McGaw J, Watson A. Case-control study of acute renal failure in patients with cystic fibrosis in the UK. Thorax. 2008;63(6):532–5.

28. Downes KJ, Patil NR, Rao MB, Koralkar R, Harris WT, Clancy JP, et al. Risk factors for acute kidney injury during aminoglycoside therapy in patients with cystic fibrosis. Pediatr Nephrol. 2015;30(10):1879–88.

29. Lands LC, Milner R, Cantin AM, Manson D, Corey M. High-dose ibuprofen in cystic fibrosis: Canadian safety and effectiveness trial. J Pediatr. 2007;151(3):249–54.

30. Kerem E, Konstan MW, De Boeck K, Accurso FJ, Sermet-Gaudelus I, Wilschanski M, et al. Ataluren for the treatment of nonsense-mutation cystic fibrosis: a randomised, double-blind, placebo-controlled phase 3 trial. Lancet Respir Med. 2014;2(7):539–47.

31. Gibney EM, Goldfarb DS. The association of nephrolithiasis with cystic fibrosis. Am J Kidney Dis. 2003;42(1):1–11.
32. Hiatt RA, Dales LG, Friedman GD, Hunkeler EM. Frequency of urolithiasis in a prepaid medical care program. Am J Epidemiol. 1982;115(2):255–65.
33. Bohles H, Gebhardt B, Beeg T, Sewell AC, Solem E, Posselt G. Antibiotic treatment-induced tubular dysfunction as a risk factor for renal stone formation in cystic fibrosis. J Pediatr. 2002;140(1):103–9.
34. Dharmsathaphorn K, Freeman DH, Binder HJ, Dobbins JW. Increased risk of nephrolithiasis in patients with steatorrhea. Dig Dis Sci. 1982;27(5):401–5.
35. Knauf F, Thomson RB, Heneghan JF, Jiang Z, Adebamiro A, Thomson CL, et al. Loss of cystic fibrosis transmembrane regulator impairs intestinal oxalate secretion. J Am Soc Nephrol. 2017;28(1):242–9.
36. Perez-Brayfield MR, Caplan D, Gatti JM, Smith EA, Kirsch AJ. Metabolic risk factors for stone formation in patients with cystic fibrosis. J Urol. 2002;167(2 Pt 1):480–4.
37. Reungjui S, Prasongwatana V, Premgamone A, Tosukhowong P, Jirakulsomchok S, Sriboonlue P. Magnesium status of patients with renal stones and its effect on urinary citrate excretion. BJU Int. 2002;90(7):635–9.
38. Nouisa-Arvanitakis S, Stapleton FB, Linshaw MA, Kennedy J. Therapeutic approach to pancreatic extract-induced hyperuricosuria in cystic fibrosis. J Pediatr. 1977;90(2):302–5.
39. Hurley MN, Prayle AP, Flume P. Intravenous antibiotics for pulmonary exacerbations in people with cystic fibrosis. Paediatr Respir Rev. 2015;16(4):246–8.
40. Kidney Disease: Improving Global Outcomes (KDIGO) Acute Kidney Injury Work Group. KDIGO clinical practice guideline for acute kidney injury. Kidney Int. 2012;Supplement 2:1–138.
41. Prayle AP, Jain K, Touw DJ, Koch BC, Knox AJ, Watson A, et al. The pharmacokinetics and toxicity of morning vs. evening tobramycin dosing for pulmonary exacerbations of cystic fibrosis: a randomised comparison. J Cyst Fibros. 2016;15(4):510–7.
42. McWilliam S, Antoine D, Rosala-Hallas A, Jones A, MacLean C, Prayle A, et al. The protekt study – a phase IIA, randomised, controlled, open-label trial of rosuvastatin for the prevention of aminoglycoside-induced kidney toxicity in children with cystic fibrosis. Pediatr Pulmonol. 2017;52(s47):353.
43. Rowbotham NJ, Smith S, Leighton PA, Rayner OC, Gathercole K, Elliott ZC, et al. The top 10 research priorities in cystic fibrosis developed by a partnership between people with CF and healthcare providers. Thorax. 2018;73(4):388–90.
44. Ellis ML, Shaw KJ, Jackson SB, Daniel SL, Knight J. Analysis of commercial kidney stone probiotic supplements. Urology. 2015;85(3):517–21.
45. Miller OF, Kane CJ. Time to stone passage for observed ureteral calculi: a guide for patient education. J Urol. 1999;162(3 Pt 1):688–90; discussion 90–1.
46. Coll DM, Varanelli MJ, Smith RC. Relationship of spontaneous passage of ureteral calculi to stone size and location as revealed by unenhanced helical CT. AJR Am J Roentgenol. 2002;178(1):101–3.
47. Wang RC, Smith-Bindman R, Whitaker E, Neilson J, Allen IE, Stoller ML, et al. Effect of tamsulosin on stone passage for ureteral stones: a systematic review and meta-analysis. Ann Emerg Med. 2017;69(3):353–61. e3
48. Quon BS, Mayer-Hamblett N, Aitken ML, Smyth AR, Goss CH. Risk factors for chronic kidney disease in adults with cystic fibrosis. Am J Respir Crit Care Med. 2011;184(10):1147–52.
49. Nazareth D, Walshaw M. A review of renal disease in cystic fibrosis. J Cyst Fibros. 2013;12(4):309–17.
50. Quon BS, Mayer-Hamblett N, Aitken ML, Goss CH. Risk of post-lung transplant renal dysfunction in adults with cystic fibrosis. Chest. 2012;142(1):185–91.
51. Pedersen SS, Jensen T, Osterhammel D, Osterhammel P. Cumulative and acute toxicity of repeated high-dose tobramycin treatment in cystic fibrosis. Antimicrob Agents Chemother. 1987;31(4):594–9.
52. Abramowsky CR, Swinehart GL. The nephropathy of cystic fibrosis: a human model of chronic nephrotoxicity. Hum Pathol. 1982;13(10):934–9.

53. Al-Aloul M, Miller H, Alapati S, Stockton PA, Ledson MJ, Walshaw MJ. Renal impairment in cystic fibrosis patients due to repeated intravenous aminoglycoside use. Pediatr Pulmonol. 2005;39(1):15–20.

54. Stehling F, Buscher R, Grosse-Onnebrink J, Hoyer PF, Mellies U. Glomerular and tubular renal function after repeated once-daily tobramycin courses in cystic fibrosis patients. Pulm Med. 2017;2017:2602653.

55. Smyth A, Tan KH, Hyman-Taylor P, Mulheran M, Lewis S, Stableforth D, et al. Once versus three-times daily regimens of tobramycin treatment for pulmonary exacerbations of cystic fibrosis--the TOPIC study: a randomised controlled trial. Lancet. 2005;365(9459):573–8.

56. Yahiaoui Y, Jablonski M, Hubert D, Mosnier-Pudar H, Noel LH, Stern M, et al. Renal involvement in cystic fibrosis: diseases spectrum and clinical relevance. Clin J Am Soc Nephrol. 2009;4(5):921–8.

57. Stankovic Stojanovic K, Hubert D, Leroy S, Dominique S, Grenet D, Colombat M, et al. Cystic fibrosis and AA amyloidosis: a survey in the French cystic fibrosis network. Amyloid. 2014;21(4):231–7.

58. Mc Laughlin AM, Crotty TB, Egan JJ, Watson AJ, Gallagher CG. Amyloidosis in cystic fibrosis: a case series. J Cyst Fibros. 2006;5(1):59–61.

59. McGlennen RC, Burke BA, Dehner LP. Systemic amyloidosis complicating cystic fibrosis. A retrospective pathologic study. Arch Pathol Lab Med. 1986;110(10):879–84.

60. Bhatt N, Bhatt N. IgA nephropathy in cystic fibrosis. Clin Nephrol. 2007;67(6):403–4.

61. Stirati G, Antonelli M, Fofi C, Fierimonte S, Pecci G. IgA nephropathy in cystic fibrosis. J Nephrol. 1999;12(1):30–1.

62. Davis CA, Abramowsky CR, Swinehart G. Circulating immune complexes and the nephropathy of cystic fibrosis. Hum Pathol. 1984;15(3):244–7.

63. Melzi ML, Costantini D, Giani M, Appiani AC, Giunta AM. Severe nephropathy in three adolescents with cystic fibrosis. Arch Dis Child. 1991;66(12):1444–7.

64. Ojo AO, Held PJ, Port FK, Wolfe RA, Leichtman AB, Young EW, et al. Chronic renal failure after transplantation of a nonrenal organ. N Engl J Med. 2003;349(10):931–40.

65. Cantarovich D, Renou M, Megnigbeto A, Giral-Classe M, Hourmant M, Dantal J, et al. Switching from cyclosporine to tacrolimus in patients with chronic transplant dysfunction or cyclosporine-induced adverse events. Transplantation. 2005;79(1):72–8.

66. Group DER, de Boer IH, Sun W, Cleary PA, Lachin JM, Molitch ME, et al. Intensive diabetes therapy and glomerular filtration rate in type 1 diabetes. N Engl J Med. 2011;365(25):2366–76.

Chapter 20
Sexual and Reproductive Health in Cystic Fibrosis

Erin Crowley and Cynthia D. Brown

Patient Perspective

Every person's story is unique. This statement is especially true for those of us with cystic fibrosis (CF) who often face questions and challenges regarding reproductive health and CF. When I was diagnosed with CF at one month old in 1977, the landscape was much different regarding prognosis and life expectancy. My family celebrated each milestone I achieved. If I'm being honest, I don't think I really gave a lot of thought to whether I would be able to have children and what that would look like because I didn't really think this disease would allow me to face this decision. And yet, as a young adult, my health continued to stabilize and in my late 20's I met my husband, Brian. We dated for about two years and knew within a year that we intended to spend our lives together. We were married on May 9th, 2009.

While we were dating, we had conversations about whether children were in our future. We both agreed that we would love to have children but knew there were obstacles and challenges because of my health. At this point, it was less emotional and more scientific for us. Step one was exploring whether Brian is a carrier. We knew if he was, this would be a game changer for us. Others may view this differently, but for us, we needed this information first. We were thrilled when we found out Brian was not a carrier and knew that our child would be a carrier but would not have CF. The next step was more complicated. I had a conversation with my pulmonologist. He told me that I could carry a child and that there are women with CF who carry their own children. He indicated from his experience that some women with CF have healthy pregnancies and others struggle. Those who struggle often have difficulty getting back to their original baseline, if they ever do.

E. Crowley · C. D. Brown (✉)
Indiana University School of Medicine, Division of Pulmonary, Critical Care, Occupational and Sleep Medicine, Indianapolis, IN, USA
e-mail: cyndbrow@iu.edu

© Springer Nature Switzerland AG 2020
S. D. Davis et al. (eds.), *Cystic Fibrosis*, Respiratory Medicine,
https://doi.org/10.1007/978-3-030-42382-7_20

413

With this information came many thoughts, unanswerable questions, and emotions for me. Interestingly, I think it was much simpler for Brian and my family. They didn't want me to carry a child. They hadn't filled in the rest of the blanks but they knew they didn't want me putting my body at risk. I could certainly appreciate their perspective. I (and my family) had worked hard for over 30 years to maintain my health. I had experienced the usual bumps along the way- PICC lines, hospital stays, added treatments, medication and therapies as I got older. Do I risk this to give birth and have a child? I think it would be remiss to not point out what I feel is somewhat unique to CF in this area. When we think of reproductive health and challenges, I think we most often envision a couple who has tried to have children but for some reason cannot get pregnant. With CF, women CAN most often carry and give birth to a child, but at what cost to the mother's health? There are many complicated questions but no simple answers.

In the midst of our conversations, Brian was also talking to his family about this decision. Brian's sister Julie and her husband have two children who were 5 and 7 years old at that time. She told Brian that if carrying a baby for us as our surrogate was something we were interested in she would be happy to talk more about that option. This was also a game changer for us in this process. Our conversations quickly shifted to what this would entail for everyone involved. People often ask if we would have asked Julie to do this for us if she had not offered. While I certainly don't think she would have been offended if we did ask, I don't honestly think we would have. That she came forward, willingly, was a gift in itself. So it was decided that we would undergo in vitro fertilization (IVF) for her to carry a biological child for me and Brian.

The IVF process was a new experience for all of us. We were all on board with Julie carrying one child. When the first embryo transfer didn't take, we were disappointed but knew this was not uncommon in IVF. We had transferred a frozen embryo and thankfully had more available to transfer. Statistically, our doctor explained that frozen embryos have a lower success rate, and therefore we had a very low chance of both embryos taking if we considered transferring two. Again, approaching this from a scientific standpoint, we all agreed we should transfer two embryos in the second transfer, with the hope of one of them taking.

A few weeks later, we had our first ultrasound. We had been hoping and praying for one heartbeat. We assumed we would hear one or none. Two strong heartbeats were heard on the monitor that day. Our two healthy girls, Lily and Reagan, were born at just under 36 weeks on December 18th, 2011. Julie had a seamless pregnancy, even carrying twins which was a new experience for her. Of course the hard work for us began once we brought Lily and Reagan home. Lily and Reagan will always be our greatest gifts, and we are forever grateful to Brian's sister for giving us the gift of parenthood. Admittedly, sometimes I wonder what it would have been like to have carried them and if I would have been able to sustain this pregnancy and maintain my health. But the story would have had a different ending, and we wouldn't likely have Lily and Reagan. I can't imagine our life without them both, and the overwhelming emotion for my family and me is gratitude

—Abbie, Age 41

Sexual and reproductive health (SRH) issues are a common yet frequently under-reported problem in adolescents and adults with cystic fibrosis (CF). As the CF population continues to experience overall health gains in lung function, nutrition, and life expectancy, it is likely that SRH will become a more prevalent issue, and more research will be needed to better understand the needs of the CF population. The focus of this review is to provide an overview of the current state of the literature regarding SRH in the CF population.

Puberty and Sexual Development

Since the mid to late 1960s, the delay of both growth and onset of puberty in people with CF has been recognized. This is demonstrated by the delay in menarche in adolescent girls as well as by a delay in peak pubertal height velocity in both boys and girls [1–4]. Initially, investigators hypothesized a reason for this delay to be malnutrition, but more contemporary studies have shown delayed puberty despite good nutritional status. The current explanation for this lag in the onset of puberty—even in healthy, well-nourished individuals with CF—is a delayed hypothalamic release of gonadotropin-releasing hormone [5]. A recent study in the United States surveyed 188 young women with CF between the ages of 15 and 24 about their SRH. In this survey, the average reported age of menarche was 13.1 ± 1.3 years compared to a control group of similar-aged individuals ($n = 1997$) derived from the National Survey of Family Growth where the average age of menarche was 12.4 ± 0.05 years ($p < 0.001$). In the United Kingdom, the age of menarche was reported at 12.6 ± 0.2 years in those with CF compared to 11.5 ± 0.21 years in healthy controls [6]. Adolescent girls in Poland where CF care lags behind their western European counterparts have an even greater delay in menarche with an average age of 14.6 ± 1.21 years [7].

With the onset of puberty, adolescence is a critical period of accelerated height growth. Children with CF are at high risk for impaired pubertal growth because of the demand of increased nutritional requirements. Historically, studies confirmed the clinical observation that children with CF had delayed and attenuated pubertal growth compared to healthy children. However, these studies used data from children with CF born prior to the 1970s and few were from the United States [8]. Although there have been tremendous advances in new therapies, such as enteric-coated pancreatic enzymes and comprehensive nutrition management, pubertal growth in children born after the 1980s has only slightly improved [9]. However, despite entering puberty later, Aswani and colleagues found that most individuals will achieve a normal adult height and one that is comparable to that of their parents [10].

After puberty, women with CF are felt to have normal sex hormone levels, and women typically have reported normal menstrual cycles. Secondary amenorrhea can occur with malnutrition and worsening pulmonary health. One study from 1987 describes primary or secondary amenorrhea that occurred in approximately 26% of women and irregular cycles in 24%. Compared to the women with regular menstrual cycles, those with primary or secondary amenorrhea had lower BMI, percentage body fat, and lung function [11]. Given the advances in health since this time, it is unknown if secondary amenorrhea remains common in adult women with CF. No recent research has reported this outcome. Moreover, there is also no research regarding the experience of menopause in women with CF.

In men with CF, sex hormone levels have been demonstrated to be lower than healthy age-matched controls. In a cross-sectional study evaluating sex hormones and body composition in young men with stable CF disease (age 25 ± 5 years), circulating levels of testosterone were moderately reduced on average to the extent found in healthy elderly men [12]. The decreased level of testosterone is significant because it contributed to accelerated bone loss, and testosterone deficiency has been associated with the presence of vertebral fractures. In adult men with CF, no screening guidelines for hypogonadism exist, and there are no prospective randomized controlled trials evaluating treatment of hypogonadism. Screening for low testosterone should be considered in men with symptoms of hypogonadism and as part of the evaluation of a diagnosis of osteoporosis. Testosterone measurements should be done in the morning and can be affected by acute illness. A low testosterone level should be confirmed twice before committing a patient to testosterone therapy. Finally, prior to the initiation of testosterone, the patient should be advised that testosterone therapy will diminish spermatogenesis and adversely impact the patient's reproductive potential [13].

Male Fertility

Regardless of the severity of the respiratory or gastrointestinal disease, it is estimated that 98% of males with CF have a problem of poor development of the vas deferens. The majority of males with CF have aberrant development of Wolffian duct derivatives (Fig. 20.1). Spermatogenesis occurs normally, but men are generally azoospermic because of bilateral absence of the vas deferens (CBAVD) [14, 15]. In addition to sperm, semen contains fluid that is made by the glands called seminal vesicles. In CF, dysfunction of the seminal vesicles accounts for a low volume ejaculate—less than 1.5 mL in comparison to 3.5 mL produced by males without CF. However, in males with CF, despite lower testosterone levels as a young adult, there is no evidence that sexual performance is affected [14, 15]. Sawyer and colleagues found, in a contemporary cohort of males with CF, that 90% of adults and 60% of adolescents knew that males with CF are infertile. However, there was significant confusion and lack of knowledge about infertility versus impotence, as well as a lack of awareness of the risks of sexually transmitted infections [16].

Most men with CF are functionally sterile for the reasons discussed above, although 1–2% may be fertile. Men in whom CF has been diagnosed in adulthood who have mild mutations are more likely to be fertile. For example, patients with the 3849 + 10 kb C→T mutation, both homozygous and heterozygous, have been shown to have less severe gastrointestinal disease and are fertile [17, 18]. Because

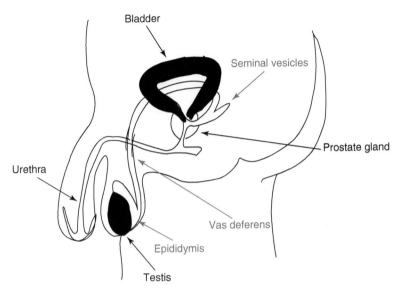

Fig. 20.1 Male reproductive tract. Sexual and reproductive health. The structures highlighted in red refer to the parts of the male reproductive tract that generally do not develop normally or are absent in males with CF

of the variable phenotypes, men with CF should not assume they are infertile. Semen analysis is recommended to determine fertility status. However, semen analysis is not routinely available in CF clinics and should not be undertaken within a few months of serious illness. In a large cohort of Australian men with CF, 95% of men stated that they would like semen analysis to occur before age 20. Also, 68% of men who had not been tested wanted semen analysis independent of their relationship status, suggesting that semen analysis should at least be offered to all men [19, 20].

Male infertility was first reported in 1968 when most children with CF did not expect to survive to reproductive age and assisted reproductive technologies (ART) did not allow for men with CF to father children. For contemporary young men, the combination of improved survival, better quality of life, and advances in ART challenge health professionals to ensure men are appropriately educated about their options for having children. Alternatives to normal conception are available and should be considered on an individual basis. Current reproductive options for men with CF are artificial insemination of their partner by donor sperm or surgical collection of their own sperm. These techniques include microsurgical epididymal sperm aspiration (MESA), percutaneous epididymal sperm aspiration (PESA), and testicular sperm extraction (TESE). These techniques are performed in consultation with an urologist, and each has associated advantages and disadvantages. MESA results in the largest numbers of sperm retrieved, but requires an open surgical procedure whereas both PESA and TESE do not require open exploration and can be repeatable. However, these procedures yield a limited sample and often do not have any additional sample for cryopreservation [21].

Historically, using standard technology at the time, *in vitro* fertilization had a low success rate in terms of both number of eggs fertilized and the ultimate birth rate. A hypothesis for the low success rates was thought to be from impaired sperm characteristics related to immaturity. In 1992, Palermo and colleagues described the technique of intracytoplasmic sperm injection (ICSI); this technique injects a single sperm into an oocyte using an extremely fine micropipette [22]. With this, success rates with surgically retrieved sperm increased dramatically. Surgically retrieved sperm are immature and incapable of fertilization by conventional means, so fertilization is achieved by injection of a selected sperm into the cytoplasm of a mature oocyte. The efficacy of ICSI gives excellent results, with high fertilization rates and pregnancies in 31–34% of treatment cycles [23]. In a study of male patients specifically with obstructive azoospermia such as CBAVD, Dohle et al. found a pregnancy rate of 41.6% [23]. In a retrospective analysis specific to CF, eight men underwent MESA, and their partners underwent one or more cycles of ICSI. The pregnancy rate was 62.5%, with four couples delivering (three sets of twins and one singleton) [24].

Female Fertility

Female fertility in CF has not been systematically studied. As noted above, most women should exhibit normal ovulatory cycles. The CFTR protein is found throughout the cells lining the cervix, endometrium and Fallopian tubes and plays a role in chloride and bicarbonate secretion in the female reproductive tract [25, 26]. There has been concern that abnormal CFTR function leads to thick and tenacious cervical mucus that acts as a mechanical barrier for conception. In addition, sperm motility and capacitation are decreased when bicarbonate is lessened in the female reproductive tract [25]. A recently published article demonstrates that women with CF have a higher prevalence of subfertility and infertility than was previously known. Out of 241 women who attempted conception, 84 women (35%) had difficulty achieving pregnancy with 28% requiring either ART or requiring more than 1 year to achieve pregnancy. Further, 17% of women in this cohort never were able to become pregnant [27]. Factors associated with subfertility and infertility in this cohort included older age and pancreatic insufficiency [27]. Despite these concerns, the number of successful pregnancies in women with CF continues to increase over time, likely correlating with the overall improved health with the CF population. In 1991, 127 pregnancies were reported in women with CF in the United States, and by 2016, this number had more than doubled to 270 [28].

Pregnancy in a Female CF Patient

Women across the spectrum of lung disease may become pregnant and bear children although those with lower lung function may have poorer maternal outcomes within 2–8 years of delivery [29]. While there have not been recommendations for definitive parameters of optimal lung function or nutrition prior to pregnancy, patients should work closely with their care teams to maximize their overall health prior to attempting to achieve pregnancy. Individualized goals for lung function and BMI are appropriate for each patient based upon recent historical values taking into account exacerbation history and general health. In addition, genetic counseling is an important part of planning prior to pregnancy. All children born to a mother with CF are obligate carriers of a CFTR mutation. The carrier frequency in the general Caucasian population is 1 in 25. Thus, the risk of a patient having a child with CF could be as high as 1 in 50 if the partner fails to undergo genetic counseling and screening [30]. It is recommended that all partners be screened for mutations in CFTR prior to pregnancy so that patients can be better informed of their risks prior to attempting pregnancy.

Currently, no standard guidelines exist regarding frequency of follow up during pregnancy. Most CF practitioners will see patients more often during a pregnancy to ensure a patient is gaining weight and maintaining lung function. Often, this averages about every other month until the last trimester and then monthly in the last trimester although this will vary based upon the patient's stability. Additional monitoring would be required for patients with lower BMI, inability to gain weight, hyperemesis gravidarum, tenuous lung function, frequent exacerbations, or CF-related or gestational diabetes mellitus. The recommended weight gain during pregnancy varies based upon pre-pregnancy BMI, and standard weight gain charts can be helpful although one should take into account the additional baseline caloric needs of CF patients. The most recent Institute of Medicine Report from 2009 recommends weight gains of 12.5–18.0 kg for patients who are underweight and 11.5–16.0 kg for patients of normal body weight [31]. In women without CF, this requires an extra 300 kcal daily to sustain growth. However, CF patients typically have caloric needs that are 110–200% of a normal individual at baseline due to malabsorption and chronic inflammation [32]. Thus, the increased caloric needs in pregnancy for a CF patient can be quite high to ensure proper weight gain, and many patients will require close nutrition monitoring throughout pregnancy. If a patient has not had an oral glucose tolerance test within the past year, one should be performed in the first trimester and again at the end of the second trimester. Alternatively, a patient planning a pregnancy should be encouraged to have an oral glucose tolerance test prior to becoming pregnant.

Medication regimens of CF patients are quite complex with most medications having limited or no testing in pregnancy. Thus, clinicians typically have to balance the clinical needs of the patient with what is known about the drug from testing in animals and prior clinical experience in pregnancy in humans. A first priority should be ensuring the health and well-being of the mother. In planning pregnancy, a medication review should be undertaken to ensure all known teratogens are stopped. As in all women, CF patients planning a pregnancy also need to supplement with additional folic acid 400 mcg daily to prevent neural tube defects, and it should be noted that this is above the amount contained in the typical CF vitamin. Another common concern when planning a pregnancy in CF is how to approach vitamin A. In animal studies, birth defects can be demonstrated with excess vitamin A, and retinoic acid derivative medications such as isotretinoin have clearly been demonstrated to be teratogenic with associated craniofacial, heart, and thymus defects. Alternatively, vitamin A deficiency also causes adverse effects in the fetus. The recommended amount of daily vitamin A in CF patients is 10,000 IU or less [30, 33].

Once pregnancy is confirmed, a close inspection of all maintenance medications should be undertaken. During time of disease stability, CF patients have a daily respiratory regimen that often includes a combination of bronchodilators, mucolytics, and inhaled antibiotics in order to prevent decline in lung function and frequent respiratory infections. Other treatments may include oral macrolide antibiotics, inhaled steroids, and, for an increasing number of patients, CFTR modulator therapies. When a patient becomes pregnant, managing the respiratory medications often becomes the most difficult part of disease management as many of the medications used have potential consequences on fetal growth and development or have very limited data available regarding fetal effects. Aminoglycosides can cause congenital deafness due to damage to the eight cranial nerve when given systemically. Because of this, some physicians try to avoid inhaled aminoglycosides as well although systemic absorption of the inhaled medication is low and is likely safe during pregnancy [30, 33]. Colistimethate is category C in pregnancy with limited human data, and inhaled colistimethate may be continued during pregnancy if a patient has frequent exacerbations due to Pseudomonas. However, as a monobactam antibiotic and category B in pregnancy, inhaled aztreonam has a better safety profile for the fetus and should be considered as an alternative for pregnancy.

Outside of inhaled antibiotics, other inhaled therapies in CF also have limited safety data, but clinical data supports their ongoing use. Extrapolating from data in asthma, the benefits of albuterol likely outweigh the potential risks in pregnant CF women [33]. Likewise, there are minimal concerns about continuing dornase or hypertonic saline during pregnancy. Macrolide antibiotics are category B in pregnancy and may be continued. Finally, if a CF patient has concomitant asthma, inhaled corticosteroids should also be continued as available data in asthmatic patients show no significant increased risk of congenital birth defects [33].

At this time, three CFTR modulators (ivacaftor, lumacaftor/ivacaftor, and tezacaftor/ivacaftor) have been FDA approved, and approximately 50% of the CF population have mutations that are potentially responsive to one of the medications [34]. Moreover, additional combinations of highly effective CFTR modulators are currently in clinical trials that will be available for up to 90% of the CF population [35, 36]. These medications pose a unique problem for the CF clinician and their patients as there is limited information about how the medications could affect pregnancy; however, the medications have the potential to greatly improve clinical stability. Ivacaftor was the first CFTR modulator approved by the FDA in 2012 [37], and currently there has been a single case report of a child delivered safely to a woman on ivacaftor throughout pregnancy [38]. In addition, newly published data suggest that there has been an abrupt increase in the pregnancy rate among women with the G551D mutation after approval of ivacaftor [39]. The exact cause of this is unknown, but could reflect several potential factors including a rebound in pregnancy rate after a suppression due to enrollment in clinical trials, improved overall health and nutrition, and possibly improved cervical mucoidity [39, 40]. Of great concern, when ivacaftor is stopped abruptly, a marked decline in health can occur that can lead to a rapid fall in lung function and death [41]. Thus, physicians must carefully consider the potential risks of stopping ivacaftor in a pregnant CF patient versus potential risks to a fetus. At this time, no definitive risks have been identified in humans, and in animal studies, no teratogenicity has been demonstrated. However, less is known about the effects of the newer combination medications. Certainly, lumacaftor/ivacaftor and tezacaftor/ivacaftor have had less dramatic effects on lung function and overall health in patients who are homozygous for the F508del mutation compared to ivacaftor in the gating mutation population [42, 43], and no dramatic declines in health have been reported upon stopping these medications at this time. Physicians caring for these patients need to make individualized decisions based upon the stability of the patient carefully considering risks and benefits, but once more highly effective therapies are available, these decisions will need to be carefully considered.

Pancreatic enzymes and vitamins other than vitamin A are typically continued without dose adjustment for pregnancy although these medications are typically classified a pregnancy category C. Given the nutritional risk to the pregnant patient with CF in the absence of these medications, the benefit is felt to outweigh any potential risks. Although there are no specific studies in pregnant women, case reports have demonstrated safe use without side effects on the fetus. The management of CF-related diabetes in pregnancy requires use of insulin and careful co-management with endocrinology.

In times of exacerbation, antibiotic management becomes more difficult as many of the usual regimens utilized are contraindicated in pregnancy. Many oral antibiotics that are commonly used cannot be given. Tetracyclines (doxycycline, minocycline) accumulate in developing long tubular bones and teeth causing permanent tooth discoloration. Trimethoprim inhibits folic acid reduction to its active form, tetrahydrafolate, and is associated with neural tube defects. Sulfmethoxazole near the time of delivery may cause kernicterus and hemolytic anemia. Fluoroquinolones have been associated with cartilage abnormalities in animals. However, in humans, the available case-control studies have not demonstrated any adverse effects. Given the uncertainty and high doses used in CF, most physicians typically avoid fluoroquinolones in pregnancy if other options are available [30]. For treatment of *Staphylococcus aureus,* an oral or intravenous penicillin or cephalosporin would be the preferred regimen if the patient has a sensitive strain. For methicillin-resistant *S. aureus* (MRSA), linezolid can be considered although the available data is primarily from treatment of pregnant women with tuberculosis [44, 45]. For intravenous therapy of MRSA, vancomycin has a good safety profile in pregnancy. While it does cross the placenta, prior case reports that have had durations of treatment as long as 28 days showed no ototoxicity or nephrotoxicity in the neonates [46]. While *Pseudomonas aeruginosa* is typically covered with two IV antibiotics in the non-pregnant CF patient, a pregnant CF patient may receive only one IV antibiotic. Preferred agents would be anti-Pseudomonal penicillins or cephalosporins given that there is more safety data with these agents. If there is resistance or allergy, meropenem could be considered as an alternative agent. Intravenous aminoglycosides can be considered if the potential benefit outweighs the risk [46]. The risk of congenital deafness is greatest in the first trimester and was specifically demonstrated with streptomycin. The inhaled route should be considered as an alternative unless the patient is critically ill.

The first successful pregnancy in a woman with pancreatic-sufficient CF was reported in 1960. In this case, the woman died 6 weeks after delivery from respiratory complications at the age of 20 years [47]. A comprehensive review of pregnancy outcomes from 1977 through 1996 at eleven care centers in the United Kingdom reported outcomes on 72 pregnancies in 55 women. In these women, 70% of pregnancies resulted in a live birth of which 46% were premature. In this cohort, there were also 14 (20%) therapeutic abortions. The average age at the time of pregnancy was 22.8 years with a mean FEV_1 of 71% predicted, generally reflecting a healthier individual than the CF population at large at the time [48]. However, pregnancy did occur in all stages of the disease with 19% of women having a $FEV_1 < 50\%$ predicted at the time of pregnancy. Overall, 12 women (22%) died during the time of follow up with a median survival after delivery of a first child of 11.9 years [48].

In the time period since this publication, many new treatments have been introduced that have improved the overall health and increased the median survival of the CF population. Contemporary studies examining the effects of pregnancy on both maternal and fetal outcomes have shown improved outcomes when compared to prior data. Most data reported are small, single-center descriptive studies. In general, infant outcomes born to mothers with CF are favorable although there is an increased risk of preterm delivery. In these studies, factors that have predicted preterm delivery include CF-related or gestational diabetes mellitus, lower baseline lung function, and lower baseline nutritional status [29, 49–51]. When compared to women without CF, patients with CF are at higher risk to deliver preterm and have a primary cesarean delivery [52]. In addition, perinatal complications are higher in women with CF compared to women without CF, including a higher risk of pneumonia (6.7% vs 0.1%), acute respiratory failure (1.2% vs. 0.04%), and death (1% vs. 0.007%) [53]. However, a recent analysis has shown no long-term effects of pregnancy on decline in lung function or BMI when compared to women with CF who did not have children in a propensity-matched analysis although they did experience more frequent exacerbations requiring intravenous antibiotics and more frequent clinic visits [54].

Successful pregnancies in CF women have been reported after lung transplantation although overall the numbers remain few at this time. In 2012, outcomes of 30 pregnancies in 21 female lung transplant recipients were reported from US transplant centers. Of these women, 10 had undergone transplant for CF. Overall, the incidence of live birth in all patients with lung transplant was 56% and was lower compared to other solid organ transplant recipients. In addition, there was a higher incidence of preterm birth in lung transplant recipients. When CF was the indication for lung transplant, there was a higher incidence of rejection during pregnancy, lower birth weight, and higher incidence of preterm birth [55].

Contraception

The female CF patient has access to the same highly efficacious choices for contraception as all women. However, many patients are not getting the proper education and counseling on sexual health and contraception options. In a recent survey of 188 women between the ages of 18 and 24 in five CF centers in the United States, less than 10% reported ever receiving contraception counseling and only 26% had undergone a pelvic exam or Pap smear. The comparison group was derived from the 2011 to 2013 National Survey of Family Growth, and among 15- to 24-year-old women in this survey ($n = 1997$), 24% had received contraceptive counseling and 57% had had a pelvic exam or Pap smear [56]. In addition, CF patients were less likely to report ever using contraception of any type (55% vs 74%) [57]. However, among current contraceptive users, CF patients were more likely to choose long-acting reversible contraception such as an IUD or subdermal implant although the sample size was low ($n = 14$, 17% vs 8%) [57].

Very little information is available about specific forms of contraception in CF. Combined oral contraceptives (OCPs) are the most common contraceptive choice in both CF and the general population. OCPs are safe and effective when taken correctly with a failure rate <1% in the general population. However, failure can be as high as 9% if OCPs are not taken correctly [58]. In CF, it is unknown if there is a difference in failure rates of OCPs although there has been concern given that most CF patients have pancreatic insufficiency and consequent malabsorption. A single study has reported pharmacokinetics in CF of combined oral contraceptives that contained higher doses of ethinyl estradiol (50 μg) than is typically used currently. In this study of six women with CF compared to six controls, the women with CF had a higher bioavailability but also a higher clearance of the estrogen component, ultimately yielding a similar area under the curve [59]. Another retrospective review of 18 women with CF on OCPs for 1 year reported no contraceptive failure, and 94% of women had pancreatic insufficiency [60]. For CF patients, concerns arise at times of antibiotic use. However, rifampin is the only antibiotic that has a definitive interaction with OCPs that decreases their effectiveness [61]. In addition, the CFTR modulator lumacaftor-ivacaftor also decreases the efficacy of OCPs. Systematic review of available data shows no concerns regarding safety. No studies have shown any deterioration in lung health with the initiation of OCPs. Indeed, some small studies have suggested a potential decrease in pulmonary exacerbations when patients were initiated on OCPs [62]. Less is known about risks and benefits of other forms of contraception in CF. Given the overall paucity of evidence, clinicians should rely on clinical judgment and consider other clinical factors when choosing contraception. Given the known risks of venous thromboembolism (VTE) with estrogen-containing contraception, these forms of contraception should be avoided in patients with prior history of VTE, particularly if there is a permanent venous access device. Medroxyprogesterone acetate has been associated with bone loss and osteoporosis, and long-term use should be carefully considered [63, 64].

There are no data regarding long-acting reversible contraceptive methods although these are felt to be generally underutilized in the CF population and the population at large. At this time, there are no specific safety concerns regarding use of these methods in CF.

Conclusion

Patients with CF are living longer and healthier lives with expected survival well into the fifth decade and beyond at this time. In the future, highly effective CFTR modulator therapy will continue to prolong survival. The sexual and reproductive health of CF patients will be expected to become a more integral part of their care in adolescence and adulthood. The CF provider needs to be able to be comfortable addressing issues associated with fertility, pregnancy, and contraception.

References

1. Boas SR, Fulton JA, Koehler AN, Orenstein DM. Nutrition and pulmonary function predictors of delayed puberty in adolescent males with cystic fibrosis. Clin Pediatr (Phila). 1998;37(9):573–6.
2. Byard PJ. The adolescent growth spurt in children with cystic fibrosis. Ann Hum Biol. 1994;21(3):229–40.
3. Johannesson M, Gottlieb C, Hjelte L. Delayed puberty in girls with cystic fibrosis despite good clinical status. Pediatrics. 1997;99(1):29–34.
4. Sawyer SM, Phelan PD, Bowes G. Reproductive health in young women with cystic fibrosis: knowledge, behavior and attitudes. J Adolesc Health. 1995;17(1):46–50.
5. Roberts S, Green P. The sexual health of adolescents with cystic fibrosis. J R Soc Med. 2005;98(Suppl 45):7–16.
6. Prasad SA, Balfour-Lynn IM, Carr SB, Madge SL. A comparison of the prevalence of urinary incontinence in girls with cystic fibrosis, asthma, and healthy controls. Pediatr Pulmonol. 2006;41(11):1065–8.
7. Umlawska W, Sands D, Zielinska A. Age of menarche in girls with cystic fibrosis. Folia Histochem Cytobiol. 2010;48(2):185–90.
8. Frayman KB, Sawyer SM. Sexual and reproductive health in cystic fibrosis: a life-course perspective. Lancet Respir Med. 2015;3(1):70–86.
9. Zhang Z, Lindstrom MJ, Lai HJ. Pubertal height velocity and associations with prepubertal and adult heights in cystic fibrosis. J Pediatr. 2013;163(2):376–82.
10. Aswani N, Taylor CJ, McGaw J, Pickering M, Rigby AS. Pubertal growth and development in cystic fibrosis: a retrospective review. Acta Paediatr. 2003;92(9):1029–32.
11. Stead RJ, Hodson ME, Batten JC, Adams J, Jacobs HS. Amenorrhoea in cystic fibrosis. Clin Endocrinol. 1987;26(2):187–95.
12. Leifke E, Friemert M, Heilmann M, Puvogel N, Smaczny C, von zur Muhlen A, et al. Sex steroids and body composition in men with cystic fibrosis. Eur J Endocrinol. 2003;148(5):551–7.
13. Blackman SM, Tangpricha V. Endocrine disorders in cystic fibrosis. Pediatr Clin N Am. 2016;63(4):699–708.
14. Denning CR, Sommers SC, Quigley HJ Jr. Infertility in male patients with cystic fibrosis. Pediatrics. 1968;41(1):7–17.

15. Kaplan E, Shwachman H, Perlmutter AD, Rule A, Khaw KT, Holsclaw DS. Reproductive failure in males with cystic fibrosis. N Engl J Med. 1968;279(2):65–9.
16. Sawyer SM, Tully MA, Dovey ME, Colin AA. Reproductive health in males with cystic fibrosis: knowledge, attitudes, and experiences of patients and parents. Pediatr Pulmonol. 1998;25(4):226–30.
17. Dreyfus DH, Bethel R, Gelfand EW. Cystic fibrosis 3849+10kb C > T mutation associated with severe pulmonary disease and male fertility. Am J Respir Crit Care Med. 1996;153(2):858–60.
18. Stern RC, Doershuk CF, Drumm ML. 3849+10 kb C-->T mutation and disease severity in cystic fibrosis. Lancet. 1995;346(8970):274–6.
19. Sawyer SM, Farrant B, Cerritelli B, Wilson J. A survey of sexual and reproductive health in men with cystic fibrosis: new challenges for adolescent and adult services. Thorax. 2005;60(4):326–30.
20. Sawyer SM, Farrant B, Wilson J, Ryan G, O'Carroll M, Bye P, et al. Sexual and reproductive health in men with cystic fibrosis: consistent preferences, inconsistent practices. J Cyst Fibros. 2009;8(4):264–9.
21. Esteves SC, Miyaoka R, Orosz JE, Agarwal A. An update on sperm retrieval techniques for azoospermic males. Clinics (Sao Paulo). 2013;68(Suppl 1):99–110.
22. Palermo G, Joris H, Devroey P, Van Steirteghem AC. Pregnancies after intracytoplasmic injection of single spermatozoon into an oocyte. Lancet. 1992;340(8810):17–8.
23. Dohle GR, Ramos L, Pieters MH, Braat DD, Weber RF. Surgical sperm retrieval and intracytoplasmic sperm injection as treatment of obstructive azoospermia. Hum Reprod. 1998;13(3):620–3.
24. McCallum TJ, Milunsky JM, Cunningham DL, Harris DH, Maher TA, Oates RD. Fertility in men with cystic fibrosis: an update on current surgical practices and outcomes. Chest. 2000;118(4):1059–62.
25. Muchekehu RW, Quinton PM. A new role for bicarbonate secretion in cervico-uterine mucus release. J Physiol. 2010;588(Pt 13):2329–42.
26. Tizzano EF, Silver MM, Chitayat D, Benichou JC, Buchwald M. Differential cellular expression of cystic fibrosis transmembrane regulator in human reproductive tissues. Clues for the infertility in patients with cystic fibrosis. Am J Pathol. 1994;144(5):906–14.
27. Shteinberg M, Lulu AB, Downey DG, Blumenfeld Z, Rousset-Jablonski C, Perceval M, et al. Failure to conceive in women with CF is associated with pancreatic insufficiency and advancing age. J Cyst Fibros. 2019;18:525.
28. Cystic Fibrosis Foundation Patient Registry 2016 annual data report. Bethesda: Cystic Fibrosis Foundation; 2017.
29. Thorpe-Beeston J, Madge S, Gyi K, Hodson M, Bilton D. The outcome of pregnancies in women with cystic fibrosis—single centre experience 1998–2011. BJOG. 2013;120(3):354–61.
30. McArdle JR. Pregnancy in cystic fibrosis. Clin Chest Med. 2011;32(1):111–20.
31. Rasmussen KMY, Ann L. Weight gain during pregnancy: reexamining the guidelines. Washington, DC: The National Academies Press; 2009.
32. Stallings VA, Stark LJ, Robinson KA, Feranchak AP, Quinton H. Evidence-based practice recommendations for nutrition-related management of children and adults with cystic fibrosis and pancreatic insufficiency: results of a systematic review. J Am Diet Assoc. 2008;108(5):832–9.
33. Edenborough FP, Borgo G, Knoop C, Lannefors L, Mackenzie WE, Madge S, et al. Guidelines for the management of pregnancy in women with cystic fibrosis. J Cyst Fibros. 2008;7:S2–S32.
34. Ren CL, Morgan RL, Oermann C, Resnick HE, Brady C, Campbell A, et al. Cystic Fibrosis Foundation pulmonary guidelines. Use of cystic fibrosis transmembrane conductance regulator modulator therapy in patients with cystic fibrosis. Ann Am Thorac Soc. 2018;15(3):271–80.
35. Davies JC, Moskowitz SM, Brown C, Horsley A, Mall MA, McKone EF, et al. VX-659–Tezacaftor–Ivacaftor in patients with cystic fibrosis and one or two Phe508del Alleles. N Engl J Med. 2018;379(17):1599–611.
36. Keating D, Marigowda G, Burr L, Daines C, Mall MA, McKone EF, et al. VX-445–Tezacaftor–Ivacaftor in patients with cystic fibrosis and one or two Phe508del Alleles. N Engl J Med. 2018;379(17):1612–20.

37. Ramsey BW, Davies J, McElvaney NG, Tullis E, Bell SC, Dřevínek P, et al. A CFTR potentiator in patients with cystic fibrosis and the G551D mutation. N Engl J Med. 2011;365(18):1663–72.
38. Kaminski R, Nazareth D. A successful uncomplicated CF pregnancy while remaining on Ivacaftor. J Cyst Fibros. 2016;15(1):133–4.
39. Heltshe SL, Godfrey EM, Josephy T, Aitken ML, Taylor-Cousar JL. Pregnancy among cystic fibrosis women in the era of CFTR modulators. J Cyst Fibros. 2017;16(6):687–94.
40. Ladores S, Kazmerski TM, Rowe SM. A case report of pregnancy during use of targeted therapeutics for cystic fibrosis. J Obstet Gynecol Neonatal Nurs. 2017;46(1):72–7.
41. Trimble AT, Donaldson SH. Ivacaftor withdrawal syndrome in cystic fibrosis patients with the G551D mutation. J Cyst Fibros. 2018;17(2):e13–e6.
42. Taylor-Cousar JL, Munck A, McKone EF, van der Ent CK, Moeller A, Simard C, et al. Tezacaftor–Ivacaftor in patients with cystic fibrosis homozygous for Phe508del. N Engl J Med. 2017;377(21):2013–23.
43. Wainwright CE, Elborn JS, Ramsey BW, Marigowda G, Huang X, Cipolli M, et al. Lumacaftor–Ivacaftor in patients with cystic fibrosis homozygous for Phe508del CFTR. N Engl J Med. 2015;373(3):220–31.
44. Marie J, Elisabeth E-A, Isabelle M, Inés De M, Nicolas V, Eric C. Bedaquiline and linezolid for extensively drug-resistant tuberculosis in pregnant woman. Emerg Infect Dis. 2017;23(10):1731–2.
45. Van Kampenhout E, Bolhuis MS, Alffenaar J-WC, Oswald LMA, Kerstjens HAM, de Lange WCM, et al. Pharmacokinetics of moxifloxacin and linezolid during and after pregnancy in a patient with multidrug-resistant tuberculosis. Eur Respir J. 2017;49(3):16017124. https://doi.org/10.1183/13993003.01724-2016.
46. Bookstaver PB, Bland CM, Griffin B, Stover KR, Eiland LS, McLaughlin M. A review of antibiotic use in pregnancy. Pharmacotherapy. 2015;35(11):1052–62.
47. Siegel B, Siegel S. Pregnancy and delivery in a patient with cystic fibrosis of the pancreas. Obstet Gynecol. 1960;16(4):438–40.
48. Edenborough FP, Mackenzie WE, Stableforth DE. The outcome of 72 pregnancies in 55 women with cystic fibrosis in the United Kingdom 1977-1996. BJOG. 2000;107(2):254–61.
49. LAU EMT, BARNES DJ, MORIARTY C, OGLE R, DENTICE R, CIVITICO J, et al. Pregnancy outcomes in the current era of cystic fibrosis care: a 15-year experience. Aust N Z J Obstet Gynaecol. 2011;51(3):220–4.
50. Renton M, Priestley L, Bennett L, Mackillop L, Chapman SJ. Pregnancy outcomes in cystic fibrosis: a 10-year experience from a UK centre. Obstet Med. 2015;8(2):99–101.
51. Reynaud Q, Poupon-Bourdy S, Rabilloud M, Al Mufti L, Rousset Jablonski C, Lemonnier L, et al. Pregnancy outcome in women with cystic fibrosis-related diabetes. Acta Obstet Gynecol Scand. 2017;96(10):1223–7.
52. Jelin AC, Sharshiner R, Caughey AB. Maternal co-morbidities and neonatal outcomes associated with cystic fibrosis. J Matern Fetal Neonatal Med. 2017;30(1):4–7.
53. Patel EM, Swamy GK, Heine RP, Kuller JA, James AH, Grotegut CA. Medical and obstetric complications among pregnant women with cystic fibrosis. Am J Obstet Gynecol. 2015;212(1):98.e1–9.
54. Schechter MS, Quittner AL, Konstan MW, Millar SJ, Pasta DJ, McMullen A. Long-term effects of pregnancy and motherhood on disease outcomes of women with cystic fibrosis. Ann Am Thorac Soc. 2013;10(3):213–9.
55. Shaner J, Coscia LA, Constantinescu S, McGrory CH, Doria C. Pregnancy after lung transplant. Prog Transplant. 2012;22(2):134–40.
56. Kazmerski TM, Sawicki GS, Miller E, Jones KA, Abebe KZ, Tuchman LK, et al. Sexual and reproductive health care utilization and preferences reported by young women with cystic fibrosis. J Cyst Fibros. 2018;17(1):64–70.
57. Kazmerski TM, Sawicki GS, Miller E, Jones KA, Abebe KZ, Tuchman LK, et al. Sexual and reproductive health behaviors and experiences reported by young women with cystic fibrosis. J Cyst Fibros. 2018;17(1):57–63.

58. Trussell J. Contraceptive failure in the United States. Contraception. 2011;83(5):397–404.
59. Stead RJ, Grimmer SF, Rogers SM, Back DJ, Orme ML, Hodson ME, et al. Pharmacokinetics of contraceptive steroids in patients with cystic fibrosis. Thorax. 1987;42(1):59–64.
60. Plant BJ, Goss CH, Tonelli MR, McDonald G, Black RA, Aitken ML. Contraceptive practices in women with cystic fibrosis. J Cyst Fibros. 2008;7(5):412–4.
61. Simmons KB, Haddad LB, Nanda K, Curtis KM. Drug interactions between non-rifamycin antibiotics and hormonal contraception: a systematic review. Am J Obstet Gynecol. 2018;218(1):88–97.e14.
62. Chotirmall SH, Smith SG, Gunaratnam C, Cosgrove S, Dimitrov BD, O'Neill SJ, et al. Effect of estrogen on pseudomonas mucoidy and exacerbations in cystic fibrosis. N Engl J Med. 2012;366(21):1978–86.
63. Roe AH, Traxler S, Schreiber CA. Contraception in women with cystic fibrosis: a systematic review of the literature. Contraception. 2016;93(1):3–10.
64. Whiteman MK, Oduyebo T, Zapata LB, Walker S, Curtis KM. Contraceptive safety among women with cystic fibrosis: a systematic review. Contraception. 2016;94(6):621–9.

Chapter 21
Mental Health in Cystic Fibrosis

Kathryn L. Behrhorst, Robin S. Everhart, and Michael S. Schechter

Patient Perspective
When Anxiety Attacks

What I thought would be a fun trip to the nail salon with my mom let me know I had a bigger problem with anxiety than I thought.

This day started out like all the rest. I woke up, did my morning treatments, ate breakfast, and got ready to go get my nails done with my mom. This is a long-running activity, and it's always a good day. We get mother-daughter time and we pick out the nail color we will wear for the next two to three weeks. That may not sound very exciting, but to me it's fun. I get to feel out my energy, my mood for that moment, and pick a color that goes with it.

Someone other than my regular guy was about to start on my nails and, in that moment, my heart began to race, my palms got sweaty. I pulled at my hands and fingers. I started biting my lips, my body shook, and water filled my eyes. For the first time, my anxiety became a disturbance to my public life. Up until this point, I thought I had everything under control. But it was in this moment I knew it had gotten out of hand. I knew something needed to change.

Growing up with cystic fibrosis, you learn about all the physical stuff that could happen. You learn about what happens when you get an infection, that hospital stays are inevitable, that doing treatments multiple times a day is meant to help keep us healthy. But I never thought that anxiety would come into my life the way it did.

K. L. Behrhorst (✉) · R. S. Everhart
Virginia Commonwealth University, Department of Psychology, Richmond, VA, USA
e-mail: behrhorstkl@vcu.edu

M. S. Schechter
Division of Pulmonary Medicine, Department of Pediatrics, Virginia Commonwealth University, Children's Hospital of Richmond at VCU, Richmond, VA, USA

© Springer Nature Switzerland AG 2020
S. D. Davis et al. (eds.), *Cystic Fibrosis*, Respiratory Medicine,
https://doi.org/10.1007/978-3-030-42382-7_21

When I heard people talk about anxiety, it was never something I thought I would deal with myself. Hospital visits started for me when I was 17. After that, I was constantly in and out of the hospital with infection after infection. I soon developed anxiety and depression. It began small with just some finger pulling and lip biting.

That day in the nail salon I knew I needed a little more help than I was giving myself, so I reached out to my care team to help me find a therapist to talk with. I am also looking into more methods of treatment like meditation and yoga. This way, I can learn new ways to control my breathing when I feel my chest get tight and my heartbeat gets faster.

I will try every single thing out there before starting any anxiety medication. Although anxiety medications work well for many of the people who take them, I just know it would not be the best fit for me. Though this was a difficult day for me, having that public anxiety attack opened my eyes and made me realize that covering up my anxiety is not solving anything.

Looking back, I'm not sure why I decided to cover it up instead of seeking more help and learning different treatments. I know now that it's no longer something I can or should cover up. It needs to be talked about more so that people who need help can find it, and also know they are not alone.

–Starr Picklesimer
from https://www.cff.org/CF-Community-Blog/Posts/2019/When-Anxiety-Attacks/,

Parent Perspective on Mental Health in CF

In aiming to better understand how mental health issues can impact CF firsthand, we interviewed a parent of a young child with CF, as well as a young adult with CF. Their experiences highlight how mental health symptoms, especially anxiety and depression, influence their ability to care for CF on a daily basis. They also offer a perspective on how they have learned to cope with their mental health issues, as well as advice for other patients with CF and their caregivers.

The parent of a young CF patient described, "For the first full year after being diagnosed, I definitely experienced increased depression. I didn't know what to expect, the feeling of the unknown was terrifying, and I spent many days of 'self-pity'. Why us? Why him? I'm not sure at what point the depression seemed to decrease but my anxiety increased and seems to remain fairly heightened. The feeling of being on constant alert with my son, trying not to miss a thing, the weight of ensuring my family/household is tended to, and the financial strain of the disease are some of my most common concerns and thoughts." A 20-year-old patient with CF described her experience when she feels depressed, "I start feeling it throughout my whole body. I feel too tired to put on my vest or get my [nebulizers] together. It makes me feel bad that I could be slowing the progression of the illness but I don't because I feel too depressed about it. I have lived my life as if I was going to die at any minute. I didn't do a whole lot of things because I wasn't sure if I would make it. Things like getting a normal job or fitting in with friends socially. If I skip treatment people don't think things are as serious as they are. It makes me pull away and lose friends because of it."

In thinking about a time when her mental health made it hard to care for her child's CF, this parent stated, "His first overnight hospital stay sticks out in my head. I was so overcome by fear, anxiety, and sadness it was almost as though I had totally forgotten how to be a mother. He was only a year and a half old, in pain, and in an unfamiliar place. I emotionally could not keep myself together, which in turn caused him to become hysterical." When having mental health symptoms, this parent noted that it helps to "take a second to step back and to look at the positive in my son and his current health. Taking a more positive approach on life overall seems to help me with the added stress of the disease daily. It helps me to know that all of the time, medications, appointments, and therapies that I put into his care allow him to be the active and 'healthy' boy that he is."

Additionally, this parent described, "I have found that, for me, going to CF events, helping other parents cope with diagnosis, raising awareness, learning more about the disease, and volunteering for events help immensely in coping with stress and mental health symptoms. This gives me purpose and allows me to share my passion of caring for my son and beating the disease with others. I am also very lucky to have friends that love our CFer as much as we do and can find the positives in the life we live. I am blessed to have a husband that understands and takes part in our daily life of caring for a CFer. Having an amazing care team for our son is also one of the biggest resources; I have knowledge at my fingertips (through phone, email, face to face) that not only know about CF but they know my son as well." Meanwhile, the adult CF patient stated that, "sometimes doing things like simply taking a shower or taking a break can be helpful. Some days I will engage in self -are and let other household tasks wait. I will get some help from my family with taking care of my son, and then I engage in self-care. Therapy has helped with my symptoms." She similarly noted that "if I lose my outpatient therapist, having my mental health coordinator and psychiatrist to talk to has also been helpful. My clinic staff is really important in giving me pep talks and being my support."

When asked what other parents should know about mental health and CF, this parent replied, "That it's normal! We have loved ones that have a terrible, potentially life-threatening disease. Don't run from it; get help, talk to people, don't be ashamed to ask questions and reach out." The adult CF patient added, "it's okay to be honest and tell the clinic when you're feeling suicidal or feeling like you don't matter in a world where healthy people are on top and we are sitting at the bottom. When I do talk about it with people, and not keep things inside, it is really helpful. Talk to people and engage with mental health care. You won't regret it."

Introduction

Background

It has long been appreciated that, in the general population, the presence of a chronic illness is a significant risk factor for the development of mental health disorders such as anxiety and depression [1–4]. Anxiety and depression are significant morbidities in themselves, but when associated with chronic somatic disease such as cystic fibrosis (CF), their importance is magnified by the challenges they pose to disease management and their impact on outcomes. Depressed patients are also more likely to engage in risky behaviors such as smoking, drinking, and drug use [5]. Depression, in particular, is also associated with nonadherence to prescribed treatments, higher rates of missed or canceled appointments, increased healthcare utilization, and higher healthcare costs [6–10].

The Impact of Stress on CF Patients and Their Caregivers

Although stress may have a negative impact on the course of some diseases by impairing immune function [11], of greater potential importance is the impact for individuals with CF. Excessive personal or parental experiences of stress may lead to depression or impaired personal and family function [12] which have a direct and specific effect on adherence. Conceptual models of adjustment to caring for a chronic disease consider both the stress of caring for the disease and the psychological and social mediators that affect how that stress is handled. A modified version of one conceptual model of adjustment to stress [13], applicable to the experience of a person with chronic disease or to the caregiver of a child with chronic disease, is shown in Fig. 21.1. Extrinsic stressors include the daily general

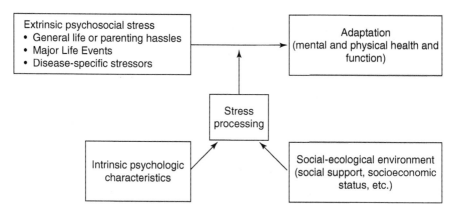

Fig. 21.1 Stress and coping model. (Modified from [13])

challenges of life common to all; those associated with major life events such as job loss or death of a loved one; and disease-specific stresses due to living with chronic illness. Disease-specific stress, which is experienced in proportion to the degree of the child's illness, has been reported to be the most important to mothers of children with CF [14]. The ability to process stress depends upon psychological characteristics (temperament, coping skills, feelings of mastery and control, resilience) and social–ecological variables (family resources and social support as well as socioeconomic status and other social determinants of health) [15]. Depression, dysfunctional behaviors (including drug and alcohol abuse), and physical illness are likely outcomes of excessive stress in the CF patient or in the CF child's caregivers. Reciprocal associations exist among components of the schema (i.e., greater disease severity is caused by but also causes more stress and decreased stress processing resources).

The Increasing Awareness of the Role of Mental Health in CF

Studies over the last few years have made it increasingly clear that depression and anxiety are common in individuals with CF as well as their parent caregivers, with estimated prevalence ranging from 10% to 30%. The International Depression Epidemiological Study (TIDES) found symptoms of depression in 10% of adolescents with CF, 19% of adults with CF, and over 30% of parent caregivers; the prevalence of symptoms of anxiety were even higher [16].

In 2013, the CF Foundation and the European Cystic Fibrosis Society invited experts to form an International Committee on Mental Health in Cystic Fibrosis (ICMH) and develop clinical care guidelines for preventing, screening, and treating anxiety and depression in individuals with CF and parent caregivers [17]. These guidelines recommend specific preventative steps, screening tools, and behavioral and medical treatment. At about that same time, a survey of mental health services available at CF centers in the USA and Europe [18] found that most centers were not adequately equipped to implement these guideline recommendations. The most important barriers, aside from a lack of experience with or training in mental health screening, were perceived limitations in staffing, time, and lack of qualified personnel to provide evidence-based interventions or referrals. The CF Foundation has subsequently funded the presence of Mental Health Coordinators as members of the core team in 138 CF programs in North America. The presence of mental health professionals on the CF team has similarly increased significantly throughout the rest of the world, and a recently published survey of center practice in Europe reported that half of all CF centers surveyed (nearly 100) had implemented mental health screening [18]. Specific aspects of mental health and behavioral care are outlined in the rest of this chapter.

Depression

Symptoms and Diagnosis

Depression is a prevalent mental health concern that impacts a large proportion of the general population as well as individuals with a chronic condition [19]. Symptoms of depression impact an individual's thoughts, feelings, and behaviors and can have a significant impact on the ability to care for oneself. Common symptoms of depression include hopelessness, anhedonia, appetite or sleep changes, concentration difficulties, and low self-esteem lasting for more than 2 weeks [20]. A number of measures have been evaluated for screening for depression in children, adolescents, and adults in the general population; the ICMH has specifically recommended the use of the Patient Health Questionnaire (PHQ-9), which is a 9-item self-reported scale of depressive symptoms that also includes an item to assess suicide risk [21]. It should be pointed out that the PHQ-9 is a screening tool that has been shown to have good sensitivity, specificity, and predictive values in tested populations. However, the validity of the PHQ-9 for screening in CF has never been formally tested and its predictive value in CF is unknown. Thus, concerns regarding the presence of depression in any given patient should not be completely allayed by a negative screen, and likewise a positive screen should be verified before specific treatment is begun.

Prevalence of Depression

The prevalence of depression in the general population varies based on age, with symptoms seen in 2–6% of children, 7–20% in adolescents, and 5–17% in adults [22]. Prevalence rates have been shown to be higher in those with chronic illnesses [16]. In the CF population, the International Depression Epidemiological Study (TIDES) found positive screens for global depression in 10% of adolescents, 19% of adults, 37% of mothers, and 31% of fathers [16]. These rates fall within the range seen in other studies assessing psychological distress in CF [23–27], and were greater than that seen in the general population across all nine countries in the TIDES study with the exception of the UK, where only 13% adolescents and <1% of adults with CF exhibited elevated screening scores [19].

Prevalence of Suicidality and Suicidal Ideation

Depressive symptoms and disorders are powerful predictors of risky behaviors (e.g., substance use and self-harm), co-morbid disorders (e.g., substance use disorders, personality disorders, anxiety disorders), school failure and absence, and later or co-occurring suicidality [28–31]. Over half of individuals in the general population with depressive mood disorders presenting during early adolescence attempt suicide at some point in life and around 22% have multiple attempts [32]. Pulmonary diseases have been associated with a two-thirds increase in the odds of lifetime suicidal ideation [33]. In the CF population, relatively little research has been reported on the prevalence of suicidal ideation or suicidality among patients. In two studies assessing rates of suicidality in adult CF clinics, between 5% and 11% of participants endorsed thoughts on the PHQ-9 of being better off dead or hurting themselves in some way [34, 35]. Although these rates are lower than those found within the general population, suicidality among CF patients is an important area for further study. The ICMH guidelines support the use of the PHQ-9 for regular screening of patients and this includes a question on suicidality; therefore, clinic staff implementing the screening tools must be properly trained to handle the endorsement of suicidal ideation. Protocol for addressing suicidal ideation, including a clinical risk assessment, safety plan, and follow-up procedures should be outlined and a toolkit for such supplements are provided by the ICMH [17].

Anxiety

Symptoms and Diagnosis

Anxiety is characterized by ongoing, excessive worry and fears that impact one's daily activities. Anxiety can present as a variety of disorders from generalized anxiety, panic disorder or obsessive-compulsive disorder (OCD) and each is defined by a different set of specific symptoms. Generalized anxiety disorder (GAD) is defined by a display of persistent cognitive (e.g., unwanted thoughts, harsh self-criticism), somatic (e.g., muscle tension, sleep disturbance), behavioral (e.g., avoidance, escape from an anxiety-provoking situation), or emotional (e.g., dread, irritability) symptoms [20]. The ICMH has recommended the use of the Generalized Anxiety Disorder 7-item (GAD-7) self-report questionnaire for screening of anxious symptoms [36].

Prevalence of Anxiety

The prevalence of anxiety in the general population is estimated to be between 25% and 32% in adolescents [37]. These rates vary based on the anxiety disorder with GAD rates around 4%, panic disorder rates around 2%, social anxiety rates around 10%, and specific phobia rates around 17% [37]. For adults, the overall prevalence of anxiety in the general population is around 31% with GAD rates around 6%, social anxiety rates around 12%, panic disorder rates around 5%, and OCD rates around 2% [38]. TIDES reported rates of anxiety symptoms in 22% of adolescents, 32% of adults, 48% of mothers, and 36% of fathers [16], close to that of the general population. Other CF studies have reported similar findings [27, 39].

Other Mental Health Considerations in CF

In addition to symptoms of depression and anxiety, individuals with CF may also experience other mental health challenges and conditions that can have an impact on an individual's overall CF care and well-being. A brief overview of several conditions is provided.

Attention-Deficit/Hyperactivity Disorder (ADHD)

ADHD is a neurodevelopmental disorder characterized by difficulties with attention, impulsivity, and hyperactivity [20]. The prevalence of ADHD in the general population is between 7% and 9% in children and between 4% and 5% in adults [40]. Studies looking at the prevalence of ADHD in children and adults with CF have found rates ranging from 9.6% to 18.9% with slightly lower rates (e.g., 9.6% and 16%) in children than in adults (e.g., 15% and 18.9%) [40–42].

Pediatric Behavioral Feeding Disorders

Diet is an emphasis of treatment for CF patients based on the established associations between better nutritional status and better lung function [43–45]. Because of this, a treatment goal for patients with CF includes higher caloric intake in order to maintain a body mass index of 22 for adult men, 23 for adult women, and at or above the 50th percentile for pediatric patients under the age of 21 [46]. Problems related to feeding behaviors are not often formally diagnosed in CF patients and frequently stem from oppositionality and defiance related to adhering to dietary recommendations for their diagnosis [47, 48]. Examples of common feeding problems seen in patients with CF include refusing to eat foods, taking longer than 20 minutes to finish a meal, spitting out food, and reluctance to be present during mealtimes [47]. One study has reported a prevalence rate of feeding challenges (based upon caregiver report) of around 32% [49].

Eating Disorders

Although disruptive behavior problems are more common in children, concerns related to body image and disordered eating are present in adolescents and adults. A 2012 systematic review of body image in CF patients found that males with CF tend to have a poorer overall body image compared to both females with CF and healthy men. One possible explanation for this finding is that males may experience greater disconnect between the traditional appearance expectations for men (i.e., larger build) and the typical low body weight and stature seen in males with CF [50].

Although females were found to have more positive body image, which is congruent with socio-cultural stereotypes for women (i.e., desire to be thin), concerns exist about females with CF being more content with a lower body mass index (BMI) and the detrimental effects this can have on lung function and CF progression [43].

For adolescents in the general population, the lifetime prevalence of any eating disorder is around 3% [30]. Estimated rates of anorexia nervosa in adolescents are around 0.3%, around 0.9% for bulimia nervosa, and around 1.6% for binge eating disorder [51]. In adults, recent lifetime estimates for anorexia nervosa are around 0.8%, 0.3% for bulimia nervosa, and 0.9% for binge eating disorder [52]. In the CF population, individuals are prone to endorsing symptoms of anorexia nervosa rather than binge eating disorder or bulimia nervosa. However, estimated prevalence rates of eating disorders in the CF population are by and large consistent with the general population [53, 54]. Differences are seen in rates of disordered eating behaviors but diagnoses of eating disorders are not significantly different [55].

Impact of Mental Health Challenges and Disorders

Adherence

The primary cause of increased CF-related morbidity and mortality caused by mental health disorders appears to be through decreased adherence to daily CF care. While difficulties with measuring adherence compromise the validity of most adherence-related studies, depression is associated with a substantially increased likelihood of nonadherence to treatment in individuals with chronic conditions [6]. Parental depression has also been found to have an important negative impact on adherence to childhood asthma treatment, resulting in worse health outcomes [56]. Mental health difficulties are associated with worse perceptions of self-efficacy and can impact self-care (e.g., disease management, diet, exercise) and concentration (i.e., making it harder to organize oneself and manage medications) [57]. On the other hand, anxiety has been shown to improve parentally reported adherence in children and adolescents with CF [58]. Parents attempting to manage disruptive child behaviors may have an even more difficult time trying to manage adherence to CF care, although systematic research has not been conducted in this area. Limited research has suggested (unsurprisingly) that eating disorders are associated with worse adherence to nutrition-related treatments [59].

Health Outcomes

In the general population, individuals with anxiety and depression exhibit worse overall health [60]. Patients with comorbid chronic medical conditions or chronic lung disease and mental health concerns (e.g., anxiety, depression, eating disorder) have worse medical symptoms and increased impairment than those without psychological disorders [61].

In CF, depression has been associated with worse lung function [25, 62], increased rate of pulmonary exacerbations and decreased health-related quality of life [25, 39] as well as increased healthcare utilization and costs [63]. A recent longitudinal study of 1005 eligible patients who participated in the US TIDES showed the 5-year hazard ratio of death associated with depression was 2.0; 95% CI (1.3, 3.0)]. When adjusted for confounders the HR was 1.4; 95% CI (0.9, 2.1). The adjusted HR was higher in adults [1.6; 95% CI (1.0, 2.4)] and those screening in the severe range [2.0; 95% CI (1.2, 3.4)]. It should be noted that the cause of death in this population did not differ by mental health status, and the number of deaths due to suicide was too small to evaluate [64].

In a handful of studies, both anxiety and disordered eating behaviors have shown significant associations with lung function. For instance, anxiety was negatively correlated with lung function in 11- to 14-year-old children and in adults [65, 66]. Anxiety and eating disorders were also associated with worse nutritional status for adults [59, 66]. The aforementioned study of mortality in TIDES subjects [64] did not find an association between anxiety and mortality.

Health-Related Quality of Life (HRQOL)

Not surprisingly, mood disorders and mental health symptoms are associated with a decrease in overall HRQOL. In adults, lower scores on the Cystic Fibrosis Questionnaire-Revised (CFQ-R), a measure of QOL, have been associated with depression, specifically in the domains of emotional functioning and eating disturbances [24, 25, 67]. Two recent studies of children and adolescents with CF found both depression and anxiety to have large effects on HRQOL across numerous domains [68, 69].

Family Functioning

Mental health not only influences the functioning of an individual with CF but also has a significant effect on family members and the overall family unit. Caregivers and other family members assisting in the care of children and adolescents with CF are faced with complicated medical timing and regimens, concerns about exposure and infection, and challenges with weight gain and growth management [70]. Although not many studies have focused on associations between specific psychological diagnoses and family functioning, broad measures have found a significant relationship between psychological and family functioning (e.g., organization, cohesiveness, expressiveness) [70–72]. Additionally, family functioning has been associated with adherence to specific components of the CF treatment regimen, such as pancreatic enzymes [73].

Delivering Mental Healthcare in CF

1. *Prevention*

While there is currently little published experience with prevention of anxiety and depression in the CF population, randomized trials targeted at other high-risk groups with chronic disease have shown success in this regard [74]. Further investigation into the types of intervention likely to be most effective in CF is necessary, but based upon experience in other areas, encouraging resilience, teaching coping skills, supporting mindfulness, and enabling self-help will likely be of benefit. Specifically, all individuals with CF and their caregivers should be educated on signs and symptoms of mental health disorders, as well as their prevalence and impact, and offered supportive interventions to promote effective coping skills, management of distress related to medical procedures [62, 75], and training in problem-solving and cognitive behavioral skills that can decrease anxiety and improve resilience. Surveillance in early childhood for behavioral feeding disorders can lead to appropriate treatment or referral, and training in effective parenting skills is likely to have a beneficial effect on both parent caregivers and maturing children [76].

2. *Screening*

The ICMH guidelines [17] make specific recommendations regarding the use of the PHQ-9 and GAD-7 for annual screening of adolescents 12 years and older and adults with CF. In addition, it is recommended that children with CF between the ages of 7 and 11 be evaluated for depression and anxiety when caregiver depression or anxiety scores are elevated, or when significant symptoms of depression or anxiety in the child are reported or observed. Furthermore, the ICMH recommends offering annual screening for depression and anxiety to at least one primary caregiver of children and adolescents with CF.

3. *Treatment*

Screening is only effective when it is done in the context of an established approach to treatment. In the USA, due to resources committed by the CF Foundation, many CF centers have mental health coordinators with the skills to provide treatment for common mental health problems, especially when they are mild. The CF care model is especially well-suited to support an approach that has been called the collaborative care model. Collaborative care is an innovative way of treating depression and anxiety, involving multiple health professionals working together to address mental health problems in the context of the medical home. Over the past 15 years, a robust evidence-base for this approach has emerged, and a recent Cochrane review found collaborative care to represent a useful addition to clinical pathways for adult patients with depression and anxiety [77]. Its use has been extended to the chronic disease setting, where integrated collaborative care has been shown to improve medical and mental health outcomes including reducing rates of hospitalizations and healthcare costs and optimizing healthcare treatments [60, 78, 79]. In collaborative care programs, care is provided by a multidisciplinary team including:

- A PCP or medical specialist.
- Mental health coordinator or care management staff. A nurse, clinical social worker, or psychologist, who is based in the medical clinic and trained to provide care coordination, brief behavioral interventions, and to support treatments such as medications initiated by the medical physician. In some models this staff also provides brief/structured psychotherapy.
- A mental health consultant, typically a psychiatrist, who advises the medical care treatment team with a focus on patients who present diagnostic or therapeutic challenges. Psychiatric consultation can be provided in person, through the use of telephone or tele-video consultation. The degree to which the consultant is needed will vary by the level of expertise available within the medical team.

Psychological Interventions

The implementation of routine screening of symptoms in CF patients was the first big step toward proper treatment of mental health conditions in this population. An important next step is to ensure that patients are able to receive appropriate referrals for treatment and intervention options after the identification of moderate or severe symptoms. Several evidence-based psychological interventions have been supported for the treatment of depression, anxiety, disruptive behaviors, and eating dysfunction/disorders. Although these interventions have received strong support from research performed in the general population, continued examination of the impact of psychological interventions within the chronic illness population and specifically within CF population is warranted.

Cognitive behavioral therapy (CBT) has received extensive support in efficacy and effectiveness research for treating both depression and anxiety. CBT in both individual and group formats has shown promise in reducing symptoms by addressing dysfunctional thoughts, emotions, and behaviors. The typical length of treatment for CBT ranges from 8 to 12 weeks and involves the teaching of coping skills, behavioral activation, and cognitive restructuring practices [80].

Interpersonal therapy (IPT) is another evidence-based treatment for depression, anxiety, and eating disorders [81–83]. IPT is targeted toward social interactions and problems such as conflicts with others, changes in social roles, and loss. Goals of IPT include assisting individuals with improving their communication skills, encouraging healthy expression of emotions, enhancing behavior patterns, and providing attention in relationships [82].

Acceptance and commitment therapy (ACT) has received specific focus alongside CBT and IPT in the CF population for treating anxiety, depression, and general social and emotional functioning [84]. The overall objective of ACT is to improve effectiveness when acting in line with long-term goals and life values and overcoming difficulties related to the presence of bodily symptoms, emotional struggles, and interfering thoughts [85]. ACT manuals have recently been adapted specifically for use in individuals with CF by incorporating a focus on poor adherence to medications which may stem from symptoms of depression and anxiety [86].

Dialectical behavior therapy (DBT) has been suggested as an alternative modality for therapeutic intervention and it has received support in targeting depression and suicidality with preliminary outcomes showing improvements in eating disorders as well [87, 88]. DBT targets emotion regulation skill building by eliciting patient goals, teaching targeted skills (e.g., mindfulness, distress tolerance), and establishing a plan to practice skills and regulate emotions [88].

Behavioral parent training (BPT) is the first line of psychological treatment for ADHD and disruptive behavior disorders. BPT and/or general behavior modification strategies have been successfully used to address concerns related to ADHD, ODD, or feeding and mealtime behaviors in CF patients [89, 90]. BPT provides parents with strategies to identify and alter antecedents and consequences of child behavior. Parents learn to target and monitor problematic behaviors and appropriate replacement behaviors, provide prosocial verbal praise and tangible rewards, and decrease unwanted behaviors through effective ignoring, time out, and instructional strategies [91].

Pharmacological Interventions

In conjunction with psychological interventions, pharmacological interventions have been supported in treating depression, anxiety, eating disorders, and ADHD. Research highlights that the most effective interventions for these disorders are a combined psychological and pharmacological approach. For treating depression and anxiety, selective serotonin reuptake inhibitors (SSRIs) such as sertraline, citalopram, escitalopram, and fluoxetine are options for adolescents and adults that are appropriate for CF [16]. Due to potential pharmacokinetic alterations in CF, it is important to closely monitor all new medications for adverse effects and therapeutic benefits [17].

When patients are not responding effectively to behavioral interventions for anxiety alone, benzodiazepines are another short-term adjunct pharmacological treatment for symptoms. Benzodiazepines are beneficial in their rapid-acting formula without the risk of serotonin syndrome [92]. However, they require very close monitoring in patients with a history or risk of substance use or depression. Some evidence has been found supporting SSRIs and mood stabilizers for treating bulimia nervosa and binge eating disorder [93], but psychotherapies remain the primary treatment of choice for eating disorders.

For treatment of ADHD, ODD, or other disruptive behavior disorders, psychological intervention is the first line of treatment, particularly in those under the age of 6 years [94]. After the age of six, approved stimulant or non-stimulant medications can be prescribed for treatment. Although most primary care physicians are more readily familiar with stimulant medication (e.g., methylphenidate, dextroamphetamine) and thus prescribe it first, they commonly cause appetite suppression, which can be a significant adverse side effect for CF patients attempting to maintain their BMI and high caloric intake [42]. Nonstimulant medications (e.g., atomoxetine, clonidine, guanfacine, bupropion, and nortriptyline) may be a better alternative for CF patients, and this should be explained during a discussion with prescribing physicians [42].

Conclusion

In sum, patients with CF and their parent caregivers experience an increased burden in caring for CF that has implications for their mental health, and specifically depression and anxiety. In CF, mental health symptoms have a direct and negative impact on adherence, which can place patients at greater risk for experiencing worse CF health outcomes, such as lung function and BMI. Notably, the CF Foundation has recognized the importance of focusing on mental health in the CF community by placing mental health coordinators at CF centers across the USA and aiming to normalize discussions of mental health between patients and their care teams. Evidence-based treatments exist to minimize mental health symptoms, with manuals being adapted to specifically target mental health symptoms among patients with CF and their families. Thus, resources exist to support individuals with CF and their families with the goal of enabling patients to manage their CF as prescribed and with fewer mental health symptoms overall.

References

1. Wells KB, Golding JM, Burnam MA. Chronic medical conditions in a sample of the general population with anxiety, affective, and substance use disorders. Am J Psychiatry. 1989;146:1440–6.
2. Herrmann C. International experiences with the hospital anxiety and depression scale: a review of validation data and clinical results. J Psychosom Res. 1997;42:17–41.
3. Riolo SA, Nguyen TA, Greden JF, King CA. Prevalence of depression by race/ethnicity: findings from the National Health and Nutrition Examination Survey III. Am J Public Health. 2005;95:998–1000.
4. Roy-Byrne PP, Davidson KW, Kessler RC, et al. Anxiety disorders and comorbid medical illness. Gen Hosp Psychiatry. 2008;30:208–25.
5. Whittemore R, Kanner S, Singleton S, Hamrin V, Chiu J, Grey M. Correlates of depressive symptoms in adolescents with type 1 diabetes. Pediatr Diabetes. 2002;3:135–43.
6. DiMatteo MR, Lepper HS, Croghan TW. Depression is a risk factor for noncompliance with medical treatment: meta-analysis of the effects of anxiety and depression on patient adherence. Arch Intern Med. 2000;160:2101–7.

7. Gorman JM. Comorbid depression and anxiety spectrum disorders. Depress Anxiety. 1996-1997;4:160–8.
8. Katon W, Ciechanowski P. Impact of major depression on chronic medical illness. J Psychosom Res. 2002;53:859–63.
9. Sherbourne CD, Wells KB, Meredith LS, Jackson CA, Camp P. Comorbid anxiety disorder and the functioning and well-being of chronically ill patients of general medical providers. Arch Gen Psychiatry. 1996;53:889–95.
10. Dowson CA, Kuijer RG, Mulder RT. Anxiety and self-management behavior in chronic obstructive pulmonary disease: what has been learned? Chron Respir Dis. 2004;1:213–20.
11. Busse WW, Kiecolt-Glaser JK, Coe C, Martin RJ, Weiss ST, Parker SR. NHLBI workshop summary: stress and asthma. Am J Respir Crit Care Med. 1995;151:249–52.
12. Patterson JM, Budd J, Goetz D, Warwick WJ. Family correlates of a 10-year pulmonary health trend in cystic fibrosis. Pediatrics. 1993;91:383–9.
13. Wallander JL, Varni JW. Adjustment in children with chronic physical disorders: programmatic research on a disability stress-coping model. In: LaGreca AM, Siegal L, Wallander JL, Walker CE, editors. Stress and coping in child health. New York: Guilford Press; 1992. p. 279–98.
14. Quittner AL, DiGirolamo AM, Michel M, Eigen H. Parental response to cystic fibrosis: a contextual analysis of the diagnosis phase. J Pediatr Psychol. 1992;17:683–704.
15. Quittner AL, DiGirolamo AM. Family adaptation to childhood disability and illness. In: Ammerman RT, Campo JV, editors. Handbook of pediatric psychology and psychiatry. Boston: Allyn & Bacon; 1998. p. 70–102.
16. Quittner AL, Goldbeck L, Abbott J, et al. Prevalence of depression and anxiety in patients with cystic fibrosis and parent caregivers: results of The International Depression Epidemiological Study across nine countries. Thorax. 2014;69(12):1090–7.
17. Quittner AL, Abbott J, Georgiopoulos AM, Goldbeck L, Smith B, Hempstead SE, Marshall B, Sabadosa KA, Elborn S. International committee on mental health. International committee on mental health in cystic fibrosis: cystic fibrosis foundation and european cystic fibrosis society consensus statements for screening and treating depression and anxiety. Thorax. 2016;71:26–34.
18. Abbott J, Havermans T, Jarvholm S, Landau E, Prins Y, Smrekar U, Staab D, Verity L, Verkleij M. ECFS Mental Health Working Group. Mental health screening in cystic fibrosis centres across Europe. J Cyst Fibros. 2019;18(2):299–303. https://doi.org/10.1016/j.jcf.2018.09.003.
19. Duff AJ. Depression in cystic fibrosis; implications of The International Depression/Anxiety Epidemiological Study (TIDES) in cystic fibrosis. Paediatr Respir Rev. 2015;16:2–5. https://doi.org/10.1016/j.prrv.2015.07.006.
20. American Psychiatric Association, editor. Diagnostic and statistical manual of mental disorders (DSM-5). 5th ed: American Psychiatric Publishing, Incorporated; 2013.
21. Kroenke K, Spitzer RL, Williams JB. The PHQ-9: validity of a brief depression severity measure. J Gen Intern Med. 2001;16(9):606–13.
22. Kessler RC, Avenevoli S, Costello EJ, et al. Prevalence, persistence, and sociodemographic correlates of DSM-IV disorders in the National Comorbidity Survey Replication Adolescent Supplement. Arch Gen Psychiatry. 2012;69(4):372–80. https://doi.org/10.1001/archgenpsychiatry.2011.160.
23. Smith BA, Modi AC, Quittner AL, et al. Depressive symptoms in children with cystic fibrosis and parents and its effects on adherence to airway clearance. Pediatr Pulmonol. 2010;45:756–63.
24. Havermans T, Colpaert K, Dupont LJ. Quality of life in patients with cystic fibrosis: association with anxiety and depression. J Cyst Fibros. 2008;7:581–4.
25. Riekert KA, Bartlett SJ, Boyle MP, et al. The association between depression, lung function, and health-related quality of life among adults with cystic fibrosis. Chest. 2007;132:231–7.
26. Latchford G, Duff AJ. Screening for depression in a single CF centre. J Cyst Fibros. 2013;12:794–6.

27. Besier T, Born A, Henrich G, et al. Anxiety, depression, and life satisfaction in parents caring for children with cystic fibrosis. Pediatr Pulmonol. 2011;46:672–82.
28. Beesdo K, Knappe S, Pine DS. Anxiety and anxiety disorders in children and adolescents: developmental issues and implications for DSM-V. Psychiatr Clin N Am. 2009;32:483–524. https://doi.org/10.1016/j.psc.2009.06.002.
29. Kessler RC, Avenevoli S, Ries Merikangas K. Mood disorders in children and adolescents: an epidemiologic perspective. Biol Psychiatry. 2001;49(12):1002–14.
30. Merikangas KR, He JP, Burstein M, Swanson SA, Avenevoli S, Cui L, Benjet C, Georgiades K, Swendsen J. Lifetime prevalence of mental disorders in U.S. adolescents: results from the National Comorbidity Survey Replication--Adolescent Supplement (NCS-A). J Am Acad Child Adolesc Psychiatry. 2010;49(10):980–9. PMID: 20855043
31. MacLean J, Kinley DJ, Jacobi F, Bolton JM, Sareen J. The relationship between physical conditions and suicidal behavior among those with mood disorders. J Affect Disord. 2011;130:245–50.
32. Weissman MM, Wolk S, Goldstein RB, et al. Depressed adolescents grown up. JAMA. 1999;281(18):1707–13. https://doi.org/10.1001/jama.281.18.1707.
33. Druss B, Pincus H. Suicidal ideation and suicide attempts in general medical illnesses. Arch Intern Med. 2000;160(10):1522–6.
34. Garcia G, Snell C, Sawicki G, et al. Mental health screening of medically admitted patients with cystic fibrosis. Psychosomatics. 2018;59(2):158–68.
35. Quon BS, Bentham WD, Unutzer J, Chan YF, Goss CH, Aitken ML. Prevalence of symptoms of depression and anxiety in adults with cystic fibrosis based on the PHQ-9 and GAD-7 screening questionnaires. Psychosomatics. 2015;56(4):345–53.
36. Spitzer RL, Kroenke K, Williams JB, Lowe B. A brief measure for assessing generalized anxiety disorder: the GAD-7. Arch Intern Med. 2006;166(10):1092–7.
37. Bennett, S., & Walkup, J. (2016). Anxiety disorders in children and adolescents: Epidemiology, pathogenesis, clinical manifestations, and course. Retrieved from http://www.uptodate.com/contents/anxiety-disorders-inchildren-and-adolescents-epidemiologypathogenesis-clinical-manifestationsand-course?source=search_result&search=Anxiety+disorders+in+children+and+adolescents%3A+Epidemiology%2C+pathogenesis%2C+clinical+manifestations%2C+and+course&selectedTitle=1~150
38. Harvard Medical School, 2007. National Comorbidity Survey (NCS). (2017, August 21). Retrieved from https://www.hcp.med.harvard.edu/ncs/index.php. Data table 1: lifetime prevalence DSM-IV/WMH-CIDI disorders by sex and cohort.
39. Yohannes AM, Willgoss TG, Fatoye FA, et al. Relationship between anxiety, depression, and quality of life in adult patients with cystic fibrosis. Respir Care. 2012;57:550–6.
40. Georgiopoulos AM, Friedman D, Porter EA, Krasner A, Kakarala SP, Glaeser BK, et al. Screening for ADHD in adults with cystic fibrosis: prevalence, health-related quality of life, and adherence. J Cyst Fibros. 2018;17(2):276–80.
41. Cohen-Cymberknoh M, Tanny T, Breuer O, Blau H, Mussaffi H, Kadosh D, et al. Attention deficit hyperactivity disorder symptoms in patients with cystic fibrosis. J Cyst Fibros. 2018;17(2):281–5.
42. Georgiopoulos AM, Hua LL. The diagnosis and treatment of attention deficit-hyperactivity disorder in children and adolescents with cystic fibrosis: a retrospective study. Psychosomatics. 2011;52:160–6.
43. Beker LT, Russek-Cohen E, Fink RJ. Stature as a prognostic factor in cystic fibrosis survival. J Am Diet Assoc. 2001;101(4):438–42.
44. Konstan M, Butler S, Wohl M, Stoddard M, Matousek R, Wagener J, et al. Growth and nutritional indexes in early life predict pulmonary function in cystic fibrosis. J Pediatr. 2003;142(6):624–30.
45. Peterson ML, Jacobs DR, Milla CE. Longitudinal changes in growth parameters are correlated with changes in pulmonary function in children with cystic fibrosis. Pediatrics. 2003;112(3):588–92.

46. Stallings VA, Stark LJ, Robinson KA, Feranchak AP, Quinton H. Evidence-based practice recommendations for nutrition-related management of children and adults with cystic fibrosis and pancreatic insufficiency: results of a systematic review. J Am Diet Assoc. 2008;108:832e9.
47. Crist W, McDonnell P, Beck M, Gillespie C, Barrett P, Mathews J. Behavior at mealtimes and the young child with cystic fibrosis. J Dev Behav Pediatr. 1994;15:157–61.
48. Stark L, Jelalian E, Opipari L, Powers S, Janicke D, Mulvihill M, et al. Child behavior and parent management strategies at mealtimes in families with a school-age child with cystic fibrosis. Health Psychol. 2005;24:274–80.
49. Ward C, Massie J, Glazner J, et al. Problem behaviours and parenting in preschool children with cystic fibrosis. Arch Dis Child. 2009;94:341–7.
50. Tierney S. Body image and cystic fibrosis: a critical review. Body Image. 2012;9(1):12–9.
51. Swanson SA, Crow SJ, Le Grange D, Swendsen J, Merikangas KR. Prevalence and correlates of eating disorders in adolescents: results from the National Comorbidity Survey Replication Adolescent Supplement. Arch Gen Psychiatry. 2011;68(7):714–23. https://doi.org/10.1001/archgenpsychiatry.2011.22.
52. Udo T, Grilo CM. Prevalence and correlates of DSM-5–defined eating disorders in a nationally representative sample of U.S. adults. Biol Psychiatry. 2018;84:345–54.
53. Raymond N, Chang P, Crow S, Mitchell J, Bieperink B, Beck M, Crosby RD, Clawson CC, Warwick WJ. Eating disorders in patients with cystic fibrosis. J Adolesc. 2000;23:359–63.
54. Bryon M, Shearer J, Davies H. Eating disorders and disturbance in children and adolescents with cystic fibrosis. Child Health Care. 2008;36:67–77.
55. Shearer J, Bryon M. The nature and prevalence of eating disorders and eating disturbance in adolescents with cystic fibrosis. J R Soc Med. 2004;97:36–42.
56. Bartlett SJ, Krishnan JA, Riekert KA, et al. Maternal depressive symptoms and adherence to therapy in inner-city children with asthma. Pediatrics. 2004;113:229–37.
57. Stewart SM, Rao U, White P. Depression and diabetes in children and adolescents. Curr Opin Pediatr. 2005;17:626–31.
58. White T, Miller J, Smith GL, McMahon WM. Adherence and psychopathology in children and adolescents with cystic fibrosis. Eur Child Adolesc Psychiatry. 2009;18:96–104.
59. Linkson L, Macedo P, Perrin FM, et al. Anorexia nervosa in cystic fibrosis. Paediatr Respir Rev. 2018;26:24–6.
60. Katon W, Lin EH, Kroenke K. The association of depression and anxiety with medical symptom burden in patients with chronic medical illness. Gen Hosp Psychiatry. 2007;29:147–55.
61. James A, Soler A, Weatherall R. Cognitive behavioural therapy for anxiety disorders in children and adolescents. Cochrane Database Syst Rev. 2005;4:CD004690.
62. Fidika A, Herle M, Goldbeck L. Symptoms of depression impact the course of lung function in adolescents and adults with cystic fibrosis. BMC Pulm Med. 2014;14:205.
63. Snell C, Fernandes S, Bujoreanu IS, Garcia G. Depression, illness severity, and healthcare utilization in cystic fibrosis. Pediatr Pulmonol. 2014;49(12):1177–81.
64. Schechter MS, Ostrenga JS, Fink AK, Barker DH, Sawicki GS, Quittner AL. Decreased survival in cystic fibrosis patients with a positive screen for depression. Thorax 2019; submitted for publication.
65. Bregnballe V, Thastum M, Schiøtz PO. Psychosocial problems in children with cystic fibrosis. Acta Paediatr. 2007;96:58–61.
66. Anderson DL, Flume PA, Hardy KK. Psychological functioning of adults with cystic fibrosis. Chest. 2001;119:1079–84.
67. Quittner AL, Buu A, Messer MA, Modi AC, Watrous M. Development and validation of the cystic fibrosis questionnaire in the United States: a health-related quality-of-life measure for cystic fibrosis. Chest. 2005;128:2347–54.
68. Cronly JA, Duff AJ, Riekert KA, Fitzgerald AP, Perry IJ, Lehane EA, Horgan A, Howe BA, Chroinin MN, Savage E. Health-related quality of life in adolescents and adults with cystic fibrosis: physical and mental health predictors. Respir Care. 2019;64(4):406–41.

69. Knudsen K, Pressler T, Mortensen L, et al. Associations between adherence, depressive symptoms and health-related quality of life in young adults with cystic fibrosis. Springer Plus. 2016;5:1216.
70. Szyndler JE, Towns SJ, van Asperen PP, McKay KO. Psychological and family functioning and quality of life in adolescents with cystic fibrosis. J Cyst Fibros. 2005;4:135–44.
71. Spieth LE, Stark LJ, Mitchell MJ, et al. Observational assessment of family functioning at mealtime in preschool children with cystic fibrosis. J Pediatr Psychol. 2001;26:215–24.
72. McClellan CB, Cohen LL. Family functioning in children with chronic illness compared with healthy controls: a critical review. J Pediatr. 2007;150:221–3.
73. Everhart RS, Fiese BH, Smyth JM, Borschuk A, Anbar RD. Family functioning and treatment adherence in children and adolescents with cystic fibrosis. Pediatr Allergy Immunol Pulmonol. 2014;27(2):82–6.
74. van Zoonen K, Buntrock C, Ebert DD, et al. Preventing the onset of major depressive disorder: a meta-analytic review of psychological interventions. Int J Epidemiol. 2014;43(2):318–29.
75. Uman LS, Birnie KA, Noel M, et al. Psychological interventions for needle-related procedural pain and distress in children and adolescents. Cochrane Database Syst Rev. 2013;10:CD005179.
76. Stark LJ, Quittner AL, Powers SW, et al. Randomized clinical trial of behavioral intervention and nutrition education to improve caloric intake and weight in children with cystic fibrosis. Arch Pediatr Adolesc Med. 2009;163(10):915–21.
77. Archer J, Bower P, Gilbody S, et al. Collaborative care for depression and anxiety problems. Cochrane Database Syst Rev. 2012;10:CD006525.
78. Walker J, Hansen CH, Martin P, et al. Integrated collaborative care for major depression comorbid with a poor prognosis cancer (SMaRT Oncology-3): a multicentre randomised controlled trial in patients with lung cancer. Lancet Oncol. 2014;15(10):1168–76.
79. Huffman JC, Mastromauro CA, Beach SR, et al. Collaborative care for depression and anxiety disorders in patients with recent cardiac events: the Management of Sadness and Anxiety in Cardiology (MOSAIC) randomized clinical trial. JAMA Intern Med. 2014;174(6):927–35.
80. Rachman S. The evolution of cognitive behaviour therapy. In: Clark DF, Fairburn CG, Gelder MG, editors. Science and practice of cognitive behaviour therapy. Oxford, UK: Oxford University Press; 1997. p. 1–26.
81. Markowitz JC, Lipsitz J, Milrod BL. Critical review of outcome research on interpersonal psychotherapy for anxiety disorders. Depress Anxiety. 2014;31:316–25.
82. Swartz HA, Grote NK, Graham P. Brief interpersonal psychotherapy (IPT-B): overview and review of evidence. Am J Psychother. 2014;68:443–62.
83. Kass AE, Kolko RP, Wilfley DE. Psychological treatments for eating disorders. Curr Opin Psychiatry. 2013;26:549–55.
84. Casier A, Goubert L, Huse D, et al. The role of acceptance in psychological functioning in adolescents with cystic fibrosis: a preliminary study. Psychol Health. 2008;23:629–38.
85. Wicksell RK, Kanstrup M, Kemani MK, Holmström L, Olsson GL. Acceptance and commitment therapy for children and adolescents with physical health concerns. Curr Opin Psychol. 2015;2:1–5.
86. Bennett DS, O'Hayer CV, Wolfe W, Juarascio A, Winch E. Reducing anxiety & depression among individuals with cystic fibrosis through acceptance and commitment therapy: a treatment manual including adaptation for telehealth. Department of Psychiatry: Drexel University.
87. Dimeff LA, Koerner K, editors. Dialectical behavior therapy in clinical practice: applications across disorders and settings. New York: Guilford Press; 2007.
88. Telch CF, Agras WS, Linehan MM. Dialectical behavior therapy for binge eating disorder. J Consult Clin Psychol. 2001;69(6):1061–5.
89. Stark LJ, Powers SW, Jelalian E, Rape RN, Miller DL. Modifying problematic mealtime interactions of children with cystic fibrosis and their parents via behavioral parent training. J Pediatr Psychol. 1994;19(6):751–68.

90. Powers SW, Stark LJ, Chamberlin LA, et al. Behavioral and nutritional treatment for preschool-aged children with cystic fibrosis: a randomized clinical trial. JAMA Pediatr. Published online May 01, 2015;169(5):e150636. https://doi.org/10.1001/jamapediatrics.2015.0636.

91. Chronis AM, Chacko A, Fabiano GA, et al. Enhancements to the behavioral parent training paradigm for families of children with ADHD: review and future directions. Clin Child Fam Psychol Rev. 2004;7:1. https://doi.org/10.1023/B:CCFP.0000020190.60808.a4.

92. Smith BA, Georgiopoulos AM, Quittner AL. Maintaining mental health and function for the long run in cystic fibrosis. Pediatr Pulmonol. 2016;51(S44):S71–8. https://doi.org/10.1002/ppul.23522.

93. Milano W, De Rosa M, Milano L, Riccio A, Sanseverino B, Capasso A. The pharmacological options in the treatment of eating disorders. ISRN Pharmacol. 2013;352865 https://doi.org/10.1155/2013/352865.

94. American Academy of Pediatrics, Subcommittee on Attention-Deficit/Hyperactivity Disorder, Steering Committee on Quality Improvement and Management. ADHD: clinical practice guideline for the diagnosis, evaluation, and treatment of attention-deficit/hyperactivity disorder in children and adolescents. Pediatrics. 2011;128(5):1007–22.

Chapter 22
Understanding Treatment Adherence in Cystic Fibrosis: Challenges and Opportunities

Emily F. Muther, Jennifer L. Butcher, and Kristin A. Riekert

Patient Perspective

As with any chronic illness, life seems to be based around adherence to treatment plans and medications. The goal is finding that perfect balance between living what each of us consider our own "normal" or "happy" lives, while still going the extra mile to keep our bodies healthy in order to maximize those lives. Although it is not ideal to sit and vibrate on multiple thirty minute respiratory treatments, take handfuls of pills every day of our lives and experience the more-than-occasional hospital visit, the impressive and unique quality about Cystic Fibrosis patients is our ability to adapt and persevere while maintaining radiant positivity. The interesting thing is… since we are only contagious to one another, we must figure out our own paths and endure our own struggles with little interaction with anyone like us.

My greatest struggle with my health occurred during my first semester of university. When I moved into my dorm, I was so focused on maintaining my grades, making money for myself, trying to interact with new people, and dealing with stress that my health began to fall to the wayside. On top of that, as I noticed myself feeling worse and I saw my PFT scores, I felt undoubtedly more stressed than I had at the beginning of school. As I made my way further into the semester, I had to express to

E. F. Muther (✉)
University of Colorado School of Medicine, Children's Hospital Colorado, Department of Psychiatry, Aurora, CO, USA
e-mail: Emily.muther@childrenscolorado.org

J. L. Butcher
Michigan Medicine C.S. Mott Children's Hospital, Department of Pediatrics, Ann Arbor, MI, USA
e-mail: jennbutc@med.umich.edu

K. A. Riekert
Johns Hopkins School of Medicine, Department of Medicine, Baltimore, MD, USA
e-mail: kriekert@jhmi.edu

© Springer Nature Switzerland AG 2020
S. D. Davis et al. (eds.), *Cystic Fibrosis*, Respiratory Medicine,
https://doi.org/10.1007/978-3-030-42382-7_22

my roommates that I could not handle smoking in the room (a normal college activity) and initially I felt alone and embarrassed that I had to ask them to stop. I had to reassure myself that this was not a situation that made me a prude, and that my own health and well-being is something in which I am allowed to be selfish. It is then when I identified the people who loved me for who I am.

If I could give any advice to others my age or younger who are dealing with Cystic Fibrosis, it is that your health is your first priority. Anyone or anything that does not align with that is detrimental to your time, your energy, and your body. Do not ever feel insecure about standing up for yourself and your needs. People who are worth being in your life will do anything they can to help or at least understand you. Come up with a way to make your treatments more enjoyable. Personally, I love music. My vest treatments were a way for me to zone out and to listen to my favorite songs. When I am with my friends, they enjoyed the back massage that came with sitting behind me. Or, if I had an important paper to write or needed a study session for an exam: I knew I would have to be in the same place for at least thirty minutes, so it was the perfect allotted time to begin studying or writing.

When you are open and honest about your CF, the people in your life will try to help you stay happy and healthy. It may seem irritating initially, considering doctors or family members already ask you these same questions ... although, in retrospect, having your boyfriend ask you if you have done your vest, roommates ask if you have taken your pills, or friends make sure you are alright to join them after you have just been sick is deeply comforting... as you know you have a team of people to support you in your efforts to stay on top of your health, even though they have no experience with the disease themselves.

My advice to healthcare professionals when dealing with Cystic Fibrosis is to be clear, open, and honest when it comes to our care. The single thing that causes me the most anxiety and frustration is when I feel like something about my own body is being kept from me or I feel like I am not getting an honest answer. Communication is key, even if you are worried it will be difficult to hear.

As I mentioned, the incredible thing about Cystic Fibrosis patients is that we are able to see through our hardships. Even though we may live differently than others, we are still willing and able to do what we wish, live our lives to the fullest, and use our negative experiences as lessons. With every breath, we are thankful for life and look forward to a bright future.

– Lauren Gray, Age 18

Introduction

While the development of new treatments for cystic fibrosis (CF) has led to a significant improvement in life expectancy and overall outcomes for those living with this disease, daily management of CF is time intensive, complex, and burdensome. With the development of new therapies, high treatment adherence is often necessary in order for patients to experience the clinical benefit [1, 2]. Adolescence is a time that is typically characterized by a decline in lung function for individuals with CF, with epidemiologic data suggesting that the steepest decline in pulmonary function, measured by forced expiratory volume in 1 second (FEV_1), occurs during the adolescent and young adult ages of 13–21 years [3]. While the foundations for successful daily management of CF begin at an early age, learning how to manage one's health is important throughout the lifespan. Adolescence and young adulthood is a time when the responsibility of management of daily CF-related care typically begins to shift, and noted difficulties with adherence to the medical regimen are common. Many challenges to adherence with CF treatments exist, including the developmental task of increasing autonomy and decreased parental involvement, competing demands and lack of effective time management skills, treatment complexity and the disruption of daily routine and the adolescent perceptions of illness and importance of required treatments.

Defining the Problem

Complexity of CF care The daily clinical management of CF involves time-intensive interventions that are complex and tedious [4, 5]. The treatments for CF fall into multiple categories and differ in terms of their impact on the symptoms of this disease as well as the time and effort required to adhere to the therapy. These include pancreatic enzyme replacement, fat-soluble vitamin replacement; high-caloric density and high-fat diets; inhaled treatments such as muculytics, bronchodilators, antibiotics, and corticosteroids; chest physiotherapy and airway clearance; exercise; oral antibiotics; insulin for CF-related diabetes; and most recently, CF transmembrane conductance regulator (CFTR) modulators [1, 6–9]. Most individuals living with CF are asked to incorporate a combination of many of the abovementioned treatments into their daily routines. This daily treatment schedule may take up to several hours per day, frequently disrupting typical routines and activities [10]. The major goals of treatment are to promote good nutrition and optimize growth, to delay or decelerate the development of lung disease by treating infections and clearing mucus from the lungs, and to recognize and treat the complications of CF [11].

Over the past two decades, new treatments have emerged as advances in drug development and technology have occurred, which has increased the perceived burden of treatment on patients [12]. Interview data from youth with CF revealed that the amount of time devoted to adhering to treatments, specifically inhaled medications, is experienced as a significant challenge [10]. Furthermore, both objective and perceived complexity with daily therapeutic requirements have been shown to be a significant barrier to adherence in CF treatment for adolescents and young adults [1, 10]. Rates of adherence to treatments for CF vary depending on the type of treatment [13–15], age and gender of the patient [16, 17], and the method of assessment [18].

Treatment adherence Treatment adherence is defined as the extent to which a patients' behavior is consistent with healthcare recommendations and the degree to which they actively participate in these medical recommendations and plans provided by the CF care team [7]. Rates of nonadherence are known to be high in children and adolescents with chronic illness, and adolescents with CF have demonstrated poorer adherence than younger children [5, 19, 20].

Studies of adherence rates in individuals living with CF have utilized both direct and indirect techniques and measures. Despite the incredible advances and benefits of CF treatments, medication adherence among those with this disease remains low, ranging from 33% to 76% based on pharmacy dispensing records and electronic medication monitors [13, 21, 22]. Rates of adherence differ within and between the various CF treatments included in the common daily care routine. In general, adherence rates tend to be highest for oral antibiotic treatments; lower rates are seen for nebulized therapies and pancreatic enzymes and yet even lower for vitamin therapy, dietary changes, exercise, and airway clearance [13, 23–27].

Adherence Measurement

Tools to measure adherence are becoming more common and feasible, especially given the increase of available electronic information exchange. Yet, the reliability and usefulness of the various measures available vary greatly, and selection of the most appropriate tool is largely dependent on convenience and ease of data access [28]. The increasing importance of measuring adherence to improve healthcare and reduce costs has resulted in a surplus of pharmacy claims and refill data that can result in adherence interpretations that may not be quantitatively or qualitatively beneficial to healthcare providers or patients. Therefore, it is important to understand the goal of obtaining information related to an individual's adherence, which will inform the type of measurement that will be most helpful. In the absence of a "gold standard" measurement, the choice must take into account the purpose of each assessment and the desired outcome [28]. For example, if one is trying to learn more about an individual's daily habits and barriers to completing treatments, pharmacy refill history will provide more of an epidemiological picture, but will not assist in helping to reduce barriers to adherence for that individual.

Evidence suggests that adherence in CF decreases as children get older, particularly in adolescence and during transition to young adulthood [29–31]. Methods for measuring adherence in CF include electronic monitoring devices, pharmacy refill data, administrative claims data, pill counts, and self-report [32]. In general, self-report measures of adherence are known to be the least reliable compared to other methods, with individuals with CF regularly over-reporting frequency of treatments [33]. Conversely, while there is no widely accepted standard for measuring treatment adherence, techniques such as those that utilize microelectronic devices to measure the data and time when a bottle is opened (i.e., MEMS Smart Caps,

AARDEX, Inc., Union City, California, USA) or the date and time that a nebulizer is active, provide more objective measures of treatment adherence [27].

Adherence rates vary widely depending on measurement type, target medication/ behavior, time frame, and age studied. Given concerns about the overestimation of adherence with self-report, recent research has focused on objective measurement methods [34]. When attempting to capture adherence, it is recommended that a multi-method approach be employed, including both a self-report instrument and an objective measurement tool [35]. Given the limitations of self-report, measurements of adherence should ideally be triangulated with more than one method [33]. Researchers have sought to examine the efficacy of composite adherence rates, especially when examining associations with health outcomes.

Adherence Prevalence Rates

Using composite medication possession ratios from pharmacy refill data, median adherence rates in CF are generally described at around 50% [36, 37] with variation between 48% (37) and 63% [29] in two larger studies of individuals with CF between school age and adulthood. Studies of individuals across ages (toddler to adult) with CF that specifically examined adherence to high-frequency chest wall oscillation (HFCWO) vest therapy using electronic monitoring found adherence rates ranging between 61% [34] and 69% [38].

Although most studies examine adherence in a cross-sectional manner, a few have sought to examine patterns of adherence across time [9, 39, 40]. Using electronic data logs from nebulizers, McNamara and colleagues measured average monthly adherence to inhaled antibiotics. They reported rates of 60–70% adherence over 1 year among children aged 2–15 years. Modi and colleagues [40] used group-based trajectory modeling to establish three adherence groups that they labeled as low, medium, and high. Across 18 months, those with the lowest and highest adherence demonstrated little change, but those in the medium adherence group displayed significant variability.

One of the most consistent findings related to adherence prevalence is a reported decline as children move into adolescence [37, 41]. However, adherence even in young childhood appears suboptimal. Studies in children from infancy to the age of 5 years demonstrate adherence rates of 76–83% for inhaled and oral medication based on pharmacy refill history [9], 50.6% adherence for pancreatic enzymes using electronic pill cap monitoring [42], and 11% adherence to the recommended daily allowance of calories (RDA recommendation of 120%) measured using dietary diaries [43].

During school age, overall rates of adherence using pharmacy refill and electronic monitoring appear to range between 50% (23)and 73% [9]. However, studies measuring nutritional adherence have demonstrated lower rates of adherence. Adherence to pancreatic enzymes measured using electronic pill cap was reported to be 37.5% [42], and adherence to the RDA of daily calories (120%) measured using dietary diaries was reported to range between 20 and 34% [44, 45]. Parents of young children endorse nutritional adherence as one of their greatest challenges [35, 46].

In adolescence, prevalence of adherence varies between studies, but continues to be suboptimal. Based on pharmacy refill history, Shakkottai and colleagues [9] demonstrated rates between 46% and 67% depending on the medication. Another study reported slightly higher rates for dornase alfa and hypertonic saline of 86% and 74%, respectively, using pharmacy refill history [47]. Adherence remains suboptimal during adulthood. Using pharmacy refill history in a study of individuals between ages 16 and 63 years, average adherence to pulmonary medications was reported to be 44.4% [48]. Using data from a nebulizer with an electronic monitor, even lower rates of adherence at 36% were reported [33]. Even self-report data demonstrated low adherence to medications in 74% of adults [49].

Barriers to Managing Daily CF Care

Given the difficulty with maintaining optimal medical regimen adherence, researchers have sought to identify barriers. Along with age, longer therapy time [38], treatment burden [32], poor disease knowledge [47], and lower socioeconomic status [50] are the most likely crosscutting barriers. Specific barriers for the youngest children with CF (ages 0–5 years) remain understudied. However, studies on parental coping at the time of a child's diagnosis support that engaging in active coping (information and social support seeking) and tailoring education may aid in overall adjustment, thereby setting the stage for a parent's ability to assist with adherent behaviors for their child [51, 52].

During school-age years, parents have endorsed oppositional behaviors in their children, forgetting, and time-management as barriers [35]. More recently, parental mental health concerns, especially depression, have been identified as a barrier. Barker and Quittner [42] reported rates of enzyme adherence at 34.8% for children with parents endorsing depressive symptoms versus 48.5% for children of parents not endorsing symptoms. Parental mental health concerns may have a long-lasting impact as those who endorsed these concerns when their children were between the ages of 3 and 8 years reported lower chest physiotherapy adherence 3 years later [53].

During adolescence, self-reported depressive symptoms become an area of concern. Children between the ages of 7 and 17 years endorsing these symptoms were reported to have significantly lower rates of adherence to airway clearance measured using daily phone diaries [54]. Furthermore, in the same study, poor parent-child relationship quality was significantly associated with worse adherence to airway clearance [54].

Questionnaires and semi-structured interviews are two methods that have been used to elicit an adolescent's subjective perspective on adherence barriers. Themes that have emerged include barriers related to time pressure, competing priorities, lack of perceived consequences or doubts about treatment necessity, privacy concerns, increased awareness of disease progress, intentional and unintentional forgetting, and losing medications [55, 56]. Adolescents who reported doubts about the necessity of chest physiotherapy and antibiotics also had worse self-reported adherence [57]. Finally, symptoms of pain are another potential barrier. Adolescents who endorse higher daily pain ratings demonstrated lower adherence based on prescription refill history [58].

During adulthood, similar barriers have been identified (treatment burden, forgetting, no perceived benefit) [59] with depressive symptoms being a continued concern. Self-reported depressive symptoms have been negatively correlated with self-reported adherence [49] and pharmacy refill data history [48]. Furthermore, medication beliefs have been found to mediate the relationship between depression and adherence with higher depressive symptoms being associated with less positive medication beliefs, which were also associated with lower medication adherence [48]. Finally, being uninsured as an adult has been associated with poor adherence to clinic visits, acquisitions of respiratory cultures, and completion of pulmonary function testing [60]. Additionally, difficulty in understanding treatment recommendations is related to poorer self-reported adherence to provider recommendations [61].

Protective Factors

Along with an understanding of the barriers to adherence, studying factors that promote optimal medical regimen adherence is also crucial. In childhood, two important factors that promote adherence are the development of routines and positive family relationships/functioning. In interviews with parents, the establishment of routines has emerged as an important theme. Parents endorse the challenges with establishing and maintaining routines and often do this over time through trial and error [62]. Social support has been identified as important in assisting parents with this task [62]. A study using electronic data capture from nebulizer use reported that adherence during weekdays while school was in session was higher compared to weekends or school holidays, supporting the value of predictable daily routines on adherent behaviors [63]. Similarly, Barker and Quittner (2016) found that children had higher adherence to pancreatic enzymes at school than at home (94.4% vs. 42.3%), which may be related to predictable scheduling. However, when schedules become too hectic, adherence may suffer as shown through a study of inhaled antibiotics using electronic data capture that reported worse adherence in the morning (58%) than the evening (75%). Routine schedules may continue to facilitate adherence into adulthood. Self-reported beliefs about strong habits related to nebulizer use were found to predict adherence over 3 months using electronic data capture from nebulizers [64].

In childhood, positive family relationships and functioning have been identified as a likely facilitator of adherence. Parents who strongly believe that treatments are necessary [41] and have higher feelings of self-efficacy, or a belief in their ability to be successful with managing certain tasks and/or situations [65], have children with better adherence. Positive family relationships have been reported to be associated with improved adherence [66, 67], and the strength of the parent-adolescent relationship has been found to influence an adolescent's thoughts and behaviors around adherence [68].

Positive family functioning may promote adherence in an indirect manner by contributing to parents staying involved in daily CF care for a longer amount of time. Studies have found that children whose parents assist with starting HFCWO vest therapy demonstrate better adherence [38]. Furthermore, parents who were present and demonstrated prosocial behaviors during their children's respiratory treatments had children with higher 3-month adherence [69]. Adherence has been shown to remain higher for the adolescents who are supervised when completing treatments [70].

Using semi-structured interviews with adolescents and adults, additional protective themes have been identified. These include recognition of the importance of therapies, social support/care team support, structured routines/organizational strategies, self-efficacy, disclosure, easier/faster treatments, prioritizing treatments, understanding the negative effects of poor adherence, and gradual and thoughtful transition of responsibility from parent to child [10].

Given the wide variety of barriers and facilitators to optimal medical regimen adherence that have been identified, it is likely that a tailored approach will be needed in adherence assessment to identify the factors influencing a specific individual. Indeed, research has clearly demonstrated that, "there is no one-size fits all intervention for adherence to medication in cystic fibrosis" [71].

Evidence-Based and Promising Interventions to Address Adherence

There have been very few evaluations of the efficacy of adherence promotion interventions for any age group. The one area that has the strongest evidence is providing education plus behavior management interventions targeting nutrition and growth in children (2–12 years) for increasing calorie intake and weight [43, 72, 73]. Meta-analyses have concluded that beyond these studies, there have been minimal studies of sufficient quality to conclude if any adherence or self-management intervention is effective [74, 75]. However, given the growing evidence of the importance of adherence, the past few years have seen an increasing number of intervention studies targeting adherence.

In the largest study of adherence in CF, Quittner et al. (in press) conducted a pragmatic evaluation of a brief problem-solving plus education intervention delivered during the course of a CF clinic visit compared to standard care with 607 adolescents (mean age = 15 years). Unfortunately, no group differences were found for medication adherence or secondary outcomes including lung function, body mass index, or pulmonary exacerbations. The authors hypothesized several factors may have contributed to a lack of efficacy including that the number of sessions delivered ($M = 2.5$) may have been too low and behavioral coaches often did not deliver the problem-solving sessions as designed. Similarly, Knudsen [76] found no change in self-reported medication adherence using a coaching intervention for young adults ($N = 40$ 18–30 years old) that included goal setting and identifying and addressing adherence barriers.

In contrast, researchers in the UK are evaluating how to integrate adherence monitoring and a standardized, theory-driven multidisciplinary intervention approach into regular CF care. The intervention includes adherence self-monitoring, goal setting, and problem-solving. Their single-site pilot study ($N = 64$ mean age = 27 years) demonstrated a 10% improvement in nebulized medication adherence and a multi-site, randomized controlled trial is planned [77]. Similarly, in a promising pilot study of 38 adolescents (mean age = 16 years), Shakkottai et al. [78] reported that weekly home monitoring of lung function via spirometry resulted in a 5% increase in overall refill adherence compared to the year before the intervention. However, adherence did not statistically improve for any of the individual drugs monitored (dornase alfa, hypertonic saline, pancreatic enzymes, and vitamins). Together these studies suggest that self-monitoring of symptoms, lung function or behavior may be key for improving adherence.

Electronic reminders, such as text messages, are often proposed as a solution to the ubiquitous barrier of forgetting. A meta-analysis involving several chronic illnesses reported that reminders are associated with a significant, yet small, improvement in medication adherence [79]. In CF, Morton et al. [80] provided 13 children (mean age = 12 years) with text message reminders for 6 months and compared their adherence, using electronic recording from a nebulizer, to the 6 months prior. For eight of the children, their baseline adherence was ≥80% and remained stable, while 2 of the 3 that reported a baseline adherence of 50–80% improved. Surprisingly, however, the two children with <50% adherence at baseline demonstrated a dramatic *decline* during the reminder message period. While not definitive, these results remind us that interventions cannot be one-size-fits-all and need to be tailored to an individual's unique challenges.

Enhanced pharmacist support (e.g., medication reconciliation and education, assistance with accessing treatments, counseling to address barriers) may be a critical first step to address access to medications and knowledge deficits that may be contributing to nonadherence. An observational study evaluating the change in refill adherence at a single pediatric CF center during the implementation of integrated pharmacy services revealed a 17% increase in adherence to dornase alfa (the only drug evaluated) 2 years after implementation [81]. A large national pharmacy chain with a CF-specific support program matched 202 individuals (mean age = 20.5 years) using their program to similar individuals not using their program and reported a statistically significant improvement in inhaled tobramycin refill adherence, but not dornase alfa, ivacaftor, or aztreonam [82]. These results show that while access to medications is essential, it doesn't address all barriers, and filling a prescription does not ensure that the medication is taken daily.

Future Directions to Optimize Adherence for People with CF

The era of developing and testing innovative adherence interventions is just beginning and holds great promise. Given the vast number of adherence barriers faced by individuals with CF, a large toolbox of strategies is needed. Indeed, it is well established across chronic illnesses that multifaceted interventions are more effective than those using a single strategy [83, 84]. In CF, to be most effective, interventions will likely need to be delivered by different members of the multidisciplinary care team with specific training and expertise in addressing the identified barriers such as accessing treatments (e.g., insurance and financial issues) and addressing psychosocial barriers (e.g., motivation, confidence, and mental health). Pharmacists or behavioral counselors are important for these interventions [85–87]. Arden et al. [71] reported that all people with CF experience barriers, but people with low adherence (e.g., <25%) may have different barriers than people with high adherence (e.g., >75%), which reinforces the need for personalized intervention. Regular and systematic assessments of adherence barriers will not only allow for early identification of challenges, it will also permit more efficient and effective intervention delivery by tailoring to an individual.

Infection control challenges as well as the distance many individuals with CF live from their care center makes mobile health (mHealth) interventions, such as telehealth and Smartphone applications, highly appealing. Indeed, there are tens of thousands of adherence applications already available, including at least 35 that are specific for CF [88]. Unfortunately, few, if any, have demonstrated improved adherence, and they do not include the content or functionality that individuals with CF desire [88, 89]. A core theme is the desire for a single application to offer all needed functions including assisting with enzyme calculation, visualization of data, automated refill assistance and provision of social support, as well as the importance of including those most impacted in the design of the application [88].

Adherence monitoring technology and analytic techniques for use of big data are now sophisticated enough that patterns of medication use can be studied. This advancement can allow for the early detection of adherence declines; thereby, intervening before bad habits are formed. There is emerging evidence that having established habits is associated with higher adherence [64]. Thus, another innovative direction is studying how to help people with CF establish positive habits around completing treatments.

There are developmental time points where habits and routines are likely to be disrupted; therefore, requiring great attention from the care team. One core time is during adolescence where primary responsibility for treatment transitions from parent to the individual with CF. Another key transition point is during young adulthood. During normal development, young adults face many changes involving their social support (e.g., moving out of the parental home), living situation, peer relationships, academic or work settings, and health insurance status. These changes can have profound impact on an individual's ability and motivation to complete daily CF treatments. These transition periods are yet another time point to consider for targeting preventative interventions and may require individual tailoring. After identifying efficacious interventions, the next challenge is to determine how to best help CF Centers implement them. Indeed, even within the scope of a research study [86], it is challenging to provide enough of an intervention to result in benefit. To that end, using quality improvement strategies may improve a CF team's approach for addressing nonadherence [87, 90].

Conclusion

In the era of personalized medicine with highly effective treatments, adherence becomes all the more important to ensure that every individual with CF can achieve their maximum health and quality of life. The need to understand how individuals are interacting with their own health and healthcare team becomes more critical as the cost and complexity of available CF interventions and treatments increases. Additionally, poor adherence is associated with greater adverse clinical outcomes in CF. Data from the first generation of CFTR modulators shows that even when treatment delivery is easy (i.e., it's "just" a pill), adherence can be suboptimal. Immense resources have been dedicated to developing these medical treatments; it is imperative that similar resources and efforts be allocated to determining how to ensure people with CF maximally benefit from these life-changing treatments. While prevalence rates, measurement strategies, and implications for health outcomes are clear, the known impact of a complex treatment regimen and life with a chronic illness like CF is also well understood. Factors such as accessibility of healthcare services, health beliefs and disease knowledge, social support and networking, and specific demographic variables are also related to adherence. Efforts geared toward improving adherence in CF must address these critical variables as well.

References

1. Sawicki GS, Sellers DE, Robinson WM. High treatment burden in adults with cystic fibrosis: challenges to disease self-management. J Cyst Fibros. 2009;8(2):91–6.
2. Johnson KB, Ravert RD, Everton A. Hopkins Teen Central: assessment of an internet-based support system for children with cystic fibrosis. Pediatrics. 2001;107(2):E24.
3. Preston W. Highlights of the 2014 patient registry data. https://www.cff.org/Our-Research/CF-Patient-Registry/Highlights-of-the-2014-Patient-Registry-Data/: Cystic Fibrosis Foundation Yearly Publication; 2015.
4. Sanders MR, Gravestock FM, Wanstall K, Dunne M. The relationship between children's treatment-related behaviour problems, age and clinical status in cystic fibrosis. J Paediatr Child Health. 1991;27(5):290–4.
5. Smith BA, Wood BL. Psychological factors affecting disease activity in children and adolescents with cystic fibrosis: medical adherence as a mediator. Curr Opin Pediatr. 2007;19(5):553–8.

6. Cheng J, Purcell HN, Dimitriou SM, Grossoehme DH. Testing the feasibility and acceptability of a chaplaincy intervention to improving treatment attitudes and self-efficacy of adolescents with cystic fibrosis: a pilot study. J Health Care Chaplain. 2015;21(2):76–90.
7. Kettler LJ, Sawyer SM, Winefield HR, Greville HW. Determinants of adherence in adults with cystic fibrosis. Thorax. 2002;57(5):459–64.
8. Savage E, Beirne PV, Ni Chroinin M, Duff A, Fitzgerald T, Farrell D. Self-management education for cystic fibrosis. Cochrane Database Syst Rev. 2011;(7):Cd007641.
9. Shakkottai A, Kidwell KM, Townsend M, Nasr SZ. A five-year retrospective analysis of adherence in cystic fibrosis. Pediatr Pulmonol. 2015;50(12):1224–9.
10. Sawicki GS, Heller KS, Demars N, Robinson WM. Motivating adherence among adolescents with cystic fibrosis: youth and parent perspectives. Pediatr Pulmonol. 2015;50(2):127–36.
11. Colin AA, Wohl ME. Cystic fibrosis. Pediatr Rev. 1994;15(5):192–200.
12. Sawicki GS, Ren CL, Konstan MW, Millar SJ, Pasta DJ, Quittner AL. Treatment complexity in cystic fibrosis: trends over time and associations with site-specific outcomes. J Cyst Fibros. 2013;12(5):461–7.
13. Zindani GN, Streetman DD, Streetman DS, Nasr SZ. Adherence to treatment in children and adolescent patients with cystic fibrosis. J Adolesc Health. 2006;38(1):13–7.
14. White H, Morton AM, Peckham DG, Conway SP. Dietary intakes in adult patients with cystic fibrosis--do they achieve guidelines? J Cyst Fibros. 2004;3(1):1–7.
15. Chappell F, Williams B. Rates and reasons for non-adherence to home physiotherapy in paediatrics: pilot study. Physiotherapy. 2002;88(3):138–47.
16. Masterson TL, Wildman BG, Newberry BH, Omlor GJ. Impact of age and gender on adherence to infection control guidelines and medical regimens in cystic fibrosis. Pediatr Pulmonol. 2011;46(3):295–301.
17. Patterson JM, Wall M, Berge J, Milla C. Gender differences in treatment adherence among youth with cystic fibrosis: development of a new questionnaire. J Cyst Fibros. 2008;7(2):154–64.
18. Quittner AL, Modi AC, Lemanek KL, Ievers-Landis CE, Rapoff MA. Evidence-based assessment of adherence to medical treatments in pediatric psychology. J Pediatr Psychol. 2008;33(9):916–36; discussion 37-8.
19. DiMatteo MR. Variations in patients' adherence to medical recommendations: a quantitative review of 50 years of research. Med Care. 2004;42(3):200–9.
20. Lin AH, Kendrick JG, Wilcox PG, Quon BS. Patient knowledge and pulmonary medication adherence in adult patients with cystic fibrosis. Patient Prefer Adherence. 2017;11:691–8.
21. Burrows JA, Bunting JP, Masel PJ, Bell SC. Nebulised dornase alpha: adherence in adults with cystic fibrosis. J Cyst Fibros. 2002;1(4):255–9.
22. Modi AC, Lim CS, Yu N, Geller D, Wagner MH, Quittner AL. A multi-method assessment of treatment adherence for children with cystic fibrosis. J Cyst Fibros. 2006;5:177.
23. Modi AC, Lim CS, Yu N, Geller D, Wagner MH, Quittner AL. A multi-method assessment of treatment adherence for children with cystic fibrosis. J Cyst Fibros. 2006;5(3):177–85.
24. Myers LB, Horn SA. Adherence to chest physiotherapy in adults with cystic fibrosis. J Health Psychol. 2006;11(6):915–26.
25. Nasr SZ, Chou W, Villa KF, Chang E, Broder MS. Adherence to dornase alfa treatment among commercially insured patients with cystic fibrosis. J Med Econ. 2013;16(6):801–8.
26. White D, Stiller K, Haensel N. Adherence of adult cystic fibrosis patients with airway clearance and exercise regimens. J Cyst Fibros. 2007;6(3):163–70.
27. White T, Miller J, Smith GL, McMahon WM. Adherence and psychopathology in children and adolescents with cystic fibrosis. Eur Child Adolesc Psychiatry. 2009;18(2):96–104.
28. Whalley Buono E, Vrijens B, Bosworth HB, Liu LZ, Zullig LL, Granger BB. Coming full circle in the measurement of medication adherence: opportunities and implications for health care. Patient Prefer Adherence. 2017;11:1009–17.
29. Eakin MN, Bilderback A, Boyle MP, Mogayzel PJ, Riekert KA. Longitudinal association between medication adherence and lung health in people with cystic fibrosis. J Cyst Fibros. 2011;10:258.

30. Arias Llorente RP, Bousono Garcia C, Diaz Martin JJ. Treatment compliance in children and adults with cystic fibrosis. J Cyst Fibros. 2008;7(5):359–67.
31. Conway SP, Pond MN, Hamnett T, Watson A. Compliance with treatment in adult patients with cystic fibrosis. Thorax. 1996;51(1):29–33.
32. Bishay LC, Sawicki GS. Strategies to optimize treatment adherence in adolescent patients with cystic fibrosis. Adolesc Health Med Ther. 2016;7:117–24.
33. Daniels T, Goodacre L, Sutton C, Pollard K, Conway S, Peckham D. Accurate assessment of adherence: Self-report and clinician report vs electronic monitoring of nebulizers. Chest. 2011;140:425.
34. Oates GR, Stepanikova I, Rowe SM, Gamble S, Gutierrez HH, Harris WT. Objective versus self-reported adherence to airway clearance therapy in cystic fibrosis. Respir Care. 2019;64:176.
35. Modi AC, Quittner AL. Barriers to treatment adherence for children with cystic fibrosis and asthma: what gets in the way? J Pediatr Psychol. 2006;31:846.
36. Eakin MN, Riekert KA. The impact of medication adherence on lung health outcomes in cystic fibrosis. Curr Opin Pulm Med. 2013;19:687.
37. Quittner AL, Zhang J, Marynchenko M, Chopra PA, Signorovitch J, Yushkina Y, et al. Pulmonary medication adherence and health-care use in cystic fibrosis. Chest. 2014;146:142.
38. Mikesell CL, Kempainen RR, Laguna TA, Menk JS, Wey AR, Gaillard PR, et al. Objective measurement of adherence to out-patient airway clearance therapy by high-frequency chest wall compression in cystic fibrosis. Respir Care. 2017;62:920.
39. McNamara PS, Mccormack P, Mcdonald AJ, Heaf L, Southern KW. Open adherence monitoring using routine data download from an adaptive aerosol delivery nebuliser in children with cystic fibrosis. J Cyst Fibros. 2009;8:258.
40. Modi AC, Cassedy AE, Quittner AL, Accurso F, Sontag M, Koenig JM, et al. Trajectories of adherence to airway clearance therapy for patients with cystic fibrosis. J Pediatr Psychol. 2010;35:1028.
41. Goodfellow NA, Hawwa AF, Reid AJ, Horne R, Shields MD, McElnay JC. Adherence to treatment in children and adolescents with cystic fibrosis: a cross-sectional, multi-method study investigating the influence of beliefs about treatment and parental depressive symptoms. BMC Pulm Med. 2015;15:43.
42. Barker DH, Quittner AL. Parental depression and pancreatic enzymes adherence in children with cystic fibrosis. Pediatrics. 2016;137:e20152296.
43. Powers SW, Stark LJ, Mitchell MJ, Byars KC, Mulvihill MM, Hovell MF, et al. Caloric intake and eating behavior in infants and toddlers with cystic fibrosis. Pediatrics. 2004;109:E75.
44. Stark LJ, Jelalian E, Mulvihill MM, Powers SW, Bowen AM, Spieth LE, et al. Eating in preschool children with cystic fibrosis and healthy peers: behavioral analysis. Pediatrics. 1995;95(2):210–5.
45. Stark LJ, Mulvihill MM, Jelalian E, Bowen AM, Powers SW, Tao S, et al. Descriptive analysis of eating behavior in school-age children with cystic fibrosis and healthy control children. Pediatrics. 1997;99(5):665–71.
46. Stark LJ, Powers SW. Behavioral aspects of nutrition in children with cystic fibrosis. Curr Opin Pulm Med. 2005;11:539.
47. Faint NR, Staton JM, Stick SM, Foster JM, Schultz A. Investigating self-efficacy, disease knowledge and adherence to treatment in adolescents with cystic fibrosis. J Paediatr Child Health. 2017;53(5):488–93.
48. Hilliard ME, Eakin MN, Borrelli B, Green A, Riekert KA. Medication beliefs mediate between depressive symptoms and medication adherence in cystic fibrosis. Health Psychol. 2015;34:496.
49. Knudsen KB, Pressler T, Mortensen LH, Jarden M, Skov M, Quittner AL, et al. Associations between adherence, depressive symptoms and health-related quality of life in young adults with cystic fibrosis. Springerplus. 2016;5:1216.

50. Oates GR, Stepanikova I, Gamble S, Gutierrez HH, Harris WT. Adherence to airway clearance therapy in pediatric cystic fibrosis: socioeconomic factors and respiratory outcomes. Pediatr Pulmonol. 2015;50:1244.
51. Havermans T, Tack J, Vertommen A, Proesmans M, de Boeck K. Breaking bad news, the diagnosis of cystic fibrosis in childhood. J Cyst Fibros. 2015;14:540.
52. Jessup M, Douglas T, Priddis L, Branch-Smith C, Shields L. Parental experience of information and education processes following diagnosis of their infant with cystic fibrosis via newborn screening. J Pediatr Nurs. 2016;31:e233.
53. Sheehan J, Massie J, Hay M, Jaffe A, Glazner J, Armstrong D, et al. The natural history and predictors of persistent problem behaviours in cystic fibrosis: a multicentre, prospective study. Arch Dis Child. 2012;97:625.
54. Smith BA, Modi AC, Quittner AL, Wood BL. Depressive symptoms in children with cystic fibrosis and parents and its effects on adherence to airway clearance. Pediatr Pulmonol. 2010;45:756.
55. Dziuban EJ, Saab-Abazeed L, Chaudhry SR, Streetman DS, Nasr SZ. Identifying barriers to treatment adherence and related attitudinal patterns in adolescents with cystic fibrosis. Pediatr Pulmonol. 2010;45(5):450–8.
56. Sawicki GS, Heller KS, Demars N, Robinson WM. Motivating adherence among adolescents with cystic fibrosis: youth and parent perspectives. Pediatr Pulmonol. 2015;50:127.
57. Bucks RS, Hawkins K, Skinner TC, Horn S, Seddon P, Horne R. Adherence to treatment in adolescents with cystic fibrosis: the role of illness perceptions and treatment beliefs. J Pediatr Psychol. 2009;34(8):893–902.
58. Blackwell LS, Quittner AL. Daily pain in adolescents with CF: effects on adherence, psychological symptoms, and health-related quality of life. Pediatr Pulmonol. 2015;50:244.
59. George M, Rand-Giovannetti D, Eakin MN, Borrelli B, Zettler M, Riekert KA. Perceptions of barriers and facilitators: Self-management decisions by older adolescents and adults with CF. J Cyst Fibros. 2010;9:425.
60. Li SS, Hayes D, Tobias JD, Morgan WJ, Tumin D. Health insurance and use of recommended routine care in adults with cystic fibrosis. Clin Respir J. 2018;12:1981.
61. Pakhale S, Baron J, Armstrong M, Tasca G, Gaudet E, Aaron SD, et al. Lost in translation? How adults living with cystic fibrosis understand treatment recommendations from their healthcare providers, and the impact on adherence to therapy. Patient Educ Couns. 2016;99:1319.
62. Grossoehme DH, Filigno SS, Bishop M. Parent routines for managing cystic fibrosis in children. J Clin Psychol Med Settings. 2014;21:125.
63. Ball R, Southern KW, McCormack P, Duff AJ, Brownlee KG, McNamara PS. Adherence to nebulised therapies in adolescents with cystic fibrosis is best on week-days during school term-time. J Cyst Fibros. 2013;12(5):440–4.
64. Hoo ZH, Gardner B, Arden MA, Waterhouse S, Walters SJ, Campbell MJ, et al. Role of habit in treatment adherence among adults with cystic fibrosis. Thorax. 2019;74(2):197–9.
65. Grossoehme DH, Szczesniak RD, Britton LL, Siracusa CM, Quittner AL, Chini BA, et al. Adherence determinants in cystic fibrosis: cluster analysis of parental psychosocial, religious, and/or spiritual factors. Ann Am Thorac Soc. 2015;12:838.
66. DeLambo KE, Ievers-Landis CE, Drotar D, Quittner AL. Association of observed family relationship quality and problem-solving skills with treatment adherence in older children and adolescents with cystic fibrosis. J Pediatr Psychol. 2004;29(5):343–53.
67. Everhart RS, Fiese BH, Smyth JM, Borschuk A, Anbar RD. Family functioning and treatment adherence in children and adolescents with cystic fibrosis. Pediatr Allergy Immunol Pulmonol. 2014;27(2):82–6.
68. Nicolais CJ, Bernstein R, Saez-Flores E, McLean KA, Riekert KA, Quittner AL. Identifying factors that facilitate treatment adherence in cystic fibrosis: qualitative analyses of interviews with parents and adolescents. J Clin Psychol Med Settings. 2019;26:530.
69. Butcher JL, Nasr SZ. Direct observation of respiratory treatments in cystic fibrosis: parent-child interactions relate to medical regimen adherence. J Pediatr Psychol. 2015;40:8.
70. Modi AC, Marciel KK, Slater SK, Drotar D, Quittner AL. The influence of parental supervision on medical adherence in adolescents with cystic fibrosis: developmental shifts from pre to late adolescence. Child Health Care. 2008;37(1):78–92.

71. Arden MA, Drabble S, O'Cathain A, Hutchings M, Wildman M. Adherence to medication in adults with cystic fibrosis: an investigation using objective adherence data and the theoretical domains framework. Br J Health Psychol. 2019;24(2):357–80.
72. Stark LJ, Quittner AL, Powers SW, Opipari-Arrigan L, Bean JA, Duggan C, et al. Randomized clinical trial of behavioral intervention and nutrition education to improve caloric intake and weight in children with cystic fibrosis. Arch Pediatr Adolesc Med. 2009;163(10):915–21.
73. Stark LJ, Opipari-Arrigan L, Quittner AL, Bean J, Powers SW. The effects of an intensive behavior and nutrition intervention compared to standard of care on weight outcomes in CF. Pediatr Pulmonol. 2011;46(1):31–5.
74. Goldbeck L, Fidika A, Herle M, Quittner AL. Psychological interventions for individuals with cystic fibrosis and their families. Cochrane Database Syst Rev. 2014;(6):Cd003148.
75. Savage E, Beirne PV, Ni Chroinin M, Duff A, Fitzgerald T, Farrell D. Self-management education for cystic fibrosis. Cochrane Database Syst Rev. 2014;(9):Cd007641.
76. Knudsen KB, Pressler T, Mortensen LH, Jarden M, Boisen KA, Skov M, et al. Coach to cope: feasibility of a life coaching program for young adults with cystic fibrosis. Patient Prefer Adherence. 2017;11:1613–23.
77. Hind D, Drabble SJ, Arden MA, Mandefield L, Waterhouse S, Maguire C, et al. Supporting medication adherence for adults with cystic fibrosis: a randomised feasibility study. BMC Pulm Med. 2019;19(1):77.
78. Shakkottai A, Kaciroti N, Kasmikha L, Nasr SZ. Impact of home spirometry on medication adherence among adolescents with cystic fibrosis. Pediatr Pulmonol. 2018;53(4):431–6.
79. Tao D, Xie L, Wang T. A meta-analysis of the use of electronic reminders for patient adherence to medication in chronic disease care. J Telemed Telecare. 2015;21(1):3–13.
80. Morton RW, Elphick HE, Edwards E, Daw WJ, West NS. Investigating the feasibility of text message reminders to improve adherence to nebulized medication in children and adolescents with cystic fibrosis. Patient Prefer Adherence. 2017;11:861–9.
81. Zobell JT, Schwab E, Collingridge DS, Ball C, Nohavec R, Asfour F. Impact of pharmacy services on cystic fibrosis medication adherence. Pediatr Pulmonol. 2017;52(8):1006–12.
82. Kirkham HS, Staskon F, Hira N, McLane D, Kilgore KM, Parente A, et al. Outcome evaluation of a pharmacy-based therapy management program for patients with cystic fibrosis. Pediatr Pulmonol. 2018;53(6):720–7.
83. Nieuwlaat R, Wilczynski N, Navarro T, Hobson N, Jeffery R, Keepanasseril A, et al. Interventions for enhancing medication adherence. Cochrane Database Syst Rev. 2014;(11):Cd000011.
84. Pai AL, McGrady M. Systematic review and meta-analysis of psychological interventions to promote treatment adherence in children, adolescents, and young adults with chronic illness. J Pediatr Psychol. 2014;39(8):918–31.
85. Abraham O, Morris A. Opportunities for outpatient pharmacy services for patients with cystic fibrosis: perceptions of healthcare team members. Pharmacy (Basel). 2019;7(2):34.
86. Quittner AL, Eakin MN, Alpern AN, Ridge AK, McLean KA, Bilderback A, et al. Clustered randomized controlled trial of a clinic-based problem-solving intervention to improve adherence in adolescents with cystic fibrosis. J Cyst Fibros. 2019;
87. Riekert KA, Eakin MN, Bilderback A, Ridge AK, Marshall BC. Opportunities for cystic fibrosis care teams to support treatment adherence. J Cyst Fibros. 2015;14(1):142–8.
88. Floch J, Zettl A, Fricke L, Weisser T, Grut L, Vilarinho T, et al. User needs in the development of a Health App ecosystem for self- management of cystic fibrosis: user-centered development approach. JMIR Mhealth Uhealth. 2018;6(5):e113.
89. Hilliard ME, Hahn A, Ridge AK, Eakin MN, Riekert KA. User preferences and design recommendations for an mHealth App to promote cystic fibrosis self-management. JMIR Mhealth Uhealth. 2014;2(4):e44.
90. Gardner AJ, Gray AL, Self S, Wagener JS. Strengthening care teams to improve adherence in cystic fibrosis: a qualitative practice assessment and quality improvement initiative. Patient Prefer Adherence. 2017;11:761–7.

Part V
Therapies Directed at the Basic Defect

Chapter 23
Molecular Genetics of Cystic Fibrosis

Sangwoo T. Han and Garry R. Cutting

Cystic fibrosis is an autosomal recessive condition caused by loss of function of the Cystic Fibrosis Transmembrane conductance Regulator (CFTR). Many different DNA sequence variants can cause CF by affecting a variety of molecular mechanisms. Identifying, classifying, and understanding the mechanistic consequences of pathogenic *CFTR* variants have long been the primary goals of CF molecular genetics research. The functional consequences of many *CFTR* variants have been studied utilizing epidemiological studies, detailed clinical studies, and various model organisms and model systems. Capitalizing on the mechanistic understanding of specific pathogenic variants enabled development of small molecule modulators of mutant forms of CFTR. Future modulators will likely also rely on understanding the functional consequences of pathogenic variants to deliver effective molecular therapies to more individuals with CF. At the same time, research into gene therapy continues to progress with the promise of delivering long-term treatment for all individuals with CF. However, CF can be highly variable and individuals with the same *CFTR* genotype may present with differing severity of phenotype or therapeutic response. Thus, a significant portion of the variability underlying CF lies separate from the disease-causing variant, hidden among *cis* variation within *CFTR* as well as *trans* variation at genetic loci distinct from *CFTR*. Understanding the total variation contained in the genome of CF patients will allow for a complete understanding of their phenotype, enabling development and delivery of precise medical care for every individual living with CF.

S. T. Han · G. R. Cutting (✉)
Johns Hopkins University School of Medicine, Institute of Genetic Medicine, Baltimore, MD, USA
e-mail: gcutting@jhmi.edu

© Springer Nature Switzerland AG 2020
S. D. Davis et al. (eds.), *Cystic Fibrosis*, Respiratory Medicine,
https://doi.org/10.1007/978-3-030-42382-7_23

467

Pathogenic DNA Sequence Variants Cause CF

Individuals who inherit two defective copies of the Cystic Fibrosis Transmembrane conductance Regulator (*CFTR*) gene develop cystic fibrosis (CF). *CFTR* was identified in 1989 and is a relatively large gene, encompassing approximately 190 kb and 27 exons that encode 1480 amino acids [1]. Cystic fibrosis affects at least 70,000 individuals worldwide [2] although it has markedly different incidence among populations. Individuals who carry a single defective copy of *CFTR* are asymptomatic carriers, although other genes have been identified which can cause phenotypes similar to CF; chronic bronchiectasis with or without elevated sweat chloride concentrations may be caused by mutations in *ENaC* [3] or *CA12* [4]. However, the complete CF phenotype, including elevated sweat chloride, impaired GI motility, obstructed small and large airways, and obstruction of exocrine pancreatic ducts, has only been attributed to loss of CFTR function. The highest incidence of CF exists in white individuals of Northern European descent, where the carrier frequency is estimated at approximately 1 in 25 and a disease incidence of approximately 1 in 2,500 [5]. In contrast, the incidence of CF in Japan is estimated at approximately 1 in 350,000 due to a much lower estimated carrier frequency of 1 in 591 [6]. Multiple theories have been proposed to explain the high carrier frequency of CF in whites of European ancestry but none have achieved universal acceptance, including selective advantage [7].

To date, more than 2,000 variants have been identified in *CFTR* as documented by the CF Mutation Database (CFMD, www.genet.sickkids.on.ca), and many, but not all, of these variants are likely to be pathogenic. However, one variant p.Phe508del (F508del) is found on 70% of CF causing alleles and individuals homozygous for this allele account for approximately half of all individuals who have CF [8]. In addition to F508del, a few dozen variants exist at lower worldwide frequency, and they too exhibit allele frequencies that can vary considerably between populations, as is the case for p.Trp1282Ter (W1282X) [9]. In 2001, the American College of Medical Genetics (ACMG) released guidelines for testing for CF in the general population that included a list of 23 CF causing variants, including F508del [10]. These 23 variants account for approximately 87% of CF causing alleles worldwide, and both CF causing variants in 75% of individuals with CF. Since the total number of variants to test was only 23, they could be assayed by commercially available genotyping assays or by direct sequencing of the *CFTR* exons containing those variants [11]. Identifying both CF causing variants in the remaining individuals with CF requires identifying and classifying very rare variants. This decreases the utility of genotyping assays making DNA sequencing the diagnostic method of choice. Sequencing offers the advantage of being able to assay all single nucleotide variants (SNVs) and small insertions and deletions without having to design a test for each variant individually, allowing for a single streamlined laboratory workflow. Furthermore, sequencing can identify known variants as well as novel variants. Consequently, sequencing uncovers variants that are not pathogenic as well as variants of unknown significance (VUS), which shifts the challenge from the discovery of variants to the interpretation of variants.

To understand which *CFTR* variants cause CF and which ones do not, the U.S. CF Foundation funded a project entitled the Clinical and Functional Translation of CFTR or CFTR2 (www.cftr2.org). CFTR2 has collected clinical and genotype information from approximately 90,000 individuals from around the world who are followed by a CF clinic or are enrolled in CF Patient Registry [2]. The individuals carry 1,641 variants in *CFTR* of varying molecular consequences (Fig. 23.1a). Separately, databases that catalog genetic variation across the entire human genome have been useful in characterizing the pathogenicity of disease-causing variants due to their enrichment in affected populations. Currently, the largest of these databases is the gnomAD database [12] which currently contains whole exome or whole genome sequence data of approximately 140,000 individuals (http://gnomad.broadinstitute.org). As of November 2018, gnomAD had identified 2,842 variants at the *CFTR* locus (Fig. 23.1b) in individuals who do not have CF. CFTR2 and gnomAD demonstrate different distributions of classes of variants due to their differing methods of ascertainment. CFTR2 consists of individuals with CF or CF-related symptoms, and so is enriched for deleterious variants. Conversely, the majority of individuals

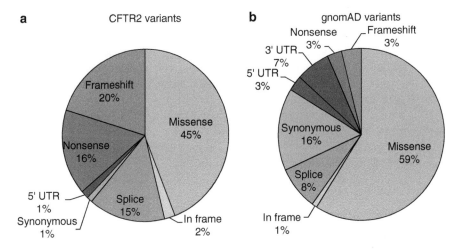

Fig. 23.1 Distribution of CFTR variants found in coding sequence
Distribution of 1,641 DNA sequence variants identified in individuals with CF as reported to CFTR2 from CF patient registries and 2,842 variants reported in gnomAD. Sequence variants identified in these individuals are primarily identified by sequencing only the coding regions and canonical splice sites, although whole genome and deep intronic sequencing is performed for a minority of samples. Both databases show diverse distributions of types of sequence variants, however in different proportions. The proportion of premature termination codon-generating variants (nonsense, frameshift, and splice) are over-represented in CFTR2 compared to gnomAD, which represents the general population. This enrichment for deleterious variants in CFTR2 is due to sampling primarily affected individuals while individuals in gnomAD are not affected by CF or CF-related diseases. Missense variants are the largest category of variant in both populations, although they represent a higher proportion in unaffected individuals, suggesting many missense variants are neutral and not deleterious

represented in gnomAD do not have CF or CF-related symptoms, and thus the database represents the carrier frequencies of CF-causing variants in the general population. This difference is demonstrated by the significantly greater portion of nonsense and frameshift variants and decreased fraction of synonymous variants in CFTR2 compared to gnomAD. The diversity of CF-causing variants illustrates why the ACMG 23 variant panel is of insufficient sensitivity for genetic diagnosis. The challenge for optimal genetic testing is the identification and classification of every *CFTR* variant, allowing for more precise diagnosis and clinical care.

Studying CFTR Function

Epidemiological and natural history studies can accurately assess the impact of sequence variants in *CFTR* but are often severely underpowered due to the extremely rare frequency of most CF-causing variants. Animal models offer the ability to study the pathophysiology of CF in an entire organism, but are unable to fully recapitulate the human phenotype and orthologous mutations [13, 14], while also being time-consuming and expensive. Cellular models offer the ability to reproducibly measure a very specific parameter (e.g., channel conductance or protein folding) of human CFTR protein, but interpretation is limited to the robustness of the assay and the correlation of functional measures with clinical outcomes. While informatic tools hold great promise, they are not yet reliable enough to make accurate predictions of pathogenicity [15, 16].

Cell-based systems have been used extensively to predict the functional consequence of sequence variants, especially those that are rare. Cellular models using Fischer rat thyroid (FRT) [2, 17, 18] and CF bronchial epithelial (CFBE) cell lines [16, 19] have demonstrated considerable utility for studying individual variants and assigning disease liability, but have limited ability to test large numbers of variants. New CRISPR-based techniques have allowed for saturation mutagenesis to test every possible nucleotide substitution in parallel for the cancer predisposition genes *BRCA1* [20] and *PTEN* [21]. While the functional assays utilized in those studies are not as specialized as those used to study CFTR, it is possible that similar high-throughput studies could be applied to *CFTR* in the near future. Robust model systems have the potential to aid in the interpretation of all genetic variants and their continued improvement will bring accurate diagnoses to all individuals with CF.

There are a number of known molecular mechanisms that can be affected by *CFTR* variants and assays used to measure their effects are detailed here (Table 23.1). However, complicating functional studies of *CFTR* variants is that single variants may have multiple molecular effects, such as a nonsynonymous variant that also affects messenger RNA (mRNA) splicing [22]. Missplicing is especially complex and difficult to predict as it can occur by several different mechanisms and result in

Table 23.1 Functional consequences of DNA sequence variants

Molecular defect	Description	Example functional assay
DNA sequence deletion or duplication	*CFTR* gene is partially or wholly deleted or duplicated, preventing transcription of mRNA	Multiplex ligation-dependent probe amplification (MLPA) of genomic DNA
Promoter	Promoter activity is impaired, decreasing or abolishing transcription of *CFTR* mRNA	Dual luciferase reporter assay using cultured cells
Premature termination	PTC triggers nonsense-mediated decay of the mRNA transcript, abolishing or minimizing translation of CFTR peptide	RT-PCR from primary cells
mRNA splicing	Occlusion or aberrant activation of a splice site result in aberrant mRNA transcripts with retention of intronic sequence, skipping of whole exons, truncation of exons, or inclusion of additional pseudo-exons	RT-PCR from primary cells
Translation efficiency	Nucleotide substitution does not alter peptide sequence but utilizes a codon recognized by a different tRNA, which may alter the kinetics of peptide translation	Pulse chase
Protein folding or processing	Amino acid substitution results in a peptide sequence that is unable to fold properly and is degraded by cellular quality control processes	Western blot of protein lysate from cultured or primary cells
Protein localization	Amino acid substitution alters epitopes of the CFTR peptide, causing it to be directed to improper parts of the cell such as the basolateral membrane	Immunofluorescence of cultured cells
Channel activation and gating	Amino acid substitution that prevents the ATP-mediated opening of the CFTR channel	Patch clamp of cultured or primary cells
Channel conductance	Amino acid substitution that interferes with the ability of chloride ions to pass through the open CFTR channel	Patch clamp of cultured or primary cells
Protein turnover	Amino acid substitution that increases the speed at which CFTR is recycled from the cell membrane	Pulse chase

several different effects on the mRNA transcript (Fig. 23.2); moreover, splicing variants may or may not also affect the amino acid code. Splicing variants that alter the protein code add a significant complication of having to understand the mechanistic consequences of that variant on both splicing and protein function. Thus *in vitro* studies of nonsynonymous splicing variants using cDNA constructs need to accommodate the effect of the variant on splicing and protein function. For example, the p.Ile1234Val (I1234V) variant is associated with a severe phenotype even though the amino acid substitution does not affect protein function because it results in a severe splicing defect [23], while the p.Gln831Ter (E831X) premature termination codon (PTC) variant is associated with a milder phenotype due to a missplicing event that removes the PTC from the mature mRNA transcript [24]. However,

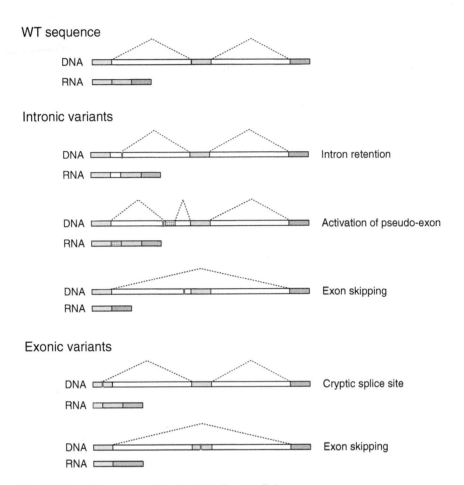

Fig. 23.2 Possible outcomes of variants that disrupt splicing

WT-CFTR splices across introns (white boxes), connecting adjacent exons (colored boxes) together to form a *CFTR* mRNA molecule containing all exons and no introns. Splice variants (red marks) can occur within introns or exons and affect mRNA transcripts in several different ways.

Intronic splice variants can negatively impact mRNA splicing by one of three mechanisms, depending on their location within the intron. Intronic variants near splice sites may generate a new splice site that is stronger than the nearby native splice site. This new, stronger, splice sequence causes splicing to occur at the variant location instead of at the exon-intron junction, following the path drawn by the dashed line. This leads to retention of intronic sequence in the mature mRNA. Secondly, variants deep within the intron may activate a pseudo-exon; a stretch of DNA that has characteristics of a real exon but is normally unable to be spliced in a normal transcript, represented by the spotted box. Splice variants that activate a cryptic splice site may lead to inclusion of the pseudo-exon in the mature mRNA. Lastly, alteration of the intronic portion of the native splice site itself may cause the cellular splicing machinery to miss this exon entirely, leading to loss of that exon in the mature mRNA.

Exonic variants that impact splicing may be synonymous or nonsynonymous, the concurrent effect on amino acid sequence is inconsequential with regards to splicing. A variant within an exon may create or activate a cryptic splice site that is stronger than the native splice site. This would truncate the exon at the site of the cryptic splice site, leading to a mature mRNA missing a portion of that exon. Alternatively, an exonic variant may disrupt the binding of splicing protein to an exonic splice enhancer, causing the entire exon to be neglected during splicing and resulting in exon skipping variants with multiple molecular processes are not limited to splicing, as even the common F508del variant results in multiple molecular defects, impairing protein biogenesis and chloride transport [25]. To draw firm conclusions that aid in patient care, functional assays are only useful if they are sufficiently robust to accurately measure total effect of a variant upon CFTR.

Development of Genotype-Specific CFTR Modulators

Treatment of CF has made remarkable strides in recent years, beginning with the development of the compound VX-770 (ivacaftor, Kalydeco®) to treat individuals carrying the p.Gly551Asp (G551D) variant [26]. Ivacaftor, a compound known as a potentiator, is an effective therapy because it targets CFTR dysfunction caused by variants that affect channel gating [26–28]. A second class of compounds, correctors act by stabilizing CFTR biogenesis, allowing the peptide to fold sufficiently to escape protein degradation [29]. Correctors have been shown to be effective in treating the common F508del variant by correcting CFTR folding. In combination with ivacaftor, the correctors VX-809 (lumacaftor) [30], VX-661 (tezacaftor) [31], VX-445 [32], and VX-659 [33] have been shown to be effective for individuals homozygous for F508del as well as heterozygous for F508del with a number of other residual function [34] or minimal function [32] variants. These compounds have revolutionized care for individuals with CF and should prove effective for treating the vast majority of individuals with CF by providing therapy to individuals who carry at least one copy of F508del [32], leaving less than 5% of CF patients without effective molecular therapy.

Developing modulator therapies for variants that disrupt other aspects of CFTR activity will likely require more detailed understandings of the functional mechanisms underlying those defects. The most significant of those variants might be the p.Asn1303Lys (N1303K) variant, which trails only F508del, p.Gly542Ter (G542X), G551D, and p.Trp1282Ter (W1282X) in frequency [9]. N1303K disrupts multiple molecular processes, including protein folding [35], but has been shown to be minimally responsive to corrector compounds [36, 37]. However, recent work has shown that N1303K exhibits a gating defect similar in magnitude to G551D [38] which can be improved if enough protein is expressed at the cell surface [19]. Similar to F508del, the strategy for achieving effective therapy for N1303K is likely to require treatment by a combination of compounds targeting multiple molecular mechanisms [39], but will require development of a modulator capable of increasing the number of protein molecules at the cell surface. Although the number of variants known to cause CF and the number of potential variants that might cause CF seems impractically high to study, the number of molecular mechanisms affected by those variants appears to be manageable. While the development of each modulator requires significant effort, it appears that almost all variants fall into a few mechanisms of CFTR dysfunction. Indeed, recent clinical [34] and cellular studies [19] suggest that most, if not all, individuals with residual CFTR function would benefit from the already available modulator therapies.

Developing therapy to address variants that disrupt production and stability of *CFTR* mRNA has yet to be as successful as protein binding modulators, but progress is being made. Variants that introduce a premature termination codon (PTC), such as W1282X, often result in nonsense-mediated decay [40], making them mechanistically very similar across genetic diseases. Treatment for PTC variants is of significant interest as variants of this type are among the most common disease-causing variants in loss of function (i.e., recessive) genetic conditions [41]. Duchenne muscular dystrophy (DMD) is most often caused by *de novo* PTC variants and so treatment for PTC variants is of particular interest in DMD research. Currently, the most promising therapies are nonsense suppression by PTC readthrough by compounds such as PTC-124 [42] and antisense oligonucleotides (ASO) that promote skipping of deleterious exons and the restore reading frame [43]. The mechanisms and therapeutic strategies underlying these therapies are not unique to DMD and have the potential to inform and expedite development of their corollary CF therapies.

Large deletions require utilization of therapeutic strategies aimed at replacing defective *CFTR* with an exogenous copy, and the most prominent of these strategies is viral gene replacement therapy [44–46]. If successful, gene replacement therapy could provide the ultimate long-term treatment for CF as it could be administered to all individuals with CF agnostic to their genotype, including those with large deletions. However, gene therapy trials have faced significant obstacles in treating CF as well as other Mendelian disorders. For example, insertional mutagenesis caused by retroviral gene therapy vectors resulted in the development of lymphoblastic leukemia [47]. Additional challenges specific to CF have also prevented development of effective gene therapy. Prominent among these is the thick mucus typically found in the airways of individuals with CF which prevents efficient transduction of the underlying epithelial cells [48]. However, newer technologies and newer strategies continue to be developed [44–46] with the hope of one day delivering effective gene therapy for CF.

It is currently an exciting time in CF research, as small molecule modulators have the potential to treat greater than 90% of individuals who have CF. Significant progress has been made in recent years to treat the remaining individuals, most of whom carry PTC and deletion variants that were previously thought to be molecularly untreatable.

Genetic Variability Underlies the Clinical Variability of CF

Up to this point in time, molecular genetics studies have focused almost exclusively on the identification and characterization of individual sequence variants. However, it has been known for many years that many different versions (alleles) of every gene exist in the human population [49], even if those different alleles cannot be physiologically distinguished. Moreover, additional variation exists outside of *CFTR*, in modifier genes or modifier loci which control key aspects of CF clinical presentation [50]. The results of this variation are significant variability in disease and interaction with environmental factors, even among individuals with the same *CFTR* genotype [51].

Most variation within *CFTR* is assumed to be neutral with respect to clinical presentation because the majority of those sequence variants are found within intronic sequences. However, several alleles of *CFTR* have been observed which contain multiple functional variants in the same gene, i.e., *in cis*, and are called complex alleles [52]. Complex alleles can influence the pathogenicity of variant and therapeutic decisions (Fig. 23.3, *upper panel*). The best-studied complex allele of *CFTR* is the p.Arg117His (R117H) variant *in cis* with the 5 T allele. R117H exhibits variable penetrance based on which polythymidine (poly T) tract variant in intron 9 is found *in cis*. When R117H is found *in cis* with the 5 T version of the poly T tract, the combination of variants generally causes CF. However, when R117H is found *in cis* with the 7 T or 9 T version of the poly T tract, CF is rarely observed [53]. The explanation is that the poly T tract influences the splicing efficiency of the *CFTR* mRNA transcript by affecting the interaction with the polypyrimidine tract binding protein that is required for efficient splicing [54]. Thus, R117H in combination with the 5 T variant is sufficiently deleterious to consistently cause CF since the amino acid substitution paired with the splicing variant yields a reduced quantity of CFTR protein that has reduced function. Complex alleles can also impact therapeutic response in cases when multiple disease-causing variants are found *in cis*. The p.Arg1070Gln (R1070Q) variant, which has been shown to respond well to ivacaftor [18] and was approved for treatment based on cellular studies, is sometimes found *in cis* with the p.Ser466Ter (S466X) nonsense variant [55], which will abolish response to ivacaftor (Fig. 23.3, *lower panel*). Although many *in cis* variants may be neutral with respect to patient care, there are examples when understanding the complete *CFTR* allele is necessary for delivering effective care.

While *cis* elements within *CFTR* may explain a portion of variability associated with certain variants, there are additional causes of variability that are incompletely understood. *Trans* genetic elements are those that exist at loci distinct from *CFTR* and are inherited separately from *CFTR* located on distinct chromosomes or far enough away from *CFTR* that they are genetically unlinked (i.e., can be independently inherited). Modifier genes are examples of *trans* elements that can influence CF phenotype independent of *CFTR* genotype. Genome-wide association studies (GWAS) have successfully identified genetic modifiers of clinical outcomes such as lung disease [56, 57] and CF-related diabetes [58]. Genes *TGFB1* [59] and *SLC26A9* [58] have been implicated in modifying the severity of CF and response to modulators. However, it appears that more extensive studies such as whole-genome sequencing of individuals with CF will be required to fully understand the extent of variation, its effect on clinical outcomes and aid in the identification of the DNA variants responsible for disease modification. Although *CFTR* is the single most important determinant in the diagnosis and treatment of CF, understanding non-*CFTR* variability will allow for the prediction of clinical outcomes and fine tuning of therapy to deliver a precisely tailored therapy to every individual with CF.

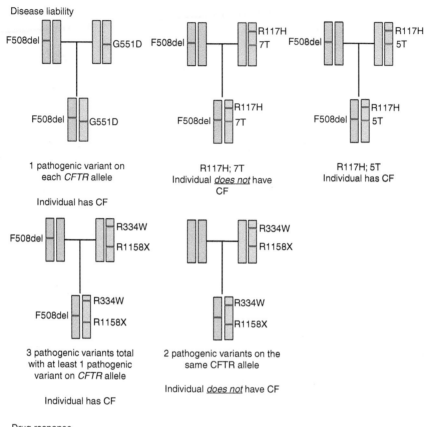

Disease liability

1 pathogenic variant on each *CFTR* allele

Individual has CF

R117H; 7T
Individual *does not* have CF

R117H; 5T
Individual has CF

3 pathogenic variants total with at least 1 pathogenic variant on *CFTR* allele

Individual has CF

2 pathogenic variants on the same CFTR allele

Individual *does not* have CF

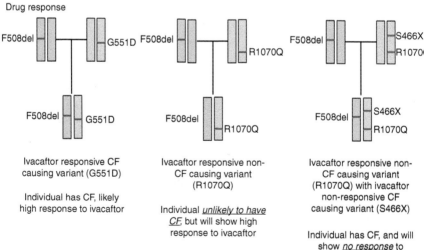

Drug response

Ivacaftor responsive CF causing variant (G551D)

Individual has CF, likely high response to ivacaftor

Ivacaftor responsive non-CF causing variant (R1070Q)

Individual *unlikely to have CF*, but will show high response to ivacaftor

Ivacaftor responsive non-CF causing variant (R1070Q) with ivacaftor non-responsive CF causing variant (S466X)

Individual has CF, and will show *no response* to ivacaftor

←

Fig. 23.3 Understanding complete alleles is crucial for diagnosis and therapeutic decisions
CFTR function is determined by the quality of the CFTR allele based on the variants present on that allele. F508del and G551D are two fully penetrant pathogenic variants, the presence of one of these variants on an allele of CFTR is sufficient to disrupt CFTR activity of that allele. R117H is a mildly deleterious variant that does not cause disease when it is found *in cis* with a 7 T variant, but when it is found *in cis* with a 5 T variant, CFTR function is impaired enough to cause disease. In some cases, multiple severe variants can exist on the same allele, such as R334W and R1158X. Independently, R334W and R1158X are sufficient to disrupt the function of a *CFTR* allele. However, because they can exist on the same allele, it is important to know their phase because when they are *in cis*, a variant must be identified on the opposite allele in that individual. Prediction of therapeutic response is dependent on knowing the molecular characteristics of CFTR expression from each allele. Most importantly, this entails knowing whether CFTR protein will be generated or not. F508del and G551D are the primary variants for which CFTR modulators were developed, in part because they are known to allow production of protein, albeit in a defective form. R1070Q is a rare missense variant that is approved for treatment with ivacaftor; however, individuals with R1070Q alone are unlikely to have CF. R1070Q is known to exist *in cis* with the PTC-generating variant S466X and an allele containing S466X will not make protein for a modulator drug to act on

Looking Forward

Pursuing accurate diagnosis, effective modulator therapies, and detailed understanding of the underlying causes of variability in CF will move the CF field forward. Accurate assignment of disease liability can be achieved by knowing what sequence variants exist in the CF population as well as the general population. Several effective modulator therapies have been developed that may be able to treat 90–95% of individuals with CF. Treatment of the remaining individuals requires tackling other molecular mechanisms of CFTR dysfunction. Assessing the genetic variability of individuals with CF beyond the *CFTR* locus has historically been impractical and limited by the cost of genome sequencing, but recent technological advances have made genome-wide investigation a realistic goal. As gene sequencing becomes more routine in the diagnosis of CF, all *CFTR* variants will be available to aid in interpreting the role of CFTR in disease severity. Additionally, genetic studies of the general population will catalog CFTR variants and their frequency in the general population. It is likely that in the near future *all* individuals with CF will know what their disease-causing *CFTR* variants are.

The development of potentiators and correctors that target the molecular basis of CF has revolutionized treatment in less than 10 years. Developing additional CFTR modulators promises to deliver effective therapy to individuals whose variants affect molecular mechanisms beyond gating and folding. The key challenge will be developing therapies for individuals who are unable to produce any CFTR protein due to deficiencies in mRNA production or stability, such as individuals carrying deletion or PTC variants. Therapy for those alleles may employ RNA-targeted or gene therapy technologies, which are in development for CF as well as several other Mendelian conditions. An unanswered question is the ability of CFTR modulator therapy to fully recover lung or pancreatic function as it is possible that loss of CFTR may cause irreversible damage. Beginning treatment at a younger age should prevent significant disease progression [60], further increasing quality of life and lifespan for individuals born with CF today.

The effects of common genomic variants across the genome are not as well understood as the effects of rare variants with large effect that cause monogenic diseases like CF. However, inter-individual variation may play a significant role in predicting disease severity, progression, and optimal treatment. GWAS targeting various aspects of CF pathophysiology have been undertaken and represent the first steps in addressing the role of genome variation [61]. The next steps will include whole-genome sequencing of individuals with CF combined with deep phenotyping and longitudinal studies to understand how underlying genetic variation contributes to variation in disease severity and clinical outcomes.

These advances in CF genetics have had a significant impact on the CF community, allowing individuals with CF to live longer healthier lives. Molecular genetics research in CF has shown the promise and utility of understanding the consequences of DNA sequence variants for developing therapy targeted not only to the defective gene but to the specific molecular defect conferred by specific variants.

References

1. Riordan JR, Rommens JM, Kerem B, Alon N, Rozmahel R, Grzelczak Z, et al. Identification of the cystic fibrosis gene: cloning and characterization of complementary DNA. Science. 1989;245:1066–73. https://doi.org/10.1126/science.2475911.
2. Sosnay PR, Siklosi KR, Van Goor F, Kaniecki K, Yu H, Sharma N, et al. Defining the disease liability of variants in the cystic fibrosis transmembrane conductance regulator gene. Nat Genet. 2013;45. https://doi.org/10.1038/ng.2745.
3. Azad AK, Rauh R, Vermeulen F, Jaspers M, Korbmacher J, Boissier B, et al. Mutations in the amiloride-sensitive epithelial sodium channel in patients with cystic fibrosis-like disease. Hum Mutat. 2009;30:1093–103. https://doi.org/10.1002/humu.21011.
4. Lee M, Vecchio-Pagán B, Sharma N, Waheed A, Li X, Raraigh KS, et al. Loss of carbonic anhydrase XII function in individuals with elevated sweat chloride concentration and pulmonary airway disease. Hum Mol Genet. 2016;25:1923–33. https://doi.org/10.1093/hmg/ddw065.
5. Brock DJH. Carrier screening for cystic fibrosis. Prenat Diagn. 1994;14:1243–52. https://doi.org/10.1002/pd.1970141309.
6. Yamashiro Y, Shimizu T, Oguchi S, Shioya T, Nagata S, Ohtsuka Y. The estimated incidence of cystic fibrosis in Japan. J Pediatr Gastroenterol Nutr. 1997;24:544–7.
7. O'Donald P. The evolution of selective advantage in a deleterious mutation. Genetics. 1967;56:399–404.
8. Kerem B-S, Rommens JM, Buchanan JA, Markiewicz D, Cox TK, et al. Identification of the cystic fibrosis gene: genetic analysis. Science. 1989;245:1073.
9. Bobadilla JL, Macek M, Fine JP, Farrell PM. Cystic fibrosis: a worldwide analysis of CFTR mutations—correlation with incidence data and application to screening. Hum Mutat. 2002;19:575–606. https://doi.org/10.1002/humu.10041.
10. Grody WW, Cutting GR, Klinger KW, Richards CS, Watson MS, Desnick RJ. Laboratory standards and guidelines for population-based cystic fibrosis carrier screening. Genet Med. 2001;3:149–54. https://doi.org/10.1097/00125817-200103000-00010.

11. Strom CM, Crossley B, Buller-Buerkle A, Jarvis M, Quan F, Peng M, et al. Cystic fibrosis testing 8 years on: lessons learned from carrier screening and sequencing analysis. Genet Med. 2011;13:166–72. https://doi.org/10.1097/GIM.0b013e3181fa24c4.

12. Lek M, Karczewski KJ, Minikel EV, Samocha KE, Banks E, Fennell T, et al. Analysis of protein-coding genetic variation in 60,706 humans. Nature. 2016;536:285–91. https://doi.org/10.1038/nature19057.

13. Keiser NW, Engelhardt JF. New animal models of cystic fibrosis: what are they teaching us? Curr Opin Pulm Med. 2011;17:478–83. https://doi.org/10.1097/MCP.0b013e32834b14c9.

14. Lavelle GM, White MM, Browne N, McElvaney NG, Reeves EP. Animal models of cystic fibrosis pathology: phenotypic parallels and divergences. Biomed Res Int. 2016;2016:e5258727. https://doi.org/10.1155/2016/5258727.

15. Ghosh R, Oak N, Plon SE. Evaluation of in silico algorithms for use with ACMG/AMP clinical variant interpretation guidelines. Genome Biol. 2017;18:225. https://doi.org/10.1186/s13059-017-1353-5.

16. Raraigh KS, Han ST, Davis E, Evans TA, Pellicore MJ, McCague AF, et al. Functional assays are essential for interpretation of missense variants associated with variable expressivity. Am J Hum Genet. 2018;0. https://doi.org/10.1016/j.ajhg.2018.04.003.

17. Yu H, Burton B, Huang C-J, Worley J, Cao D, Johnson JP, et al. Ivacaftor potentiation of multiple CFTR channels with gating mutations. J Cyst Fibros. 2012;11:237–45. https://doi.org/10.1016/j.jcf.2011.12.005.

18. Van Goor F, Yu H, Burton B, Hoffman BJ. Effect of ivacaftor on CFTR forms with missense mutations associated with defects in protein processing or function. J Cyst Fibros. 2014;13:29–36. https://doi.org/10.1016/j.jcf.2013.06.008.

19. Han ST, Rab A, Pellicore MJ, Davis EF, McCague AF, Evans TA, et al. Residual function of cystic fibrosis mutants predicts response to small molecule CFTR modulators. JCI Insight. 2018;3:pii: 121159. https://doi.org/10.1172/jci.insight.121159.

20. Findlay GM, Daza RM, Martin B, Zhang MD, Leith AP, Gasperini M, et al. Accurate classification of BRCA1 variants with saturation genome editing. Nature. 2018;562:217. https://doi.org/10.1038/s41586-018-0461-z.

21. Mighell TL, Evans-Dutson S, O'Roak BJ. A saturation mutagenesis approach to understanding PTEN lipid phosphatase activity and genotype-phenotype relationships. Am J Hum Genet. 2018;102:943–55. https://doi.org/10.1016/j.ajhg.2018.03.018.

22. Lee M, Roos P, Sharma N, Atalar M, Evans TA, Pellicore MJ, et al. Systematic computational identification of variants that activate exonic and intronic cryptic splice sites. Am J Hum Genet. 2017;100:751–65. https://doi.org/10.1016/j.ajhg.2017.04.001.

23. Molinski SV, Gonska T, Huan LJ, Baskin B, Janahi IA, Ray PN, et al. Genetic, cell biological, and clinical interrogation of the *CFTR* mutation c.3700 A>G (p.Ile1234Val) informs strategies for future medical intervention. Genet Med. 2014;16:625–32. https://doi.org/10.1038/gim.2014.4.

24. Hinzpeter A, Aissat A, Sondo E, Costa C, Arous N, Gameiro C, et al. Alternative splicing at a NAGNAG acceptor site as a novel phenotype modifier. PLoS Genet. 2010;6:e1001153. https://doi.org/10.1371/journal.pgen.1001153.

25. Dalemans W, Barbry P, Champigny G, Jallat S, Jallat S, Dott K, et al. Altered chloride ion channel kinetics associated with the ΔF508 cystic fibrosis mutation. Nature. 1991;354:526–8. https://doi.org/10.1038/354526a0.

26. Van Goor F, Hadida S, Grootenhuis PDJ, Burton B, Cao D, Neuberger T, et al. Rescue of CF airway epithelial cell function in vitro by a CFTR potentiator, VX-770. Proc Natl Acad Sci U S A. 2009;106:18825–30. https://doi.org/10.1073/pnas.0904709106.

27. De Boeck K, Munck A, Walker S, Faro A, Hiatt P, Gilmartin G, et al. Efficacy and safety of ivacaftor in patients with cystic fibrosis and a non-G551D gating mutation. J Cyst Fibros. 2014;13:674–80. https://doi.org/10.1016/j.jcf.2014.09.005.

28. Ronan NJ, Fleming C, O'Callaghan G, Maher MM, Murphy DM, Plant BJ. THe role of ivacaftor in severe cystic fibrosis in a patient with the r117h mutation. Chest. 2015;148:e72–5. https://doi.org/10.1378/chest.14-3215.

29. Van Goor F, Hadida S, Grootenhuis PDJ, Burton B, Stack JH, Straley KS, et al. Correction of the F508del-CFTR protein processing defect in vitro by the investigational drug VX-809. Proc Natl Acad Sci U S A. 2011;108:18843–8. https://doi.org/10.1073/pnas.1105787108.

30. Wainwright CE, Elborn JS, Ramsey BW, Marigowda G, Huang X, Cipolli M, et al. Lumacaftor–ivacaftor in patients with cystic fibrosis homozygous for Phe508del CFTR. N Engl J Med. 2015;0:null. https://doi.org/10.1056/NEJMoa1409547.

31. Donaldson SH, Pilewski JM, Griese M, Cooke J, Viswanathan L, Tullis E, et al. Tezacaftor/ivacaftor in subjects with cystic fibrosis and F508del/F508del-CFTR or F508del/G551D-CFTR. Am J Respir Crit Care Med. 2017;197:214–24. https://doi.org/10.1164/rccm.201704-0717OC.

32. Keating D, Marigowda G, Burr L, Daines C, Mall MA, McKone EF, et al. VX-445–tezacaftor–ivacaftor in patients with cystic fibrosis and one or two Phe508del alleles. N Engl J Med. 2018;379:1612–20. https://doi.org/10.1056/NEJMoa1807120.

33. Davies JC, Moskowitz SM, Brown C, Horsley A, Mall MA, McKone EF, et al. VX-659–tezacaftor–ivacaftor in patients with cystic fibrosis and one or two Phe508del alleles. N Engl J Med. 2018;379:1599–611. https://doi.org/10.1056/NEJMoa1807119.

34. Rowe SM, Daines C, Ringshausen FC, Kerem E, Wilson J, Tullis E, et al. Tezacaftor–ivacaftor in residual-function heterozygotes with cystic fibrosis. N Engl J Med. 2017;377:2024–35. https://doi.org/10.1056/NEJMoa1709847.

35. Veit G, Avramescu RG, Chiang AN, Houck SA, Cai Z, Peters KW, et al. From CFTR biology toward combinatorial pharmacotherapy: expanded classification of cystic fibrosis mutations. Mol Biol Cell. 2016;27:424–33. https://doi.org/10.1091/mbc.E14-04-0935.

36. Awatade NT, Uliyakina I, Farinha CM, Clarke LA, Mendes K, Solé A, et al. Measurements of functional responses in human primary lung cells as a basis for personalized therapy for cystic fibrosis. EBioMedicine. 2015;2:147–53. https://doi.org/10.1016/j.ebiom.2014.12.005.

37. Rapino D, Sabirzhanova I, Lopes-Pacheco M, Grover R, Guggino WB, Cebotaru L. Rescue of NBD2 mutants N1303K and S1235R of CFTR by small-molecule correctors and transcomplementation. PLoS One. 2015;10:e0119796. https://doi.org/10.1371/journal.pone.0119796.

38. DeStefano S, Gees M, Hwang T-C. Physiological and pharmacological characterization of the N1303K mutant CFTR. J Cyst Fibros. 2018;17:573–81. https://doi.org/10.1016/j.jcf.2018.05.011.

39. Noel S, Sermet-Gaudelus I, Sheppard DN. N1303K: leaving no stone unturned in the search for transformational therapeutics. J Cyst Fibros. 2018;17:555–7. https://doi.org/10.1016/j.jcf.2018.07.009.

40. Shieh PB. Emerging strategies in the treatment of Duchenne muscular dystrophy. Neurotherapeutics. 2018; https://doi.org/10.1007/s13311-018-00687-z.

41. Frischmeyer PA, Dietz HC. Nonsense-mediated mRNA decay in health and disease. Hum Mol Genet. 1999;8:1893–900.

42. Welch EM, Barton ER, Zhuo J, Tomizawa Y, Friesen WJ, Trifillis P, et al. PTC124 targets genetic disorders caused by nonsense mutations. Nature. 2007;447:87–91. https://doi.org/10.1038/nature05756.

43. Aartsma-Rus A, Janson AAM, Kaman WE, Bremmer-Bout M, den Dunnen JT, Baas F, et al. Therapeutic antisense-induced exon skipping in cultured muscle cells from six different DMD patients. Hum Mol Genet. 2003;12:907–14.

44. Steines B, Dickey DD, Bergen J, Excoffon KJDA, Weinstein JR, Li X, et al. CFTR gene transfer with AAV improves early cystic fibrosis pig phenotypes. JCI Insight. 2016;1. https://doi.org/10.1172/jci.insight.88728.

45. Cooney AL, Alaiwa MHA, Shah VS, Bouzek DC, Stroik MR, Powers LS, et al. Lentiviral-mediated phenotypic correction of cystic fibrosis pigs. JCI Insight. 2016;1. https://doi.org/10.1172/jci.insight.88730.

46. Alton EWFW, Beekman JM, Boyd AC, Brand J, Carlon MS, Connolly MM, et al. Preparation for a first-in-man lentivirus trial in patients with cystic fibrosis. Thorax. 2017;72:137–47. https://doi.org/10.1136/thoraxjnl-2016-208406.

47. Hacein-Bey-Abina S, Kalle CV, Schmidt M, McCormack MP, et al. LMO2-associated clonal T cell proliferation in two patients after gene therapy for SCID-X1. Science. 2003;302:415–9.
48. Prickett M, Jain M. Gene therapy in cystic fibrosis. Transl Res. 2013;161:255–64. https://doi.org/10.1016/j.trsl.2012.12.001.
49. Harris H. Enzyme and protein polymorphism in human populations. Br Med Bull. 1969;25:5–13.
50. Boyle MP. Strategies for identifying modifier genes in cystic fibrosis. Proc Am Thorac Soc. 2007;4:52–7. https://doi.org/10.1513/pats.200605-129JG.
51. Vecchio-Pagán B, Blackman SM, Lee M, Atalar M, Pellicore MJ, Pace RG, et al. Deep resequencing of CFTR in 762 F508del homozygotes reveals clusters of non-coding variants associated with cystic fibrosis disease traits. Hum Genome Var. 2016;3:16038. https://doi.org/10.1038/hgv.2016.38.
52. Claustres M, Thèze C, des Georges M, Baux D, Girodon E, Bienvenu T, et al. CFTR-France, a national relational patient database for sharing genetic and phenotypic data associated with rare CFTR variants. Hum Mutat. 2017; https://doi.org/10.1002/humu.23276.
53. Kiesewetter S, Jr MM, Davis C, Curristin SM, Chu C-S, Graham C, et al. A mutation in CFTR produces different phenotypes depending on chromosomal background. Nat Genet. 1993;5:274–8. https://doi.org/10.1038/ng1193-274.
54. Chu C-S, Trapnell BC, Curristin S, Cutting GR, Crystal RG. Genetic basis of variable exon 9 skipping in cystic fibrosis transmembrane conductance regulator mRNA. Nat Genet. 1993;3:151–6. https://doi.org/10.1038/ng0293-151.
55. Krasnov KV, Tzetis M, Cheng J, Guggino WB, Cutting GR. Localization studies of rare missense mutations in cystic fibrosis transmembrane conductance regulator (CFTR) facilitate interpretation of genotype-phenotype relationships. Hum Mutat. 2008;29:1364–72. https://doi.org/10.1002/humu.20866.
56. Gu Y, Harley ITW, Henderson LB, Aronow BJ, Vietor I, Huber LA, et al. Identification of *IFRD1* as a modifier gene for cystic fibrosis lung disease. Nature. 2009;458:1039–42. https://doi.org/10.1038/nature07811.
57. Corvol H, Blackman SM, Boëlle P-Y, Gallins PJ, Pace RG, Stonebraker JR, et al. Genome-wide association meta-analysis identifies five modifier loci of lung disease severity in cystic fibrosis. Nat Commun. 2015;6:8382. https://doi.org/10.1038/ncomms9382.
58. Blackman SM, Commander CW, Watson C, Arcara KM, Strug LJ, Stonebraker JR, et al. Genetic modifiers of cystic fibrosis–related diabetes. Diabetes. 2013;62:3627–35. https://doi.org/10.2337/db13-0510.
59. Drumm ML, Konstan MW, Schluchter MD, Handler A, Pace R, Zou F, et al. Genetic modifiers of lung disease in cystic fibrosis. 2009; https://doi.org/10.1056/NEJMoa051469.
60. Davies JC, Cunningham S, Harris WT, Lapey A, Regelmann WE, Sawicki GS, et al. Safety, pharmacokinetics, and pharmacodynamics of ivacaftor in patients aged 2–5 years with cystic fibrosis and a CFTR gating mutation (KIWI): an open-label, single-arm study. Lancet Respir Med. 2016;4:107–15. https://doi.org/10.1016/S2213-2600(15)00545-7.
61. Cutting GR. Modifier genes in Mendelian disorders: the example of cystic fibrosis. Ann N Y Acad Sci. 2010;1214:57–69. https://doi.org/10.1111/j.1749-6632.2010.05879.x.

Chapter 24
Targeting the Underlying Defect in CFTR with Small Molecule Compounds

Jennifer S. Guimbellot and Steven M. Rowe

Patient Perspective

CFTR Modulator Drug Trials, A Patient's Perspective

As a 28-year-old adult CF *patient, I participated in numerous* CF *trials to improve treatment for* CF *patients over the course of my life. Over the past several years I've been fortunate enough to participate in multiple studies with dramatic results in both my emotional and physical health. My perspective and swing of emotions is chronicled below.*

Several years ago, I was asked to participate in an early CFTR trial, but after going through a rigorous screening process, was not eligible. To put it mildly, I was devastated. Why not, I wondered? Was I too sick, maybe the doctors made a mistake, surely they knew how sick I was? I was mad, scared, angry, hurt and depressed. As it turned out the trial was ineffective and cancelled – perhaps the Lord was protecting me from even greater disappointment.

J. S. Guimbellot
Department of Pediatrics, Division of Pediatric Pulmonary and Sleep Medicine, Gregory Fleming James Cystic Fibrosis Research Center, University of Alabama at Birmingham (UAB), Birmingham, AL, USA
e-mail: jguimbellot@peds.uab.edu

S. M. Rowe (✉)
Department of Medicine, Department of Pediatrics, Department of Cell Developmental and Integrative Biology, Gregory Fleming James Cystic Fibrosis Research Center, University of Alabama at Birmingham (UAB), Birmingham, AL, USA
e-mail: srowe@peds.uab.edu

© Springer Nature Switzerland AG 2020   483
S. D. Davis et al. (eds.), *Cystic Fibrosis*, Respiratory Medicine,
https://doi.org/10.1007/978-3-030-42382-7_24

Shortly after this trial I was asked to participate in another CFTR trial, and this time I was enrolled in the study. I was excited, anxious and hopeful wanting so bad for this new drug to work. Unfortunately, like the previous trial, this drug proved ineffective at addressing the core defect with the CF gene. While disappointed, I was also encouraged that we, the CF community, were getting closer to something big and I wanted to be part of it. I worked with my doctors at UAB and made sure they knew I was interested, and anxious, to participate in any new trials as we all searched for a "cure".

In the spring of 2017 I was approved to participate in the Phase 2, 2 week VX-152-101 study. After just two doses of the trial drug I knew something had changed, I felt different. My routine morning cough had dramatically decreased, I breathed deeper and more easily than I had in years. I couldn't believe it! Was this really the "cure" my family and I had been hoping and praying for, for years? My older brother had a double lung transplant due to his CF 15 years ago and now, perhaps this drug would help me and others avoid that fate. I felt better than I had since I was 10 years old.

I felt great, but then the trial ended and my doctors warned that I may "crash" and all of my CF realities would return: neuropathy, CF related asthma, sinus infections, lung infections and congestion, lack of energy, and so on. The doctors were right and while the physical impacts of my "crash" were terrible; the emotional and mental impacts were equally bad. My depression, anger and frustrations escalated as my physical health deteriorated. I was unable to work consistently due to health issues and I generally felt lousy all the time. I had to wait patiently for the Phase 3 of the VX-659 trial, knowing there was a drug that would make me feel better.

And then it happened, the Phase 3 Trial was announced, my hope returned, and my family and I prayed I would get the "drug", not the placebo. The trial began and just like in Phase 2, I knew almost immediately that I was receiving the drug. My PFT's improved dramatically in just 72 hours and all my terrible CF realities began to go away again. I felt better, breathed easier, gained weight, had more energy and even my neuropathy began to go away (completely over time). It truly was, and is the miracle we have been hoping and praying for!

While the drug goes through the FDA approval process, I'm fortunate to remain on it, hopeful and excited about my future without all the terrible physical and emotional challenges of CF. My perspective would not be complete without expressing my sincere thanks and deep gratitude to all the Doctors and caregivers at UAB and around the world that have invested so much time and energy to get us to this point. Also, I need to thank the CF Foundation and their tireless pursuit of a Cure, along with Vertex Pharmaceuticals for taking a chance and partnering with the CF Foundation on this incredible, life changing journey.

–Mark Sleeper

Introduction

Cystic fibrosis (CF), or mucoviscidosis, is an autosomal recessive disease that presents when a patient has two variant alleles of the *Cystic Fibrosis Transmembrane conductance Regulator (CFTR)* protein. Currently, 2031 genetic variants have been identified in *CFTR* [1], of which 312 are known to be disease causing [2]. Variants for which the functional effects on CFTR are known have been sorted into six general molecular classes based on their underlying cell biology (Fig. 24.1) [3]. It is important to note that although the class system is a useful construct, the properties of individual mutations often overlap significantly, with many variants having features of multiple classes [4]. For example, the most common variant in the United States, F508del, found in over 70% of patients, has features of Class II (altered protein maturation) and Class III (altered channel function) [4].

Based on the molecular defects in CFTR, several small molecules have been successfully developed to address the underlying defect caused by particular mutations [5–9]. CFTR potentiators act on CFTR that has reached the surface of epithelial cells in a variety of tissues by potentiating cAMP-mediated channel gating and

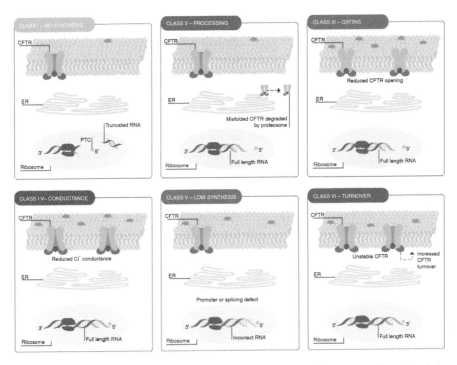

Fig. 24.1 Six general mutation classes for variants in CFTR. Modulators are selected by their mechanism of action to correct the specific defect caused by each mutation. Many mutations have overlapping defects, requiring a combination of different modulators to rescue CFTR. (Reproduced from Quon and Rowe [128], with permission from BMJ Publishing Group Ltd.)

increasing the open probability of the channel [8, 10, 11]. CFTR correctors act to promote CFTR trafficking and allow more properly folded CFTR to reach the cell surface [6, 12]. Of these, three are currently in clinical use and approved for patients with eligible variants: the potentiator ivacaftor (approved in 2012), and the corrector-potentiator combination therapies lumacaftor/ivacaftor (approved in 2015), and tezacaftor/ivacaftor (approved in 2018). Many more compounds are in development (https://www.cff.org/Trials/Pipeline). In addition to correctors and potentiators, CFTR amplifiers act to increase the total pool of CFTR protein available for correction and potentiation [13], and translational readthrough agents induce suppression of premature termination codons [14–16]. This chapter will summarize progress in small molecule therapies that address aspects of the molecular defects that occur in CFTR, and are hastening in a new era of CF therapy in which the overwhelming majority of patients with CF will ultimately have access to highly effective CFTR modulator therapy, and with it a substantial change in long-term prognosis.

CFTR Potentiators

The CFTR protein is an ABC transporter, and shares similarities with other members of this family, including two transmembrane domains that comprise the channel, and two nucleotide-binding domains (NBD) that reside in the cytosol [17]. One key distinction is the presence of a unique regulatory domain (R domain), which requires phosphorylation of serine residues in a protein kinase A-dependent manner. Once this phosphorylation takes place, binding of adenosine triphosphate (ATP) to the NBDs results in NBD dimerization, controlling the gating (opening and closing) of the channel [18]. Genetic variants that impair this process, such as the *G551D* mutation which changes an amino acid at the ATP-binding site, reduce open probability (P_o, the fraction of time that the channel is open and capable of conducting ions), thus blocking channel gating [18]. Potentiators act on the mutant CFTR to increase the open probability, thus increasing (or potentiating) the time the channel spends in an open conformation, and subsequently increasing the amount of chloride and bicarbonate that is transported through the cell surface [8].

The development of ivacaftor is an exceptional story of drug development, from first report of the compound in 2007 to FDA approval in 2012. Small molecule compounds (over 228,000) that had been developed for drug-like properties were screened using a novel, cell-based fluorescence assay that detected potentiation of F508del CFTR based on changes in membrane potential [9]. Compounds that were identified as potential hits were further screened with a variety of secondary assays, such as electrophysiology assays (including short-circuit current measurements and patch-clamp). One compound was selected as a "scaffold" for further medicinal chemistry approaches to improve the compound's structure and increase potentiator activity, target selectivity, and predicted in vivo pharmacokinetics. After multiple rounds of synthesis, the compound that would eventually be known as ivacaftor (VX-770) was identified as an orally bioavailable, potent potentiator of CFTR in

2007 [19]. By 2008, a Phase II clinical trial establishing safety and tolerability was underway [20, 21] and further confirmatory testing in cultured bronchial epithelial cells with G551D/F508del *CFTR* showed that ivacaftor increased chloride channel activity of CFTR by approximately 50% compared to cells from healthy volunteers, reduced sodium absorption by the epithelial sodium channel (ENaC), and increased the volume of the airway surface liquid (ASL).

A Phase III randomized, double-blind, placebo-controlled trial was initiated in patients with CF age 12 years and up with at least one *G551D* allele, who had percent predicted forced expiratory volume in 1 second (ppFEV1) between 40% and 90% [22]. Treatment effects showed clinically relevant improvements in the cohort taking ivacaftor: change in ppFEV1 was a maximum of 10.6 percentage points and was sustained throughout the 48 weeks of the trial; sweat chloride was reduced by 48.1 mmol/l; weight increased by 2.7 kg, and there was a 55% reduction in the risk of experiencing a pulmonary exacerbation. Subjective measures of respiratory symptoms were also improved. A clinical trial for children aged 6–11 years [23] showed similar treatment effects that were also sustained over 48 weeks, with an absolute change in ppFEV1 of 12.5 percentage points, decrease in sweat chloride of 53.5 mmol/l, and an increase in weight of 2.8 kg. The drug was well tolerated with few side effects, although liver function test monitoring was recommended on the basis of mild elevation of transaminases. In January of 2012, ivacaftor was approved by the FDA for patients with at least one *G551D* allele.

Subsequently, indication for the use of ivacaftor has extended to patients with at least one of 37 other variants, including eight other gating mutations shown to respond both in vitro [24] and in clinical trials [25, 26]. These studies of patients with at least one non-*G551D* gating mutations revealed improvements of similar magnitude to those of patients with *G551D*. In patients with the R117H mutation, which exhibits both gating and conductance abnormalities and exhibits residual CFTR function, ivacaftor was also shown to be beneficial, although the absolute change in ppFEV1 was substantially lower in this population (2.1 percentage points). Because the in vitro results predicted the clinical outcomes of patients with non-*G551D* gating mutations, the FDA then began accepting in vitro data as suggestive of clinical response to ivacaftor for an additional 27 mutations over the next 4 years (Table), and additional mutations are presently being studied.

There has been a concerted effort to bring ivacaftor, and ultimately other CFTR modulators, to younger populations, before the onset of irreversible organ injury. In the KIWI trial conducted in children aged 2–5 years with any gating mutation, sweat chloride was reduced by 46.9 mmol/l, and weight, height, BMI, and z-score all significantly improved [27]. Lung clearance index (LCI), an early marker of small airways obstruction, was subsequently shown to improve with ivacaftor treatment in this age group [28]. Children aged 12–24 months with any gating mutation were also evaluated [29]. In these patients, an even greater improvement in sweat chloride (73.5 mmol/l) was reported as compared to older children and adults; there was also an increase in fecal elastase, a marker of exocrine pancreatic function, indicating that ivacaftor restored pancreatic sufficiency in some patients. These results have raised the promise that organ preservation may be possible with highly effective CFTR modulator therapy, if instituted early in life. In the younger age groups, pharmacokinetic studies showed similar overall exposures compared to older children and adults, and a similar safety profile with the exception that children 5 years and under had a slightly higher rate of adverse events including elevated transaminases, prompting more frequent monitoring of liver tests in young children. Ivacaftor is now approved by the FDA for any patient 2 years and up with a mutation in *CFTR* that is predicted to be responsive to ivacaftor on the basis of clinical or in vitro data. For patients with mild disease, defined as those with ppFEV1 >90%, studies have also confirmed efficacy, principally using LCI [30].

At the other end of the disease severity spectrum, ivacaftor has also been studied in patients with severe lung disease (ppFEV1 < 40%). In this group, ivacaftor resulted in significant improvements in lung function, weight, sweat chloride, pulmonary exacerbations, and treatment burden [31–37]; in some cases, patients listed for transplant significantly improved, and no longer require consideration for transplant [34]. In patients with established bronchiectasis, structural lung disease improved by serial CT scan, although this has largely been associated with changes in mucus plugging and decreased peribronchial thickening, whereas established bronchiectasis did not improve [38, 39]. Acute changes in air trapping have also been reported [40].

Since the introduction of ivacaftor in 2012, there have been many studies of long-term outcomes using the Cystic Fibrosis Foundation Patient Registry database, local cohorts, and long-term observational trials. These studies have confirmed ivacaftor's safety and effectiveness. For example, patients have been found to have a lower risk of CF-related complications including transplantation, hospitalization, death, and pulmonary exacerbation [41–43]; reduced isolation of *Pseudomonas aeruginosa* and *Staphylococcus aureus* [44–48]; long-term maintenance of lung function and weight gain even without obvious initial improvement with ivacaftor treatment [49]. Prominent effects have also been demonstrated beyond the lung, including improved gastrointestinal pH [50], improved hepatic steatosis [51], and accelerated linear growth of children [52]. Safety has also been confirmed by these studies, with few reported adverse events. Some patients with severe lung disease have had increased cough and mucus production that is often transient during induction of treatment [33], and transaminitis is a relatively common adverse event that rarely results in discontinuation and may be related to underlying CF [53]. The development of cataracts, suggested by studies in rats given ivacaftor, prompted ophthalmologic exams in pediatric patients undergoing treatment with ivacaftor. In at least one study [54], approximately 17% of children were found to have non-visually significant cataracts in association with ivacaftor use, although ivacaftor was not determined as the definitive cause. Because of this, routine baseline and periodic ophthalmologic exams are recommended in children prescribed ivacaftor.

One point to consider with ivacaftor use is due to pharmacologic factors, including drug-drug interactions (DDIs) [53, 55, 56]. Ivacaftor is extensively metabolized in humans by CYP3A4/5 to the less active metabolites [53]. Ivacaftor is a weak inhibitor of CYP3A4 and P-glycoprotein, a drug transporter common in many tissues; many clinically available drugs are substrates of these proteins. Metabolism is induced by CYP3A4 inducers, including rifampin, which is indicated for antimycobacterial therapy; clinically significant pulmonary symptoms have resulted from the concomitant use of rifampin and ivacaftor in an other wise stable CF patient [57]. The rapid metabolism after cessation of therapy has also been implicated in ivacaftor withdrawal syndrome, which can result in severe pulmonary exacerbation after ivacaftor is abruptly discontinued [58]. Careful consideration of the need for therapy cessation or concomitant use with CYP3A4 inducers is recommended. To overcome some of the problems associated with metabolism of ivacaftor, a deuterated form of ivacaftor, which reduces metabolism of the parent compound and increases overall drug exposure is in clinical trials [59].

Although ivacaftor potentiates the F508del CFTR protein and other processing mutations to a small degree in vitro [60], studies in patients homozygous for F508del showed no significant clinical improvement [61]. Interestingly, approximately 15% of these patients showed a small decrease in sweat chloride, substantiating in vitro results and suggesting that in some patients mature protein reaches the apical membrane and can be potentiated by ivacaftor. Nevertheless, the results established that for most F508del homozygotes, potentiation would not be sufficient to elicit clinical benefit, and a corrector would be needed for most patients. The findings also began to establish thresholds of CFTR activity necessary to impart clinical benefit.

Because of the extensive in vitro and in vivo studies of ivacaftor showing safety, tolerability, and effectiveness, it has been rapidly expanded to younger children and those with mutations expected to respond. Ivacaftor is an essential component in two other combination therapies, lumacaftor/ivacaftor and tezacaftor/ivacaftor, and is an important component of other combination therapies in development. Other potentiators are currently in the pipeline, including experimental potentiators PTI-808, GLP1837, and QBW251, which may act similarly to ivacaftor in that they principally effect P_o [62]. New potentiators may help overcome destabilization of mature F508del reported for ivacaftor in vitro [63], although the clinical significance of this effect remains uncertain. New potentiators may also help expand CFTR-targeted therapy to all CF patients, and if differential activity is demonstrated, help match the best drug combination to each individual patient.

CFTR Correctors

During translation of the normal protein, CFTR is folded into an appropriate conformation in the endoplasmic reticulum (ER) and trafficked through the Golgi apparatus, modified via glycosylation into its mature form, and delivered to the apical membrane [64]. The common *F508del* mutation is not properly folded in the ER and is directed to the proteasome for degradation [65]. This results in little to no CFTR protein delivered to the apical membrane. The first step in this process requires the trafficking of mature CFTR protein to the apical surface by using a corrector, a pharmacologic agent that promotes proper folding of F508del CFTR. The second step is correction of its gating abnormality, a second consequence of the

F508del mutation. Because over 70% of patients have at least one copy of the *F508del* variant, it has been the target of intense effort to correct this misfolding. F508del CFTR is a complex mutant protein, with more than one defect that must be addressed.

Correctors that act as chaperones (proteins that assist with the folding and post-translational modification process) were successful in vitro, such as 4-phenylbutyrate, 8-cyclopentyl-1,3-dipropylxanthine, but not in clinical trials [66, 67]. Other early compounds that directly acted on the CFTR protein, such as curcumin, were not found to be effective in vivo [68, 69]. With the advent of novel high-throughput screening for CFTR chloride channel activity, new correctors were identified [6, 9, 70] that have subsequently resulted in significant improvements in patients [71–78]. A major advance that enabled the translation was experience with primary human bronchial epithelial cells, which provided a more stringent and faithful model system as compared to heterologous over-expression systems that often did not translate [8].

The first corrector to demonstrate benefit in patients was lumacaftor (previously known as VX-809), shown to elicit modest improvements in sweat chloride, but not in lung function, intestinal CFTR maturation, or patient-reported outcomes (PROs), reaffirming knowledge regarding efficacy thresholds [79]. Because of the known gating defect in F508del CFTR, combination therapy with both a potentiator and corrector was studied in two large Phase III clinical trials. Statistically significant improvements in lung function (ppFEV1 ~3.5% over placebo), weight gain, and frequency of pulmonary exacerbations were all observed, in addition to modest improvements in sweat chloride [80, 81], but noting that these improvements were substantially lower than for patients with *G551D* taking ivacaftor. In long-term observational studies involving patients prescribed lumacaftor/ivacaftor therapy for clinical use, these results have remained consistent [76, 77]. However, limited efficacy and a higher rate of patient intolerance due to respiratory adverse events, such as chest tightness, that lead to discontinuation has limited the use of this combination therapy somewhat [76, 82]. In addition, lumacaftor was found to be a potent inducer of cytochrome p450 3A4, which increased likelihood of drug-drug interactions (DDIs) and significantly reduced exposure of ivacaftor in patients [56, 83]. Ivacaftor/lumacaftor was not found to be helpful in patients with only one copy of F508del [73], indicating a gene-dose effect and confirming therapeutic thresholds.

In part because of the limitations posed by lumacaftor, a second, related corrector, tezacaftor (VX-661) was developed. Tezacaftor does not induce the metabolism of ivacaftor and exhibits substantially fewer drug-drug interactions [84, 85], and was evaluated in several CF populations. Tezacaftor/ivacaftor was efficacious and well-tolerated in patients homozygous for F508del CFTR, improving $ppFEV_1$ by 4%, a magnitude that resembled lumacaftor/ivacaftor [72, 85]. In patients heterozygous for F508del and a residual function mutation known to respond to ivacaftor in vitro, the combination was also effective, improving $ppFEV_1$ by 7%, and superior to the benefit posed by ivacaftor monotherapy (5%) [71]. In contrast, tezacaftor/ivacaftor was not efficacious in patients heterozygous for F508del and a mutation that does not respond to tezacaftor or ivacaftor in vitro (a so-called minimal function allele [86, 87]), nor in patients with a gating mutation in which tezacaftor/ivacaftor was compared to ivacaftor monotherapy [88]. Overall, these studies indicated improved corrector therapy would be needed to impart benefit to a single F508del allele, or to achieve efficacy that rivaled ivacaftor treatment of gating mutations. Studies have demonstrated tezacaftor/ivacaftor is well tolerated and similarly efficacious in F508del homozygous individuals that discontinued lumacaftor/ivacaftor; however, head-to-head study comparisons have not been conducted, and evidence to support the selection of one combination therapy for a given patient with two copies of *F508del CFTR* is not available. Given tezacaftor's improved tolerability, decreased likelihood for DDIs, and its amenability as a corrector for triple combination corrector therapy, tezacaftor/ivacaftor is a reasonable first-line agent for naïve patients.

Other CFTR correctors have shown promising results in early phase trials. GLPG2222, a novel corrector, was well tolerated with few adverse events, and efficacy on par with that of tezacaftor, when used in combination with ivacaftor in patients with a gating mutation [89] or homozygous for F508del [90]. PTI-801, another novel corrector, has also shown tolerability and efficacy in ongoing trials [91]. While not a corrector, CFTR amplifiers are a new class of modulators that enhance translation of the *CFTR* mRNA and increase available substrate for other CFTR modulators to act upon. PTI-428, a CFTR amplifier, is well tolerated and improved ppFEV1 [92], suggesting potential for use as an adjunct to a variety of other modulators. The corrector PTI-801 is currently in clinical trials in combination with a novel potentiator, PTI-808, and a CFTR amplifier PTI-428 [93].

Acknowledging that greater efficacy must be achieved for patients with one or more copies of F508del, the community has searched vigorously for second-generation correctors that exceed efficacy established for tezacaftor or lumacaftor. While a single corrector has yet to reach the threshold set by ivacaftor in G551D in vitro, a combination of a novel and mechanistically distinct corrector combined with tezacaftor, when also added to ivacaftor, has exceeded this benchmark, in cells derived from either F508del homozygous or F508del heterozygous individuals. Thus tezacaftor/ivacaftor is also the basis for two triple combination therapies currently in development. Phase 2 results have been extremely promising, inducing marked improvements in spirometry (~14% $ppFEV_1$ with 4 weeks of treatment), respiratory symptoms, and sweat chloride in patients heterozygous for F508del and a minimal function allele, and 10% improvement in $ppFEV_1$ in patients homozygous for F508del already using tezacaftor/ivacaftor [94, 95]. Phase III results have been consistent with the published Phase 2 results [96]. One of these triple combination CFTR modulator therapies, including ivacaftor, tezacaftor, and elexacaftor, was selected to submit for regulatory approval for patients with at least one F508del mutation and a second, minimal function mutation. The expansion of such a highly successful therapy could be transformative for the vast majority of patients with CF.

While lumacaftor and tezacaftor are thought to act directly on the CFTR protein to promote maturation [97], other correctors are in development, some with similar mechanisms, but others with distinct modes of action. For example, some identified correctors are less specific to the CFTR protein and instead, act on the chaperone machinery to reduce degradation of the F508del protein. For example, F508del CFTR is known to have a shorter half-life at the apical membrane than wild-type CFTR [98]. To address this problem, certain agents improve surface recycling [99] and endocytosis [100]. Others also bind to CFTR and improve channel activity or conformational stability [101, 102]. As additional correctors are developed and approved, patients and clinicians will have more choices in selecting agents in a personalized fashion.

Translational Readthrough

A common minority of mutations in *CFTR* are considered Class I, a heterogeneous group of mutations that result in little to no CFTR protein produced by the cell due to nonsense mutations, frameshifts, deletions, or other major variants. Among them are premature termination codons (PTCs), representing approximately 10% of all patients, and are particularly prevalent in certain populations (up to 45% in Israel) [103]. In addition to foreshortened and dysfunctional polypeptides produced by PTCs, they result in interruption of normal ribosomal activity, activating nonsense-mediated decay (NMD) and causing mRNA degradation. PTC mutations are the underlying problem in a variety of genetic diseases other than CF, and significant attention has been directed to develop agents that induce translational readthrough via insertion of near-cognate amino acids [104, 105]. Readthrough compounds interact with the ribosomal RNA, interrupting the normal cessation of translation when the ribosome reaches the mutant PTC, which confers a weaker signal for termination than the native stop codon present at the normal 3′ end of the mRNA. Interestingly, these compounds do not readthrough native stop codons [106–109], as they have more faithful translational termination machinery conferred by local mRNA context. Translational readthrough as a therapeutic strategy exploits this difference, but also relies upon stabilization of mRNA induced during the pioneer round of translation to augment available mRNA for translation [110–112].

Aminoglycosides, a class of antimicrobials that target the ribosome, were discovered to induce readthrough in *E. coli* [113], yeast and humans in vitro [114]. Both intravenous and topical gentamicin have been shown to promote the production of full-length CFTR protein in patients with CF and a nonsense mutation, but not in other mutations such as *F508del* [106–109, 115]. No significant clinical improvement was detected in these studies, which may indicate heterogeneity of the protein phenotype and need for additional modulation of the abnormal protein due to the missense mutations that result from near-cognate insertion [116]. In addition, aminoglycosides have undesirable pharmacologic properties, including poor bioavailability necessitating inhaled or systemic administration, as well as a narrow therapeutic window to avoid toxicity. Therefore, compounds with readthrough capability but with improved pharmacologic profiles are of interest for treatment of this population. Synthetic aminoglycosides have been developed with favorable preclinical results, and are presently in development [117–119].

Another approach is to identify novel small molecules to induce readthrough. Ataluren, formerly PTC124, was identified by high-throughput screening using reporters [120] and ultimately was found to enhance the ribosome's use of near-cognate tRNAs [121]. Because of promising preclinical results and implications for many diseases caused by nonsense mutations, it has been extensively studied, but did not have consistent beneficial effects on outcomes in clinical trials for CF, likely due to marginal efficacy [14–16, 122]. One reason for the poor outcome in vivo may be related to quantitatively low *CFTR* mRNA expression due to NMD, resulting in a smaller pool of mRNA available for translational readthrough, a covariate for treatment response [111, 123]. The failure of Ataluren despite early encouraging results has also highlighted the need for better preclinical models, including primary human bronchial epithelial cells with two premature termination codons and improved animal models with native tissue expression of nonsense mutations [124]. Efforts are underway to identify new compounds that exhibit greater readthrough of common CFTR nonsense alleles and can be augmented by corrector/potentiator therapy, and incorporate our latest knowledge of CFTR-dependent functional assays [116]. Several FDA-approved compounds were identified in an early variant of this study, prior to medicinal chemistry, but probably do not have sufficient efficacy to warrant further development on their own [125]. Another nonsense-specific approach includes transduction of tRNAs that insert amino acids into the PTC site, which is natively more efficient but also requires efficient delivery of the tRNA coding sequence [126].

Matching Therapies to Patients

While there has been considerable progress in advancing CFTR modulators due to specific groups of CFTR mutations, many of which are relatively common, challenges remain for less common mutations in which the molecular defect is unknown, or the population too small to be tested prospectively. Presently, only ~65% of patients in the United States are currently eligible for any modulator therapy based on mutation alone (2017 CFFPR Highlights). Identifying a treatment to target the underlying CFTR defect in any given patient is extremely challenging due to the many possible disease-causing variants and the unique defects of each on the expression, maturation, and function of CFTR. Complicating this further, 40% of patients carry more than one variant in *trans* (meaning, one variant on each allele, also called compound heterozygotes), further complicating the implementation of a global treatment strategy for all patients with CF.

Despite the challenge, CF care is on the forefront of the implementation of precision medicine, which is the practice of matching a precise treatment strategy with an individual patient, taking into account the specifics of their disease, genetic background, and/or demographics, among other factors. As a prime example, while randomized clinical trials were conducted prior to FDA approval of ivacaftor, lumacaftor/ivacaftor and tezacaftor/ivacaftor [23, 25–27, 71–74, 77, 81, 127], since then mutations have been identified that also respond to ivacaftor or ivacaftor/tezacaftor based on in vitro data alone, allowing extension of approved labeling in the United States [60] (Table 24.1). In other cases, a "theratyping" approach will be needed, in which therapeutic response to one or more CFTR modulators is evaluated for an individual patient based on a cell-based response, and appropriate therapy determined or optimized.

Table 24.1 Mutations conferring eligibility for FDA-approved CFTR modulator therapies

Variant	Ivacaftor	Tezacaftor/ivacaftor	Lumacaftor/ivacaftor
Requires only one allele			
G551D	✓		
G178R	✓		
G551S	✓		
G1244E	✓		
G1349D	✓		
S549N	✓		
S549R	✓		
S1251N	✓		
S1255P	✓		
R117H	✓		
G1069R	✓		
R1070Q	✓		
711 + 3A → G	✓	✓	
2789 + 5G → A	✓	✓	
3272-26A → G	✓	✓	
3849 + 10kbC → T	✓	✓	
A455E	✓	✓	
A1067T	✓	✓	
D110E	✓	✓	
D110H	✓	✓	
D579G	✓	✓	
D1152H	✓	✓	
D1270N	✓	✓	
E56K	✓	✓	
E193K	✓	✓	
E831X	✓	✓	
F1052V	✓	✓	
F1074L	✓	✓	
K1060T	✓	✓	
L206W	✓	✓	
P67L	✓	✓	
R74W	✓	✓	
R117C	✓	✓	
R347H	✓	✓	
R352Q	✓	✓	
R1070W	✓	✓	
S945L	✓	✓	
S977F	✓	✓	
Requires two alleles			
F508del/F508del		✓	✓

References

1. Cystic Fibrosis Centre at the Hospital for Sick Children. Cystic fibrosis mutation database 2011. Available from: http://www.genet.sickkids.on.ca/cftr/Home.html.
2. The Clinical and Functional TRanslation of CFTR (CFTR2) http://cftr2.org2018. Updated 8/31/2018. Available from: http://cftr2.org.
3. Oliver KE, Han ST, Sorscher EJ, Cutting GR. Transformative therapies for rare CFTR missense alleles. Curr Opin Pharmacol. 2017;34:76–82.
4. Veit G, Avramescu RG, Chiang AN, Houck SA, Cai Z, Peters KW, et al. From CFTR biology toward combinatorial pharmacotherapy: expanded classification of cystic fibrosis mutations. Mol Biol Cell. 2016;27(3):424–33.
5. Galietta LV, Jayaraman S, Verkman AS. Cell-based assay for high-throughput quantitative screening of CFTR chloride transport agonists. Am J Physiol Cell Physiol. 2001;281(5):C1734–42.
6. Pedemonte N, Lukacs GL, Du K, Caci E, Zegarra-Moran O, Galietta LJ, et al. Small-molecule correctors of defective DeltaF508-CFTR cellular processing identified by high-throughput screening. J Clin Invest. 2005;115(9):2564–71.
7. Van Goor F, Hadida S, Grootenhuis PD, Burton B, Stack JH, Straley KS, et al. Correction of the F508del-CFTR protein processing defect in vitro by the investigational drug VX-809. Proc Natl Acad Sci U S A. 2011;108(46):18843–8.
8. Van Goor F, Hadida S, Grootenhuis PD, Burton B, Cao D, Neuberger T, et al. Rescue of CF airway epithelial cell function in vitro by a CFTR potentiator, VX-770. Proc Natl Acad Sci U S A. 2009;106(44):18825–30.
9. Van Goor F, Straley KS, Cao D, Gonzalez J, Hadida S, Hazlewood A, et al. Rescue of DeltaF508-CFTR trafficking and gating in human cystic fibrosis airway primary cultures by small molecules. Am J Physiol Lung Cell Mol Physiol. 2006;290(6):L1117–30.
10. Jih KY, Hwang TC. Vx-770 potentiates CFTR function by promoting decoupling between the gating cycle and ATP hydrolysis cycle. Proc Natl Acad Sci U S A. 2013;110(11):4404–9.
11. Eckford PD, Li C, Ramjeesingh M, Bear CE. Cftr potentiator Vx-770 (ivacaftor) opens the defective channel gate of mutant Cftr in a phosphorylation-dependent but Atp-independent manner. J Biol Chem. 2012;287:36639.
12. Farinha CM, King-Underwood J, Sousa M, Correia AR, Henriques BJ, Roxo-Rosa M, et al. Revertants, low temperature, and correctors reveal the mechanism of F508del-CFTR rescue by VX-809 and suggest multiple agents for full correction. Chem Biol. 2013;20(7):943–55.
13. Molinski SV, Ahmadi S, Ip W, Ouyang H, Villella A, Miller JP, et al. Orkambi(R) and amplifier co-therapy improves function from a rare CFTR mutation in gene-edited cells and patient tissue. EMBO Mol Med. 2017;9(9):1224–43.
14. Wilschanski M, Miller LL, Shoseyov D, Blau H, Rivlin J, Aviram M, et al. Chronic ataluren (PTC124) treatment of nonsense mutation cystic fibrosis. Eur Respir J. 2011;38(1):59–69.
15. Kerem E, Konstan MW, De Boeck K, Accurso FJ, Sermet-Gaudelus I, Wilschanski M, et al. Ataluren for the treatment of nonsense-mutation cystic fibrosis: a randomised, double-blind, placebo-controlled phase 3 trial. Lancet Respir Med. 2014;2(7):539–47.
16. Sermet-Gaudelus I, Boeck KD, Casimir GJ, Vermeulen F, Leal T, Mogenet A, et al. Ataluren (PTC124) induces cystic fibrosis transmembrane conductance regulator protein expression and activity in children with nonsense mutation cystic fibrosis. Am J Respir Crit Care Med. 2010;182(10):1262–72.
17. Zhang Z, Liu F, Chen J. Molecular structure of the ATP-bound, phosphorylated human CFTR. Proc Natl Acad Sci U S A. 2018;115(50):12757–62.
18. Hwang TC, Yeh JT, Zhang J, Yu YC, Yeh HI, Destefano S. Structural mechanisms of CFTR function and dysfunction. J Gen Physiol. 2018;150(4):539–70.
19. Abstracts of the 21st annual North American cystic fibrosis conference, October 3–6, 2007, Anaheim, California, USA. Pediatr Pulmonol Suppl. 2007;30:99–412.

20. Abstracts of the 21st annual North American cystic fibrosis conference, October 23–25, 2008, Orlando, Florida, USA. Pediatr Pulmonol Suppl. 2008;31:105–483.

21. Accurso FJ, Rowe SM, Clancy JP, Boyle MP, Dunitz JM, Durie PR, et al. Effect of VX-770 in persons with cystic fibrosis and the G551D-CFTR mutation. N Engl J Med. 2010;363(21):1991–2003.

22. Ramsey BW, Davies J, McElvaney NG, Tullis E, Bell SC, Drevinek P, et al. A CFTR potentiator in patients with cystic fibrosis and the G551D mutation. N Engl J Med. 2011;365(18):1663–72.

23. Davies JC, Wainwright CE, Canny GJ, Chilvers MA, Howenstine MS, Munck A, et al. Efficacy and safety of ivacaftor in patients aged 6 to 11 years with cystic fibrosis with a G551D mutation. Am J Respir Crit Care Med. 2013;187(11):1219–25.

24. Yu H, Burton B, Huang CJ, Worley J, Cao D, Johnson JP Jr, et al. Ivacaftor potentiation of multiple CFTR channels with gating mutations. J Cyst Fibros. 2012;11(3):237–45.

25. De Boeck K, Munck A, Walker S, Faro A, Hiatt P, Gilmartin G, et al. Efficacy and safety of ivacaftor in patients with cystic fibrosis and a non-G551D gating mutation. J Cyst Fibrosis. 2014;13(6):674–80.

26. Guimbellot J, Solomon GM, Baines A, Heltshe SL, VanDalfsen J, Joseloff E, et al. Effectiveness of ivacaftor in cystic fibrosis patients with non-G551D gating mutations. J Cyst Fibrosis. 2019;18(1):102–9.

27. Davies JC, Cunningham S, Harris WT, Lapey A, Regelmann WE, Sawicki GS, et al. Safety, pharmacokinetics, and pharmacodynamics of ivacaftor in patients aged 2-5 years with cystic fibrosis and a CFTR gating mutation (KIWI): an open-label, single-arm study. Lancet Respir Med. 2016;4(2):107–15.

28. Ratjen F, Klingel M, Black P, Powers MR, Grasemann H, Solomon M, et al. Changes in lung clearance index in preschool-aged patients with cystic fibrosis treated with ivacaftor (GOAL): a clinical trial. Am J Respir Crit Care Med. 2018;198(4):526–8.

29. Rosenfeld M, Wainwright CE, Higgins M, Wang LT, McKee C, Campbell D, et al. Ivacaftor treatment of cystic fibrosis in children aged 12 to <24 months and with a CFTR gating mutation (ARRIVAL): a phase 3 single-arm study. Lancet Respir Med. 2018;6(7):545–53.

30. Davies J, Sheridan H, Bell N, Cunningham S, Davis SD, Elborn JS, et al. Assessment of clinical response to ivacaftor with lung clearance index in cystic fibrosis patients with a G551D-CFTR mutation and preserved spirometry: a randomised controlled trial. Lancet Respir Med. 2013;1(8):630–8.

31. Barry PJ, Plant BJ, Nair A, Bicknell S, Simmonds NJ, Bell NJ, et al. Effects of ivacaftor in patients with cystic fibrosis who carry the G551D mutation and have severe lung disease. Chest. 2014;146(1):152–8.

32. Carter S, Kelly S, Caples E, Grogan B, Doyle J, Gallagher CG, et al. Ivacaftor as salvage therapy in a patient with cystic fibrosis genotype F508del/R117H/IVS8-5T. J Cyst Fibrosis. 2015;14(4):e4–5.

33. Hebestreit H, Sauer-Heilborn A, Fischer R, Kading M, Mainz JG. Effects of ivacaftor on severely ill patients with cystic fibrosis carrying a G551D mutation. J Cyst Fibrosis. 2013;12(6):599–603.

34. Polenakovik HM, Sanville B. The use of ivacaftor in an adult with severe lung disease due to cystic fibrosis (DeltaF508/G551D). J Cyst Fibrosis. 2013;12(5):530–1.

35. Ronan NJ, Fleming C, O'Callaghan G, Maher MM, Murphy DM, Plant BJ. The role of ivacaftor in severe cystic fibrosis in a patient with the R117H mutation. Chest. 2015;148(3):e72–e5.

36. Taylor-Cousar J, Niknian M, Gilmartin G, Pilewski JM. Investigators VX. Effect of ivacaftor in patients with advanced cystic fibrosis and a G551D-CFTR mutation: safety and efficacy in an expanded access program in the United States. J Cyst Fibrosis. 2016;15(1):116–22.

37. Wood ME, Smith DJ, Reid DW, Masel PJ, France MW, Bell SC. Ivacaftor in severe cystic fibrosis lung disease and a G551D mutation. Respirol Case Rep. 2013;1(2):52–4.

38. Chassagnon G, Hubert D, Fajac I, Burgel PR, Revel MP. Investigators. Long-term computed tomographic changes in cystic fibrosis patients treated with ivacaftor. Eur Respir J. 2016;48(1):249–52.

39. Ronan NJ, Einarsson GG, Twomey M, Mooney D, Mullane D, NiChroinin M, et al. CORK study in cystic fibrosis: sustained improvements in ultra-low-dose chest CT scores after CFTR modulation with ivacaftor. Chest. 2018;153(2):395–403.
40. Adam RJ, Hisert KB, Dodd JD, Grogan B, Launspach JL, Barnes JK, et al. Acute administration of ivacaftor to people with cystic fibrosis and a G551D-CFTR mutation reveals smooth muscle abnormalities. JCI Insight. 2016;1(4):e86183.
41. Bessonova L, Volkova N, Higgins M, Bengtsson L, Tian S, Simard C, et al. Data from the US and UK cystic fibrosis registries support disease modification by CFTR modulation with ivacaftor. Thorax. 2018;73(8):731–40.
42. McKone EF, Borowitz D, Drevinek P, Griese M, Konstan MW, Wainwright C, et al. Long-term safety and efficacy of ivacaftor in patients with cystic fibrosis who have the Gly551Asp-CFTR mutation: a phase 3, open-label extension study (PERSIST). Lancet Respir Med. 2014;2(11):902–10.
43. Volkova N, Moy K, Evans J, Campbell D, Tian S, Simard C, et al. Disease progression in patients with cystic fibrosis treated with ivacaftor: data from national US and UK registries. J Cyst Fibrosis. 2020;19(1):68–79.
44. Hubert D, Dehillotte C, Munck A, David V, Baek J, Mely L, et al. Retrospective observational study of French patients with cystic fibrosis and a Gly551Asp-CFTR mutation after 1 and 2years of treatment with ivacaftor in a real-world setting. J Cyst Fibrosis. 2018;17(1):89–95.
45. Strang A, Fischer AJ, Chidekel A. Pseudomonas eradication and clinical effectivness of Ivacaftor in four Hispanic patients with S549N. Pediatr Pulmonol. 2017;52(7):E37–E9.
46. Rowe SM, Heltshe SL, Gonska T, Donaldson SH, Borowitz D, Gelfond D, et al. Clinical mechanism of the cystic fibrosis transmembrane conductance regulator potentiator ivacaftor in G551D-mediated cystic fibrosis. Am J Respir Crit Care Med. 2014;190(2):175–84.
47. Heltshe SL, Mayer-Hamblett N, Burns JL, Khan U, Baines A, Ramsey BW, et al. Pseudomonas aeruginosa in cystic fibrosis patients with G551D-CFTR treated with ivacaftor. Clin Infect Dis. 2015;60(5):703–12.
48. Millar BC, McCaughan J, Rendall JC, Downey DG, Moore JE. Pseudomonas aeruginosa in cystic fibrosis patients with c.1652GA (G551D)-CFTR treated with ivacaftor-changes in microbiological parameters. J Clin Pharm Ther. 2018;43(1):92–100.
49. Heltshe SL, Rowe SM, Skalland M, Baines A, Jain M. Network GIotCFFTD. Ivacaftor-treated patients with cystic fibrosis derive long-term benefit despite no short-term clinical improvement. Am J Respir Crit Care Med. 2018;197(11):1483–6.
50. Gelfond D, Heltshe S, Ma C, Rowe SM, Frederick C, Uluer A, et al. Impact of CFTR modulation on intestinal pH, motility, and clinical outcomes in patients with cystic fibrosis and the G551D mutation. Clin Transl Gastroenterol. 2017;8(3):e81.
51. Hayes D Jr, Warren PS, McCoy KS, Sheikh SI. Improvement of hepatic steatosis in cystic fibrosis with ivacaftor therapy. J Pediatr Gastroenterol Nutr. 2015;60(5):578–9.
52. Stalvey MS, Pace J, Niknian M, Higgins MN, Tarn V, Davis J, et al. Growth in prepubertal children with cystic fibrosis treated with ivacaftor. Pediatrics. 2017;139(2). pii: e20162522.
53. McColley SA. A safety evaluation of ivacaftor for the treatment of cystic fibrosis. Expert Opin Drug Saf. 2016;15(5):709–15.
54. Dryden C, Wilkinson J, Young D, Brooker RJ. Scottish Paediatric Cystic Fibrosis Managed Clinical N. The impact of 12 months treatment with ivacaftor on Scottish paediatric patients with cystic fibrosis with the G551D mutation: a review. Arch Dis Child. 2018;103(1):68–70.
55. Robertson SM, Luo X, Dubey N, Li C, Chavan AB, Gilmartin GS, et al. Clinical drug-drug interaction assessment of ivacaftor as a potential inhibitor of cytochrome P450 and P-glycoprotein. J Clin Pharmacol. 2015;55(1):56–62.
56. Jordan CL, Noah TL, Henry MM. Therapeutic challenges posed by critical drug-drug interactions in cystic fibrosis. Pediatr Pulmonol. 2016;51(S44):S61–70.
57. Guimbellot JS, Acosta EP, Rowe SM. Sensitivity of ivacaftor to drug-drug interactions with rifampin, a cytochrome P450 3A4 inducer. Pediatr Pulmonol. 2018;53(5):E6–8.
58. Trimble AT, Donaldson SH. Ivacaftor withdrawal syndrome in cystic fibrosis patients with the G551D mutation. J Cyst Fibrosis. 2018;17(2):e13–e16.

59. Harbeson SL, Morgan AJ, Liu JF, Aslanian AM, Nguyen S, Bridson GW, et al. Altering metabolic profiles of drugs by precision deuteration 2: discovery of a deuterated analog of ivacaftor with differentiated pharmacokinetics for clinical development. J Pharmacol Exp Ther. 2017;362(2):359–67.

60. Van Goor F, Yu H, Burton B, Hoffman BJ. Effect of ivacaftor on CFTR forms with missense mutations associated with defects in protein processing or function. J Cyst Fibrosis. 2014;13(1):29–36.

61. Flume PA, Liou TG, Borowitz DS, Li H, Yen K, Ordonez CL, et al. Ivacaftor in subjects with cystic fibrosis who are homozygous for the F508del-CFTR mutation. Chest. 2012;142(3):718–24.

62. Yeh HI, Sohma Y, Conrath K, Hwang TC. A common mechanism for CFTR potentiators. J Gen Physiol. 2017;149(12):1105–18.

63. Phuan PW, Veit G, Tan JA, Finkbeiner WE, Lukacs GL, Verkman AS. Potentiators of defective DeltaF508-CFTR gating that do not interfere with corrector action. Mol Pharmacol. 2015;88(4):791–9.

64. Qu BH, Strickland E, Thomas PJ. Cystic fibrosis: a disease of altered protein folding. J Bioenerg Biomembr. 1997;29(5):483–90.

65. Thibodeau PH, Richardson JM 3rd, Wang W, Millen L, Watson J, Mendoza JL, et al. The cystic fibrosis-causing mutation deltaF508 affects multiple steps in cystic fibrosis transmembrane conductance regulator biogenesis. J Biol Chem. 2010;285(46):35825–35.

66. Rubenstein RC, Egan ME, Zeitlin PL. In vitro pharmacologic restoration of CFTR-mediated chloride transport with sodium 4-phenylbutyrate in cystic fibrosis epithelial cells containing delta F508-CFTR. J Clin Invest. 1997;100(10):2457–65.

67. Rubenstein RC, Zeitlin PL. A pilot clinical trial of oral sodium 4-phenylbutyrate (Buphenyl) in deltaF508-homozygous cystic fibrosis patients: partial restoration of nasal epithelial CFTR function. Am J Respir Crit Care Med. 1998;157(2):484–90.

68. McCarty NA, Standaert TA, Teresi M, Tuthill C, Launspach J, Kelley TJ, et al. A phase I randomized, multicenter trial of CPX in adult subjects with mild cystic fibrosis. Pediatr Pulmonol. 2002;33(2):90–8.

69. Egan ME, Pearson M, Weiner SA, Rajendran V, Rubin D, Glockner-Pagel J, et al. Curcumin, a major constituent of turmeric, corrects cystic fibrosis defects. Science. 2004;304(5670):600–2.

70. Van Goor F, Hadida S, Grootenhuis PD, Burton B, Stack JH, Straley KS, et al. Correction of the F508del-CFTR protein processing defect in vitro by the investigational drug VX-809. Proc Natl Acad Sci U S A. 2011;108(46):18843–8.

71. Rowe SM, Daines C, Ringshausen FC, Kerem E, Wilson J, Tullis E, et al. Tezacaftor-ivacaftor in residual-function heterozygotes with cystic fibrosis. N Engl J Med. 2017;377(21):2024–35.

72. Taylor-Cousar JL, Munck A, McKone EF, van der Ent CK, Moeller A, Simard C, et al. Tezacaftor-ivacaftor in patients with cystic fibrosis homozygous for Phe508del. N Engl J Med. 2017;377(21):2013–23.

73. Boyle MP, Bell SC, Konstan MW, McColley SA, Rowe SM, Rietschel E, et al. A CFTR corrector (lumacaftor) and a CFTR potentiator (ivacaftor) for treatment of patients with cystic fibrosis who have a phe508del CFTR mutation: a phase 2 randomised controlled trial. Lancet Respir Med. 2014;2(7):527–38.

74. Cholon DM, Esther CR Jr, Gentzsch M. Efficacy of lumacaftor-ivacaftor for the treatment of cystic fibrosis patients homozygous for the F508del-CFTR mutation. Expert Rev Precis Med Drug Dev. 2016;1(3):235–43.

75. Elborn JS, Ramsey BW, Boyle MP, Konstan MW, Huang X, Marigowda G, et al. Efficacy and safety of lumacaftor/ivacaftor combination therapy in patients with cystic fibrosis homozygous for Phe508del CFTR by pulmonary function subgroup: a pooled analysis. Lancet Respir Med. 2016;4(8):617–26.

76. Hubert D, Chiron R, Camara B, Grenet D, Prevotat A, Bassinet L, et al. Real-life initiation of lumacaftor/ivacaftor combination in adults with cystic fibrosis homozygous for the Phe508del CFTR mutation and severe lung disease. J Cyst Fibrosis. 2017;16(3):388–91.

77. Konstan MW, McKone EF, Moss RB, Marigowda G, Tian S, Waltz D, et al. Assessment of safety and efficacy of long-term treatment with combination lumacaftor and ivacaftor therapy in patients with cystic fibrosis homozygous for the F508del-CFTR mutation (PROGRESS): a phase 3, extension study. Lancet Respir Med. 2017;5(2):107–18.

78. Wainwright CE, Elborn JS, Ramsey BW, Marigowda G, Huang X, Cipolli M, et al. Lumacaftor–ivacaftor in patients with cystic fibrosis homozygous for Phe508del CFTR. N Engl J Med. 2015;373(3):220–31.

79. Clancy JP, Rowe SM, Accurso FJ, Aitken ML, Amin RS, Ashlock MA, et al. Results of a phase IIa study of VX-809, an investigational CFTR corrector compound, in subjects with cystic fibrosis homozygous for the F508del-CFTR mutation. Thorax. 2012;67(1):12–8.

80. Wainwright CE, Elborn JS, Ramsey BW, Marigowda G, Huang X, Cipolli M, et al. Lumacaftor-ivacaftor in patients with cystic fibrosis homozygous for Phe508del CFTR. N Engl J Med. 2015;373(3):220–31.

81. Milla CE, Ratjen F, Marigowda G, Liu F, Waltz D, Rosenfeld M, et al. Lumacaftor/ivacaftor in patients aged 6-11 years with cystic fibrosis homozygous for F508del-CFTR. Am J Respir Crit Care Med. 2017;195(7):912–20.

82. Jennings MT, Dezube R, Paranjape S, West NE, Hong G, Braun A, et al. An observational study of outcomes and tolerances in patients with cystic fibrosis initiated on lumacaftor/ivacaftor. Ann Am Thorac Soc. 2017;14(11):1662–6.

83. Schneider EK. Cytochrome P450 3A4 induction: lumacaftor versus ivacaftor potentially resulting in significantly reduced plasma concentration of ivacaftor. Drug Metab Lett. 2018;12:71.

84. The 30th annual North American cystic fibrosis conference, Orange County Convention Center, Orlando, Florida, October 27–29, 2016. Pediatr Pulmonol. 2016;51(S45):S1–S507.

85. Donaldson SH, Pilewski JM, Griese M, Cooke J, Viswanathan L, Tullis E, et al. Tezacaftor/Ivacaftor in subjects with cystic fibrosis and F508del/F508del-CFTR or F508del/G551D-CFTR. Am J Respir Crit Care Med. 2018;197(2):214–24.

86. A study to evaluate the efficacy and safety of VX-661 in combination with ivacaftor in subjects aged 12 years and older with cystic fibrosis, heterozygous for the F508del-CFTR mutation clinicaltrials.gov2018 [updated 6/12/2018. NCT02516410]. Available from: https://clinicaltrials.gov/ct2/show/results/NCT02516410?term=vx-661&rank=5.

87. ClinicalTrials.gov Identifier: NCT02516410.

88. ClinicalTrials.gov Identifier: NCT02412111.

89. Bell S, De Boeck K, Drevinek P, Plant B, Barry P, Elborn S, et al. WS01.4 GLPG2222 in subjects with cystic fibrosis and the F508del/class III mutation on stable treatment with ivacaftor: results from a phase II study (ALBATROSS). J Cyst Fibros. 2018;17:S2.

90. van der Ent KC, Minic P, Verhulst S, Van Braeckel E, Flume P, Boas S, et al. EPS3.05 GLPG2222 in subjects with cystic fibrosis homozygous for F508del: results from a phase II study (FLAMINGO). J Cyst Fibros. 2018;17:S42.

91. The 32nd annual North American cystic fibrosis conference, Colorado Convention Center, Denver, Colorado, October 18–20, 2018. Pediatr Pulmonol. 2018;53(S2):S1–S481.

92. Flume P, Sawicki G, Pressler T, Schwarz C, Fajac I, Layish D, et al. WS01.2 phase 2 initial results evaluating PTI-428, a novel CFTR amplifier, in patients with cystic fibrosis. J Cyst Fibros. 2018;17:S1–2.

93. ClinicalTrials.gov NCT03251092, NCT03500263.

94. Keating D, Marigowda G, Burr L, Daines C, Mall MA, McKone EF, et al. VX-445-tezacaftor-ivacaftor in patients with cystic fibrosis and one or two Phe508del alleles. N Engl J Med. 2018;379(17):1612–20.

95. Davies JC, Moskowitz SM, Brown C, Horsley A, Mall MA, McKone EF, et al. VX-659-tezacaftor-ivacaftor in patients with cystic fibrosis and one or two Phe508del alleles. N Engl J Med. 2018;379(17):1599–611.

96. Two phase 3 studies of the triple combination of VX-445, tezacaftor and ivacaftor met primary endpoint of improvement in lung function (ppFEV1) in people with cystic fibrosis [press release]. http://investors.vrtx.com: Vertex Pharmaceuticals, Inc. 2019.

97. Eckford PD, Ramjeesingh M, Molinski S, Pasyk S, Dekkers JF, Li C, et al. VX-809 and related corrector compounds exhibit secondary activity stabilizing active F508del-CFTR after its partial rescue to the cell surface. Chem Biol. 2014;21(5):666–78.
98. Cholon DM, O'Neal WK, Randell SH, Riordan JR, Gentzsch M. Modulation of endocytic trafficking and apical stability of CFTR in primary human airway epithelial cultures. Am J Physiol Lung Cell Mol Physiol. 2010;298(3):L304–14.
99. Varga K, Goldstein RF, Jurkuvenaite A, Chen L, Matalon S, Sorscher EJ, et al. Enhanced cell-surface stability of rescued DeltaF508 cystic fibrosis transmembrane conductance regulator (CFTR) by pharmacological chaperones. Biochem J. 2008;410(3):555–64.
100. Young A, Gentzsch M, Abban CY, Jia Y, Meneses PI, Bridges RJ, et al. Dynasore inhibits removal of wild-type and DeltaF508 cystic fibrosis transmembrane conductance regulator (CFTR) from the plasma membrane. Biochem J. 2009;421(3):377–85.
101. Kim Chiaw P, Wellhauser L, Huan LJ, Ramjeesingh M, Bear CE. A chemical corrector modifies the channel function of F508del-CFTR. Mol Pharmacol. 2010;78(3):411–8.
102. Wellhauser L, Kim Chiaw P, Pasyk S, Li C, Ramjeesingh M, Bear CE. A small-molecule modulator interacts directly with deltaPhe508-CFTR to modify its ATPase activity and conformational stability. Mol Pharmacol. 2009;75(6):1430–8.
103. De Boeck K, Zolin A, Cuppens H, Olesen HV, Viviani L. The relative frequency of CFTR mutation classes in European patients with cystic fibrosis. J Cyst Fibrosis. 2014;13(4):403–9.
104. Bedwell DM, Kaenjak A, Benos DJ, Bebok Z, Bubien JK, Hong J, et al. Suppression of a CFTR premature stop mutation in a bronchial epithelial cell line. Nat Med. 1997;3(11):1280–4.
105. Howard M, Frizzell RA, Bedwell DM. Aminoglycoside antibiotics restore CFTR function by overcoming premature stop mutations. Nat Med. 1996;2(4):467–9.
106. Sermet-Gaudelus I, Renouil M, Fajac A, Bidou L, Parbaille B, Pierrot S, et al. In vitro prediction of stop-codon suppression by intravenous gentamicin in patients with cystic fibrosis: a pilot study. BMC Med. 2007;5:5–14.
107. Clancy JP, Bebok Z, Ruiz F, King C, Jones J, Walker L, et al. Evidence that systemic gentamicin suppresses premature stop mutations in patients with cystic fibrosis. Am J Respir Crit Care Med. 2001;163(7):1683–92.
108. Wilschanski M, Yahav Y, Yaacov Y, Blau H, Bentur L, Rivlin J, et al. Gentamicin-induced correction of CFTR function in patients with cystic fibrosis and CFTR stop mutations. N Engl J Med. 2003;349(15):1433–41.
109. Wilschanski M, Famini C, Blau H, Rivlin J, Augarten A, Avital A, et al. A pilot study of the effect of gentamicin on nasal potential difference measurements in cystic fibrosis patients carrying stop mutations. Am J Respir Crit Care Med. 2000;161(3 Pt 1):860–5.
110. Keeling KM, Wang D, Dai Y, Murugesan S, Chenna B, Clark J, et al. Attenuation of nonsense-mediated mRNA decay enhances in vivo nonsense suppression. PLoS One. 2013;8(4):e60478.
111. Linde L, Boelz S, Nissim-Rafinia M, Oren YS, Wilschanski M, Yaacov Y, et al. Nonsense-mediated mRNA decay affects nonsense transcript levels and governs response of cystic fibrosis patients to gentamicin. J Clin Invest. 2007;117(3):683–92.
112. Kerem E, Konstan MW, De Boeck K, Accurso FJ, Sermet-Gaudelus I, Wilschanski M, et al. Ataluren for the treatment of nonsense-mutation cystic fibrosis: a randomised, double-blind, placebo-controlled phase 3 trial. Lancet Respir Med. 2014;2:539.
113. Gorini L, Kataja E. Phenotypic repair by streptomycin of defective genotypes in E. Coli. Proc Nat Acad Sci United States of America. 1964;51:487–93.
114. Martin R, Mogg AE, Heywood LA, Nitschke L, Burke JF. Aminoglycoside suppression at UAG, UAA and UGA codons in Escherichia coli and human tissue culture cells. Mol Gen Genet. 1989;217(2–3):411–8.
115. Sermet-Gaudelus I, De Boeck K, Casimir GJ, Vermeulen F, Leal T, Mogenet A, et al. Ataluren (PTC124) induces CFTR protein expression and activity in children with nonsense mutation cystic fibrosis. Am J Respir Crit Care Med. 2010;182(10):1262–72.
116. Xue X, Mutyam V, Thakerar A, Mobley J, Bridges RJ, Rowe SM, et al. Identification of the amino acids inserted during suppression of CFTR nonsense mutations and determination of their functional consequences. Hum Mol Genet. 2017;26(16):3116–29.

117. Rowe SM, Sloane P, Tang LP, Backer K, Mazur M, Buckley-Lanier J, et al. Suppression of CFTR premature termination codons and rescue of CFTR protein and function by the synthetic aminoglycoside NB54. J Mol Med. 2011;89(11):1149–61.

118. Xue X, Mutyam V, Tang L, Biswas S, Du M, Jackson LA, et al. Synthetic aminoglycosides efficiently suppress cystic fibrosis transmembrane conductance regulator nonsense mutations and are enhanced by ivacaftor. Am J Respir Cell Mol Biol. 2014;50(4):805–16.

119. Nudelman I, Glikin D, Smolkin B, Hainrichson M, Belakhov V, Baasov T. Repairing faulty genes by aminoglycosides: development of new derivatives of geneticin (G418) with enhanced suppression of diseases-causing nonsense mutations. Bioorg Med Chem. 2010;18(11):3735–46.

120. Welch EM, Barton ER, Zhuo J, Tomizawa Y, Friesen WJ, Trifillis P, et al. PTC124 targets genetic disorders caused by nonsense mutations. Nature. 2007;447(7140):87–91.

121. Roy B, Friesen WJ, Tomizawa Y, Leszyk JD, Zhuo J, Johnson B, et al. Ataluren stimulates ribosomal selection of near-cognate tRNAs to promote nonsense suppression. Proc Natl Acad Sci U S A. 2016;113(44):12508–13.

122. Shoseyov D, Cohen-Cymberknoh M, Wilschanski M. Ataluren for the treatment of cystic fibrosis. Expert Rev Respir Med. 2016;10(4):387–91.

123. Kerem E, Hirawat S, Armoni S, Yaakov Y, Shoseyov D, Cohen M, et al. Effectiveness of PTC124 treatment of cystic fibrosis caused by nonsense mutations: a prospective phase II trial. Lancet. 2008;372(9640):719–27.

124. McHugh DR, Steele MS, Valerio DM, Miron A, Mann RJ, LePage DF, et al. A G542X cystic fibrosis mouse model for examining nonsense mutation directed therapies. PLoS One. 2018;13(6):e0199573.

125. Mutyam V, Du M, Xue X, Keeling KM, White EL, Bostwick JR, et al. Discovery of clinically approved agents that promote suppression of CFTR nonsense mutations. Am J Respir Crit Care Med. 2016;194(9):1092–103.

126. Keeling KM, Xue X, Gunn G, Bedwell DM. Therapeutics based on stop codon readthrough. Annu Rev Genomics Hum Genet. 2014;15:371–94.

127. Rehman A, Baloch NU, Janahi IA. Lumacaftor-ivacaftor in patients with cystic fibrosis homozygous for Phe508del CFTR. N Engl J Med. 2015;373(18):1783.

128. Quon BS, Rowe SM. New and emerging targeted therapies for cystic fibrosis. BMJ. 2016;352:i859.

Chapter 25
Gene Editing for CF

Mitchell L. Drumm

Unmet Needs for CF Therapeutics

Cystic fibrosis (CF) was first recognized as a specific disorder in the 1930s, and until recently treatment of clinical manifestations has been restricted to symptomatic therapy. CF is a systemic disease, affecting virtually every organ system in the body, requiring therapeutics to treat gastrointestinal, pulmonary, immune, endocrine, metabolic, pancreatic and liver complications, just to name a few. Consequently, the regimen of drugs and other treatments a given patient must endure is extensive and burdensome.

Identification of the gene responsible for CF, *CFTR*, encoding the cystic fibrosis transmembrane conductance regulator [1], an anion channel, has allowed therapeutic development that targets the source of the disease, absent or reduced CFTR function. In the early 1990s, transgenes encoding functional CFTR were introduced into CF cells and demonstrated that the ion transport defects of CF could be restored [2, 3]. Attempts to treat the disease by delivering CFTR transgenes were subsequently conceived and executed, but were unsuccessful at providing disease relief [4]. However, another strategy, to improve or restore CFTR function in cells by pharmacologic means was also pursued [5, 6] and with the aid of high-throughput screening this approach resulted in a new drug that increased activity of one CFTR mutation, G551D, and appeared to have very positive clinical effects [7]. This initial CFTR-modulating drug was just the first, and a panel of new drugs with impressive, positive impact on many persons with CF is now available.

Despite the successes of these "CFTR modulator" drugs, there is still a significant proportion of persons afflicted with CF who do not benefit from these

M. L. Drumm (✉)
Case Western Reserve University, Department of Genetics and Genome Sciences,
Cystic Fibrosis Research Center, Cleveland, OH, USA
e-mail: Mitchell.drumm@case.edu

© Springer Nature Switzerland AG 2020
S. D. Davis et al. (eds.), *Cystic Fibrosis*, Respiratory Medicine,
https://doi.org/10.1007/978-3-030-42382-7_25

therapies. A large percentage of individuals with CF carry mutations that make no CFTR protein (null mutations) or mutations that are not responsive to the drugs, and there are others who carry mutations predicted to respond to these drugs based on their genotype, but for unknown reasons are not responsive. For all of these individuals, other approaches are needed.

Genome Editing and Its Evolution

Strategies to repair or circumvent disease-causing mutations continue to be discovered and developed, and current methods being pursued for CF are described below and outlined in Fig. 25.1.

Targeting DNA Cleavage in Mammalian Cells New technologies have emerged over the past decade or so that allow one to manipulate the genome in very precise and specific ways. The term "genome editing" has been used to aptly describe these technologies. The first of these precision editing systems applied to mammalian cells utilized engineered fusion proteins called zinc-finger nucleases (ZFNs) that harnessed the sequence-recognition properties of certain DNA-binding proteins and

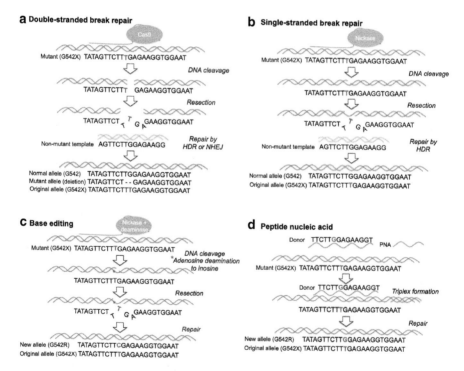

Fig. 25.1 Schematic of various strategies. (**a**) Double-stranded break repair. (**b**) Single-stranded break repair. (**c**) Base editing. (**d**) Peptide nucleic acid

linked them to a peptide with nuclease activity. These DNA-binding proteins that could cleave the DNA at, or near, their binding site were effectively sequence-specific enzymes that could break DNA at user-defined, specific sites [8]. The zinc-finger motifs that provide the DNA sequence specificity were found to be modular, and by mixing and matching them, one could create peptides that would recognize sequences found only once in the genome, setting the stage for custom-designed nucleases.

Harnessing Repair of Double-Strand Breaks The utility of this targeted nuclease system was quickly recognized and many permutations and adaptations were developed. Among the uses, it was recognized that the DNA repair processes of the cell could be manipulated to create specific sequence changes at, or near, the DNA break. Among the observations made was that when a DNA template was provided to the cells during repair, a significant proportion of the breaks would utilize the template sequences during repair and incorporate them into the chromosome. This observation had obvious application to molecular therapeutics, where one might damage the DNA at, or near, a disease-causing mutation and provide a function-restoring sequence as a template to eliminate the mutation during repair. Subsequently, another peptide-based, sequence-recognizing system was developed based on prokaryotic DNA-binding proteins [9]. This system, called TALENs (transcription activator-like effector nucleases) [10], was also modular and appeared to be more flexible than ZFNs.

However, 2013 saw reports of a new system composed of prokaryotic elements, called CRISPR/Cas9, that described the use of a short RNA molecule to target a bacterial nuclease, Cas9, to nearly any DNA sequence of a user's choice [11, 12]. This provided a fast, inexpensive method to modify specific sequences at almost any site in the genome. A target site to be modified appeared to require only the presence of a pair of adjacent guanines for the nuclease to recognize. This sequence is called the protospacer-adjacent motif, or PAM, and dictates the site and activity of Cas9 cleavage. The genomic target is recognized by a RNA molecule, called a guide RNA (gRNA). In bacteria, the gRNA is actually composed of two different RNA molecules: one to recognize the target and the other to tether Cas9 so it can be brought to the target DNA sequence. Synthetic gRNAs used for eukaryotic gene editing are single RNA molecules containing the two functional domains for finding a target in the genome and delivering Cas9 to those genomic sequences where it is intended to cut. Once the complex of gRNA, Cas9, and genomic DNA is formed, the Cas9 recognizes the "GG" guanine pair and cleaves the DNA at a position 4–5 nucleotides away, 5′ of the GG. As a GG pair is expected to occur, on average, about every 16 base pairs; most regions of the genome will have at least one GG pair sufficiently close to a desired target site.

"Nicking" One Strand of DNA As described above, there are several platforms that have properties desirable for altering specific sites in the genome, all of which involve provision of a DNA template containing the desired sequence. This template is used by the repair machinery to copy and incorporate it into the genome, rather than recombination and physical exchange of DNA strands. The first iterations of this homology-dependent repair process involved targeting double-strand breaks at the site of a mutation to be repaired, but concerns arose regarding safety if the nuclease functions were to alter DNA at other positions in the genome. To address this, the ability to edit DNA by cleaving only one strand was pursued along with strategies for chemically altering a nucleotide, a method referred to as base editing.

Zinc-finger nucleases consist of a pair of peptide modules with a Fok1 nuclease domain that cuts one of the two strands of DNA. While Fok1 monomers must be paired with a second Fok1 nuclease domain to be catalytically active, both need not be catalytically active. By inactivating the catalytic site of one of the two Fok1 domains, only one strand of DNA is cleaved, creating what is termed a "nickase." Nicking the DNA in this way still stimulates repair pathways that can be harnessed for editing, but is less likely to create frame-shifting mutations at on- or off-targeting sites. This same strategy has been applied to CRISPR/Cas9 by inducing mutations that inactivate one of the two cleavage domains of Cas9. These nickases appear to have fewer off-target effects in the genome.

Base Editing The homology-directed repair strategies require multiple components, a gRNA for targeting, Cas9 for cleavage, and a nucleic acid template with the desired sequence. To reduce the complexity, another approach to editing was developed with the intent to provide a system that could be applied without the need for a template, or donor sequence, yet still achieve precise, targeted changes in genomic sequences. It has long been recognized that many single-nucleotide variants in our genome are the consequence of a cytosine, or in some cases, adenine, deamination to uracil or inosine, respectively, that led to misincorporation of nucleotides during DNA repair or replication. A strategy referred to as base editing utilizes this process to alter mutations in a template-free way [13], reducing the number of components needed for an editing strategy and lowers the potential for unwanted mutations occurring from double-strand breaks.

As discussed above, gRNAs of the CRISPR/Cas9 system facilitate delivery of proteins to specific sequences in the genome by tethering them to Cas9, even if the Cas9 is rendered catalytically inactive [14–16]. By fusing bacterial deaminases to Cas9 it has been possible to deaminate cytosine and adenosine residues in a small window of sequences near the PAM site. If the cytosine of a C:G pair is deaminated, it creates an I (inosine):G pair that, upon repair or replication, will either restore the C:G if the G is used as the template or create a T:A pair if inosine is the template. Similarly, an A:T pair that undergoes adenosine deamination to inosine will be repaired to A:T or converted to G:C. While not comprehensive, it provides opportunities to alter all four nucleotides by virtue of the fact that either strand of DNA can be modified (the complementary base to T on one strand is A on the other strand, for example).

As may be apparent, base editing requires careful consideration of the strand on which the deaminated base will reside and also a way to ensure that the strand carrying the deaminated base will be used as the template strand during replication or repair, otherwise the modified base will be replaced with the original mutation. This has been addressed by using a Cas9 molecule in which one of the cleavage domains is inactivated, making it a nickase [17]. By nicking the strand opposite the deaminated strand, DNA repair is targeted to the desired strand and the converted or reverted residue incorporated.

The base editing technology continues to evolve, broadening its scope by engineering variants that will target deamination to different distances from the PAM sequence and using different Cas proteins that recognize a number of different PAM sequences [18]. With these permutations available, the number of sites that can be edited continues to grow.

Protein Nucleic Acids   More recently, an approach that does not require exogenous enzymatic activity was reported in which the ribose backbone of a nucleic acid is replaced with glycines to create a hybrid molecule called a peptide nucleic acid, or PNA [19]. The PNA sequence is designed so it will form a triplex with corresponding sequences in the genome at or adjacent to a sequence to be changed. The PNA/DNAtriplex stimulates recombination or repair pathways and thus when used in conjunction with a non-PNA "donor" DNA molecule containing the desired sequence at that site, the donor sequence is incorporated into the chromosomal DNA sequence. This approach has been applied to the F508del mutation and demonstrated its ability to repair CFTR mutations [20].

Inserting DNA Sequences   The ability to target DNA cleavage to specific sequences opened up numerous possibilities for genome editing. Double-stranded breaks are repaired in several ways, including a process referred to as non-homologous end joining (NHEJ), and homology-dependent repair (HDR), but it was discovered that these sites are also prone to insertion of small DNA fragments as well. Consequently, the idea of inserting CFTR coding sequences upstream of a mutation is under consideration as a therapeutic strategy. By introducing the entire coding sequence into a single exon, one could conceivably provide a universal strategy to treat all, or nearly all, persons with CF.

The *CFTR* Gene and CF Mutations

Shortly after the *CFTR* gene was identified, the Hospital for Sick Children developed a website, the CF mutation inserting DNA sequences database (http://www.genet.sickkids.on.ca/), to catalog variants in the gene as they were discovered from analyses of patient DNA. This publicly available resource shows that there are currently over 2000 mutations documented in the CFTR gene likely to cause CF. Mutations of every type are found in this database, including complete loss of function (premature stop codons, substitutions at splice sites, and frame-shifting insertions and deletions), mutations that produce protein that is not active under physiologic conditions, and partial function mutations (promoter mutations, amino acid substitutions, and some splice site variants) that produce either less CFTR or produce CFTR that has reduced function.

A second web-based resource was generated, called CFTR2 (https://www.cftr2.org/), that provides information on a large subset of mutations, but only those that have been reported in a large number of individuals so that disease phenotypic information can be linked to specific mutations. CFTR2 provides information in formats accessible to patients and their families as well as formats useful for caregivers and researchers. Together, the CF mutation database and CFTR2 are rich resources for anyone wishing to learn about specific mutations, but also illustrate the difficulties for finding a singular, therapeutic approach targeting the basic defect by addressing all mutations.

Genome Editing Strategies to Repair or Circumvent CFTR Mutations

The vast number of mutations referred to above presents logistical issues with regard to therapeutic strategies. For example, each modulator drug corrects a specific step in CFTR's biosynthesis or function. The first drug of its type, Ivacaftor (Kalydeco), augments activity of mutations like G551D by increasing their response to stimuli like cAMP. A second drug, Lumacaftor, was discovered for its ability to correct folding of mutant F508del CFTR, and when combined with Ivacaftor it provides a clinically effective drug for patients carrying a certain panel of mutations. This approach has shown that effective therapies targeting the basic defect can be found and developed, but a singular therapy likely does not exist due to the diversity of mutations and their specific effects.

For gene editing, a similar conundrum presents itself, as there are technologies that could be brought to bear for individual mutations, but the idea of engineering roughly 2000 variations of a technology for clinical use is likely not a practical one. Consequently, strategies that would effectively treat all mutations, or a small number of strategies that would treat most patients (half of persons with CF carry two different mutations) are at the top of the list currently. For example, a strategy that could repair the F508del 3-nucleotide deletion would effectively treat 90% of individuals with CF, as roughly 50% of this population carry two copies of F508del and about 40% carry F508del in combination with another mutation. Figure 25.2 outlines the different approaches for mutation-specific and mutation-agnostic CF gene editing.

To illustrate the context of this issue, the CFTR gene spans 190,298 base pairs on chromosome 7, with the vast majority of mutations in, or closely flanking, the exons where the 4440 base pairs of protein coding sequences reside. In other words, the vast majority of the 2000 disease-causing mutations are found within stretches of the gene that account for only about 4500 base pairs, corresponding to only 2.5% of

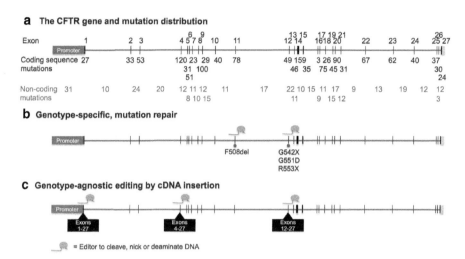

Fig. 25.2 Genome editing to address the many mutations in *CFTR*. (**a**) The CFTR gene and mutation distribution. There are over 2000 mutations spread across the 190-kilobase *CFTR* gene. Mutations in exons are given in black, listed below the respective exon. Those in the promoter, 5′ untranslated region, or introns are in blue, below their respective gene region. (**b**) Genotype-specific, mutation repair. Strategies that would involve repair of specific mutations, such as F508del, may only be able to address a single mutation, but others may located in clusters that can be repaired by a single strategy, such as G542X, G551D, and R553X that are proximate to each other and might be targeted by a single gRNA. (**c**) Genotype-agnostic editing by cDNA insertion. Examples of strategies to treat many mutations with a single editing event. Insertion of a cDNA in exon 1, such that it would be under transcriptional control of the CFTR promoter, would circumvent all mutations but the small number in the promoter and 5' UTR. Similar strategies could be used by inserting partial cDNAs upstream of mutation-rich regions, creating "super exons" that would be translated and generate functional CFTR

the gene. Because the cleavage site for editing mutations must be close to the mutation, this clustering of mutations may allow for multiple mutations to be repaired by a single editor.

Challenges in Applying Genome Editing to Cystic Fibrosis: Where, When, How and How Much?

CF is typically referred to as an epithelial disorder, but CFTR is expressed in both epithelial and non-epithelial cells. The role of each CFTR-expressing cell type in disease is not clear and thus there is not a singular cell type one can point to as "the target." Rather, implementation of genome editing for CF will require simultaneous consideration of a cell type's role in disease pathophysiology, the proportion of those cells that will need to be edited to achieve clinical benefit, when those cells need to be edited and with delivery systems that will provide to those cells a particular editing platform.

Where? Identifying Target Cells Functional studies (ion transport), in situ hybridization and immunohistochemistry have suggested cellular targets in various epithelia. For example, expressing CFTR throughout the GI epithelium prevents intestinal disease in CF mice [21, 22]. While these experimental observations were consistent with a pan-epithelial role for CFTR, recent single-cell RNA sequencing has provided evidence that there are very specific, low abundance cell types that express high levels of CFTR [23, 24]. While the functional significance of these so-called ionocytes is quite unclear at this point, their high level of CFTR expression warrants investigation for their role in disease pathogenesis to determine if they are critical targets for therapeutic approaches [25].

Non-epithelial targets are not as well understood as epithelia, but there is substantial evidence for their role in disease. For example, conditional expression of CFTR in both myeloid [26] and lymphoid [27] cells in mice implicates these cell types as contributing to the impaired innate defense and inflammation seen in CF. Other cell types also express CFTR, including neurons in the brain, smooth muscle and adipocytes, and these too may become targets once their role in CF pathophysiology is better understood.

Whether the cells requiring functional CFTR are epithelial or not, it is their progenitor cells that must be targeted if genome editing is to provide long-term benefit. The stem cells of the airway epithelium are yet to be clearly identified, but lineage tracing and single-cell analysis methods are making substantial progress in that regard. If one were to target the immune system, the stem cells of the bone marrow are much better understood and perhaps provide a rational place to start, as these cells have the additional benefit in that they could be edited ex vivo, selected for appropriately edited cells and reintroduced as in other bone marrow transplant procedures.

When? Disease Progression and Developmental Stage When one would need to have their cells edited is likely to be a complex question. Data from CFTR modulator studies indicate that early intervention is prophylactic, preventing damage. As disease progression continues, the barriers to delivery increase, particularly for the airways, as mucus and microbiome become increasingly problematic for direct delivery to the airway surface. As stem cells are the ultimate target, one must also consider the developmental stage of the patient, as the stem cell niche is proportionately larger during early development and thus the most effective time to treat would be prenatal.

How? Delivering DNA Editing Components to Cells in the Body One of the most significant challenges for gene editing is how to get the components of an editing platform to the appropriate target cells and into the nuclei of those cells to modify their genomic DNA. This challenge has two main components: identification of the appropriate target cells and development of systems that will deliver the functional editing cargo to those cells. The specific details of these challenges differ from organ to organ, as one might expect. For example, delivery to relevant cells in the airway has different physical, anatomical, and biological issues than delivery to intestines, ductal structures of pancreas or liver, or even immune cells.

For epithelial cells, there are opportunities to deliver to the apical (luminal) or basolateral sides, allowing one to think about topical delivery and systemic delivery, respectively. While the surface epithelium would be directly targeted by apical delivery, it is not clear whether the stem cell population would be reached by this route.

How Much? The Proportion of Cells Successfully Edited That Are Needed to Achieve Clinical Benefit The CFTR modulator studies have suggested thresholds of CFTR activity needed to achieve clinical effects. However, these drugs reach most, if not all cells in the body and thus one cannot discern the effects of specific cell types. As discussed above, the relative roles of different cell types are not clear. If, for example, the airway ionocytes are critically important, one may need to repair a large proportion given their rare abundance, whereas a relatively small proportion of the remaining epithelium may need to be edited for detectable benefit.

Delivery Systems and Their Cargo To date, editing platforms consist of one or more molecular species, including DNA, RNA, or protein. Delivery vehicles, such as viruses, have evolved to carry nucleic acids and thus may only be capable of transporting one species, and thus if they are to be used, the cargo must be tailored to the delivery system. Other strategies, lipid nanoparticles and other polymer-based systems, may be more amenable to chemical modifications that allow the delivery system to be custom designed for the cargo.

Numerous strategies to deliver DNA, RNA, and/or protein have been developed, such as viral particles, or hybrid viral/non-viral particles, cell penetrating peptides, lipid-based nanoparticles, and others. Their development is evolving alongside that of editing systems so that the most effective delivery system can be coupled with a compatible, optimized editing system.

Progress Toward Toward CFTR Editing

CRISPR/Cas9-mediated CFTR editing in primary cells was first shown by repairing the F508del mutation in intestinal stem cells that, after selection for corrected cells, showed functional correction as determined by organoid swelling [28]. More recently, induced pluripotent stem cells from a F508del homozygous person with CF were used for editing and the F508del mutation was repaired in vitro at high efficiency, correcting ~20% of mutant alleles [29]. These cells, differentiated to airway epithelial lineages, showed functional correction as well.

Cas9 has proven to be a versatile tool for editing, but it does not allow targeting every position in the genome. Additional Cas proteins have been examined, and one, AsCas12a, was used to correctly edit a pair of intronic mutations that affect RNA splicing and able to do so in primary cells ex vivo in human intestinal cells, providing these cells with functional CFTR [30]. While these in vitro and ex vivo approaches are encouraging and provide proof of principle, strategies to efficiently edit in vivo are yet to be developed, but hopefully on the horizon soon.

Safety Concerns

DNA editing is a permanent modification that will last the life of edited cells and, for stem cells, their daughter cells. Consequently, there are concerns about safety, as one cannot reverse, or terminate an editing therapy as one might do with traditional, pharmacologic treatments.

Some of the safety concerns revolve around unintended editing events. One that is generic to editing for any application is "off-target" DNA breaks occurring in tumor suppressor genes or other genes that may cause harm. The other that is currently unique to CF is unintended, on-target changes, as these have the potential to create inactivating mutations in an allele that may be responsive to a CFTR modulator. When NHEJ occurs to repair a double-strand break (see Fig. 25.1a), there are often small insertions or deletions that occur and create inactivating frame shifts in the coding sequence. If editing is not allele-specific, there is a risk of inactivating a drug-treatable mutation if such events happen at high frequency.

Other concerns involve immune responses of various types. If a single editing application is insufficient and multiple administrations are needed, the components of the delivery system must be non-immunogenic. This is of particular concern for viral delivery systems. Another conceptual concern is immunogenicity of CFTR and the production of neutralizing antibodies if a null mutation were corrected. Earlier gene therapy trials suggest this will not be a major issue, but is still one deserving attention. A fundamental concern with any new therapeutic strategy, such as toxicity of the therapeutic itself. For editing, there are several aspects of this, including off-target, and even on-target, unintended DNA alterations, immune responses, and toxicity to the components delivered.

References

1. Rommens JM, Iannuzzi MC, Kerem B, Drumm ML, Melmer G, Dean M, Rozmahel R, Cole JL, Kennedy D, Hidaka N, et al. Identification of the cystic fibrosis gene: chromosome walking and jumping. Science. 1989;245:1059–65.
2. Rich DP, Anderson MP, Gregory RJ, Cheng SH, Paul S, Jefferson DM, McCann JD, Klinger KW, Smith AE, Welsh MJ. Expression of cystic fibrosis transmembrane conductance regulator corrects defective chloride channel regulation in cystic fibrosis airway epithelial cells. Nature. 1990;347:358–63.
3. Drumm ML, Pope HA, Cliff WH, Rommens JM, Marvin SA, Tsui LC, Collins FS, Frizzell RA, Wilson JM. Correction of the cystic fibrosis defect in vitro by retrovirus-mediated gene transfer. Cell. 1990;62:1227–33.
4. Alton EW, Boyd AC, Davies JC, Gill DR, Griesenbach U, Harrison PT, Henig N, Higgins T, Hyde SC, Innes JA, et al. Genetic medicines for CF: hype versus reality. Pediatr Pulmonol. 2016;51:S5–S17.
5. Drumm ML, Wilkinson DJ, Smit LS, Worrell RT, Strong TV, Frizzell RA, Dawson DC, Collins FS. Chloride conductance expressed by delta F508 and other mutant CFTRs in Xenopus oocytes. Science. 1991;254:1797–9.

6. Kelley TJ, Al-Nakkash L, Cotton CU, Drumm ML. Activation of endogenous deltaF508 cystic fibrosis transmembrane conductance regulator by phosphodiesterase inhibition. J Clin Invest. 1996;98:513–20.

7. Ramsey BW, Davies J, McElvaney NG, Tullis E, Bell SC, Drevinek P, Griese M, McKone EF, Wainwright CE, Konstan MW, et al. A CFTR potentiator in patients with cystic fibrosis and the G551D mutation. N Engl J Med. 2011;365:1663–72.

8. Kim YG, Cha J, Chandrasegaran S. Hybrid restriction enzymes: zinc finger fusions to Fok I cleavage domain. Proceed Nat Acad Sci United States Am. 1996;93:1156–60.

9. Boch J, Scholze H, Schornack S, Landgraf A, Hahn S, Kay S, Lahaye T, Nickstadt A, Bonas U. Breaking the code of DNA binding specificity of TAL-type III effectors. Science. 2009;326:1509–12.

10. Boch J. TALEs of genome targeting. Nat Biotechnol. 2011;29:135–6.

11. Mali P, Yang L, Esvelt KM, Aach J, Guell M, DiCarlo JE, Norville JE, Church GM. RNA-guided human genome engineering via Cas9. Science. 2013;339:823–6.

12. Jinek M, East A, Cheng A, Lin S, Ma E, Doudna J. RNA-programmed genome editing in human cells. elife. 2013;2:e00471.

13. Gaudelli NM, Komor AC, Rees HA, Packer MS, Badran AH, Bryson DI, Liu DR. Programmable base editing of A∗T to G∗C in genomic DNA without DNA cleavage. Nature. 2017;551:464–71.

14. Cheng AW, Wang H, Yang H, Shi L, Katz Y, Theunissen TW, Rangarajan S, Shivalila CS, Dadon DB, Jaenisch R. Multiplexed activation of endogenous genes by CRISPR-on, an RNA-guided transcriptional activator system. Cell Res. 2013;23:1163–71.

15. Maeder ML, Linder SJ, Cascio VM, Fu Y, Ho QH, Joung JK. CRISPR RNA-guided activation of endogenous human genes. Nat Methods. 2013;10:977–9.

16. Gilbert LA, Larson MH, Morsut L, Liu Z, Brar GA, Torres SE, Stern-Ginossar N, Brandman O, Whitehead EH, Doudna JA, et al. CRISPR-mediated modular RNA-guided regulation of transcription in eukaryotes. Cell. 2013;154:442–51.

17. Ran FA, Hsu PD, Lin CY, Gootenberg JS, Konermann S, Trevino AE, Scott DA, Inoue A, Matoba S, Zhang Y, et al. Double nicking by RNA-guided CRISPR Cas9 for enhanced genome editing specificity. Cell. 2013;154:1380–9.

18. Huang TP, Zhao KT, Miller SM, Gaudelli NM, Oakes BL, Fellmann C, Savage DF, Liu DR. Circularly permuted and PAM-modified Cas9 variants broaden the targeting scope of base editors. Nat Biotechnol. 2019;37:626–31.

19. Ricciardi AS, Quijano E, Putman R, Saltzman WM, Glazer PM. Peptide nucleic acids as a tool for site-specific gene editing. Molecules. 2018;23:632.

20. McNeer NA, Anandalingam K, Fields RJ, Caputo C, Kopic S, Gupta A, Quijano E, Polikoff L, Kong Y, Bahal R, et al. Nanoparticles that deliver triplex-forming peptide nucleic acid molecules correct F508del CFTR in airway epithelium. Nat Commun. 2015;6:6952.

21. Zhou L, Dey CR, Wert SE, DuVall MD, Frizzell RA, Whitsett JA. Correction of lethal intestinal defect in a mouse model of cystic fibrosis by human CFTR. Science. 1994;266:1705–8.

22. Hodges CA, Grady BR, Mishra K, Cotton CU, Drumm ML. Cystic fibrosis growth retardation is not correlated with loss of Cftr in the intestinal epithelium. Am J Physiol Gastrointest Liver Physiol. 2011;301:G528–36.

23. Plasschaert LW, Zilionis R, Choo-Wing R, Savova V, Knehr J, Roma G, Klein AM, Jaffe AB. A single-cell atlas of the airway epithelium reveals the CFTR-rich pulmonary ionocyte. Nature. 2018;560:377–81.

24. Montoro DT, Haber AL, Biton M, Vinarsky V, Lin B, Birket SE, Yuan F, Chen S, Leung HM, Villoria J, et al. A revised airway epithelial hierarchy includes CFTR-expressing ionocytes. Nature. 2018;560:319–24.

25. Hawkins FJ, Kotton DN. Pulmonary ionocytes challenge the paradigm in cystic fibrosis. Trends Pharmacol Sci. 2018;39:852–4.

26. Bonfield TL, Hodges CA, Cotton CU, Drumm ML. Absence of the cystic fibrosis transmembrane regulator (Cftr) from myeloid-derived cells slows resolution of inflammation and infection. J Leukoc Biol. 2012;92:1111–22.

27. Mueller C, Braag SA, Keeler A, Hodges C, Drumm M, Flotte TR. Lack of cystic fibrosis transmembrane conductance regulator in CD3+ lymphocytes leads to aberrant cytokine secretion and hyperinflammatory adaptive immune responses. Am J Respir Cell Mol Biol. 2011;44:922–9.
28. Schwank G, Koo BK, Sasselli V, Dekkers JF, Heo I, Demircan T, Sasaki N, Boymans S, Cuppen E, van der Ent CK, et al. Functional repair of CFTR by CRISPR/Cas9 in intestinal stem cell organoids of cystic fibrosis patients. Cell Stem Cell. 2013;13:653–8.
29. Ruan J, Hirai H, Yang D, Ma L, Hou X, Jiang H, Wei H, Rajagopalan C, Mou H, Wang G, et al. Efficient gene editing at major CFTR mutation loci. Mol Ther Nucl Acids. 2019;16:73–81.
30. Maule G, Casini A, Montagna C, Ramalho AS, De Boeck K, Debyser Z, Carlon MS, Petris G, Cereseto A. Allele specific repair of splicing mutations in cystic fibrosis through AsCas12a genome editing. Nat Commun. 2019;10:3556.

Index

© Springer Nature Switzerland AG 2020
S. D. Davis et al. (eds.), *Cystic Fibrosis*, Respiratory Medicine,
https://doi.org/10.1007/978-3-030-42382-7